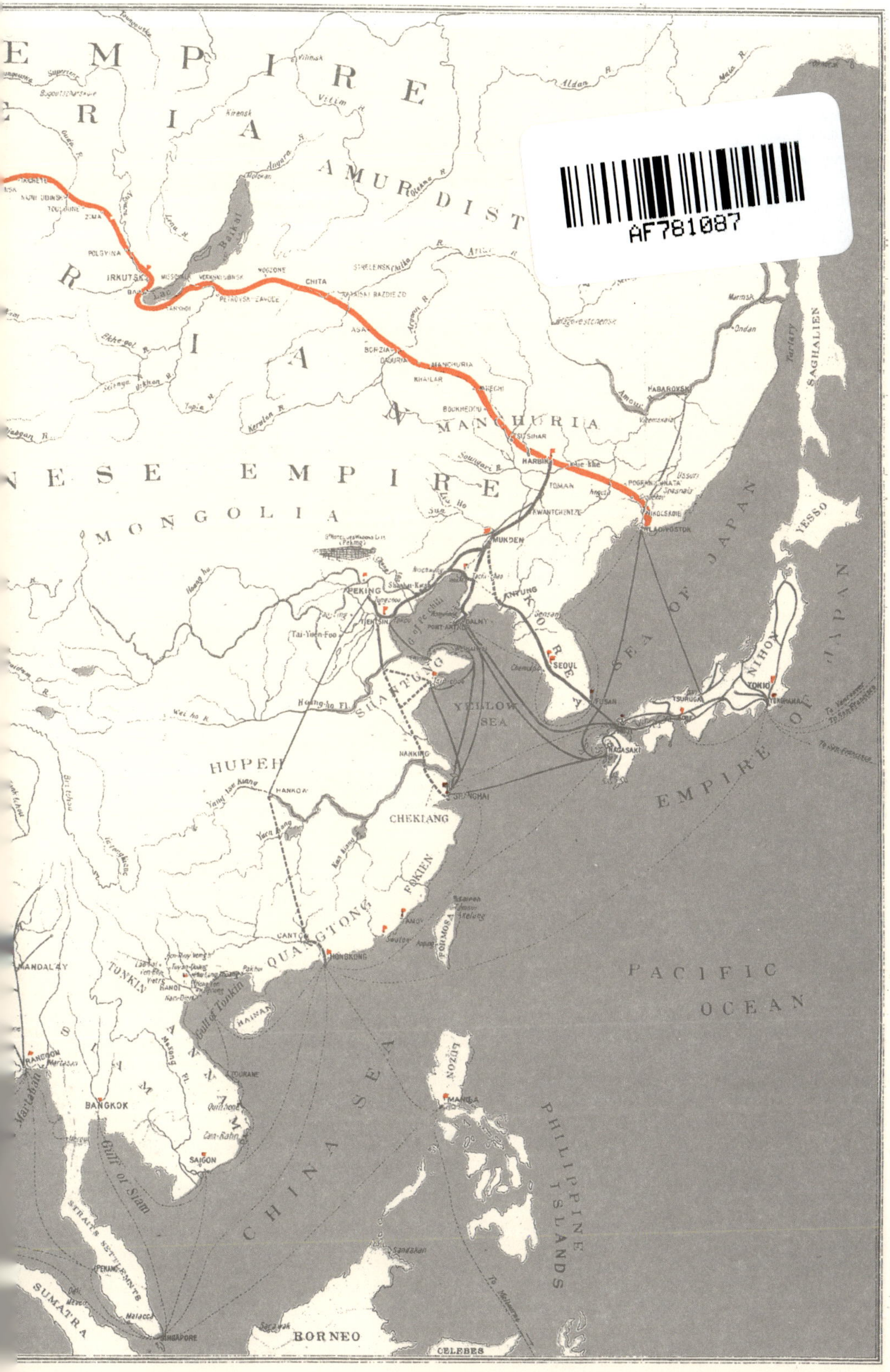
EMPIRE
AMUR DIST
MANCHURIA
MONGOLIA
IRKUTSK
CHITA
HARBIN
MUKDEN
PEKING
TIENTSIN
PORT ARTHUR
DALNY
SEOUL
FUSAN
NAGASAKI
TSURUGA
YOKIO
YOKOHAMA
VLADIVOSTOK
KHABAROVSK
SAGHALIEN
YESSO
NIHON
KOREA
SEA OF JAPAN
EMPIRE OF JAPAN
YELLOW SEA
SHANTUNG
HUPEH
HANKOW
NANKING
SHANGHAI
CHEKIANG
FOKIEN
QUANGTONG
CANTON
HONGKONG
AMOY
FORMOSA
HAINAN
TONKIN
HANOI
Gulf of Tonkin
MANDALAY
RANGOON
BANGKOK
SAIGON
Gulf of Siam
STRAITS SETTLEMENTS
PENANG
Malacca
SINGAPORE
SUMATRA
BORNEO
CELEBES
LUZON
MANILA
CHINA SEA
PHILIPPINE ISLANDS
PACIFIC OCEAN
NESE EMPIRE

WITH STETHOSCOPE IN ASIA: KOREA

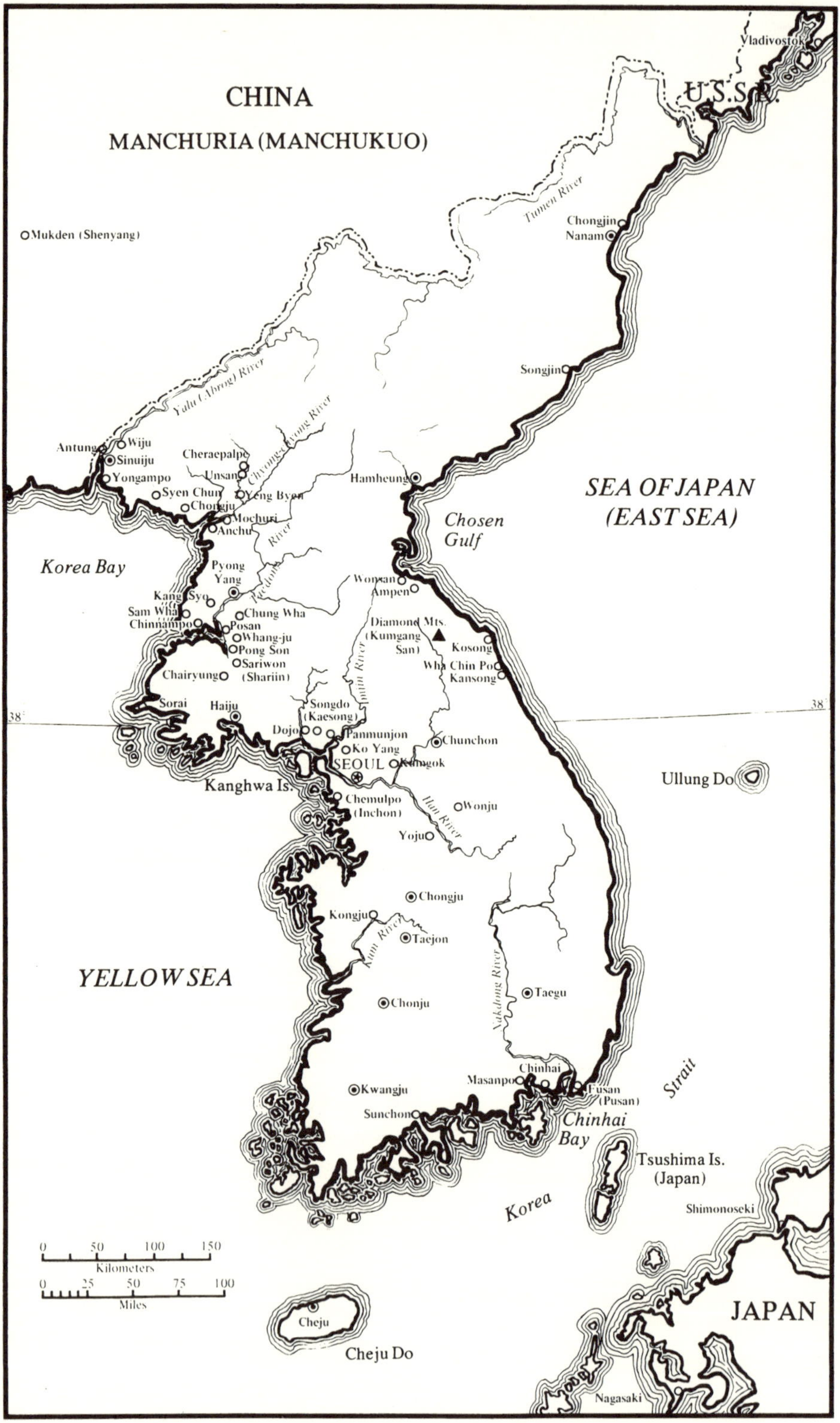

Map of Korea Showing Localities Mentioned in the Text.

WITH STETHOSCOPE IN ASIA: KOREA

SHERWOOD HALL, M.D., F.A.C.C.P.

MCL ASSOCIATES
P.O. Box 26, McLean, Virginia
2010

Printed in the United States of America

Library of Congress Catalog Number: 77-81765

ISBN: 978-0-0930696-01-6

First Edition. First Printing, 1978, Second Printing, 1981, Third Printing 2010.

Materials from the following sources are reprinted by permission:

Conrow, Marion L., from mimeographed memorandum to the Foreign Department of the Woman's Foreign Missionary Society of the Methodist Church, 1940. Used by permission of the Women's Division, Board of Global Ministries, The United Methodist Church.

Haskins, Minnie Louise, from *Gate of the Year* by kind permission of Christy & Moore, London.

Ryang, Rev. J. S., from *Within the Gate*, Charles A. Sauer, Editor, published by the Korean Methodist News Service, Seoul, 1934.

Wirt, Sherwood E., from "Korea: God's Loving Cup" from DECISION, copyright © 1973 by the Billy Graham Evangelistic Association.

Photo credits:

Black and white photograph of the U.S.A. 1932 TB Christmas Seal reproduced with permission from the American Lung Association, New York, N.Y.

Color transparencies for Korea TB Christmas Seals, 1932-1940, supplied from the collection of the Division of Postal History, Smithsonian Institution, Washington, D.C. and by their courtesy.

Black and white photograph of Drs. Sherwood and Marian Hall with stethoscope, opposite Preface, by permission of Mickey Carlton–*Richmond Review* (Canada).

To My Daughter, Phyllis

Foreword

by

Bishop Herbert Welch

Here is a book—*With Stethoscope in Asia: Korea*—but more than a book. Here is a man, Dr. Sherwood Hall, of rare and life-long devotion, not simply to the ideal in general but to a particular form of service in which he might render his utmost to our Lord.

A man of unconquerable persistence, of divine ingenuity, who would be preaching the Gospel by his character while he created medical centers that welcomed in Korea, and later in India, needy groups to the very fount of healing.

Here is a book—and I am proud, as well as happy to be able to say, here is a man even greater than his book. God bless him!

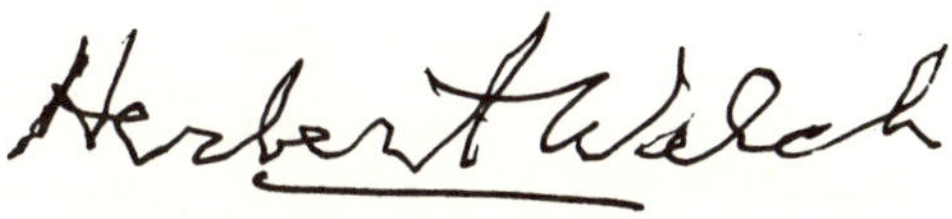

New York, May 28, 1968

Editor's Note: Dr. Sherwood Hall served directly under Bishop Herbert Welch when the latter was resident Bishop of Japan and Korea (1916-1928) for the Methodist Episcopal Church. Bishop Welch died at the age of 106 and remained active until his death on April 4, 1969. He was reputed to be until then the oldest U.S. college alumnus and the oldest bishop of any church in the world. Dr. Welch served as President of Ohio Wesleyan University from 1905 to 1916.

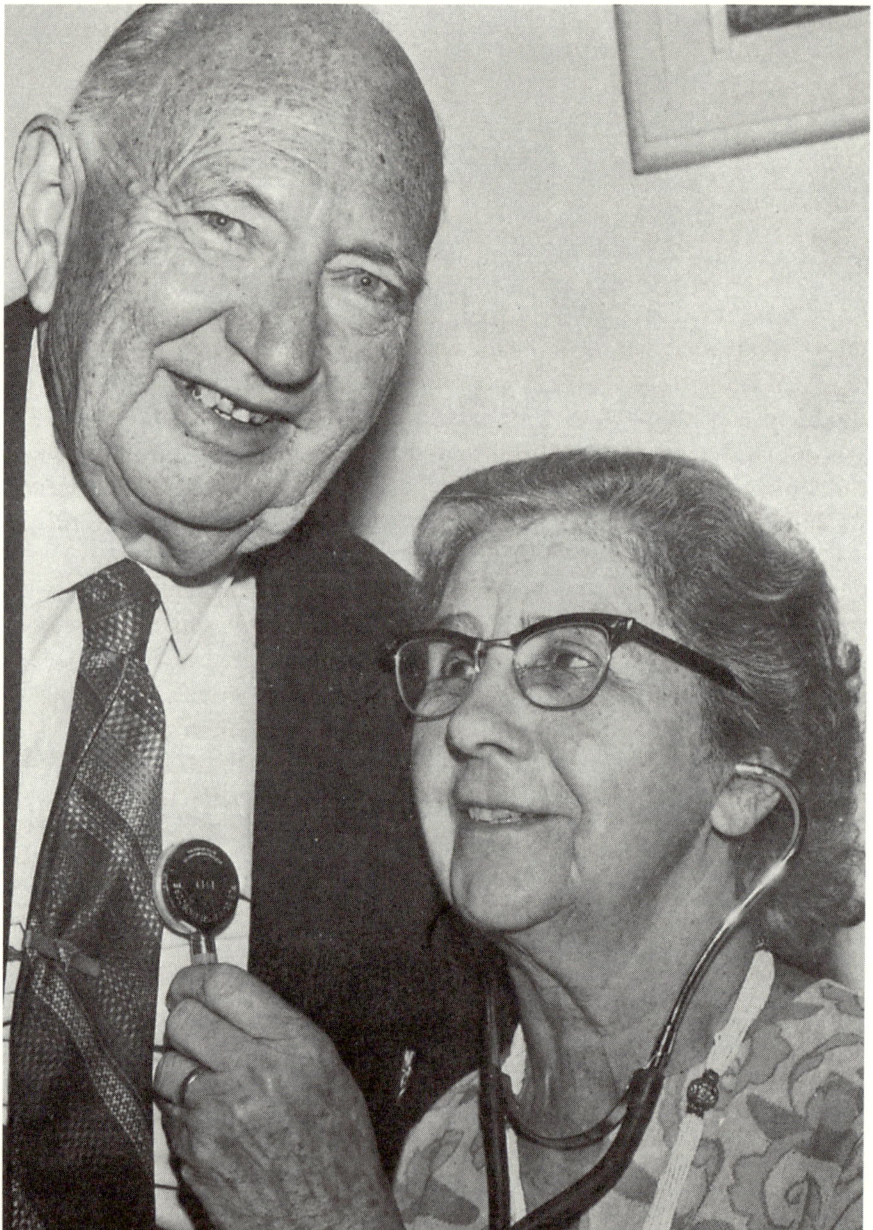

BY COURTESY OF MICKEY CARLTON – "RICHMOND REVIEW" (CANADA)

Drs. Sherwood and Marian Hall

Preface

The pioneer service of my physician parents in Korea, my birth and boyhood there, and later, the sixteen years that my doctor-wife and I spent assigned as medical missionaries to that country provided me with subject matter for many stories.

Often I had occasion to speak of the trials, sorrows, inspiration, and fulfillment that composed this unique background. My audiences were always rewardingly attentive and full of eager questions. Many generously declared that these experiences contained "a message for young and old alike," a message that "uplifted the spirit and rekindled faith in the goodness and nobility of man." They urged me to write a book so that my recollections could be shared with a larger circle of friends.

But consideration of writing that story had to wait until my wife and I set aside stethoscopes for more leisurely pursuits. The time eventually came with our retirement from thirty-nine years of medical missionary service in Asia. On my seventy-third birthday, I accepted the challenge.

Sherwood Hall, M.D.

Richmond, British Columbia
Canada

The men scattered to find sticks for the fire, while her mother was busy preparing the food. Pobai was told that she need not help but was free to gather the wild azaleas on the mountain slopes.

When everything was ready, someone called for Pobai, but there was no response. They found her clutching the beautiful azalea blooms to her bosom, a sweet and happy smile on her face. They knew then that she had gone to be with her ancestors.

* * * * * * *

Many years later, near this beautiful site, the first tuberculosis sanatorium in Korea would be erected. Its founding would help prevent the young and the promising of that land from being snatched from life before they had a chance to realize their dreams and potentialities.

Acknowledgements

It is my pleasure to acknowledge the encouragement and assistance I have received in the preparation of this book. Friends of long standing, as well as new friends with whom I have been blessed, have been generous in sharing their time, talents and suggestions, and in loaning me supplementary materials to make my task easier. Especially helpful in this regard were: Ruth Noble Appenzeller, Constance M. Ellison, Velma French, Maud K. Jensen, Charlotte M. Knutson, Kathy Lee, Frederick M. Pyke, and the late Norman L. Trott. I am indebted to many more than I could possibly name in the space allotted to me.

James W. Kerr, Philatelic Consultant to the Division of Postal History at the Smithsonian Institution, Washington, D.C., developed an interest in philately dating from his own youth in Korea. His interest in stamps, in Korea, and in me led to the donation to the Smithsonian Institution on December 15, 1972 of my original record collection of TB Christmas Seals of Korea and India. He also kindly read an early draft of the manuscript and offered much helpful guidance.

Betty Quinn graciously shared her typing and other secretarial skills at an hour of need, although we had never met. Photographic assistance was rendered by J. David Clem, who had the challenging task of restoring some of the aged and faded photographs of another era to present-day clarity.

An author's family makes its own unique contribution. I am especially grateful to my wife, Marian, for her practical assistance, patient understanding, and the partnership which helped to create my story. My son, William, helped to confirm the accuracy of some of the historical data. His interest and that of my son, Joseph, have meant much to me. I am appreciative of the enthusiasm for this project shown by my daughter, Phyllis, and of the persistent prodding with which she kept me writing. To her and to her husband,

Edward G. King, Jr., goes the credit for shepherding this book to completion.

The extended family system of the Orient has often been held up by sociologists as having advantages over the nuclear family structure of the Occident. I feel that I have had the best of both worlds. My son-in-law's mother, Cecilia B. King, has been most supportive in her belief that this story should be written. Her invaluable coaching along the way allowed me to benefit from her expertise as a staff correspondent for the *Newark Evening News* for many years. Ed's sister, Peggy Van Duyne, and brothers, Ted and Mike, gave welcome encouragement and useful advice on design and presentation. For their time and helpfulness, I am most appreciative.

My grandchildren—Marcia, Clifford and Laurie King, and Karen and Julia Hall—persuaded me to include some of their favorite Korean tales, which, like *Pobai*, they enjoyed hearing their grandfather tell. The Prologue, "'*Pobai*' (Jewel)—A Tale of the Hermit Kingdom," is dedicated to them, with fond memories of many happy "story hours" together.

Contents

PROLOGUE

"Pobai" (Jewel) A Tale of the Hermit Kingdom

Our tale begins long, long ago in the peaceful secluded "Hermit Kingdom" of Asia, known as the "Land of the Morning Calm." Neither explorers nor warfare had yet brought this little nation into the consciousness of the Western World.

Once upon a time in the Korean coastal town of Haiju (Haeju) on the Yellow Sea there lived a merchant. His mud-walled, tiled-roof dwelling also housed his elderly parents, his three sons, Yung-ke, Chang-sung, and Yong-tu, his wife, and his daughter. It was the custom of that day that girls remained nameless until they married and had sons. Then they were known as the "mother of . . ." whatever the son's name might be.

This merchant's daughter proved to be an exception, for her bright eyes and winning smiles soon endeared her to the hearts of her parents and grandparents. They began to call her *Pobai*, which in Korean means "jewel."

She was indeed the precious jewel of this household, particularly to her grandfather to whom she became especially attached. In fact, he treated her as he would one of his grandsons! At an early age he taught her the folklore of the land, and even gave her lessons in the Chinese Classics to which very few girls were ever introduced.

The northern part of Korea abounded in tigers. Pobai never tired of listening to her grandfather's seemingly endless repertoire of tiger stories. Many a winter evening they spent together, huddled beside the smoky brazier, while her grandfather recounted the folk tales she loved to hear.

One such story went something like this:

"A Korean farmer and his wife had decided one morning to leave their son and daughter at home in their straw-thatched hut while they went to market to sell their produce. While the parents were gone, the children were assigned the task of pounding bags of rice into flour. The rice-pounding contraption was somewhat like a see-saw. The pounding hammer was located at one end and the children perched on the other. Attached to the ceiling was a rope and by holding on to this, they could pull themselves up. When they did so, the hammer end dropped onto the rice, crushing it to a fine powder. As the children lowered themselves, the hammer would rise in preparation for the next drop. This proved to be such fun that the children did not view their assignment as at all laborious.

"While their parents were away, a huge tiger came prowling around the hut. The doors were bolted shut, and so the tiger jumped up on the straw roof and started to paw its way through. You can imagine the feelings of the children!

"Suddenly, a happy idea struck the young girl. She said, 'Brother, just take this bit of rope and make a lasso of it so that you can easily slip it over the tiger's paw when it claws through the ceiling. Then, fasten the other end of the rope to this rice pounder and we shall have a lot of rice pounded into flour by the time papa and mama come home!'

"'That is a wonderful idea!' responded the boy.

"This was no sooner said, than done. The tiger felt the rope tighten about its paw. Naturally the beast pulled back and in so doing, jerked up the hammer. He soon grew tired of keeping his paw raised and let it fall back which, in turn, dropped the hammer on the rice. In the meantime, the children were shoveling the rice under the hammer at a great rate and this process was repeated again and again.

"Toward evening, the boy happened to look out and saw his father aiming a gun at the tiger. He yelled, 'Papa, please don't shoot yet! We are safe and have only one more bag of rice left to pound!'"

Pobai was delighted at this story and begged her grandfather to tell her another. This he pledged to do sometime, and you may be sure she would not let him forget his promise.

In those years, girls in Korea were engaged at a very tender age to boys who were even younger. Pobai was no exception and found herself engaged to a neighbor's son whom she had never seen. She knew that at the wedding ceremony, which would take place when she reached the age of thirteen, her eyes would be pasted shut, so that she would not be able to see the groom till after she was married.

Pobai inwardly objected to the idea of not being permitted to see her groom. Although she was a girl of modesty, she was also a girl of resource and so devised a way to at least get a glimpse of her husband-to-be.

In the spring of the year, one of the most popular forms of sport for young Korean girls was to swing on long rope swings in a standing position. Pobai cleverly conceived the idea of having her father so erect the swing, that on swinging high, she could catch a glimpse of her future husband, as well as afford him an opportunity of seeing her graceful figure. The outcome of this ingenious maneuver was a complete success. Pobai in her colorful holiday attire flew high in the air. She cast furtive glances at her young swain without compromising her maidenly modesty.

After one such glimpse, Pobai ran all excited to her mother and exclaimed, "I have seen my future husband, and he is just right!"

Her mother replied, "Shame! That will bring you bad luck. I never saw your father until after we were married. See what luck it has brought me: a large tiled-roof home and a big family."

Pobai's father, who had overheard the conversation, gently chided his wife for reproving their daughter. With a sly wink at Pobai he said, "Contrary to custom, I was able to get a glimpse of your mother before we were married, and you see it has brought me good luck: a large tiled-roof home and a big family, and in you, the loveliest daughter in the land!"

Pobai, anxious to change the subject, ran to her grandfather and begged him to tell another tiger story as he had promised.

"Very well, " he agreed. "This is quite appropriate, for just today there was a rope-pulling tug-of-war contest and our side won. The story I shall tell you is based on such a contest.

"One village had challenged the village in the next valley to a game of tug-of-war. As you know, Pobai, there is a famous rope-pulling yell which each team shouts so that they can all pull in unison, '*Oo-ya-cha, oo-ya-cha, yen-ru-ye-ya, oo-ya-cha, yen-ru-ye-ya.*'

"Now the key to the story is this yell, which please keep in mind." When the grandfather gave the yell, he had a terrible coughing spell, but was finally able to proceed.

"One of the lads from the visiting village team lingered behind to play with the boys. At last he proceeded on his homeward journey. He had almost reached the mountain pass, when darkness overtook him. Because the mountains were infested with tigers, he sought protection in a wayside shrine so common in these parts. As you know, the walls of these shrines are not solid, but are constructed of wooden slats. Soon the very tired boy fell fast asleep inside the shrine and dreamed that he was still at the rope-pulling contest of the previous day.

"Just at this time, a huge tiger came down from the mountainside and happened to seat himself outside the shrine very close to where our hero-to-be was sleeping. Somehow the tiger had not yet discovered the boy. However, it had heard the pigs squealing and the babies crying in the village below. The tiger started to wag his tail in eager anticipation, as you have seen a dog or a cat do.

"In so doing, the tail slipped between the wooden slats, brushing the boy's face. The lad was dreaming that he was at the rope-pulling contest. He grabbed the tiger's tail, and started pulling for dear life. As he pulled, he yelled, '*Oo-ya-cha, oo-ya-cha, yen-ru-ye-ya, oo-ya-cha, yen-ru-ye-ya!*'

"As the surprised tiger strained to pull free, the boy awoke to discover that the rope he was tugging was a tail! With a final cry of '*Oo-ya-cha, oo-ya-cha, yen-ru-ye-ya,*' the astonished boy let go. Through the slats he watched as the tiger fled in terror.

"The next morning the boy resumed his journey homeward. He met a group of people running pell mell down the mountainside yelling at the tops of their voices, 'A tiger is after us! A tiger is after us! Run for your life!'

"Our hero replied, 'Just calm yourselves. Do not fear. I can manage that beast.'

"They shouted back, 'Don't be silly. Where is your gun? Where is your knife?' They did not wait to find out.

"Sure enough, our lad had not gone far, before he noticed a huge tiger leaping down the mountainside, baring his teeth and looking the picture of ferocity.

"Well, Pobai, what would you have done under a similar circumstance?"

She replied, "I hardly know!"

"Our hero knew exactly what to do. He calmly seated himself in the middle of the path of the onrushing tiger and yelled with all his might the rope-pulling yell, '*Oo-ya-cha, oo-ya-cha, yen-ru-ye-ya, oo-ya-cha, yen-ru-ye-ya!*'

"Upon hearing this yell, the tiger pricked up his ears. He immediately associated this yell with a terrible experience on the night before. Not eager to repeat it, the tiger bounded away as fast as his legs could carry him. Meanwhile, our hero continued on his journey. Upon reaching home he told the astounded villagers of his two encounters with the tiger."

Pobai was fascinated by this story and wanted still another one. However, Grandfather was finding talking increasingly difficult because of his cough. He suggested instead that she try to solve a difficult conundrum. Her brothers had not been able to figure it out, but he was sure that his bright granddaughter could after she had slept on it.

It seemed so simple as he phrased it:

"In the village across the river was an herb doctor who was in dire need of about three pounds of medicinal herbs for his patients. However, due to the rainy season, the bridge had been washed out and the waters were too dangerous to cross by boat.

"A flimsy temporary bridge had been thrown across the raging river, but it was so delicate that it could carry only the weight of the messenger and two additional pounds. As the matter was urgent, the messenger had to take the three pounds across in one trip. It was not feasible to drag it across by means of a cord. Listen closely now to the question: 'Under these circumstances, how did the messenger succeed in taking the extra pound of medicinal herbs across this fragile bridge in *one* trip?'"

Pobai could hardly sleep that night. She thought of various solutions, but came up against either the time factor, or the width of the river (which was too wide to throw the parcel across).

By morning, Pobai approached her grandfather with a tired though happy face. She said, "I think I have solved the problem. You know I am considered to be a good juggler. Well, I think the messenger must have juggled his way across the bridge, keeping one pound always in the air for the whole length of the bridge."

Her grandfather, very pleased with Pobai, proudly patted her head. "Yes, that is correct. I knew you were a bright girl."

In view of Pobai's impending marriage, her mother said to her, "It is now high time for you to learn some essential household tasks. You have had a longer time for play than most girls around here. You will soon be in your teens and you don't even know how to make *kimchie* (cabbage pickle). What will your mother-in-law say?"

Pobai replied, "I am not worrying about her, but I do want to please my husband."

Her mother scoffed, "He does not count at this stage for he is so young. You will have to comb his hair and perhaps even wash his face and send him off to school to study the Chinese Classics."

"Oh, I can teach him the Chinese Classics, as my grandfather taught me," Pobai responded.

Her mother laughed. "What little you know of men! Do you suppose that he would want to learn from a mere woman? You better learn your proper place in the scheme of things. Never appear to know as much as a man or that would soon be your undoing."

Pobai sighed. She did not voice her thoughts aloud but felt sure that a brighter and better day would dawn for the women of her land.

In the meantime, Pobai worked diligently. The everlasting washing and ironing were the hardest. She had to pound out the buttonless clothes on a smooth stone in a nearby stream. She worked long into the night to iron these clothes by also pounding them with a rounded smooth stick. It took her some time to catch on to the rhythm of pounding that suited her best. Often she found herself either too tired to sleep or she found her sleep interrupted by her own violent coughing spells like those of her grandfather. When the coughing did not disturb her slumbers, the typical night sounds of a Korean village did. There could always be heard the ceaseless barking of the dogs, the "rat-a-tat-tat" of the pounding sticks ironing out the clothes, and the incessant beating of the drums or "tom-toms" by the *mudongs* (Korean-style witch doctors), attempting to scare away the evil spirits or to cure the sick.

Eventually Pobai's wracking cough became worse, and she began to grow thinner and weaker. One day her parents decided that it might do her some good if they all went for a spring outing on the slopes of South Mountain. Pobai was delighted at the prospect, especially as the beautiful purple wild azaleas would now be covering the mountainside like a rich velvet carpet. Pobai was always fond of this mountain location. Between twisted Oriental pine trees she could look out on the so-called Yellow Sea, which here was really azure blue, and watch the quaint and colorful fishing boats sailing on the waters.

Pobai dressed in her gayest clothes. She was happy to reach the beautiful spot and felt as carefree as a lark. Here she did not have to think of the possibility of the *wesang* (native doctor) doing acupunctures in so-called "safe areas" of her body. Here, the even worse threat of the *mudongs* with their terrifying demoniacal dances and frenzied beating of drums was silenced. Here were only peace, sweet bird songs, beautiful flowers and her precious family.

CHAPTER 1

Beginnings

Although given no choice as to the date and place of my arrival, I could hardly have been born in a more enchanting country nor during a more dynamic period in its four thousand year history.

Korea is a six hundred mile long peninsula extending south from Chinese Manchuria and positioned between the Sea of Japan on the East and the Yellow Sea on the West. Southeast, one hundred miles across the Korea Strait lies Japan. West, about two hundred miles is mainland China. The peninsula averages two hundred miles in width and covers an area roughly the size of the state of Utah. More than thirty-two hundred offshore islands dot the country's five thousand miles of rocky indented coastline.

Racially, Koreans are distinct from both the Chinese and the Japanese. They are thought to have descended from the Caucasians of Western Asia and the nomadic tribes of Mongolia. As only one-fifth of Korea's mountainous terrain is arable, survival has always been a struggle for its inhabitants. The strategic location of the country has made political survival a major struggle as well. Korean history is one account after another of the attempts by foreign nations to dominate the Korean peninsula. Because of the persistent efforts of the Korean people to maintain the distinctive character of their country against the influence and intrusion of other nations, Korea became known as the "Hermit Kingdom."

Korea was just beginning to emerge from her proud isolation to join the family of nations when I made my appearance in Seoul on November 10, 1893. I became the first white child to be taken to live in the northern interior of the country at a time when foreigners had long been prohibited from taking up residence in that region.

A ban on Christianity and Christian proselytizing which had been in effect for one hundred years was about to be challenged by my parents, an event that was to signify a turning point for religious toleration in Korea. Early missionaries found in the center of the city of Seoul a stone tablet, erected in 1871, which bore the inscription:

> "Foreign barbarians invade the country; we either wage war or make peace with them. Making peace will mean the betrayal of the country. We warn our descendents for ten thousand years. Made in 1866 and erected in 1871."[1]

Only twenty years later, my parents, Dr. William James Hall and Dr. Rosetta Sherwood Hall, found themselves in Korea, serving as medical missionaries under the American Methodist Board of Foreign Missions. Their story begins my own.

* * * * * * *

William James Hall was born in a log cabin on January 16, 1860, at Glen Buell, Ontario, Canada. He was to be the first of five children. Known as Jimmy to his intimates, he early showed signs of being a serious and persevering student, albeit not brilliant. Aware that he had no penchant for farming, when presented with the opportunity to learn the cabinet and carpentry trade in the nearby town of Athens, he accepted, and left school at the age of seventeen in January, 1877.

However, after less than two years, his health began to fail. With a severe cough, fever and weakened body he left the carpentry shop and returned home to die of consumption. Having been converted to Christianity when he was fourteen, the now nineteen-year-old Jimmy fretted that he might die without having been of service in his faith. But, contrary to expectation, his health improved.

The thought that remained with Jimmy was, "I have one short life to live. How best can I employ it?" He found his education lacking, his means limited, but undaunted, he at once set about to equip himself for a life of usefulness.

Jimmy returned to the old one-room schoolhouse at Glen Buell and diligently applied himself to his studies. His teacher, Miss Karley,

---

[1] Harry A. Rhodes, A.M., D.D., ed., *History of the Korea Mission Presbyterian Church U.S.A. 1884-1934*, Facing p. 64.

recalled that her former pupil made astonishing progress and passed into Athens High School by Christmas, 1880. She wrote:

> "There was something endearing about Jimmy's disposition. He had no enemies—everyone loved him, and those who knew him best loved him most. I boarded at Mr. Gilroy's, and Jimmy frequently used to come there to get help in his lessons, and to visit the sick room of Mrs. Gilroy's mother, who was an invalid for several years. She was a pious Quaker lady and was quite well-versed in simple healing arts. She took an especial interest in Jimmy, and many an hour he spent gathering herbs for her and making them into simple decoctions and syrups. People often urged him to aim at becoming a minister of the Gospel, and I believe his inclination strongly led him that way. Perhaps his mother's wishes, together with the advice of this dear old Quaker friend, had an influence upon him to become a doctor. 'Thou wast born to be of great use to mankind, William James,' she would say. 'Nature has made thee a physician; thou must minister to both body and soul.'"[2]

Jimmy obtained his teacher's certificate in 1883 and spent the next two years teaching. With his earnings from that and from selling books and life insurance in his spare time, he was able to enter Medical College at Queens University, Kingston, Ontario, in 1885.

As there was no Y.M.C.A. at the Medical College, one of Jimmy's first projects was to organize a branch there. This successful undertaking exemplified his desire to serve and his gift for organization.

The great turning point in Jimmy's life came in the spring term at the college in 1887. The Reverend John Forman of India, a representative of the "Student Volunteer Movement for Foreign Missions," visited Queens. Jimmy was one of the first of 22 students to sign up for missionary service. Together they formed the local "Student Volunteer Band."

During summer vacation, Jimmy organized a contingent of Canadian students to attend the Dwight L. Moody Summer School at

---

[2] Rosetta Sherwood Hall, M.D., ed., *The Life of Rev. William James Hall, M.D.*, p. 27.

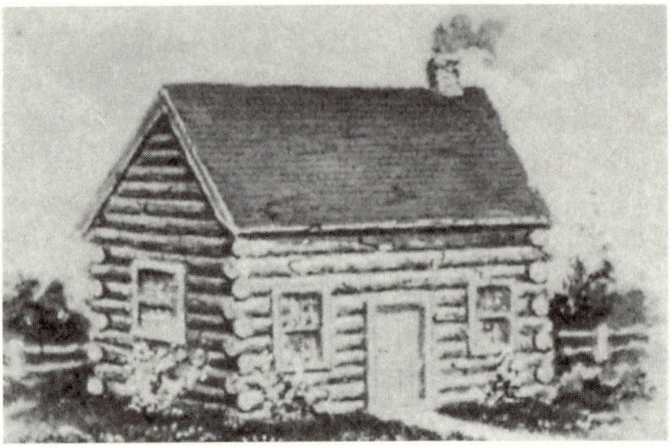

Birthplace, 1860

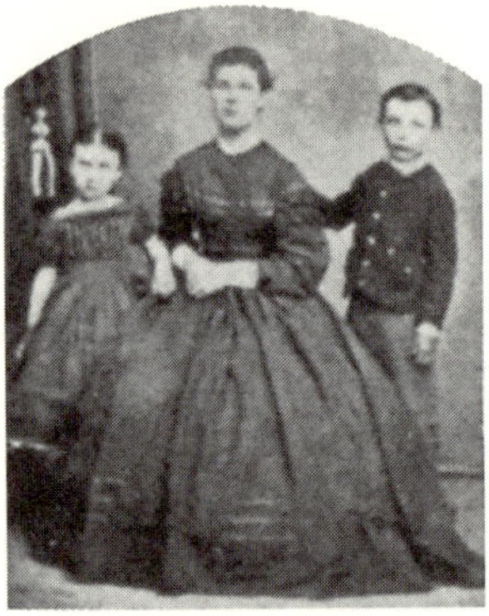

With Aunt Jane and Sister Alice

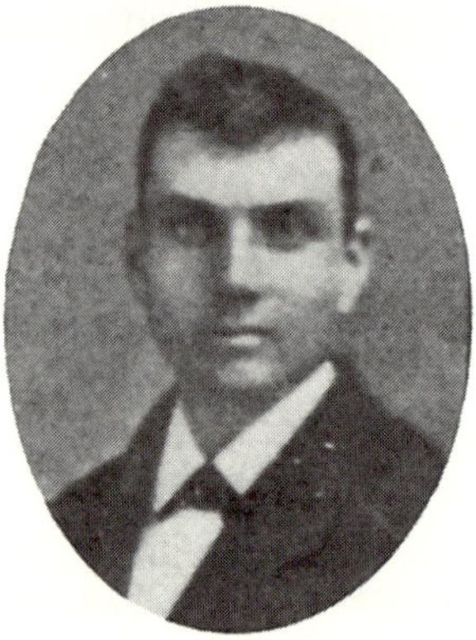

At seventeen

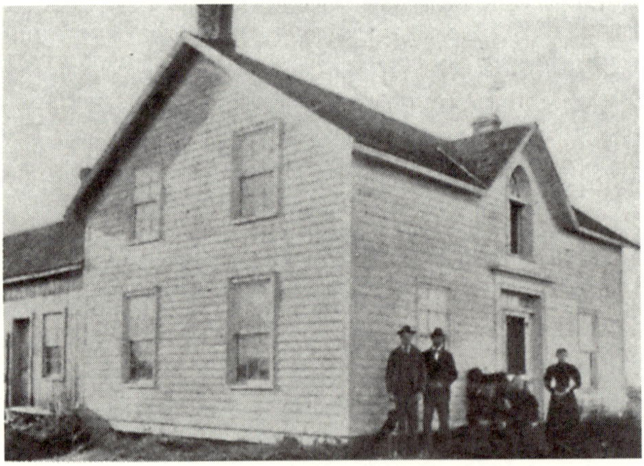

Home built in 1872

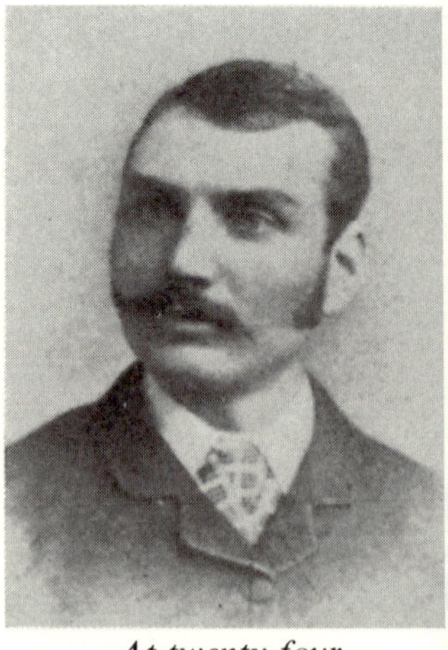

At twenty-four

WILLIAM JAMES HALL

Northfield, Massachusetts (Moody's birthplace). While there, they visited the nearby Mount Hermon School where the worldwide Student Volunteer Movement had been founded.

At Northfield, Jimmy met Dr. George D. Dowknott, Director of the International Medical Missionary Society, and a speaker at the Northfield Conference of Christian Workers. From him Jimmy learned of the opportunity which the Society offered for obtaining medical missionary training in New York City. Thus it came about that Jimmy took his third and fourth year of medical school in New York City, graduating with an M.D. degree from Bellevue Hospital Medical College in 1889.

While at the college, Dr. Hall did so well in home missionary work under Dr. Dowknott that, soon after graduation, he was appointed Medical Superintendent at the Madison Street Medical Mission under the Methodist Episcopal Church.

Dr. J. Sumner Stone, who was on the Board of Managers of the Medical Mission, later wrote of the service rendered by Dr. Hall at the time:

> "Dr. Hall, the beloved physician, a brother born for adversity, went as an angel of light among the sick and dying in the densely packed districts of lower New York. His work was a romance of grace. Without money and without price he went at the call of anyone, at any hour of the day or night, his delight being to relieve suffering and alleviate pain. None were too poor or vicious for him to serve. No cellar too damp, no garret too high for him to visit. Among murderers, thieves, thugs, harpies of vice and crime, he went in his gentle, health-giving Gospel ministry."[3]

Dr. Hall was then staying in the gracious home of Dr. and Mrs. Stone of New Rochelle, and from there he commuted daily to his work in the New York slums. The Stones had been in medical missionary work in India but had been forced to return due to poor health. They retained a deep interest in home and foreign missions and were officers of the Methodist Mission Board.

---

[3] *The Life of W. J. Hall*, p. 66.

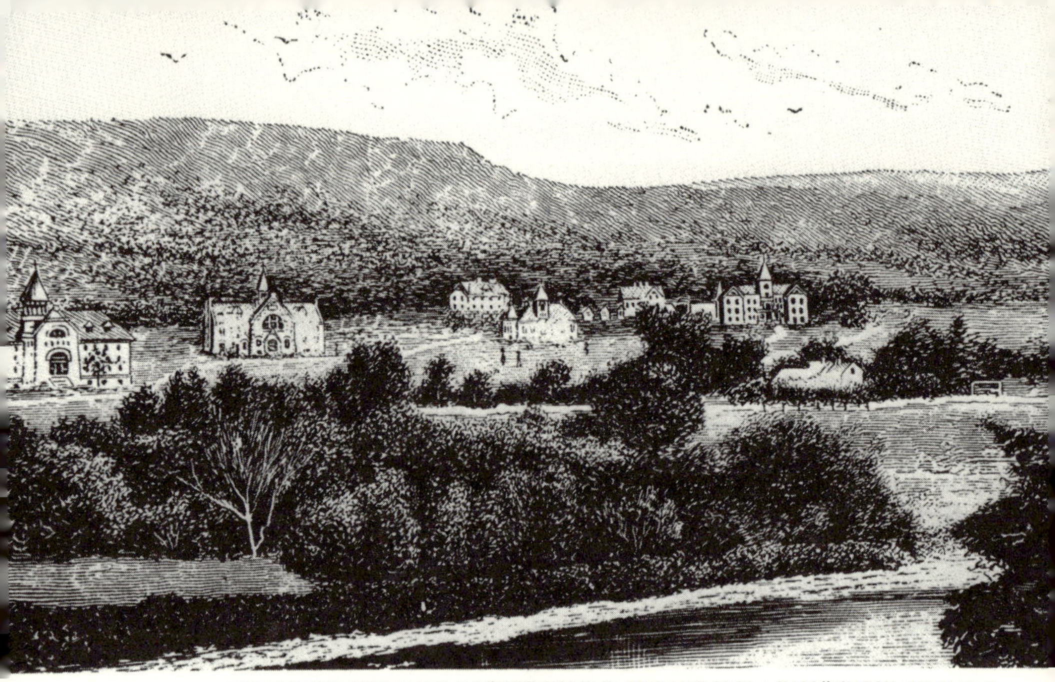

FROM "THE CHRISTIAN HERALD" (NEW YORK) IN "THE LIFE OF W. J. HALL" (EATON AND MAINS)

Dwight L. Moody School at Northfield, Massachusetts

The Stones grew very fond of Dr. Hall and treated him like a son. The strong bond between them is shown by Dr. Stone's own words:

> "The shortest biography ever written of Jesus Christ was, 'He went about doing good.' Like his Master, Dr. Hall wrought daily to lighten men's burdens, ease their pain, alleviate their sufferings, dry their tears, and open for them the gates into a brighter, better, larger life.
>
> "He wasted no time philosophizing or theorizing; he was not full of words on social, labor, or religious problems. He was a man of deeds–gentle, loving, golden deeds–not vague, wild, impracticable theories. While others questioned, he worked."[4]

W. A. Noble, a student from Drew Theological Seminary who helped out at the Madison Street Mission, confirmed this observation of Dr. Hall:

> "He possessed a rare faculty of coming in contact with the masses. He was ever evolving plans for the final evangeliza-

---

[4] *The Life of W. J. Hall*, pp. 76-77.

> tion of our great cities—plans that in extension and practicability of character were equaled only by Mr. Booth, [William Booth, founder and "general" of the Salvation Army] of England . . .
>
> "He possessed a mind that comprehended great things . . . yet the minutia of everyday life received his careful attention."[5]

One busy day in November, 1889, Nurse H. L. Jenkins stepped into the consulting room of the New York City Mission Dispensary. She announced, "Dr. Hall, I have brought our newly arrived physician, Dr. Rosetta Sherwood, to help you."

The doctor looked up from the little patient he was examining and, he afterwards claimed, fell in love at first sight with the young woman doctor who stood in the doorway.

Dr. Sherwood of Liberty, New York, a recent graduate of the Women's Medical College of Pennsylvania, all unconscious of what was going on in Dr. Hall's mind, presented him her credentials. Eager to show the Medical Superintendent in charge of the Mission that she was professionally well qualified to give him the help he needed, she handed to him her M.D. diploma, certificates, and testimonials. These indicated that following her graduation from medical school, she had served a successful internship in the Nursery and Child's Hospital on Staten Island and her diploma was endorsed by President Austin Flint, M.D. for the faculty of Bellevue Medical College.

Dr. Hall carefully read these certificates and gravely returned them to Dr. Sherwood. In later years, he teased her about the way she so highly recommended herself to him when first they met.

Rosetta Sherwood was born at Liberty, Sullivan County, New York on September 19, 1865. She grew up on the farm of her parents, Rosevelt Sherwood and Phoebe Gildersleeve Sherwood, and received her elementary education at the Chestnut Ridge School in Liberty. After attending the Liberty Normal Institute and later, the State Normal School at Oswego, New York, she was licensed to teach both elementary school and high school subjects. She taught at the Chestnut Ridge School for a year before entering the Women's Medical College of Pennsylvania in 1886. She had been inspired to do medical missionary work by hearing talks about medical and evange-

[5] *The Life of W. J. Hall*, p. 325.

listic needs in India from Mrs. Kennard Chandler, who had visited that country, and from the doctor-wife of Bishop James M. Thoburn (missionary in India at the time).

Upon completion of her medical training, Dr. Sherwood was assigned to medical welfare work in the New York slums under the auspices of the Methodist Deaconess Home. It was in this capacity that she had reported for work to Dr. Hall at the Madison Street Dispensary.

The two doctors worked well together in the rough district in which the dispensary was located. Both of them shared a dedication to full-time Christian service and both were candidates for foreign mission work in China. That Christmas, Dr. Hall asked Dr. Sherwood to be his wife. He was disappointed, but not defeated, when she put him off.

In truth, Dr. Sherwood held Dr. Hall in such high esteem that she felt she needed time to seek God's guidance in this matter. Marriage, for one thing, had not figured in her plans for a life of missionary service. From childhood she had had a pronounced curvature of the spine which remained uncorrected despite several operations. With this background, she had doubts as to her own physical stamina. Furthermore, she had undergone surgery for the removal of tubercular glands in her neck while in medical school. Should her health not prove equal to the rigors of life as a missionary, she did not want to cause Dr. Hall to give up his dreams on her account. Reasoning that a trial period on the mission field would prove her mettle in this regard, Dr. Sherwood submitted her application to the Woman's Foreign Missionary Society of the American Methodist Church.

The following Easter, Dr. Hall again proposed marriage. However, by then Dr. Sherwood had already received her overseas appointment. She was to be sent to the relatively new and unknown mission field of Korea and not to China as she had hoped. Her sailing date had been set for August. Although Dr. Hall anticipated being appointed eventually to China by the Canadian Methodist Mission Board, his assignment was contingent upon their being able to raise his salary.

Dr. Sherwood's commitment with the Woman's Foreign Missionary Society would not free her to marry for five years. She therefore felt compelled to suggest to Dr. Hall that he might prefer to marry someone else. She helpfully pointed out that by his marrying another worker, three new missionaries would be sent abroad instead

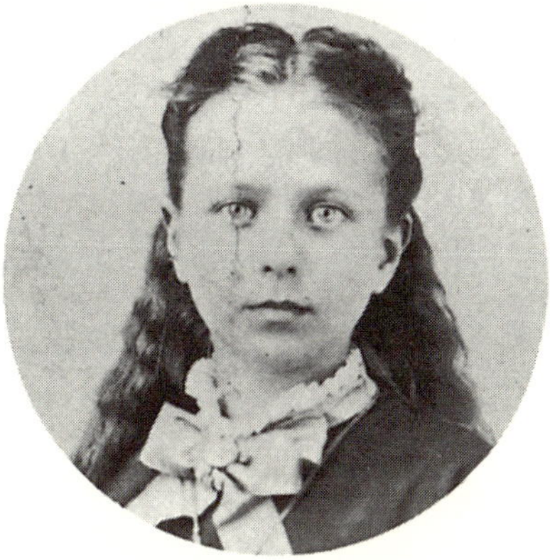

Rosetta at 10 years

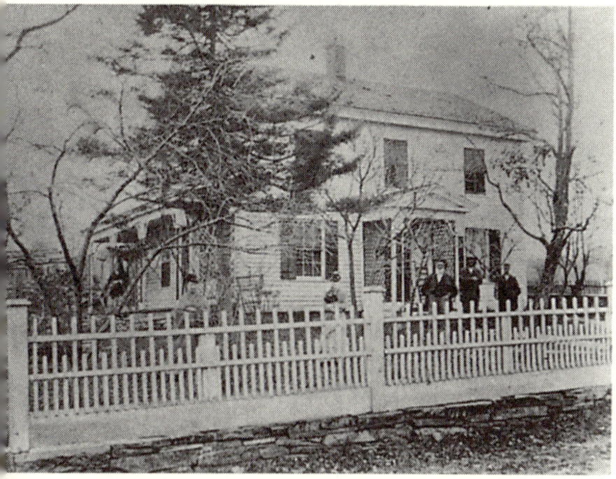

Sherwood home at Liberty, N.Y.

Dr. Hall and Dr. Sherwood at New York City Mission, 1890

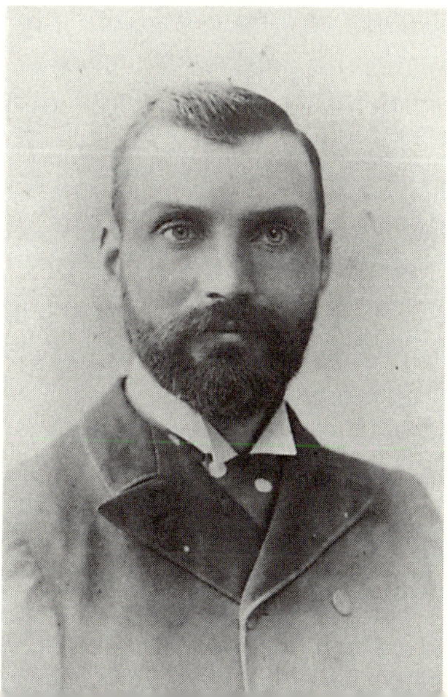

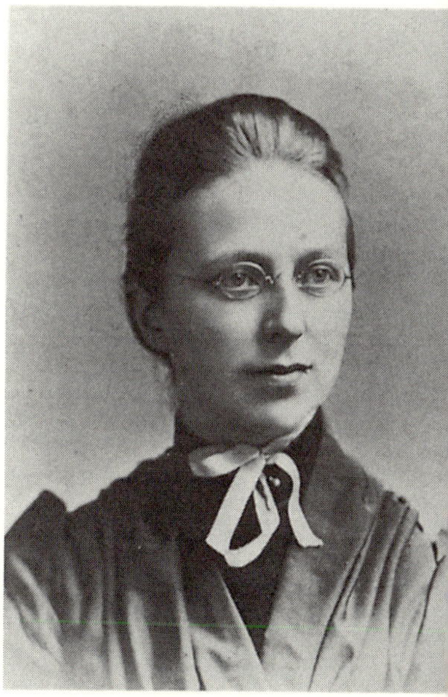

of only two. Dr. Hall did not believe in long engagements, but he decided that no one could take Dr. Sherwood's place in his affections. They became engaged.

On August 22, 1890, Dr. Sherwood left her home in Liberty for assignment in Korea. However much pain the separation caused him, Dr. Hall rejoiced that Rosetta was doing what she believed to be God's will. His new affection gave color to his whole subsequent life, although he soon discovered how very much he missed his beloved. He wrote to her:

> "I suppose now you are on the great Pacific. How often I think of you, and although you are being wafted farther and farther from me, each successive day, still in my heart you are daily nearer.
>
> "My love for you is developing a part of my character which had hitherto remained dormant. It has touched a heartstring which never vibrated before. You were never more precious to me than today.
>
> "It has been hard for me to see the one I love with all my heart going off to a strange land to fight alone in the battle of life. Though I realize you are not really alone, for He is with you. I am upholding you by my prayers. I used to think I might never meet the one I could love, as I love you, but I was mistaken. Just to think, in the most unlikely of all places, the slums of New York City, I should have discovered my heart's desire, my love! How dearly I love you, Rosetta, with a love that grows deeper and stronger each day.
>
> "The work at Madison Street Dispensary continues to move along gloriously. Many ask about you and express how they miss you. We have a girls' and boys' meeting weekly. Dear youths, how I love them! It would do you good to hear them speak and pray."

The months went by, but the Canadian Methodist Mission Board was unable to raise the money to send Dr. Hall to China. He continued his healing ministry to the poor of New York, patiently and expectantly trusting God to guide his future, and remaining open to whatever direction that might lead.

His letters to his fiancée reflected the constantly shifting possibilities that confronted and tested him. He wrote of the visit of the missionary from India, Bishop James M. Thoburn, whose wife had helped to inspire Dr. Sherwood to become a medical missionary:

"We had a glorious time on Sunday. Bishop Thoburn was at Asbury; he preached on the street in the evening, and afterward inside. I had a good visit with him at Dr. Stone's. He wants me for India, but I think that is not my place. But the needs and claims of the foreign field are pressing upon me with greater force than ever, and the probability is that I will start for China in about a year."

In a letter dated March 3, 1891 he wrote:

"Our Board doesn't expect to be able to send out any medical missionaries this year. I have an offer to go to China to treat some Europeans in the government employ, with the privilege of doing all the missionary work I choose. There is no missionary in that place at all. In this way I could get to the field without any expense to the Missionary Society and be self-supporting. The engagement would be for five years. The New York City Church Extension and Missionary Society have engaged my services another year, but I told them there was a possibility of my going to the foreign field next fall."

On June 3 he reported:

"I received a letter from Dr. Baldwin, stating that they wished to see me at the Secretaries' rooms. I went up, and they asked me if I would be willing to go to Korea in case they had to send a man to take Dr. Scranton's work. I said I would. But now they can't settle anything until Bishop Goodsell returns. But I have given up the Chinese government offer entirely in view of going to Korea under our own Board."

Dr. Baldwin was Executive Secretary of the American Methodist Episcopal Mission Board. Dr. William B. Scranton, to whom Dr. Hall referred, had gone to Korea in May, 1885, soon after the first Methodist missionaries to Korea, Mr. and Mrs. Henry G. Appenzeller, along with Dr. Horace G. Underwood of the Presbyterian Church, had set foot on Korean soil Easter Sunday, April 5, 1885. Dr. Scranton began the first resident medical work of the Methodist Mission in Korea and subsequently became a District Superintendent as well as Superintendent of the Mission.

Dr. Scranton's mother, Mrs. Mary F. Scranton, had accompanied her son and his wife as the first missionary to be sent to Korea by the Woman's Foreign Missionary Society (W.F.M.S.). Mrs. M. F. Scranton served as the "Lady Bishop" of the Society. She was, therefore, Dr. Sherwood's "boss" in 1890 when the new missionary arrived in Korea.

It was because the Scrantons were returning to the United States on furlough in 1891 that Dr. Hall was being considered to fill Dr. Scranton's position in the medical work of the Mission. However, when Bishop Goodsell returned to New York in August, he apparently did not favor sending another doctor to Korea just then. He rejected the suggestion that Dr. Hall be sent as Dr. Scranton's replacement.

Dr. Hall took this turn of events as God's leading. He wrote to his sweetheart:

> "The way to the foreign field at present appears to be hedged, and God is marvelously opening up my way here and giving me the hearts of the people. Indications point strongly as though He wanted me in New York. He knows best, and I am glad to have Him choose for me. I don't lay nearly so many plans as I used to. I am just resting passive in His hands."

Not long after he had written this, another letter followed, on August 27:

> "The Canadian Methodist Board have been urging me very strongly for the past two weeks to go out under them to China, and went to work and raised the money to send me, without receiving any encouragement from me, as I hoped to go out under the Board here; but the Lord has hedged up the way here and opened it wide there."

Naturally, the doctor longed to receive his appointment to Korea, but with him it was not a question of choice, but obedience. His prayer had been, "Lord, open the way and I shall follow." He prepared to leave, shipping his goods with the Canadian party assigned to go to China with him. Two of its members had been converted to Christianity by Dr. Hall during their high school days, Dr. Omar Kilborn (who was also at Queens with him), and the Reverend G. E. Hartwell who had received his training at Drew Theological Seminary in Madison, New Jersey.

Resigned to the events that seemed to have shut the door for him to Korea, Dr. Hall wrote to his fiancée on September 2, 1891:

> "As long as our life work is to be in China, why not both get there as soon as possible? Why not come now if the Board will release you? We are spending our best years apart when I am sure we could do much more efficient work for God if united."

He went on to tell of his plan to see Mrs. H. B. Skidmore of the Woman's Foreign Missionary Society in New York to see if Rosetta could be released from her commitment to the Society and meet him in Shanghai on October 30. They could be married there and proceed to Western China.

Rosetta, in her turn, struggled to determine what God wanted her to do between her desire to be with Dr. Hall in China and her wish to fulfill her five-year obligation to the W.F.M.S. Her dilemma was happily resolved in the next letter she received from her fiancé.

It seemed that Dr. Scranton and Dr. Baldwin had persuaded the American Methodist Mission Board that it was not in their best interests to lose Dr. Hall to the Canadian Mission Board and to China. Dr. Hall penned the following letter to Dr. Sherwood on her 26th birthday, September 19, 1891:

> "Well, Rosetta, I have just been appointed to Korea! Yesterday I received my release from the Canadian Board, providing I was appointed by our Board to Korea. I rejoice that the Lord has opened the way. He knew I would gladly go anywhere for Him, and I feel so grateful that we are soon

to be together. I never felt His presence and power more than now. I will now take some post-graduate work. I am rooming at 118 East 45th Street with Dr. Scranton. I have also met his mother, and I like both very much. They speak highly of you. Dr. Baldwin tells me he wants me to leave Vancouver November 22. I go that way, that I may visit my dear old home . . . I expect Mrs. Skidmore would much rather I was not going to Korea. I am urged on every side to remain here, but I feel God has work for me to do."

The farewell for Dr. Hall was a heartwarming experience. Andrew Green, Esq., Comptroller of New York City, spoke with deep appreciation for the service performed by Dr. Hall at the Madison Street Mission. The Hon. James A. Seaman of the Board of Home Missions of the Methodist Episcopal Church paid tribute to Dr. Hall's ability, rare enthusiasm and his devotion.

Also in attendance were some of Dr. Hall's special younger friends. None delighted his heart more than the eager, bright eyed, confident children he had taken with him on an unprecedented camping trip to Charleston Lake, 500 miles north of New York City, near his home in Canada. To this day, residents of that farm community recall Jimmy's legendary venture with 130 children from the New York slums, many of whom had never seen a live cow or chicken. Friendly farmers had loaded the excited children onto their hay wagons to transport them from Athens, Ontario, to their campsite at Charleston Lake and a never-to-be-forgotten experience.

Perhaps the most touching tributes came from the poor and the wretched who had been served by the Dispensary. Many spoke with tears in their eyes. A Jewish patient stammered out his feelings:

> "Dr. Hall has visited us constantly for some time. He is a wonderful man; he treats us without charge; he brings us food and then gets down on his knees and prays for us all."[6]

Dr. Hall's fellow workers at the Mission attested to the comfort and strength they too had derived from his prayers. Special appreciation was expressed for the characteristic patience, tact, and cheerful

---

[6] *The Life of W. J. Hall*, p. 324.

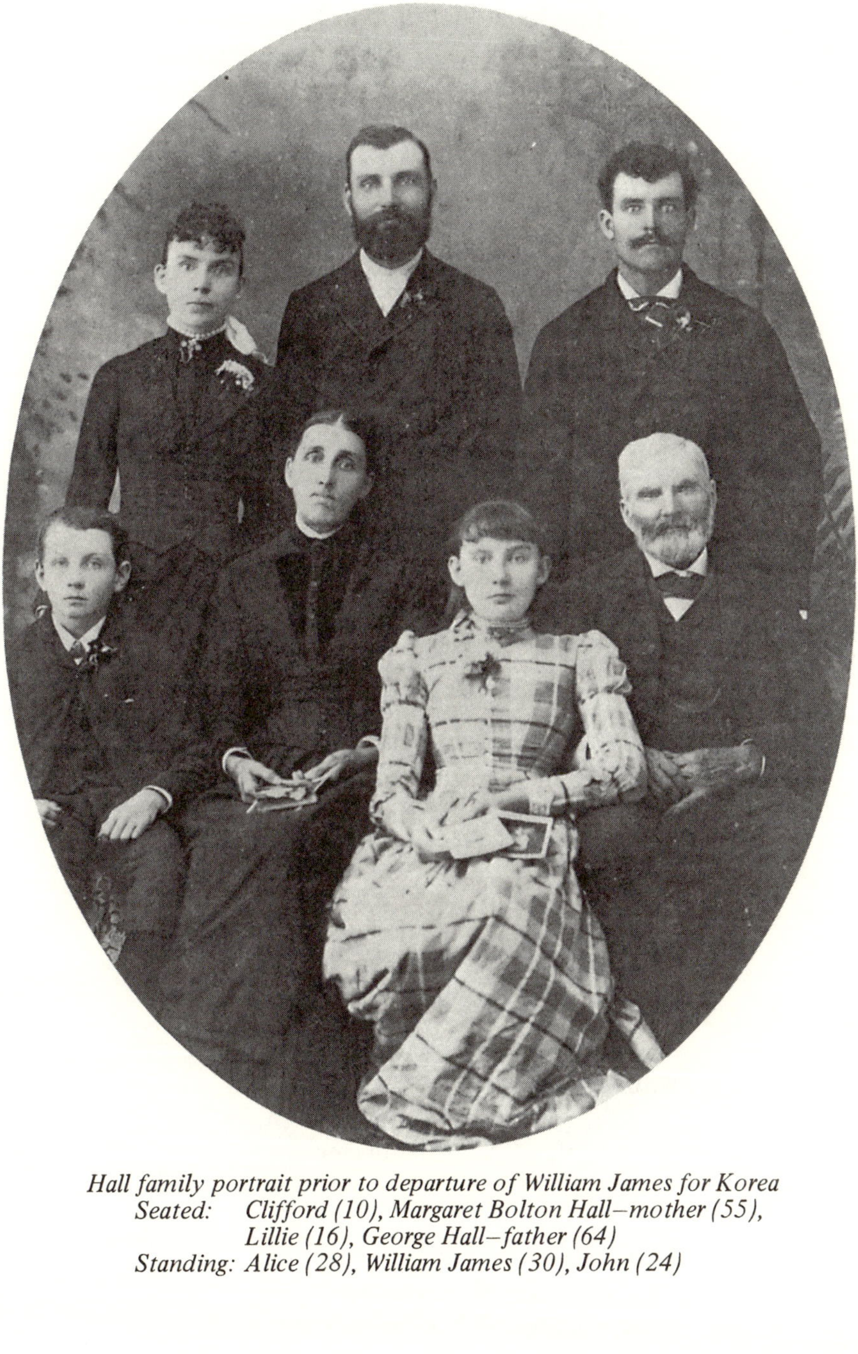

Hall family portrait prior to departure of William James for Korea
Seated: Clifford (10), Margaret Bolton Hall–mother (55), Lillie (16), George Hall–father (64)
Standing: Alice (28), William James (30), John (24)

optimism by which he led the work of the Mission. One medical student noted that Dr. Hall's constant recognition and encouragement of what was good in a person gave him the key to people's hearts. The speaker had directly experienced the way that Dr. Hall, with his great, generous heart, would overestimate a person's character for good and therefore give one the courage to try and be equal to that estimate.

At the close of the farewell speeches, the people flocked around, reluctant to let Dr. Hall go. Fanny Crosby, who had assisted Dr. Hall in the Sunday school at the Mission, was there. This renowned poet and hymn writer, blind since the age of six weeks, was now a frail and gentle lady of 71. She announced that she had composed a hymn in honor of their beloved doctor on his departure for the foreign mission field and wanted to offer it as her personal tribute of appreciation to Dr. Hall:

WHO WILL GO?

(Tune: "Hark, the voice of Jesus calling")

O'er the ruthless rolling ocean,
    Where the prince of darkness reigns,
Holding fast his countless victims,
    Crushed beneath his cruel chains;
O, the wail of bitter anguish,
    O, the deep despairing cry,
Send us light or we must perish,
    Send it quickly or we die.

To these wretched, starving millions,
    Who the bread of life will bear?
At the throne of grace and mercy,
    Who will plead with them in prayer?
Who will undertake the journey
    O'er the stormy billow's foam,
Leaving all without a murmer,
    Parents, friends, a native home?

Firmly, bravely comes the answer,
    From a loyal mission band,
That our blessed Lord is keeping,

In the hollow of His hand;
Firmly, bravely comes the answer.
Even now I hear him say,
"Gracious Master, Thou hast called me,
And Thy message I obey."

Dearest brother, you are going,
Where you oft may sow in tears,
And the fruit of earnest labor,
Be withheld perhaps for years,
Though you toil amid their changes,
Burning sun and chilling frost,
Not a seed will be forgotten,
Not a single blade be lost.

God be with you on the billows,
God protect you o'er the main,
In his tender, loving kindness,
Bring you back to us again;
But if otherwise determined,
And on earth we meet no more,
May we all sing hallelujah,
On the bright eternal shore.

—Fanny Crosby[7] (1820-1915)

[7] *The Life of W. J. Hall*, pp. 420-421.

CHAPTER 2

First Impressions of the Korean Kingdom

The Methodist Church began its missionary work in Korea in 1885. It had to reckon with a host of Korean customs, fears, and superstitions which would dictate initially the type of services the missionary could offer.

The Yi dynasty, which was the ruling power in Korea at that time, had instituted a law of seclusion for women in order to protect them and safeguard the institution of the family. Women had enjoyed great public freedom during the previous dynasty, but in the final decades of the Koryo regime they had become the special objects of violence and debauchery. These evils extended into the royal household and ultimately contributed to the destruction of the state.

To remedy the situation, the succeeding Yi dynasty withdrew women from the public eye. At the age of six or seven years, a girl was removed from all outside associations and confined to the inner apartments of her father's home. She left this protective isolation only when she married and then promptly found herself confined to the seclusion of her husband's home.

This custom made it clear that if Korean women were to receive the benefits of medical care and Christian outreach, a woman physician was needed. Consequently, Dr. Scranton had appealed to the Woman's Foreign Missionary Society to provide a hospital exclusively for the care of women and children. In response, Dr. Meta Howard was sent out in 1887 and inaugurated the first hospital for women in Korea. It was located on the same compound where Mrs. Mary Fitch Scranton had founded the first school for girls. This latter eventually developed into the great school and college for women named by Queen Min, *Ewha Haktang* (Pear Blossom Institution).

Dr. Howard treated several thousand women and children before her own health failed and she was forced to return to the United States in 1889. Dr. Rosetta Sherwood was to be her replacement.

As the *SS Oceanic* steamed its way across the Pacific toward Yokahama, Japan, it carried many missionaries who were traveling to assignments in Japan, China and Korea. Dr. Sherwood was among them and met several whose paths would cross hers again in the years to come. Dr. Isaac T. Headland, who was journeying to China, would one day be a college professor to her son.

Miss Margaret Bengel, a twenty-one year old teacher, was the only other missionary whose destination was Korea. Dr. Sherwood and she were both assigned to the W.F.M.S. compound in Seoul. Miss Bengel was to assist Miss Louise C. Rothweiler and Mrs. Scranton in the school. The two young travelers took an immediate liking to each other and became close companions for the rest of the journey.

Eighteen days and eleven hours after leaving San Francisco, the *SS Oceanic* arrived in Yokahama, a distance of some 5,477 miles. Dr. Sherwood and Miss Bengel took another vessel down the Japanese coast to Kobe and there transferred to the *SS Owari Maru* which was to take them via Nagasaki to Korea. In a long letter home, written scroll-fashion upon 34 yards of six-inch-wide Korean ricepaper, Dr. Sherwood recorded her travels and her early impressions for her family back in Liberty, New York:

> "Today, October 10, 1890, we come in sight of the coast of Korea. As we draw nearer, I look with considerable interest at this country which promises to be my home for some time to come. I can't say that it looks very inviting, though I am bound to make the best of it. The hills and mountains are irregular in outline, very steep, rocky and almost barren.
>
> "We anchored off Fusan [Pusan] for twenty-four hours. Fusan is a Japanese settlement almost entirely, so we could not form much of an opinion of Koreans. We saw a number of them however. Their village is a mile or more back behind the hills, but we can see them from the ship passing along the road that winds about the mountain. They look rather picturesque all dressed in white from head to foot. We only see the men; the women do not go out until after sunset, when the men go in. Rather a novel custom, but rather a good one

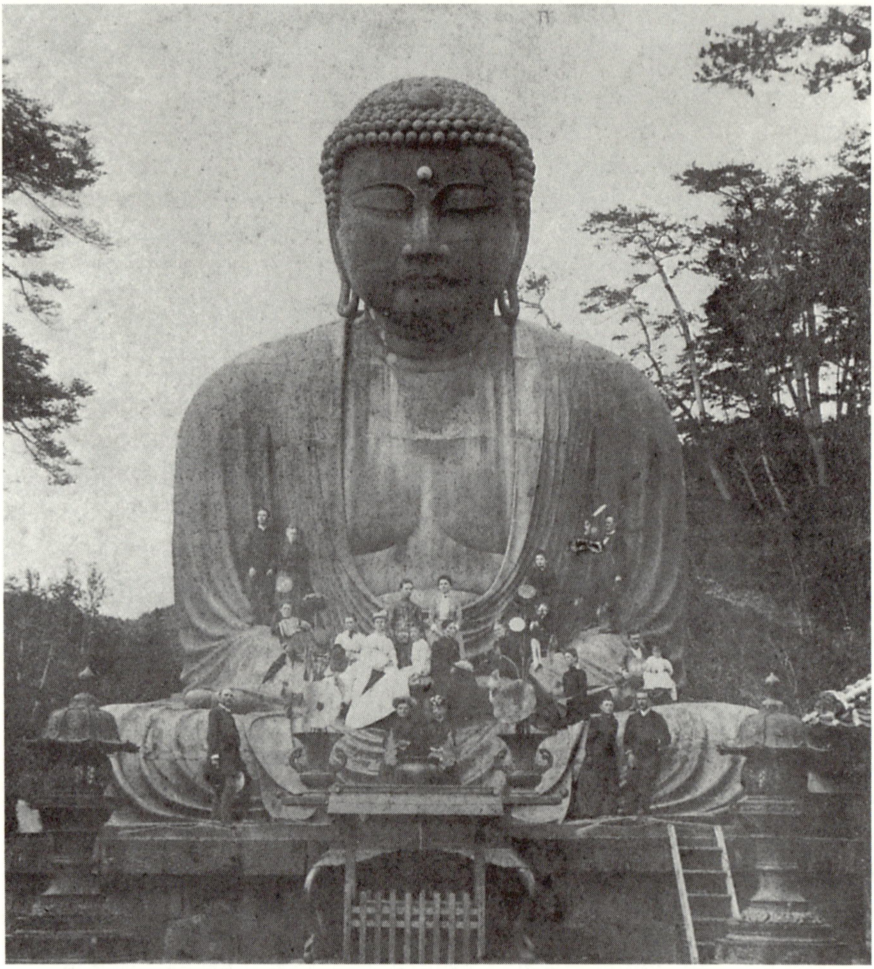

Miss Bengel (center, 2nd from left with white hat), Dr. Sherwood (standing next to Miss Bengel) and other missionaries seated on lap of the Dai-butsi at Kamakura, Japan, 1890

so far as the men are concerned it seems to me. I wonder how our American men would like it?

"All of our party went ashore in a sampan for a stroll upon land. We went first to the telegraph station, and a Korean man sent a message for Miss Bengel and me to Mrs. Scranton. He understands a little English and no doubt is well up in Chinese, as are all Korean scholars. This is the only telegraph line in Korea, from Fusan to Seoul, and there are no railroads, and no wagon roads either, for that matter. All traveling is done on foot, or in a chair carried by men, or upon horseback.

"Koreans are usually divided into three classes: the 'upper' composed of officials; the 'middle,' merchants and those able to hire labor; and the 'lower,' all who are employed in any form of manual work . . .

"The Koreans seem to me to be quite unlike either the Chinese or the Japanese. Some of the first few I saw in Fusan reminded me more of the American Indian. They are not as tall as the Indians, but are taller than the Japanese. They all have long hair.

"While unmarried they go bare-headed, parting their hair in the middle and wearing it in a long braid down the back. A Korean bachelor ranks as a boy even if he is fifty, and it is not until he is married or engaged that he is allowed to put up his hair. Then he shaves it at the crown—taking it off just where the Chinese man leaves his, and leaving it where the Chinese man shaves it off. Then he gathers the long hair left and twists it into a tight high knot to the front of the crown of his head. It is made to stand up straight by running a wooden or silver pin down through it . . . A band of horsehair about two inches wide, closely fitting the head all about the margin of the hair and closely holding all short hairs neatly back, usually completes the men's hair dressing.

"The hat seems to be worn by the Korean for ornament rather than use. They have quite wide brims but small high crowns, and they wear them perched back over their knot of hair on the crown of the head, tying them with a ribbon that passes under the chin. They are made of a thin cloth pasted smoothly over a light bamboo frame. The best ones are made of horsehair and ordinarily they are black, but just now they are white, in mourning for the King's mother, Old Queen Cho. The palace hat is different in shape—has sort of wings at the side, and the farmer's hats are quite as large as bushel baskets which they somewhat resemble.

"The Korean coat is long, some made of plain white linen, some of Korean silk, and some of coarse cotton cloth. They are not all just the same cut—some being slit up the sides; some up the back. Some have just loose sleeves, and others, the large flowing sleeve answering as a pocket like the Japanese. They all fasten by lapping over the breast a little at one side, tied in a bow with strings of the same material usually. They wear large loose trousers of a peculiar cut, bound in around the ankle. These also are white. In winter both coat and trousers are wadded with cotton, but they are always light tinted or white. Only small boys wear colored clothes. The soldiers wear black, or men of rank sometimes have a thin overdress of black. White muslin stockings and low shoes, more like slippers, pointed and turned up at the toes, complete this queer looking costume . . . If he be a literary man or a man of some rank, he usually carries a plain white fan that closes, summer and winter . . .

"One of the first things I noticed in Korea is their way of carrying burdens upon the back. They have a sort of rudely shaped easel made of crocheted sticks which they call a *jiggy*. They will carry a large trunk or any other heavy burden with apparent ease upon one of these . . .

"Soon after returning to the *Owari*, we were upon our way once more, and began plowing up the west side of Korea through the waters of the Yellow Sea . . . Most of our way a chain of islands to our east separate us from the coast of the mainland . . .

"Monday, October 13, 1890 – . . . How glad I am this bright morning. We are soon to reach Chemulpo [Inchon] the port of Seoul, and soon my long journey by land and by sea will be finished and I will be upon my field of labor in this 'Land of the Morning Brightness.' . . . We anchored off Chemulpo while eating breakfast. The tide not being in, we had to anchor some three miles out; but, by 10 A.M. Miss Rothweiler came in a boat to meet us, and soon afterwards we left with her for the shore.

"Miss Rothweiler came down from Seoul Saturday. Sunday was the day of the Queen's funeral, and everyone went to Seoul, so it was impossible yet this morning to get chair coolies to take us up in time to get in before the city gates close at 7 P.M. So we went to a hotel in Chemulpo kept by a Chinese man called 'Steward' where we were made quite comfortable till the next morning when we got an early

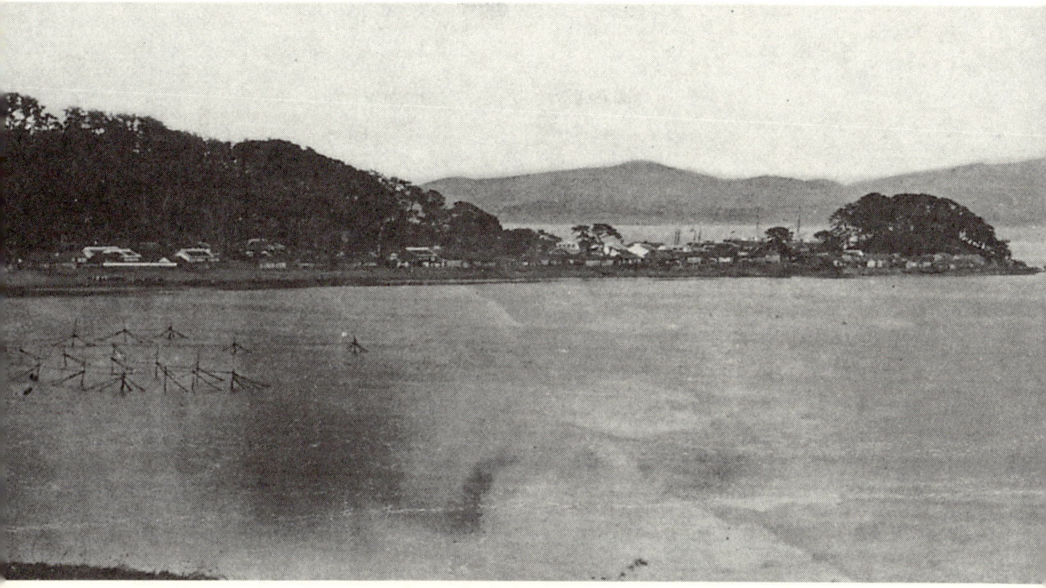

Fusan, 1890–first glimpse of Korea

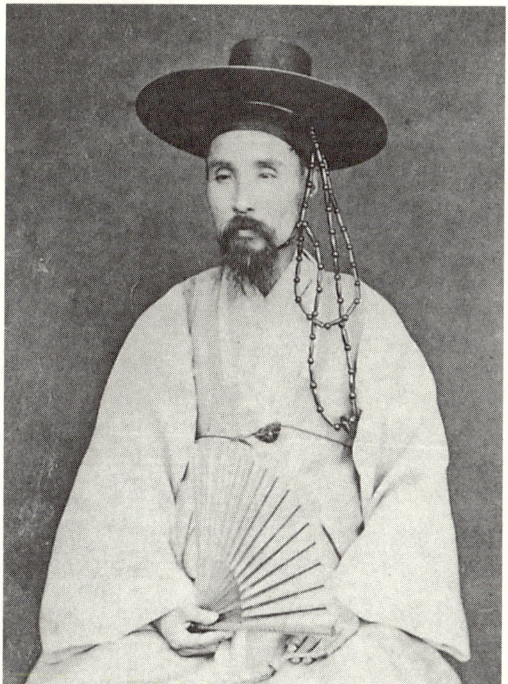

Korean of upper class

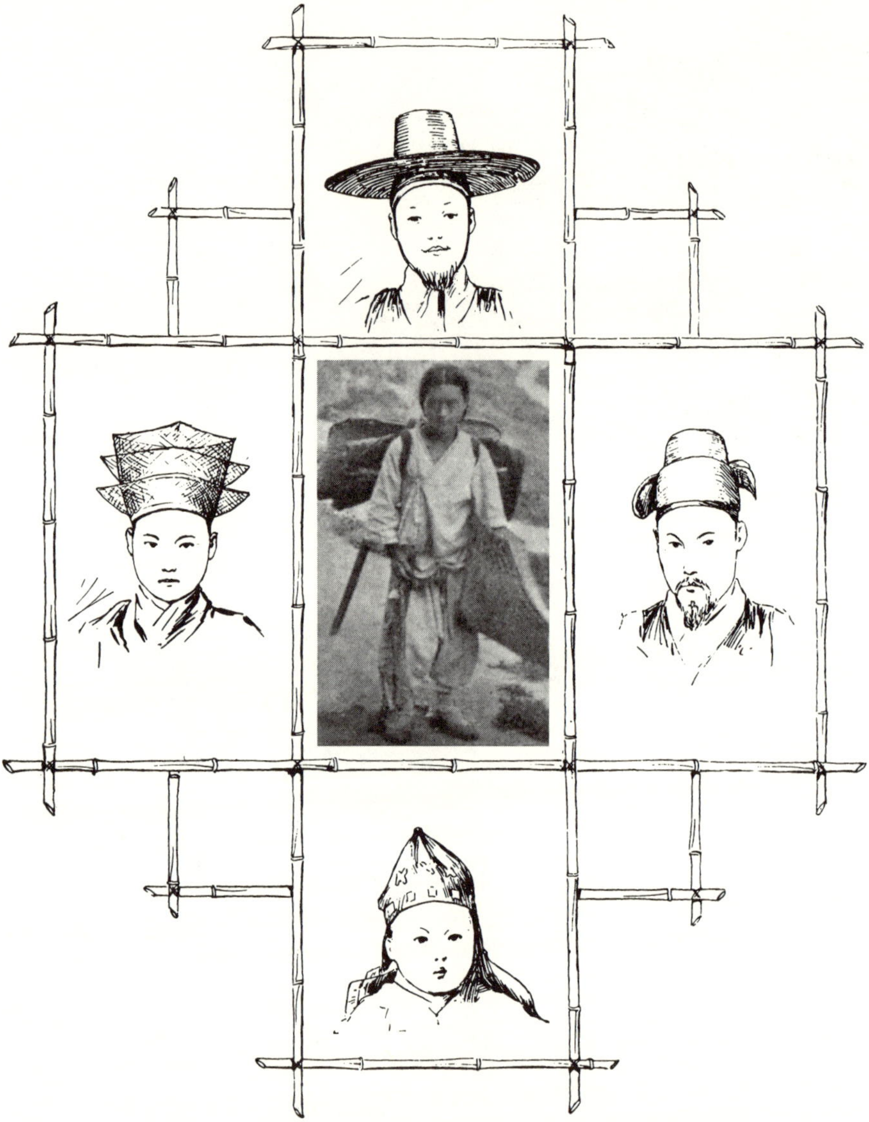

Korean hats: Top–gentleman's hat; Middle l. to r.–scholar's hat, farmer with farmer's hat, palace hat; Bottom–holiday hat

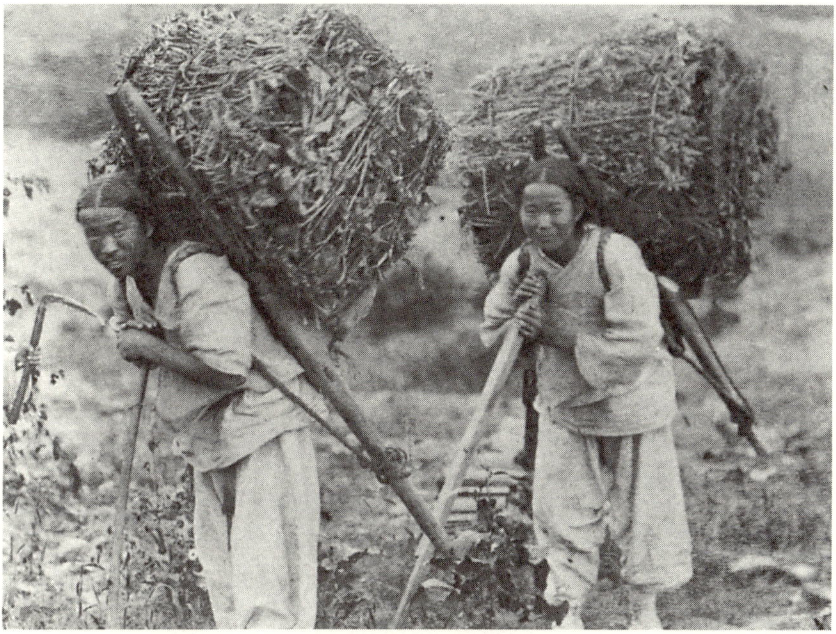

Coolies carrying brush on "jiggies"

breakfast. With the help of Mr. Gale we got our chair coolies together and started by 8:30 A.M. on the road to Seoul.

"We met Mr. Gale [James Scarth Gale] at the hotel last evening. He is one of the missionaries at Seoul, and came down yesterday to see a friend, Mr. M. C. Fenwick, off on the *Owari*. He is a Canadian sent out by the Y.M.C.A. of Toronto, I believe. We find him very pleasant company.

"It takes eight men for one chair, four carrying for a time, then the other four relieving. Native officials only have the four and some only two, but as they sit on their feet, their chairs are lighter than ours. They walk along at a pretty good rate, averaging about four miles an hour. Very often the reserve men step up and take hold of the bars, which pass one on either side of the chairs, while the others change the stick from one shoulder to the other. It is done very quickly and does not much interfere with the progress. I found by actual count that they made this change four times in five minutes! I wanted to propose their padding the stick or wearing a pad upon the shoulder, but Mr. Gale said it wouldn't do. They would not take up any *new* methods!

"We see no vehicles of any kind upon wheels. Mr. Gale rides a pony, and we meet or sometimes pass quite a little caravan upon ponies, with pack horses or an ox laden upon either side with baggage. Our valises and steamer trunks were carried on *jiggies* all the way from Chemulpo to Seoul [27 miles]!

"Noticed some quite good looking farm land as we passed along. They raise some rice, but not as much as farther south. Patches of Korean turnips, which taste much like our winter radishes and are eaten raw like them; buckwheat, millet and a sort of brown corn are about all of the crops that are out now. This has been a very good season in Korea I am told.

"Now and then upon a hillside we pass a Korean burying ground. Their graves are mounds looking like haycocks, and are unmarked as a rule.

"There are not many trees upon our way, and few to be seen upon the mountains; but I noticed a few small groves and an occasional large tree. It is said that the Korean cuts a tree while it is small because they believe if they let it be till it is large, it then has a spirit and they dare not kill it. It seems such a pity that they should thus rob themselves and the coming generations of all the beautiful young trees, which would make their country so much fairer and more valuable. They fortunately have coal fields or else I do not know what would be done for fuel by and by. They have not yet learned to make any use of coal, however.

"For a ways before reaching the Han River we crossed quite a stretch of sand. It seemed like going through a desert. At the river we had to cross in crude ferry boats. There are swarms of houses all along the river, and they are pretty thick from there to the city gate. The city wall was built in 1396. It is 13 miles long, 20 to 40 feet high and was built in six months! We have gotten glimpses of the city wall here and there for quite a ways back. It extends in some places quite a ways outside of the city, running up over the mountains on either side . . .

"A little outside of the city we were met by Rev. F. Ohlinger and Dr. W. B. McGill of our Parent Board. It seemed very pleasant to see their faces.

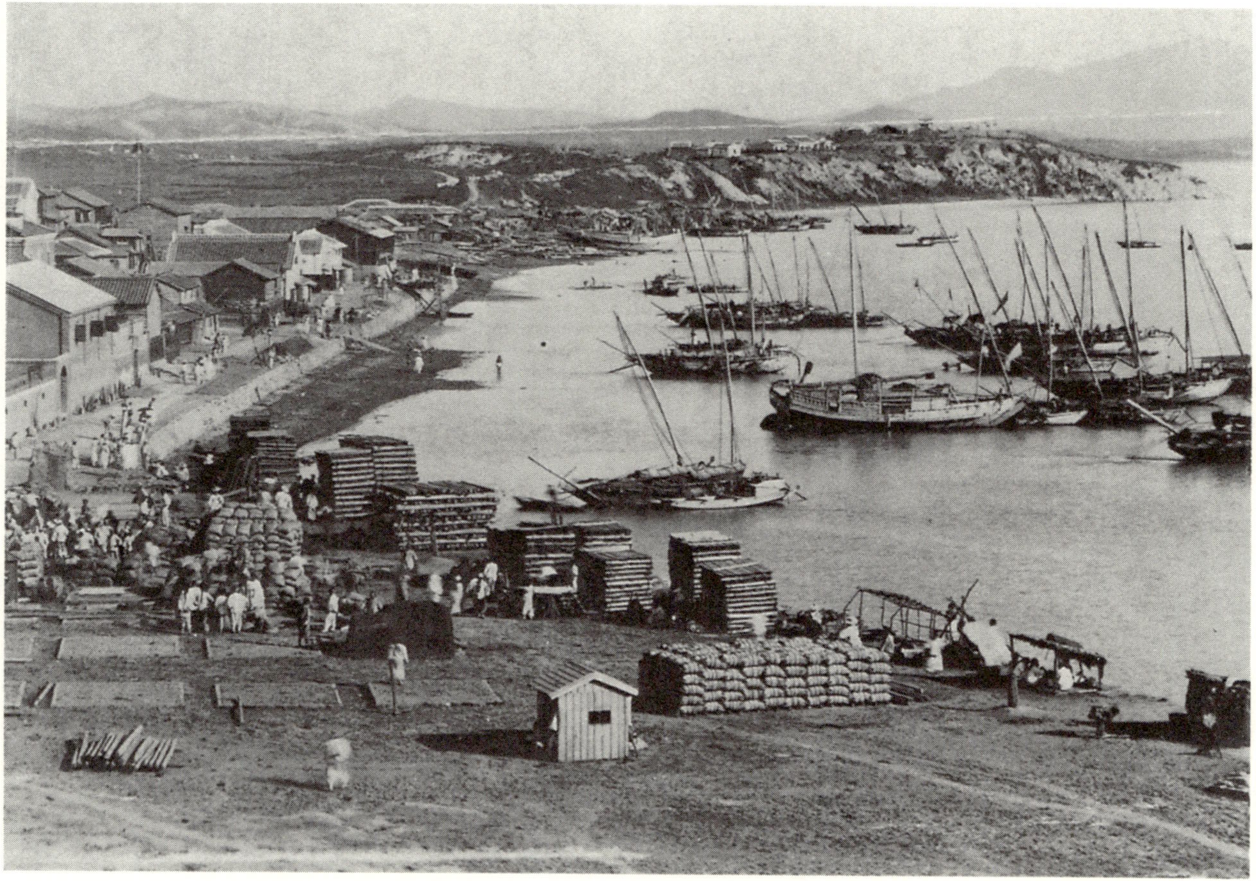

Chemulpo (Inchon) Harbor, 1890

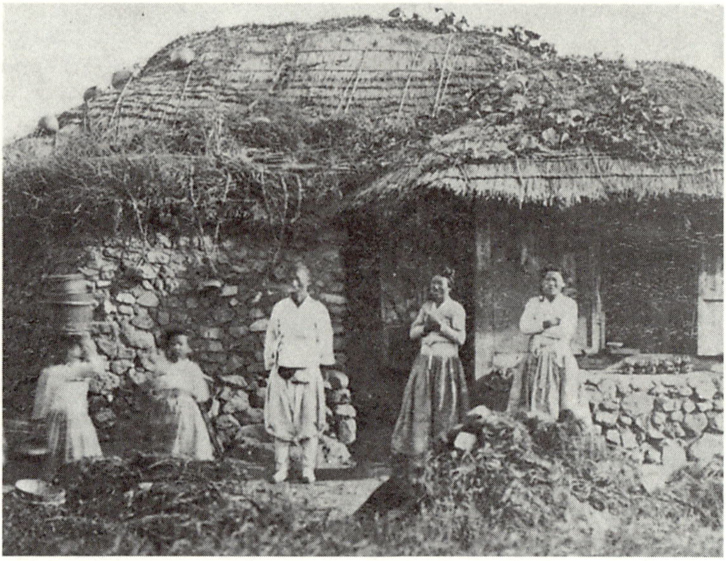

Korean farmhouse with gourd vines growing over thatched roof

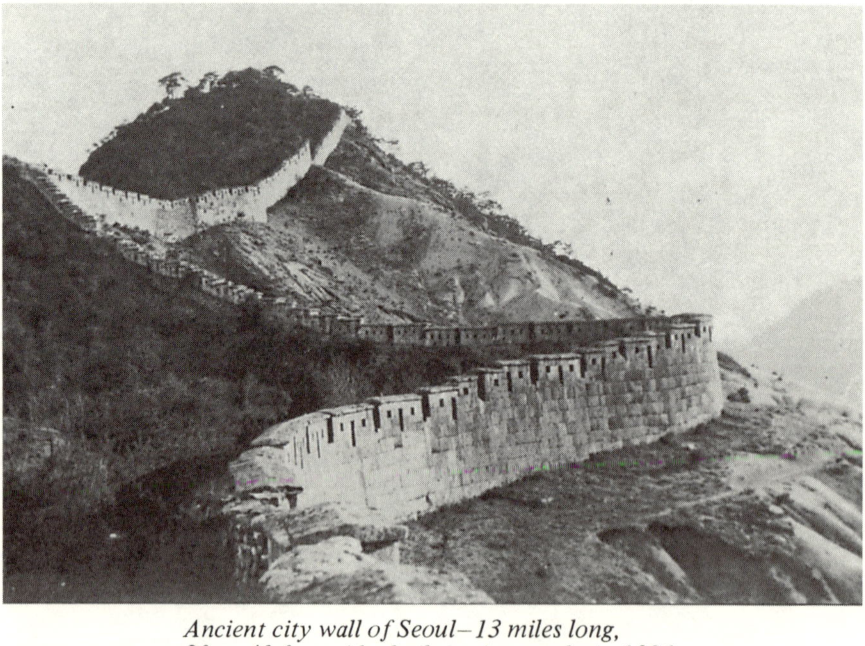

Ancient city wall of Seoul–13 miles long, 20 to 40 feet wide, built in six months in 1396

"Some after 4 P.M. we entered Seoul by what is called the West Gate. It only took us a few moments now to reach the grounds of the W.F.M.S. They extend back to the city wall, are quite high, commanding a good view of the city and the mountains around, and are really perhaps the prettiest grounds in the city. They join those of the Parent Board at one side, both being enclosed in one large compound containing our home and school, the school of the Parent Board, both hospitals and the homes of Dr. Scranton, Rev. Appenzeller and Rev. Ohlinger. The latter's home and the boys school are brick buildings, more on the American style; the others are Korean in style—framework of wood, walls of mud and tiled roofs. They are very pretty and artistic in appearance I think.

"Mrs. Scranton met us on the porch and in her own sweet graceful way bade us welcome to our new home.

"I am most agreeably surprised with our house. I had heard that it was so damp that mushrooms grew upon its walls; but I have seen nothing of the kind. Upon the contrary, the sanitary condition seems fairly good. It is well drained. Being upon high ground gives good opportunity for this.

"Like all Korean houses it is all upon the one floor, built about a sort of court. Besides three nice school-rooms and the pupils' sleeping rooms and dining room, there are three pleasant rooms for the teachers and a reception room, a dining room and kitchen. All are finished in Korean style—the rafters of small pealed logs about one foot apart, the large hewn cross beams and all the framework appearing. These are stained brown and varnished, and the mud walls are covered with paper which is carefully cut to fit in all about the rafters and beams. The effect of the whole is something I like. Since there are only rooms for one more besides Mrs. Scranton and Miss Rothweiler, it was thought best that Miss Bengel should have these rooms as they were near the school, and that I should occupy rooms in a small Korean house a few steps from the main building.

"I like my pretty little house so much. There are three rooms—the front room has three windows, an outside door, and doors opening into two small rooms. All of the rooms are sunny and the front room is very pleasant. It will be my sitting room, study, and office. It contains a nice writing desk, a table, a Korean dressing bureau and cabinet, both odd and pretty with many little nooks and drawers that are convenient for putting away things. I brought my books and revolving book case with me, and some framed pictures that I have had from a child, and so with a neat matting on the floor, a rug or two, and a few easy chairs, I have a comfortable room that seems really homelike to me. One small room I use for a clothes and trunk room—the other contains my bed, wash stand and a Korean money chest bound in brass. I didn't suppose I would ever have money enough to need such a thing as that, but here, where it takes one thousand pieces about as large as our quarter to make one dollar (gold), a little money occupies a large space. People don't carry it in pocketbooks here but in bundles on the back or if very much, on one of those *jiggies*, or a pony!

"My rooms are finished off in about the same style as those of the main building—some places the mud walls have shrunken away from the beams so you could stick your fingers through, but I have had these pasted up for winter. Like all Korean houses, I have an *on-dol* or, as the Chinese call it, a *kang*—that is a place made of stone under the floor where a fire is burned and the room heated in this way. It is very nice for cold feet and I rather like it. However, I have only used it a little as I have a coal stove also and that takes less fuel, which is very expensive in Korea . . .

"Mrs. Scranton is a nice looking woman with blue eyes and gray hair. She is so kind and good; everyone loves her dearly. I also like Miss Rothweiler very much. She is a plain-looking, plain-spoken active little woman of German descent. She and Miss Bengel come from near the same place in Ohio. Miss Bengel is our baby missionary, as I think I have mentioned. She is a pretty brunette of twenty-one, a dear earnest girl that we all love. It is so nice to have such congenial co-workers—it makes our home life so pleasant.

"And now I think I must tell about my hospital—I cannot wait any longer. It didn't take me as long as this to visit it that first day, and the very next morning I began my work there. I am delightfully surprised with the hospital and dispensary; they are so much better than I expected. To be sure,

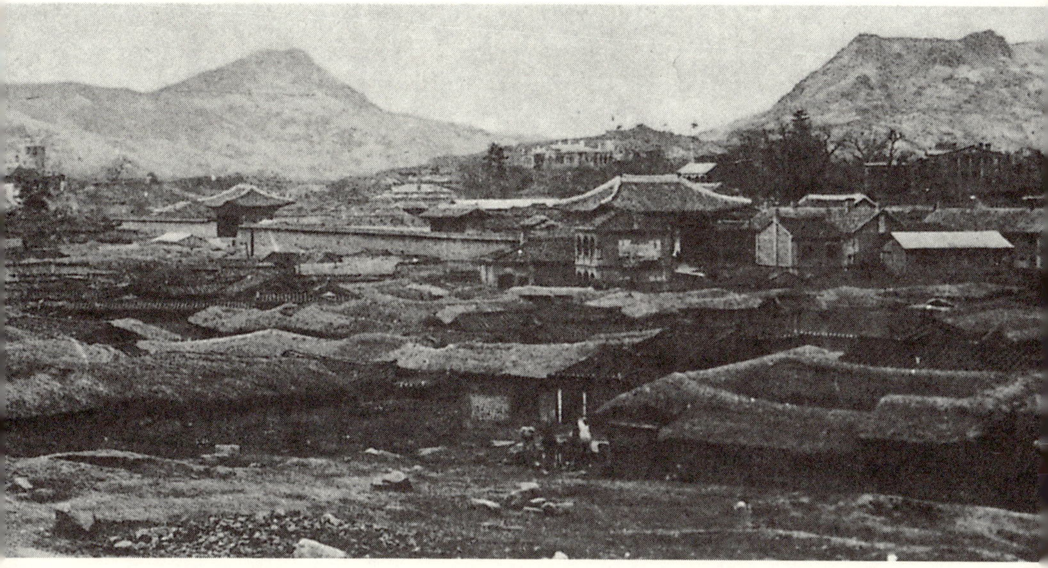

Seoul–palace at center; Russian, French, and British Legations in background

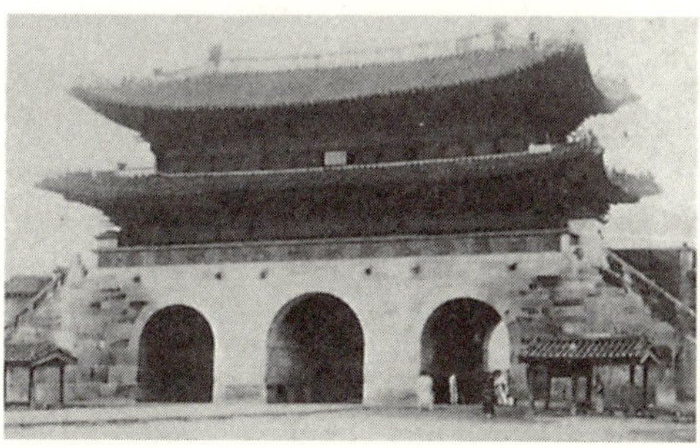

Royal Palace Gate

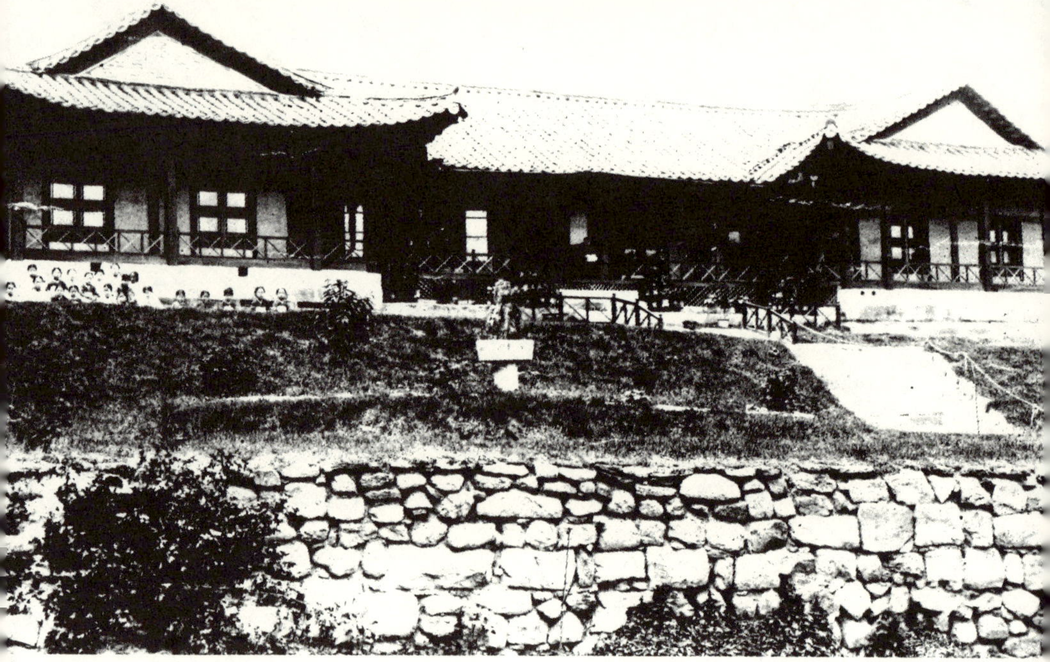

Woman's Foreign Missionary Society Home and Ewha School

they are nothing but Korean houses, modeled over a little, but they look nice and answer the purpose very well. There is a nice large drug room, with store room, and room for washing and cleaning up bottles etc. There is a good sized waiting room, and a consulting room between it and the drug room. There is a fine large front room, well lighted, that can be used as an operating room. There are five rooms for inpatients. We call them 'wards' but they are hardly large enough to be dignified by that name, though each will accommodate several patients comfortably. They are warmed by *on-dols* and the patients rest upon the warmed floors rolled up in a blanket in Korean style. We have added sheets to the outfit and that is about all. It makes it a little hard for the doctor till one gets used to it to have to get down upon the floor to take a patient's pulse or respiration, dress wounds etc., but upon the whole I believe it is the best thing. In the first place, *it is Korean*. They think our beds must be very cold, and I see no reason for trying to change customs that do no harm. As their floors are warmed, it is really a comfortable place to sleep; second, there is no danger of your patient getting out of bed when you don't want her to; third, it is clean—bed with room is easily disinfected; and last, but perhaps not least in a mission hospital, it is *economical*!

"I found quite a good stock of drugs upon hand. Dr.

Scranton of the Parent Board has done all that he could for our Woman's Hospital since Dr. Howard went home, and so things were in a much better working order than I expected. The instruments upon hand, with those I brought with me, make quite a fair supply but we need more. I sent off a drug order soon after I came that took all the money then on hand, but no doubt we will have more sent us to buy instruments with, and thanks to my Liberty friends I have a purse that will be nice to help out . . .

"But here is the picture of the hospital. Is it not pretty? I believe I am really proud of it! The lady in a gray dress is Dr. Meta Howard who began medical missionary work here in 1887 but had to return home two years later on account of ill health. Our hospital helper, 'Sara,' stands to the right in a white Korean dress. She is matron and all the nurse we have. We call her Pung Sun Omani which means Pung Sun's mother, Korean women having no names of their own. The other woman is the hospital cook. Our '*Kuisyu*' (soldier) stands in the foreground dressed in the costume of a Korean soldier. He is our right-hand man—does most of our Korean

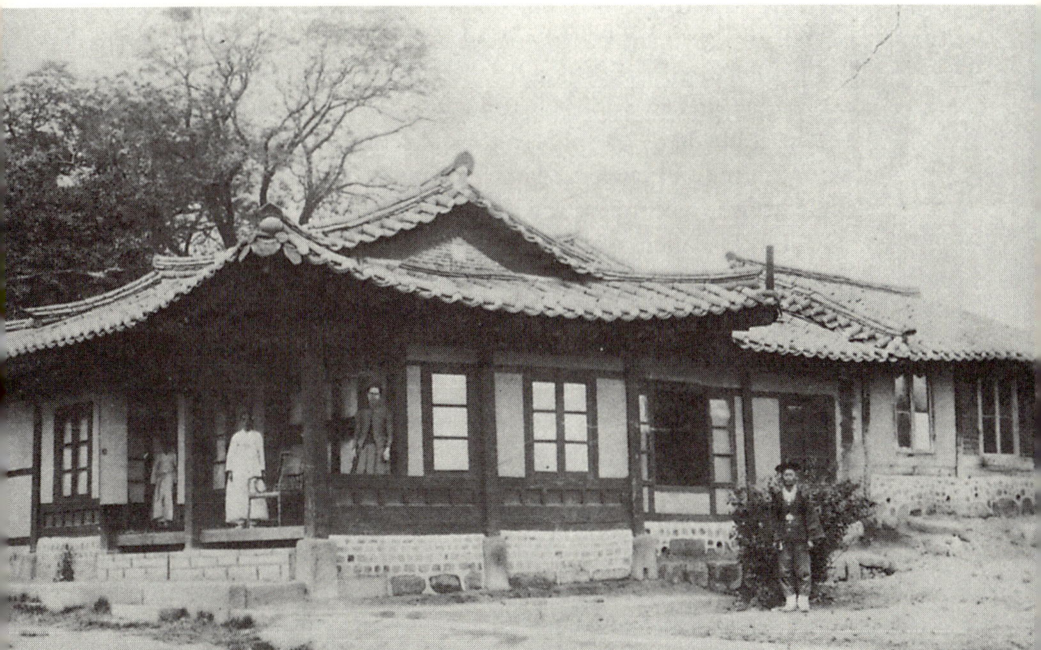

Woman's Foreign Missionary Society Hospital

marketing, shopping, money exchanging etc. He seems quite trustworthy and we would not know how to get along without him. The *Kuisyu* (Kēsū) and Pung Sun Omani are both Christians, and are earnest workers in the Lord's vineyard. Pung Sun Omani reads the Bible in Korean to the hospital patients and talks and prays with them. She is faithful in her attendance upon the religious services in our woman's church that we have recently organized here, and brings those patients who are able to come, with her.

"The first day I had four patients in the dispensary, the next day nine and in nearly three months that I have been here now, there have been 270 first visits and 279 return visits or a total of 549 cases that I have treated in the dispensary. Upon looking over the diagnoses in my record of cases, I find over 50 varieties of disease. Struma, syphilis, asceris lumbracoides, eye, ear and skin troubles predominate. Abscesses to be opened and teeth to extract are also common. Have only had eight in-patients so far, and have made but 21 professional out-calls.[1]

"The majority of my dispensary patients are from the lower class, of course, as the others must not be seen upon the street in the daytime. When I get to know the language better and don't have to spend so much time in studying, or if another doctor is sent out to the work, I would like to have a *night clinic* so that it would be proper for any woman to come–high, low, or middle class. Sometimes the better class women come in closed chairs, or they send for me to come to their house, paying for my chair coolies.

"I was called out the other day to the house of a titled Korean of the Min family. They had quite a little clinic for me. I prescribed for six people! It was a large Korean house, one of the best–built about a court–the men's apartments upon one side, the women's upon the other. There seemed to be a grandmother and several daughters-in-law, one in bride's attire. There were many children and servants. The rooms had been freshly papered. There were some nice Korean screens and cabinets. The floors were clean and very warm.

[1] Note added later: "During the ensuing three years, treated over 14,000 cases."

"We had to sit down and eat before we went or it would have offended them much. They brought in a small Korean table about one foot high on which were two brass bowls of vermicelli soup, and preserved ginger, and pears cooked in honey. The soup was quite good. We had brass chop sticks to eat it with, but as I didn't know how to manage mine very well, they brought me one of those big brass spoons. I tasted of the *kimchie*, a favorite dish with Koreans. It reminded me of sauerkraut but was so hot with red-pepper that I could only take one very small taste. We left some chapters from the Gospels, printed in Korean, with the women of this household, and I pray that some good seed will sink into their hearts and bring forth fruit for the Master.

"The Korean woman . . . is well dressed, her yoke and sleeves are made of some bright colored silk, probably purple, and the long outside skirt of perhaps a light green, though it is more often white or light blue. Young Korean women usually dress in bright colors unless in mourning when they wear white. A Korean girl parts her hair in the middle and wears it in a long braid down her back until her wedding day when it is put up in a low coil at the nape of the neck, fastened with a wooden, coral, or silver bar pin. They do not wear earrings. In fact, to all appearances, the dress of a Korean woman is very sensible. But, in truth, so many skirts fastened by bands which, though broad, have to be bound so tightly about chest and waist to keep them from slipping down make it not so hygienic as it looks. If they could be sewed to the yokes, they would do very well. The only undergarments worn are two pairs of large loose drawers, something like our divided petticoats. It takes 13 yards of muslin to make two pair. In winter one pair and the yokes are wadded with cotton . . . The skirts are not sewed together like ours, but they lap them over a foot or two—the lower class women upon the right side and the upper class on the left side.

"Korean women carry their children upon the back much the same as the Japanese or tie them to the back of an older sister or to a 'child-nurse.' Quite little girls often bring sick children to me at the dispensary this way.

"My dispensary patients always seem very grateful for the help they receive, thanking me very much, '*Mănhe kōm ăp so*.' From those that are able I have had many presents sent, such as from ten to twenty-five persimmons, a peck of chestnuts or three or four 'strings of eggs.' They always get eggs by the string in Korea—ten in a string. They are placed end to end and bound with straw and carried much as they do strings of money. One of my surgical cases sent me a rooster and three hens! I think I must tell you something of this patient.

"This young lady of sixteen came to me in a closed chair from some 30 miles away in the country, with a hand three fingers of which were grown together and bound down to the palm, the result of a burn of several years ago. It is considered a great disgrace in Korea if a girl is not married before she is sixteen, and I expect it was this hand that kept her from being sought in marriage for she is a good looking bright natured girl. I kept her in the hospital, etherized her and dissected up the fingers, bandaged them separately, then straightened them out and fastened them to a splint. I tried to have it an antiseptic operation and succeeded very nicely, as she never had a temperature of over 99° afterwards.

"Though I was careful to make the most of what skin I could dissect up and stretch over, yet there were large raw surfaces left that were rather discouraging to look at, so I tried skin grafting. As I had not an interpreter with me the first time I decided to do this, and could not make Miss Yuen, as I called her (the family name was Yuen), understand the necessity of it, I took some of the first grafts off of myself. Then I wanted to take some from the patient, but she did not see the point; neither did Pung Sun Omani who was helping me. So I was going to take more from myself but both united in preventing my every attempt. So I dressed the wounds and waited till the next time, when I could have Miss Rothweiler interpret for me that the wounds would be a very long time healing if they were not helped in this way.

"A few days after, a man came for medicine for a woman whom I had helped in a difficult labor the day before. From his description I thought she was quite sick, so I said I had better go and see her. But as it rained he thought I couldn't

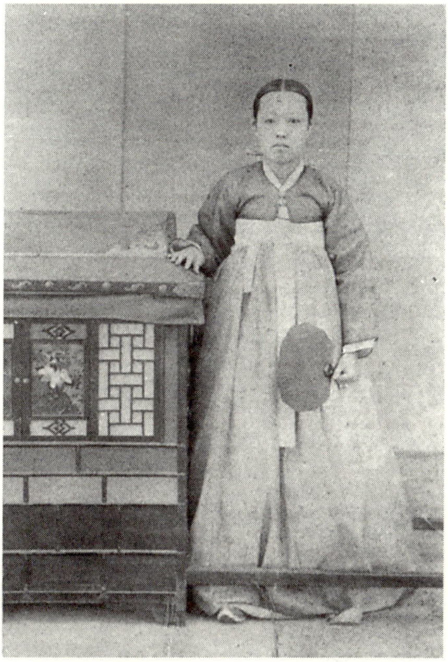

Korean woman beside her closed chair

go through the rain! Then the *Kuisyu* told him how I had even given of my skin to a Korean girl! And so the news spread and I heard of it in a number of ways afterward. Our hospital woman, Pung Sun Omani, told Mrs. Scranton she would have to read her Bible more before she could do such a thing, and altogether it seemed to be quite a little object lesson for them, though I had no such thought in the first place.

"Both Miss Rothweiler and Miss Bengel gave me some grafts, and later Pong Api, one of the wildest of the schoolgirls, *volunteered* her arm and was very brave—not once flinching. Then Miss Yuen herself let me have a few more and when her brother visited her he let me have some. So I put on three or four every time I dressed it, some twenty-five or thirty in all. Of these, some six or eight lived and did well, making little islands that reached out and met others on the margin of the skin so that by Christmas time it was nearly all healed and the day after, I allowed her to go home. They seemed much pleased with the result.

"While she was here Miss Yuen attended prayers nearly every evening in the Girls School. She went to our Sunday School and she read Luke's Gospel through twice, and I feel quite sure that seed has been sown that will bring forth fruit. One day when Pung Sun Omani was away, I found Miss Yuen sitting down in the waiting room at the dispensary reading to the patients from her Gospel. When she went home, she took Luke and some other books and tracts we have translated into Korean with her, and I believe much good will come of it.

"Dr. Scranton's Korean helper in the hospital, speaking of a successful cataract operation the doctor has had lately, says, 'He has given an eye to a blind man; and of all the professions, that of medicine is the chief first.' I might not like to make such an unqualified statement as this Korean man, yet it does seem to me that medical work is a great help, to say the least, in the mission-field, and I do thank God from the depths of my soul for giving me the privilege of helping a little this way.

"We have 26 girls in our school now–varying in age from 7 to 17. They have two Korean teachers besides our missionary teachers. One teaches Chinese which it is quite necessary to know in Korea as it is the Latin, as you might say, of the Korean language. The other teaches Korean Reading, Writing and Composition. Miss Rothweiler teaches the Bible, Geography, and Arithmetic in Korean and the more advanced girls have Arithmetic in English. Miss Bengel instructs them in English Reading, Writing and Composition, also gives them all exercises in Calisthenics. The girls take care of their own rooms and learn to sew and cook . . . All are interesting girls, and though I don't have time as yet to see much of them, except professionally when they are sick, yet I have grown to love them dearly . . .

"Our two oldest girls are soon to be married–they have both received their wedding outfit from their affianced. This is according to Korean custom. I witnessed the ceremony that attends the receival of these things and I will try and tell something of it. A servant comes bearing upon the head a large Korean box with bright brass hinges and lock and wrapped up in red silk with green tassels. This is received in the court by the mother of the girl, or in this case, in our hall by Mrs. Scranton, and it is placed upon a big stone dish full of freshly made Korean bread. Then the intended bride is brought out. According to custom, she has to be almost dragged out by main force. When she gets out, she does not look, but turns her back while the mother takes out, one by one, the pieces of bright colored silks for yokes and skirts, white silk for drawers, cotton cloth, and three or four bundles of cotton, and the silver pin to fasten up her hair with on the wedding day, and a pair of large silver rings, also an official looking document written in Chinese which answers for our marriage certificate. These things are admired, and then put back without unfolding and locked up for three days, and then they are cut and sewed and made up by the bride and her friends. A Korean girl never sees her husband until after she is married–all arrangements between them being made by the 'go between.' After marriage, she is not supposed to look at her husband or speak to him for three days, and the longer she remains in silence before him, the better it is considered.

"Our girls are to be married with the Christian ceremony; but Korean customs are otherwise quite closely observed . . . It is the custom for the groom to be married in the 'palace-going' robes and hat which are usually hired for the occasion . . .

"I want to tell you something of two more of our school-girls whom I call 'my girls' as I am training them to help me in my work, in the dispensary. One is a little Japanese girl whose father lives here in Seoul, the other is Korean, both about fourteen years old and firm friends. They have been in the school about three years. Chyom Tong, the Korean girl, speaks English very well and makes a very good interpreter, though she doesn't enjoy the drug work as well as Owaka San, who I think is going to make a good little druggist. In fact, she is quick to help in everything where she sees she can be of use and is very brave though she is such a little mite of a thing.

"She wrote me after I came saying, 'I am glad because you come to help Korean sick people. I do not speak English, but I want to help you. Miss Bengel teaches me speak English and you teach me medicine words. Then after while I know both.'

"They are already a great help to me. It is fortunate that one is a Japanese as she can go out with me when I am called outside in the daytime. Chyom Tong can only go out in the

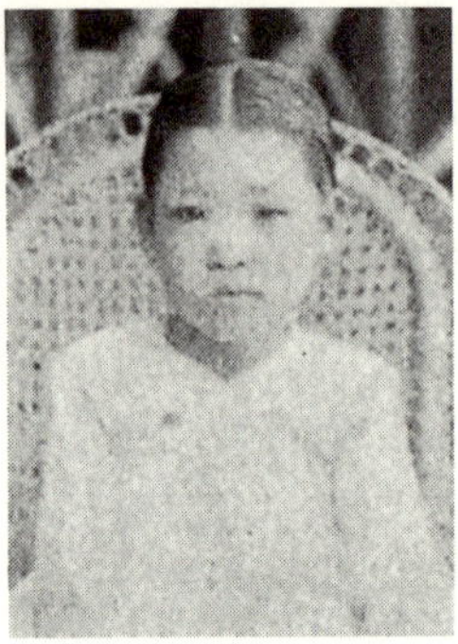

Dr. Sherwood's 14 year old assistants: Chyom Tong (top), Owaka San (bottom)

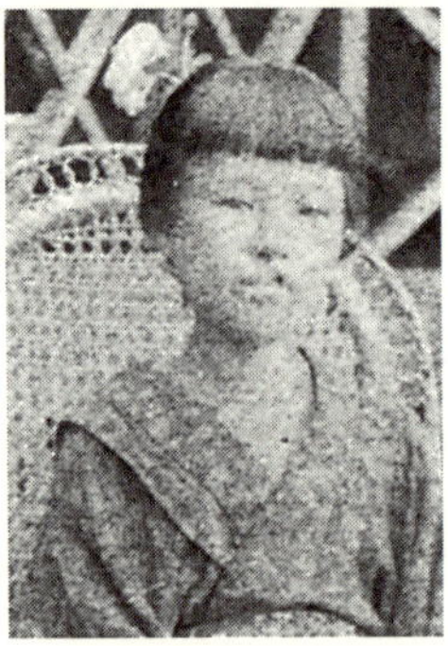

city with me at night in a closed chair. I trust that this training may not only teach them to help me but that it may be an aid to them in leading them out into larger fields of usefulness . . .

"Hearing a great pounding in the kitchen the other day that I knew meant Korean ironing, I went in to watch the operation. The Koreans rip their garments apart when they wash them; then after starching and ironing, make them over again, looking as well as new. Their method of ironing is rather strange. They sit upon the floor before a wooden framework with uprights at either end, between which rests a stone and upon this lies a round stick with the cloth to be ironed wrapped about it. This is beaten with sticks that look like ball clubs, each woman using two. The way they play these sticks in beating the cloth reminds me of threshing buckwheat with a flail. Their ironing looks nice—they beat cotton cloth until it shines like silk. As a Korean man's clothing is practically all white, it is often more than his wife can do to do his sewing for him, as every time a garment is washed and ironed it has to be made over again.

"One day since we have been here, the King went outside the city walls to receive a great Chinese ambassador. Such an occasion makes quite a *kugyang* (a sight) in Seoul which many go to see. We went with quite a number of other foreigners. The soldiers with rifles and bayonets, the flags and canopies, the rude musical instruments and the different costumes did make indeed quite a sight for us. We saw the Chinese ambassador, and caught a glimpse of our Korean King, Li H'oung. The present king is about 40 years old and succeeded to the throne in 1875. He is favorable to intercourse with other nations, and during his reign the Hermit nation has made treaties with the U.S., Japan and some European powers. The old law prohibiting the teaching of Christianity has never been repealed, but since the massacre of nine French missionaries some twenty years ago, Christian liberty has not been much interfered with.

"The city of Seoul with its suburbs has a population of about one million people. There are a few broad streets, and some good looking buildings, but upon the whole Seoul is the meanest looking most filthy city I ever saw—the dirt of the streets is something not to be described.

"A few women of the lower class are seen on the street, but they have their outside wrap up over the head and drawn about the face so that not much more than the eyes appear. They usually walk with a staff. I heard General Dye describe Korea briefly the other day as 'the land where the women carry the canes, and the men the fans.'

"It does seem as if everything went by contrary over here. When we meet in the street, we turn to the right, they turn to the left. We shake hands with each other, they shake their own hands. We wear black boots, they white.[2] When in mourning, we put on a black hat, they put on a white one. We uncover our heads as a mark of respect, they keep theirs covered. Our doors swing and our windows shove as a rule,

[2] Note added later: "They were in mourning for some time after I came to Korea, and that is why white shoes were then used."

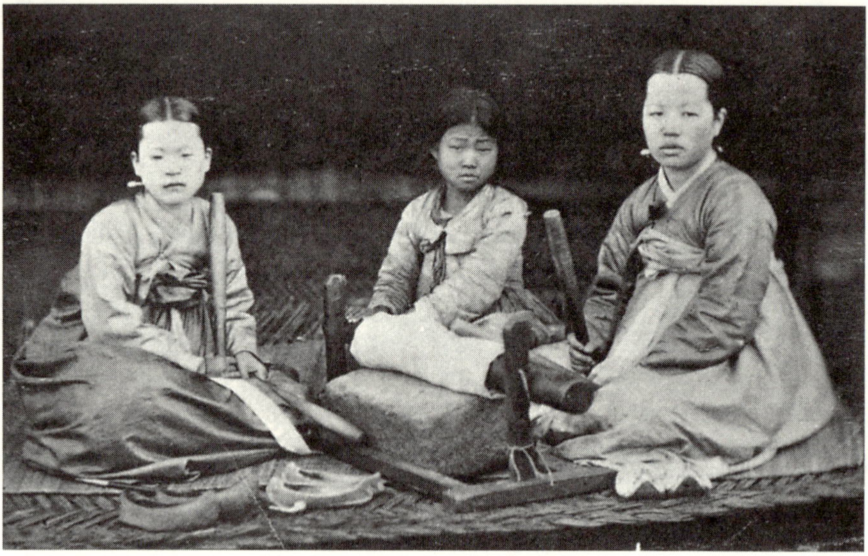

Korean women ironing

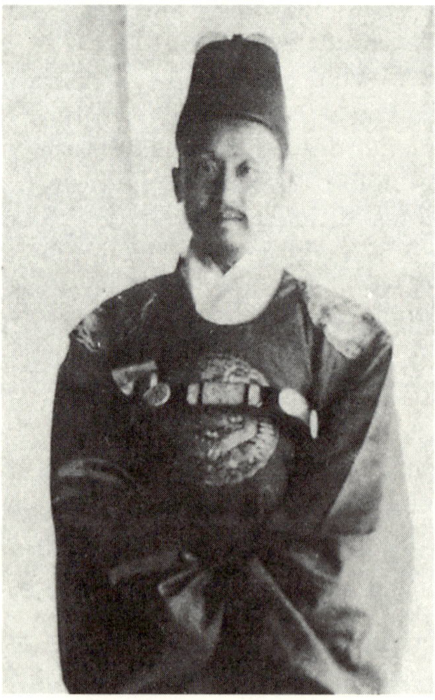

Korean King, Li H'oung

but as a rule, their doors shove and their windows swing. In reading or writing our columns run horizontally, and from left to right—theirs run perpendicularly and from right to left. We put footnotes at the bottom of a page, they at the top. We say 'North, East, South, West.' They say 'East, West, South, North.' And they consider it a great compliment to tell you that you look *old*.

"The Kingdom of Korea, embracing as it does an area as large as Great Britain, varies in climate with the latitude. Here in Seoul from October to January it has not seemed much different than in New York. The air is quite damp especially nights and mornings, so it seems much warmer in summer and colder in winter than the thermometer's register warrants. We needed fires to keep comfortable in the house in October, but the roses bloomed in the garden until Thanksgiving before the frost injured them. Have had one or two light falls of snow, but it has been an open winter so far. They usually have more snow, but it gets away in time to begin gardening in March. The summers are pretty hot, and mosquitos and fleas render them a trifle tormenting to say the least.

"The principle article of food is rice. There are also potatoes, cabbage, beans, buckwheat, onions, turnips etc. Chestnuts grow large and very abundantly. They are also an article of diet. A nut like the English walnut is also native here and there is a variety of pine nut that is very good.

"Korea has quite a variety of fruit. There are fine persimmons, fair peaches, plums and apricots. The pears are nice looking, but taste about like so much sawdust wet up in water, and there are no apples.[3] The native small fruits such as strawberries look nice but like the pears are tasteless. Foreigners, however, have introduced cultivated strawberries, black-caps, and other fruits which seem to do nicely.

"We have to depend upon condensed milk. The native cows are few and have not been trained in as milkers. Koreans never use milk. So we have Orange County milk from the

[3] Apple trees were later successfully introduced to Korea by the Reverend W. L. Swallen, D.D., Northern Presbyterian missionary to Korea, 1892-1932.

Condensery in Walden that I enjoyed a visit to once. It does very nicely except in places where one doesn't want it sweetened. Butter is 60 cents per pound. Eggs are very cheap. Water is very hard. We condense ours that we use to drink in the summer. Chicken is the most common meat though we have mutton from China and beef sometimes. The other day a Korean General made us a present of ten pheasants which are very good. This winter we make our breakfasts generally from boiled rice and Korean buckwheat cakes. We are all fond of both. Our dinners and suppers are not so much different from those at home, as we have our own garden and raise many of the home vegetables. Of course, there are some things we miss in Korea, but we have much more and much better than I expected.

"Our mail comes and goes once in two weeks as a rule, though this winter it has sometimes been three weeks. It seems quite a long time to wait from one mail day to the next and when it comes, we look so anxiously for the hoisting of the mail flag—a signal that the mail carrier has arrived from Chemulpo. I don't know what we would do without the home letters.

"Buddhism has been placed under ban by the reigning King, and though the lower class have some forms of demon worship and the upper class are influenced by Confucianism, yet Korea has no recognized religion. Her people seem waiting for the 'Good News' that the missionaries of Christ bring. Indeed you are sometimes stopped upon the street and thanked for coming so far to tell '*Chosen saram*' about God and Jesus Christ, His Son. They are an extremely grateful people, always anxious to do something in return for any favor shown them. The other day in the hospital a poor woman said she wanted to sell her body to get me a present for making her little son well.

"Though it is customary to observe a sort of formal politeness toward woman—it being a breach of good manners to speak to or even look at any woman outside of one's family—yet the Koreans believe her to be without a soul, and unworthy even of a name . . .

"As may have already been gathered from my letter, I like my work in Korea and I thank the Lord for sending me here. He is so good. In Seoul there are scarcely twenty-five missionaries, counting missionaries' wives. What are they among a million people? But among the remaining eleven millions of Korean people outside of the capital there is no missionary, though there are three ports open to foreigners . . . *The harvest truly is great, but the laborers are few.*"

CHAPTER 3

Historical Highlights

The laborers may have seemed few to the newly arrived young lady doctor. However, that few represented dramatic progress for Christians in the Hermit Kingdom over a period of less than five years. To understand the Korea of my parents' day, it is helpful to know something of the fascinating political, cultural and religious history which had shaped the country up to that time.

LEGEND OF THE FIRST KING, 2333 B.C.

Korean legend has it that the Creator wished to form a kingdom and sent his son to earth in the form of a wind. Through a virgin whom he found sitting beside a stream, he became incarnate in the person of the god-man called Tangun, the first King of Korea. Ancient writings declare that Tangun was the third person of a divine trinity: Whan-in being God, Whan-oong being the Spirit and Tangun being the God-Man.

Tangun is said to have civilized the nine wild tribes of the land in 2333 B.C. and named the country *Chosun* (Morning Calm). Pyong Yang (Pyongyang) was his capital. For years the Korean calendar was computed according to the number of years since the founding of Tangun's kingdom. The altar at which he is said to have worshipped is located on a mountain, Marisan, on the island of Kanghwa near Chemulpo.

LAND OF MORNING BRIGHTNESS

The earliest ruler of Korea who can be documented historically, however, was Kija, who founded a dynasty in 1122 B.C. that was to last nearly a thousand years. After the fall of the Shang Dynasty in China, Kija, formerly an officer of the royal court, emigrated to Korea with five thousand followers. He settled in the city of Pyong Yang which he made the capital of his newly formed kingdom of *Ch'ao Hsien* (Morning Brightness or Freshness). He is said to have been an enlightened leader who introduced his new followers to the influences of Chinese civilization in the form of a code of laws; skills in agriculture, textiles, medicine, and reading; and Chinese literature.

CHINA, THE MIDDLE KINGDOM

Civilization had developed in China much earlier than in any other part of East Asia, so that the Chinese viewed themselves as the "Middle Kingdom," the center and source of all civilization. Literacy, monarchical government and social classes had made their appearance in China before they existed among the peoples on her borders. It thus became easy for China to assume that all other nations should be subordinated to the superior Middle Kingdom and should eventually become Chinese. This policy of conquest (or conciliation where conquest failed) was to significantly affect Chinese-Korean relations, and for more than 2500 years after Kija, China was to be the dominant influence on Korea. A natural consequence of Chinese encroachment was that Korean social and political institutions were from earliest times patterned roughly along Chinese lines, although they did maintain many Korean characteristics.

Forty-two generations after Kija had founded the Kingdom of *Ch'ao Hsien*, the dynasty fell in 194 B.C. at the hands of another conqueror from China by the name of Wiman. He is said to have introduced to Korea the Chinese custom of wearing the hair in a "top knot." As we have seen from Dr.

Rosetta Sherwood's letter, even to the hairdo, the Koreans gave their own distinctive style. This custom endured in Korea until it was officially discouraged in 1895 to satisfy Japanese reform demands, precisely because it was so identified with Korean tradition.

THE FIRST CENTURIES

Culture, trade, refugees and Chinese conquerors traversed the overland trade routes between China and Korea in the first century B.C. By the first century A.D. there existed three monarchical states on the Korean peninsula which caused this era to be known as the Three Kingdoms Period. Silla, founded in 57 B.C., occupied the territory in the southeast along the Nakdong River above what is now Pusan. Koguryo was formed in 37 B.C. and for a time was the strongest of the three kingdoms. Its territory extended north from Seoul into what is presently southern Manchuria. The third kingdom, Paekche, came into being in 18 B.C. It was located in the southwest in the area of the Han River basin close to Seoul.

CHINESE CULTURAL INFLUENCE

For a span of four centuries, China was too preoccupied by turmoil within her own boundaries to pay much attention to the Korean peninsula and the periodic conflicts which erupted between the three kingdoms. In 415 A.D., however, it appeared that both Koguryo and Paekche had accepted a relationship with China which was to set a pattern for the future. They received investiture from the Chinese emperor. This did not mean any loss of autonomy for the Korean kingdoms but did acknowledge the cultural superiority of China and involved certain mutual obligations, including an annual tribute from Korea to China.

The culture in all three kingdoms reflected Chinese influence not only because of past Chinese conquests and interference, but also because the only manner of writing then available was the Chinese ideographic system. The picture-symbol characters of Chinese ideograms represented ideas rather than sounds. The highly inflected Korean language did not readily lend itself to such a system, although the latter was arbitrarily adapted to embody sounds, which accounted for the peculiarly Korean pronunciations given to Chinese words. For the most part, however, adoption of the Chinese writing system meant the adoption of the Chinese language as well for literary purposes. The thousands of Chinese characters that formed the complex Chinese system of writing limited literacy to scholars and men of leisure who were the only ones who had time for such study. Inevitably, Chinese literature and the Confucian classics came to be studied by an elitist group, for the Korean phonetic alphabet was not introduced until the fifteenth century.

CONFUCIANISM SHAPES GOVERNMENT AND SOCIETY

In this manner the basic principles of social and political philosophy espoused by Confucius (551-479 B.C.) became the dominant system of thought concerning government and society in Korea, just as it had been in China, and for the same reasons. Characteristically, Koreans shaped it to fit their own social structure which was more strongly aristocratic than the Chinese. Pride of family was so important to the Korean, for example, that the criterion for high position came to be based on one's birth, rather than on one's qualities of learning and virtue, as was the ideal espoused in China.

The basic tenets of Confucian doctrine outlined rules for five principal relationships: king and subject, husband and wife, parent and child, elder and younger brother, friend and friend. The king, husband, parent and elder brother in the first four relationships held the prerogative of "rule" which was to be exercised with righteousness and benevolence. The other side of each of these four relationships was characterized by submission which was to be righteous and sincere. In the fifth relationship, that between friend and friend, mutual faithfulness was held up as the guiding virtue.

The guidelines soon became binding law in Korea and were used to establish a code of 'justice.' Thus, if a parent killed a child, or an elder brother murdered his younger brother, it was not considered a capital offense and would be punished only with a beating and exile. But if a son killed his father or an elder brother, he would be beheaded at once, as would also be the case for a man who killed his mother-in-law.

In this system of justice, murder was usually punished by death unless the accused was an insane person or a deaf-mute. In that event, such persons would instead be exiled to a remote locality. Capital offenses were punished by decapitation or hanging, or what was considered to be the worst punishment, by being cut into six parts. Lesser forms of punishment consisted of beating, bastinado (beating on the bottom of the feet), placing in stocks, or banishment. A money commutation might be allowed in all save capital cases. Two pieces of hemp cloth or seven ounces of silver might be given as a fine instead of 100 blows; and ten pieces of hemp cloth or 35 ounces of silver in lieu of a year of exile to the remotest frontiers of the realm and so on.

Confucius was more interested in examining the guidelines for exemplary moral conduct between people than he appeared to be in formulating a religious creed, and he avoided speculation on the philosophical questions of immortality, the soul and God. He used the word "Heaven" in his writings rather than naming a specific supreme being.

In later years, neo-Confucian scholars referred to a personal God or over-ruling Providence which could be discovered through nature. However, the aspect which Koreans incorporated most significantly into their own culture was the concept of filial piety, which even extended to the dead, in the form of ancestor worship. Although there is no indication that Confucius practiced ancestor worship, this became a cornerstone of Confucianism in both China and Korea after his death (497 B.C.). It was perhaps a natural outgrowth of his view that the family was sacred. Confucius considered it a special value to have many sons to better demonstrate the virtues of filial piety. In Korea, grave mounds were carefully tended and sacrificial offerings to the dead were religiously observed on set days before graves and ancestral tablets. The latter were strips of wood, several inches long, which bore the name of the deceased and were set upright upon a wooden base.

EARLY BUDDHIST INFLUENCE

Besides the teachings of Confucius, Buddhism had an important role in Korean life for a few centuries following its introduction to the Three Kingdoms in 372 A.D. A Chinese priest, Sun Tao, is said to have been the first to bring the teachings and images of Buddha to the kingdom of Koguryo in that year.

Because of its accommodating nature, Buddhism became readily incorporated into the beliefs, customs and political order of the Koreans. The elaborate Buddhist rituals and their emphasis on man's spiritual nature and pilgrimage toward a paradise (Nirvana), added an emotional complement which had been missing from the more earthly oriented, practical philosophy of Confucianism.

Buddhism had its origins in India where it was founded by Gautama Siddartha (Circa 563-483 B.C.), an Indian prince who renounced his wealth to search for an answer to the cause of pain, death and evil he saw in the world. He received his "enlightenment" while meditating under a sacred Bodhi tree. The term Buddha is a title meaning "the enlightened one."

Gautama taught his followers that through right living, right thinking and self-denial, they too could learn to extinguish the desires and passions that caused earthly suffering. These desires only bound them to endless cycles of birth, death and reincarnation. Thus they were compelled to forever work out the cosmic law of cause and effect, *karma*, whereby virtuous conduct was rewarded in future reincarnations and evil conduct led to retribution. To this basically Hindu doctrine of the transmigration of the soul into progressively higher or lower forms of human or animal life, depending on earned merits or demerits, Gautama added his concept of Nirvana. This was a divine state of illumination which was gained through the extinction of desires, where the individual soul was released from earthly existence and the cycles of rebirth.

In the centuries following the death of Gautama, Buddhism split into two major sects. Hinayana (Lesser Vehicle) revered Buddha as a great teacher, rather than a divine being, and followed more closely his teaching that the ideal Buddhist was the holy man, or *arhat*, who attained enlightenment for himself alone. This sect moved to South India, Ceylon, Burma and Thailand. Mahayana (Greater Vehicle) was the form of Buddhism that was exported via Buddhist missionaries to Tibet, Mongolia, China, Korea and Japan. It had developed theistic characteristics that were quite distinct and differed in several respects from the religion founded by Gautama.

Gautama was known in Korea as Sakyamoni, "the sage of the Sakya clan" (which referred to his aristocratic family origins from the Indian warrior caste). Although deified as the god of gods and surrounded with a rich mythology of his doings in the various heavens, he was actually superseded in Mahayana Buddhism by a non-historical figure, the god known in Korea as Amida-Pul, or the Amida Buddha. The Amida Buddha, or the "Buddha of Infinite Light," was viewed as a redeemer to whom the prayers of the faithful were addressed and who lived in the "Great Western Paradise," or Nirvana, where all good Buddhists hoped to go.

The Mahayana Buddhist was assisted on his spiritual journey by saintly men who had already earned sufficient merits through various reincarnations to achieve Nirvana. However, these holy men, called *Bodhisattvas*, chose not to enter Nirvana until the whole human race had been helped to achieve the merits required to enter Nirvana with them. Thus, for the masses of common people who preferred not to follow the monastic disciplines, they could appeal to their favorite *Bodhisattva*, and through faith and dependence on his merit, they could attain salvation. The Mahayana concept of the path to Nirvana did not require the extinguishing of the individual soul, but saw it as continuing to a paradise, if it had earned merit, or to a hell, if its conduct deserved punishment.

In 384 A.D., twelve years after being brought to Koguryo, Buddhism was introduced to the kingdom of Paekche by an Indian Caucasian priest, Marananda. Silla was the last of the three kingdoms to embrace Buddhist teachings which were said to have been brought there in 424 A.D. by an Ethiopian Buddhist, Mukocha. One hundred and thirty years later, priests from Paekche successfully introduced Buddhism to Japan.

The elaborate Buddhist mythology of the various gods and goddesses who interceded on behalf of humans provided a rich source of material for expression in the fine arts as Buddhism spread through the Three Kingdoms. Under Buddhist influence major advances were made in temple architecture, ceramics and sculpture.

KOREAN PENINSULA UNITED, 668 A.D.

The long period of instability and internal conflict which had gripped China for about 400 years came to a close with the founding of the Sui Dynasty as rulers of all China in 589 A.D. Determined to secure their northern borders and have all people acknowledge the superiority of the Middle Kingdom, the Sui attacked Koguryo in 598. However, this and later attacks were repelled.

The T'ang Court which replaced the Sui Dynasty in 618, sought to gain control of Korea by turning the Three Kingdoms against each other. T'ang and Silla forces combined to defeat the Kingdom of Paekche. China took over the kingdom and moved against Koguryo in the north, again allied with Silla. Eight years later, Koguryo finally was defeated and China removed its main forces from the peninsula.

Revolts soon broke out in the two conquered kingdoms. However, Silla supported rather than suppressed these uprisings. A T'ang force was sent to reestablish control. Silla decisively defeated this force and a truce was negotiated in which China recognized Silla as an independent state, ruling all areas south of Pyong Yang.

For the first time, the Korean peninsula was unified as a single political identity, a goal it would again be desirous of achieving many centuries hence. Silla enjoyed a period of greatness despite further attacks from the T'ang Chinese on the one hand and Japanese pirates on the other. The arts, agriculture, mining and diplomacy all flourished. Silla exchanged envoys with Japan and eventually regained harmony with China. Through its law, language and civilization, Silla succeeded in binding into a homogeneous nation peoples who were of different racial origins and who had, heretofore, never enjoyed a common leadership.

THE 500 YEAR KORYO DYNASTY

Revolts, and the excesses of luxury, combined in time to lead to Silla's overthrow in 918. The Koryo Dynasty which followed maintained a united peninsula and remained in power until 1392. The name, Koryo, which means high hills and sparkling waters, is a shortened form of the name of the former northern kingdom of Koguryo and is the word from which the modern name, Korea, is derived. It is indeed descriptive of the mountainous terrain and the short, swift rivers and streams which extend the length and breadth of the peninsula. The Taedong River which flows past the city of Pyong Yang had marked the northern border of the kingdom of Silla. In the tenth century, under Koryo, the northern border was extended to the Abrog (Yalu) and Tumen Rivers (the present boundary of North Korea), and the capital was established at Songdo (Kaesong).

Buddhism enjoyed wide acceptance during the Koryo period and became the state religion. During this time, a system of government examinations called *Kwagu* was introduced which, for a thousand years, was the educational system used in the training of Korean young people. The means by which a man could advance in the governmental hierarchy depended upon his completion of an exacting course of study which occupied most of his time between the ages of five and twenty-five. As only *yangbans* (aristocrats) could attend these schools and become candidates to take the examinations, the majority of the people were excluded from both education and government.

TARTAR AND CHIN INVASIONS

For the first one hundred years of the dynasty, the Koryo Kingdom was beset by invasions from Khitan Tartar tribes who peopled the state of Liao in southwestern Manchuria and a portion of northern China. The T'ang Dynasty in China had given way to the Sung Dynasty and the latter shared with Korea a concern for protecting its borders from the Tartars. Both China and Liao felt that the control of Korea was vital to their ability to maintain dominance in East Asia. Although Korea tried to preserve a role of neutrality, the other nations would not permit it, as was to be the case repetitively throughout Korean history.

Although Koryo forces successfully drove out the Tartars in 1018, by the 12th century they had another enemy on their northern border formed from another group of Manchurian tribes known as the Jurched. These people had grown sufficiently powerful to form themselves into a new state to which they gave the Chinese name, Chin. Chin defeated Liao and proceeded to conquer all of North China to the Yangtze River by 1135. Koryo was forced to acknowledge Chin superiority and, therefore, resisted the appeal for help against Chin by the Sung Court in South China.

MILITARY DICTATORSHIP ESTABLISHED

Koreans were having their own internal problems which revolved primarily around contention for the throne, and rivalry between the military and civil officials. The twelfth century was marked by a series of bloody power struggles, exploitation of farmers, peasant revolts and a general weakening of the central government due to its internal discords.

General Choe Chung-hon of Koryo succeeded in eliminating all his rivals in the year 1196 and established a military dictatorship which brought about a measure of stability. For 60 years, Choe Chung-hon and his descendents ruled Korea. The kings were treated as mere figureheads, being elevated and deposed at will.

GENGHIS KHAN FORCES INVADE, 1231 A.D.

Contemporary with the establishment of the Choe dictatorship in Korea, a power was rising in the West on the steppes of Central Asia. This was the group of tribes known collectively as the Mongols. Temujin, a remarkable military leader who led his tribe to dominance over the others, became known to history as Genghis Khan, ruler for a time of one of the largest empires in the world. By the 13th century it stretched from China to eastern Europe. On their march to China, the Mongols defeated the Chin state and pursued the fleeing Khitan Tartars of Liao into Korea. The Koryo troops in 1231 were unequal to the Mongol invasion and sued for peace. In return for this the Mongols demanded an immense tribute, and then withdrew to proceed to their main objective of conquering China. However, for the next 30 years the Mongols plagued Korea with sporadic attacks.

By 1270, the Korean king had concluded that resistance to the Mongols was futile and despite opposition from the military, the king was restored to the throne, in power as well as in name, and the military dictatorship came to an end. The Mongols assured their continued control of Korea by requiring all crown princes to reside in Peking and to marry Mongols.

So it was that in 1271 the Korean Crown Prince Choong-yul married a Mongol princess, daughter of Kublai Khan, who, in 1260, had come to the throne of his famous grandfather, Genghis Khan. Choong-yul took over the Korean throne in 1274. His Mongol wife created no small stir in the kingdom, for women of the Mongols enjoyed far greater freedom than either their Chinese or Korean counterparts. The Mongol woman was not hidden behind a veil but rode openly beside her husband and was even skilled in the use of a bow and arrow.

A school for the study of the Mongol language was opened at Songdo. This language contained an alphabet of forty-one letters and is reputed to have inspired the Korean phonetic alphabet, developed two hundred years later.

Relations between Korea and China became more amicable and for a time Kublai Khan withdrew his troops from Korea and sent all captured Koreans home. With Korea now a vassal of Peking, the Mongols attempted several invasions of Japan by way of Korea, forcing Korea to provide troops, ships and supplies. These attempts to conquer Japan all failed, but Korea suffered extensive losses of lives and property. The invasion attempts were finally given up in 1281.

DECLINE OF MONGOL POWER

During the next century, the Mongols lost their grip on China. The new Ming Dynasty, which gained control in China, looked with disfavor on the continued amicable relationship between the Koryo Court and the

Mongols. In 1388, Ming forces occupied the former Mongol fortress of Chilryong on the Northern Koryo border in a move to prevent further collusion between the Mongols and the Koreans. The Koryo response to this situation was to send General Yi Song-gye on a military expedition against the Ming-held fortress.

General Yi had distinguished himself in repelling Japanese pirate raids which had been ravaging Korean coastal towns. However, he was reluctant to expose the country to their recurrence by removing troops to the North, especially during the summer rainy season, a particularly ill chosen time to launch any offensive. The Koryo regime turned a deaf ear to General Yi's counsel.

GENERAL YI TAKES CONTROL, 1388 A.D.

As the General had predicted, by the time the Koryo forces reached the northern boundary, the diseases which often accompanied the rainy season had decimated many of his soldiers. Anticipating sure defeat for his men if they were to attempt an attack on the Mings, General Yi decided that the only alternative open to him was to seize power himself and put into practice those policies which he felt would best serve the interests of Korea. He marched back to Songdo and, in a surprise move, took control of the Koryo government.

General Yi's assumption of power was supported by lower government officials who were neo-Confucianists. In order to maintain their support, General Yi did not immediately assume the throne, for this would have violated Confucian principles. Instead, he presented himself as a reformer who would restore Confucian policies, end the favor which Buddhism had so long enjoyed in political circles, break the power of the pro-Mongol faction in the government and restore the traditional relationship Korea had formerly had with China. For four years he preserved the outward appearances of Koryo rule while discretely placing his own men in positions of power. In 1392 the highest organ of the Koryo government proclaimed that the Koryo Dynasty was at an end and that Yi Song-gye was rightfully King of Korea. He was given the posthumous title, Yi Taijo, which means Grand Progenitor, and became the founder of Korea's last royal dynasty, which was to endure until the Japanese annexation of Korea in 1910.

RISE TO POWER OF THE NEO-CONFUCIANISTS

The new kingdom took an ancient name—Chosun (Land of the Morning Calm). Until this time, Buddhism and Confucianism had coexisted amicably even during the Koryo period when Buddhism was the dominant and official faith. However, during the eleventh century in China, a scholar named Chu Hsi had developed a system of thought which integrated some of his own cosmological ideas with Confucian principles and gave the system a metaphysical aspect which the Sage himself had avoided. This neo-Confucianism spread rapidly among scholars in both China and Korea and soon found itself in contradiction with Buddhist beliefs. Buddhism encouraged people to abandon their families and worldly pursuits for the sake of Nirvana, while neo-Confucianism emphasized family ties and agriculture.

The differences became further accentuated when Buddhists began to become powerful in Korean politics and looked with disdain on the lesser court officials who followed the doctrines of Chu Hsi. The inevitable conflict found expression when the move to unseat the Koryo government resulted in the rise to power of the neo-Confucianists. A period of persecution of the Buddhists followed and severe limitations were placed on the practice of their religion.

The new capital of the Yi Dynasty was moved to Hanyang (Seoul) in 1395, and the following year the walls of the city were built. Confucianism was established as the official religion. Buddhists were not permitted to reside inside the walls of the new capital because of the influences they had held in the former dynasty, now in disrepute. Their temples and priests were banished to the mountains and outlying areas, and Buddhism never regained its former power in the affairs of state.

KOREA'S GOLDEN AGE

When King Taijo abdicated in 1398, one of his sons (known by the posthumous title, Taejong) ascended the throne. In seeking to complete his father's reforms, Taejong established a strict separation between military and civilian rule. When King Taejong died in 1418, his son, King Sejong, inaugurated what is now referred to as Korea's Golden Age.

King Sejong assigned a committee of scholars to work on the creation of symbols which would represent the sounds of the Korean language. This resulted in a phonetic Korean alphabet with a system of 17 consonants (later reduced to 14) and 11 vowels. While the Confucian scholar-officials looked with scorn upon this popular language, this Korean alphabet, known as *hangul* (or in earlier days as *unmun*), was a boon to commoners and especially to women who had been largely excluded from literary education. As will be seen, it proved also a boon to the early missionary attempts to spread the gospel message in book form. The invention of movable metal type is credited to Korea long before Gutenberg, although scholars vary as to the specific date. One opinion suggests that it was during this Golden Age.

King Sejong had fortifications built along the Tumen and Yalu Rivers which protected the northern area of Korea from border raids, and so allowed for its peaceful and relatively permanent integration into the rest of the kingdom. While the first two centuries of the Yi Dynasty saw many internal problems and rivalries for control of the throne, it was a period relatively free from conflicts with other nations.

TWO CENTURIES OF PEACE END

Then Japan decided to attack China in 1592 by marching through Korea. The Koreans, after two centuries of peace, were unprepared to resist the Japanese force of 150,000 men and appealed to China for help. The Ming troops from the North, combined with the sea attack by the famous Korean Admiral Yi Sun Sin, forced the Japanese under their leader, General Hideyoshi, to retreat.

Admiral Yi had invented the "turtle ship," the first ironclad vessel in history, and it proved impervious to Japanese weapons. Iron plates decked over the galley protected the rowers and an iron ram in the bow in the shape of a turtle's head gave the ship its name. Arrows could be shot through the mouth of the turtle. Eighty of these turtle boats in Chinhai Bay were effective in sinking such large numbers of Japanese troop and supply ships as to seriously retard the Japanese invasion.

An early version of the suspension bridge was also introduced by the Koreans during this war to enable the Chinese troops to come to their aid across the Yalu river. Later Japanese attacks met with guerilla warfare from Korean peasants in the South. Finally, with the death of General Hideyoshi in 1597, the invasions by the Japanese were discontinued.

However, in 1627 and again in 1636, a confederation of Manchu tribes, bent on conquering the weakened Ming Dynasty in China, marched first into Korea from Manchuria. After achieving ascendancy over the Koreans, the Manchus went on to conquer China. They adopted the dynastic title of Ching.

Korea had had a long history of being committed to China morally, culturally and diplomatically. In time, the Chings were successful in establishing relations with Korea which were about the same in nature as those which had existed with the previous rulers of China. During this period the Koreans adopted the Chinese calendar.

JESUIT TEACHINGS REACH KOREA

It was through regular diplomatic missions to the Ching Court in Peking that Koreans began to encounter Europeans. Because powers intent on ruling China had repeatedly invaded and ravaged Korea, the latter concluded that the best policy was to shun all contacts with non-Chinese foreigners. However, Portugese Jesuit missionaries had become quite influential at the Ching court because of their willingness to impart European scientific learning and technology to the Chinese. The Koreans began to take home with them Chinese translations of technical and religious books which had been prepared by the Jesuits.

Much interest developed in Korea over these books, especially those relating to Christian teachings. However, a Papal decision in the 1700's brought an abrupt end to the freedom of the Koreans to pursue this interest. At that time, the Pope had defined certain Confucian rites as religious, and therefore forbidden to Roman Catholic Christians. This made it appear to Koreans that Christianity was hostile to centuries-old beliefs. What frightened them most was that the Christians were apparently advocating the subversion of basic Confucian principles of social order. In particular, the Roman Catholics condemned as pagan religious rites, the rituals of honoring ancestors. Since this was one of the deepest rooted and most emphasized principles of Confucian thought and practice in Korea, the Catholic stance was a direct threat to filial piety.

PERSECUTION OF CHRISTIANS BEGINS, 1785

In 1785, Christianity was banned in Korea and the import of European books of any kind was forbidden. For 100 years there followed religious persecution and intolerance, primarily directed against the Roman Catholics, who formed the bulk of Christian converts in Korea in the late 1700's and early 1800's. A Chinese priest by the name of James Chu was the first to enter Korea in 1794, but he was executed in 1801. During that year, 300 Christians were martyred.

Matters were made worse at this time when a letter to the Pope from a Korean convert, Whang Sa Yung, was intercepted. The letter had urged the Pope to send troops to Korea to force the Korean government to establish a policy of religious liberty. Such an act of treason caused not only the death of Whang, but a stricter enforcement of the edict against Christianity. This was now further justified on the grounds that Christianity was the instrument of foreign powers bent on dominating Korea. Persecution and martyrdom of the Christians continued with varying intensity every few years.

FIRST PROTESTANT INFLUENCE

The first record of a Protestant missionary attempting to preach the Gospel in Korea was the Reverend Carl Augustus Frederick Gutzlaff, M.D. He was a German missionary who was aboard the British ship, *Lord Amherst*, which entered Korean waters in July, 1832 seeking trade relations with Korea. The ship waited for a month along the coast of Whanghai (Hwanghae) province for a response to its request, during which time Gutzlaff preached among the people. Along with the gifts sent to the King, Rev. Gutzlaff included two Chinese Bibles and some tracts, but they were returned with the message that trade could not be negotiated without prior consultation with China. The ship, with the Reverend Gutzlaff on board, left without the coveted trade agreement.

PRIESTS BEHEADED

In 1836, a French Catholic priest, Pierre Maubant, was successful in entering Korea. Two others, Father Chastan and Bishop Imbert, followed the next year. In 1839, the persecution of Christians became so intense that the French missionaries gave themselves up thinking to stop it. They were tortured and beheaded near Yongsan on the banks of the Han River. Their deaths and the notorious persecutions that followed resulted in the spreading of the word of the Gospel to every section of the country. Thus, despite the atrocities visited on the Christians, the Catholics reported a following of some 13,638 converts by 1855.

With the death of King Chul Chong in 1862, Queen Cho seized the seals of state and appointed a boy king, Li H'oung (posthumously called King Kojong), naming his father as Regent. The Regent took the title Tai Won Kun (Prince of the Great House). His policy continued to be both anti-foreign and anti-Christian. Under his regime, religious persecution reached its height.

TONGHAK MOVEMENT BEGINS

In 1861, a man by the name of Choe Cheu founded the religion of *Chondokyo* (Heavenly Way Doctrine). This doctrine combined concepts from Buddhism, Confucianism,

Shamanism (animistic spirit worship), Taoism and Christianity. He used the Catholic term for God, *Chun Chu*, and is said to have had a revelation to found this new religion while he was delirious from an illness and was being nursed back to health by Catholic missionaries. To insure that his new religion would not be confused with theirs, Choe Cheu called his religion *Tonghak*, which means Eastern learning, as opposed to *Sohak*, or Western learning (a term applied to Catholicism). However, the name was insufficient to protect him from the religious persecution abroad in the land, and Choe Cheu was executed in March, 1864 for teachings that were considered heretical to Confucianism. This served only to make him a martyr, and the Tonghak movement, led by his successor, Choe Si-hyong, went underground. When it again emerged in 1871, it had developed a political aspect in its championing of the cause of the common people against their exploitation by a corrupt feudalistic system. It also had become intensely nationalistic and frankly anti-Western. Later, this was to cause Western missionaries occasions for considerable anxiety.

RELIGIOUS PERSECUTION INTENSIFIES

Just as the Tonghaks had not fared well under the Tai Won Kun, the Christians continued to find themselves hounded as the Regent made a concentrated attempt to rid the nation of them. The infamous persecution of 1866 resulted in the arrests of thousands of Christians and the torture and death of hundreds more, including two bishops and seven French priests then residing in Korea. The three remaining French Roman Catholic priests successfully fled the country that year. To protest the slaughter, the French sent a naval ship to Korea. It anchored off Kanghwa

Island but left without effecting any change in Korean government policy.

AMERICAN EXPEDITION ENDS IN TRAGEDY

A Protestant missionary, the Reverend Robert Jermain Thomas of the London Missionary Society, was aboard the American schooner, the *General Sherman*, when it made its way up the Taedong River towards Pyong Yang in August, 1866 seeking trade. Mr. Thomas had spent the previous winter distributing Scriptures and Bible tracts (translated into Chinese) off the coast of Whanghai province near Sorai Beach where the Reverend Gutzlaff had preached some 34 years before. As the *General Sherman* traveled up the river, Mr. Thomas threw some of these Scriptures and tracts to Koreans standing on the river banks. The books had been supplied to him by the Reverend A. Williamson of the National Bible Society in Chefoo, China.

Not being familiar with the unusual tides along the Korean coast (as high as 30 feet in places), and unaware that torrential rains had caused the waters of the Taedong to be abnormally high, the *General Sherman* proceeded confidently up the river. However, when the tide receded, the ship became stranded on a sand bar. Before it could be released, the alarmed residents of Pyong Yang sent a scow loaded with burning pine branches and sulphur down the Taedong directly into the American ship, which caught fire. As the crew and passengers fled to shore, they were killed. Just before Mr. Thomas was slain, he proffered a Bible to his would-be assassin who later took it home. His nephew, Lee Young Tai, years later became a Christian and participated with Dr. W. D. Reynolds, a Southern Presbyterian missionary, in his work of translating the Bible into the Korean language.

The next American ship to visit Korean waters came in 1871. It also met a hostile reception as it anchored off Kanghwa Island. After destroying some forts, the Americans withdrew as the French had done previously.

These events contributed to the Regent's feeling of superiority to and invincibility from Westerners and the persecutions intensified. Death was the penalty for anyone who called himself a Christian or owned a Christian book. Although an estimated 2,000 Christians had laid down their lives by 1868, in 1884 the converts to Roman Catholicism were said to number 17,577.

KOREAN ISOLATION ENDS, 1876

In 1874, the regency of the Tai Won Kun ended when the young king, Li H'oung, came of age. Thinking to secure his continued control of the government, the Tai Won Kun arranged for his son to marry a young woman of the Min family, the orphaned niece of his wife. Queen Min, however, proved to be a match for her father-in-law and far from keeping him in power, she insured that her own relatives were placed in positions of authority.

The new regime broke the traditional isolation of Korea, and made a treaty of friendship with Japan in 1876 which opened the port of Fusan to settlement and trade. By 1880 two additional ports, Wonsan and Chemulpo, were opened to Japan.

China learned of the attempts which an American representative, Commodore Robert W. Shufeldt, was making to negotiate a treaty with Korea through the Japanese foreign office. Concerned over the possibility of Japan and the United States working in concert, the Chinese foreign policy director, Li Hung Chang, invited Commodore Shufeldt to Tientsin to discuss the matter. The result was to be the signing of the first treaty ever made between Korea and a Western nation. This was accomplished at Chemulpo on May 22, 1882.

The original agreement that had been worked out at Tientsin specifically ruled out missionary work. However, this provision was not mentioned in the final treaty signed at Chemulpo, which permitted American citizens to trade and reside in the open ports and recognized the independence of Korea. Great Britain and Germany concluded like treaties with Korea on November 26, 1883. In the next decade most of the European nations had formed treaties with Korea, thus ending her long status as a "Hermit Nation."

BIBLICAL TRANSLATIONS INTO KOREAN SCRIPT

The early Protestant introduction of the Scriptures into Korea had the effect of spreading Christianity simply by the persuasion of the written word, which was then passed along to others by those who had read it. Two missionaries of the Presbyterian Church of Scotland who were working in Manchuria, the Reverend John Ross and his brother-in-law, the Reverend John McIntyre, were responsible for the earliest Biblical translations into Korean script.

When the Ross translation of the Gospel of Luke was printed in 1882, a Korean peddler took copies with him to sell along with his medicines on his travels in eastern Manchuria. These Gospels of Luke subsequently were smuggled over the border into Korea.

One of the Bible smugglers was a Korean Christian, Soh Sang Yun, who lived in the border town of Wiju (Uiju). When he was discovered with a package of Bibles, he was immediately imprisoned. A relative in the government helped him to escape with a few of the Bibles. Soh Sang Yun fled to Sorai, the same area visited by Gutzlaff and Thomas earlier. Here he shared his copies of the Gospel and preached. Soon a sizeable group of Christians were meeting together regularly. From this group came the first seven Koreans to be ordained to the ministry of the Presbyterian church, causing Sorai to be called by some "the cradle of Protestant Christianity in Korea."

While the Bible translations in the North were primarily the Gospel of Luke, in the South the Korean translations used by the early missionaries were almost exclusively the Gospel of Mark. The reason for this was that only two years after the Ross translation of Luke was printed in Manchuria in 1882, the American Bible Society in Japan published the Rijutei translation of Mark. Rijutei (a Japanese name) was a Korean refugee to Japan. He was apparently an official of high rank who had been forced to flee from Korea in 1882 at the time the Tai Won Kun had attempted to regain the power of the Korean throne. Rijutei took a Japanese name. He became a Christian through reading a Chinese translation of the Bible. Later he studied under the Reverend R. S. Maclay and the Reverend G. W. Knox, both missionaries in Japan. It is significant to our story that this contact lead Rijutei to appeal to the churches in America asking them to send missionaries to Korea. With the help of Mr. Henry Loomis in Japan, Rijutei undertook to translate Mark into Korean. When the first missionaries did come to Korea, this Korean edition of Mark came with them.

CHINA AND JAPAN VIE FOR INFLUENCE

The internal revolt in Korea which had caused Rijutei to flee to Japan in 1882 had been sparked by the dishonest handling of soldiers' pay by the Min Court. The soldiers mutinied, Queen Min was sent into exile, and the Tai Won Kun was recalled to take over the leadership of the country. The pro-Min Chinese, however, soon came to the aid of the exiled Queen and with 3000 troops rapidly regained control of the palace. In the process, the Japanese legation was destroyed. The Chinese sent the Tai Won Kun into exile at Tientsin, where he remained for three years.

Reparations were made to the Japanese for the loss of their Legation, but from this point, the dual presence of China and Japan in Korea was to form the foundation for later conflicts. The continued rivalry between Queen Min and her father-in-law, the Tai Won Kun, allowed both to be used by China and Japan to seek their own ends. Into this political tinder-box the first Protestant resident missionaries gingerly made their way.

1884-1885, METHODIST AND PRESBYTERIAN MISSIONS ESTABLISHED

On September 12, 1883 the nephew of Queen Min, Prince Min Young Ik, was assigned to head the first Korean embassy to the United States. While on a train en route to Washington to present his credentials to President Arthur, he met Dr. Goucher, President of Goucher College in Baltimore. The Korean Prince deeply impressed Dr. Goucher, who promptly urged the Methodist Church to explore the possibilities for opening mission work in Korea with the assurance of his initial financial backing.

The Superintendent of the Methodist Mission in Japan, Dr. R. S. Maclay, was sent to Seoul to make inquiries. He arrived on June 24, 1884 and working through the Minister to the American Legation, General Lucius Foote, secured permission to open schools and hospitals. Christianity was still under ban, and so no open evangelistic work was yet permitted. Nevertheless, Dr. Maclay made arrangements for the purchase of sites for the educational and medical work of the

Methodist Foreign Missionary Society. They, in turn, sent out to Korea the Reverend Henry G. Appenzeller, the Reverend William B. Scranton, M.D. and Dr. Scranton's mother, Mrs. Mary F. Scranton in 1885.

Meanwhile, a Presbyterian missionary, Dr. Horace N. Allen, who had been serving in China, requested his Mission Board's permission to receive assignment to Korea. This was granted and he arrived in Seoul on September 20, 1884 where he was at once appointed physician to the U.S. Legation and later, to the British, Chinese and Japanese Legations. Since the treaties did not provide for missionary work, these appointments allowed Dr. Allen to establish legal residence in Seoul, not as a missionary, but as a physician. He purchased a house to which he brought his family in late October, 1884.

ASSASSINATION ATTEMPT LEADS TO ROYAL HOSPITAL

Only a few months after his arrival, Dr. Allen was to find himself in a position to make a significant contribution to the opening of Protestant mission work in Korea. The Min government, although considered quite conservative, had agreed to institute a postal service for Korea on July 17, 1884. Postage stamps were issued and the son of the Prime Minister, Hong Yong Sik, was made Postmaster General.

A group of young Koreans, who had been away in Japan to study, returned to their own country with many new ideas and attitudes. They favored the extension of foreign contacts and the use of foreign methods and became known as the Progressionists. The new Postmaster General, Hong Yong Sik, who had accompanied the first Korean embassy to America, was in sympathy with their ideas. However, when he was given his new government position, his compatriots excluded him from their plans for a coup d'état. Instead, they discussed with the Japanese their plan to assassinate some of the conservative leaders in the Min government and were assured of support.

When it was learned that a banquet was to be given December 4, 1884 at the Changdok Palace to celebrate the opening of the new postal system, the Progressives saw their opportunity. They were to set fire to the new post office and a nearby building, and when the guests poured out of the banquet hall, the selected victims would be slain. Everything went according to plan, and in the exodus from the banquet hall, Prince Min Yong Ik (who had returned from his visit to the United States) was dangerously wounded.

Dr. Allen had been dining across the city with two visitors to Korea, Messrs. Townsend and Barnadou of the Smithsonian Institution. Upon being notified of the Prince's desperate need for medical attention, Dr. Allen rushed to the scene. When he arrived, Korean doctors were deliberating on the use of bread, cobwebs or pitch to stop the Prince's bleeding. While they were diplomatically ushered out of the room to consult on the appropriate care of Prince Min, Dr. Allen ligated the severed arteries.

Meanwhile, the Progressive reformers were proceeding with their plan. They took possession of the palace and told the King that the Chinese had set fire to the post office. A letter, purportedly from the King, was then delivered to the Japanese Legation asking for their assistance. This was immediately provided.

The coup lasted only three days, for Chinese troops commanded by Yuan Shi Kai came to the defense of the palace. They outnumbered the Japanese and the King was soon reinstated. The Japanese fled back to Japan by way of Chemulpo and their Legation in Seoul was again destroyed. The Progressives also left Korea and tried to persuade Hong Yong Sik to take flight with them. However, he asserted that one ought to remain to demonstrate that their cause was based on sound principles and that the Progressives were not mere rebels. The Chinese soldiers found Hong Yong Sik in the palace and publicly executed him.

Fighting continued in the weeks that followed. Dr. Allen found himself not only caring for Prince Min, whose life hung in the balance, but also for the victims of the battle. The hostilities came to an end at last and an agreement was reached on April 18, 1885 between Japan and China that neither side would send troops into Korea without notifying the other. Both sides withdrew their soldiers and Korea agreed to pay 400,000 yen in compensation for the destruction of the Japanese Legation.

Dr. Allen, who had saved the life of Prince Min and served so faithfully in caring for the wounded, was in high favor with the King and Queen. When he therefore asked to be given a building to use as a Government Hospital, supported by Government funds, his request was granted. He further indicated to the King that he would be willing to serve there without salary, since he was supported by a "benevolent society in America." The home of the former Postmaster General, Hong Yong Sik, whom the Chinese had executed, became the new Royal Hospital which was formally opened on April 10, 1885. It was named by the King, *Kwang Hei Won* (Widespread Relief House).

Messrs. Horace Underwood and Henry Appenzeller, of the Presbyterian and Methodist Missions respectively, had arrived at Chemulpo only five days before, on Easter Sunday. They and Dr. Scranton, who arrived the next month, all began their work in Korea that spring by helping Dr. Allen in either a medical or educational capacity at the Royal Hospital. From this beginning they were able to gradually establish the early educational and medical work of their respective Missions and to purchase property. Thus, the confidence which the royal family had in Dr. Allen paved the way for the opening work of his fellow missionaries.

TESTING THE WIND

Those initial five years, during which the foundations were laid for the first mission schools and hospitals, were not without periodic episodes of tension. Centuries old distrust of foreigners and lack of familiarity with their strange ways made the Koreans view every action of the foreign community with a wariness that easily erupted into rumor and panic. Further, the 100 year persecution of the Roman Catholic Christians had established a realistic fear of the consequence of coming into too close association with Westerners who were also Christians.

It therefore was necessary for the foreign missionaries to move with care as they began their work of evangelizing Korea. Because there were so few missionaries in Korea at the outset, and because of the anti-Christian edicts, the work centered in Seoul. By the fall of 1887, however, Mr. Underwood set forth on an exploratory itinerating trip which took him to the northern Korean border town of Wiju and back by way of the western coastal town of Sorai. The following spring Mr. Appenzeller accompanied Mr. Underwood as far as Pyong Yang. On these initial trips, it became evident that the work of the early Roman Catholic and Protestant Christians, both in terms of converts and the distribution of Chinese and Korean translations of the Bible, had prepared the soil for the future growth of Christianity. The early itinerating missionaries found groups of Koreans waiting to be baptized and eager to receive them. It would seem that the century of martyrdom had not succeeded in stamping out Christianity. Even so, religious toleration was not yet at hand.

NEW EDICT AGAINST CHRISTIAN TEACHING

Messrs. Underwood and Appenzeller were called back to Seoul from Pyong Yang on April 28, 1888 by a communication from the American Minister at Seoul, Mr. Hugh A. Dinsmore, who informed them that he had received a dispatch from the Korean Foreign Office and went on to state that:

> "... it is well known to the Korean government that Americans residing in Korea are engaged in different ways in disseminating the doctrines of the Christian religion; citing the fact that it is objectionable to the government, not authorized by the treaty, and demanding that it shall cease. My aid, as the minister of the United States, being invoked to this end, it becomes my duty to request that you will refrain from teaching the Christian religion and administering its rites and ordinances to the Korean people."[1]

The missionaries held no religious meetings for several months following this prohibition.

[1] H. A. Rhodes, ed., *History of the Korea Mission Presbyterian Church U.S.A. 1884-1934*, p. 22.

The intervention of the Korean government was attributed to Catholic defiance of a royal edict which declared that no two-story building should be erected in Korea, because then it would be possible to look down over the wall which surrounded the royal palace. In violation of this decree, the French Roman Catholics had purchased an elevated site where they planned to erect a cathedral which would overlook the palace. The purchase had been made secretly and without government approval. This action had caused the immediate response from the Korean Court in the form of the interdict against Christian teaching. Although Protestants did not feel that the decree had been directed against them, the distinction between a Roman Catholic Christian and a Protestant Christian was a fine one to Koreans who viewed Christianity generally as a threat to their own venerated traditions. Korean acceptance of Westerners was to remain a delicate matter, not always entirely understood by missionaries who were eager to be about the calling that had brought them to Korea.

U.S. MARINES PROVIDE PROTECTION

Between June 10 and 25, 1888, another problem plagued the new missionaries. A rumor spread contagiously through the Korean community in Seoul that the foreigners were kidnapping Korean children in order to butcher them at the hospital for use of the body parts. It was said that some of the organs were used for medicine, the eyes for photography and the flesh was being eaten at the legations. Angry mobs made it unsafe for foreigners to be seen on the streets for a period, and American marines from Chemulpo were sent to provide extra protection to the legations. It was even reported that one or two Koreans had been killed because they were thought to be helping the foreigners obtain the children for their evil purposes. Finally, the Korean government was able to quell the rumors, but for a time, mission staff made their trips to the hospital in the company of guards.

FIRST FOREIGN WOMAN IN THE INTERIOR

On March 13, 1889, four years after his arrival in Korea, Mr. Underwood married Miss Lillias Horton, M.D., also of the Presbyterian Mission in Seoul. Dr. Horton had arrived the year before and had been serving as the women's doctor at the hospital and as physician to the Queen. The Underwoods' honeymoon was a two month long, 1000 mile trip through the northern interior. Mrs. Underwood was the first foreign woman to make such a journey.

The Underwoods had taken the precaution to get written permission for their trip from the Korean government. This served to protect them and give them authority to secure help. Upon reaching Wiju, the Underwoods found 100 applicants for Christian baptism. Thirty-three of these Mr. Underwood baptized in a service across the Yalu River in Manchuria.

MISSIONARY "MUSICAL CHAIRS"

After this, the missionaries resumed their itinerating trips, taking with them simple medicines and selling Christian books and tracts. These dangerous travels could be likened to a game of "musical chairs." The missionaries had to be careful to stay on the move, for they could never be sure when the pleasant music of a welcome reception would stop, and they would be caught standing at the mercy of an angry mob. Nonetheless, these pioneers faithfully moved forward, supported by an unquestioning belief that God would provide for every contingency and that their task was to help in the evangelization of the world.

CHAPTER 4

Pioneer Adventures

An exuberant entry was recorded in Rosetta Sherwood's journal on "Mail Day"–October 27, 1891:

> "Some very good news that makes me happy came in the mail today. Dr. Hall writes under date of *September 19th* that he has just been appointed to Korea! So, though unrealized at the time, I have this best of all birthday remembrances. It seems to me that my Heavenly Father must have planned it Himself . . . My heart is too full of thankfulness to express it in words . . .
>
> "I love Korea, and the Koreans, and my work here so much, that it does indeed seem a wonderful blessing that Dr. Hall should be sent here. I know he will do so much more for them than I ever can. Indeed I feel that it is the greatest thing that I could do for mission work in Korea, to have been instrumental in bringing Dr. Hall here, and I do thank God for the privilege."

Dr. Sherwood's future, which for a year had fluctuated uncertainly with each change in Dr. Hall's plans, was at last steadied upon a definite course. She looked forward to being reunited with him in mid-December.

The weeks before Dr. Hall was due to arrive were busy ones for Dr. Sherwood and she tackled her work with fresh enthusiasm. The number of patients treated in this time was triple the number seen in the same months the previous year. She continued teaching her little class of girls in physiology and *materia medica*.

While Dr. Sherwood had been in Chefoo, China for her vacation the previous summer, she had spent time in planning the lessons to train her young medical assistants. What she had not planned on, however, was that the sessions on the human skeleton for the physiology section of her course would develop into a problem.

She casually remarked to her fellow missionaries that she was going to introduce the girls to the study of human bones by showing them some real ones that she had found outside the city wall by Nam San (South Mountain) the previous spring. Quickly Dr. Sherwood was cautioned about the possible repercussions of using these human bones because of the old rumors that had once circulated about the foreigners using Korean babies for food and medicine. Dr. Sherwood listened to the stories of the "Baby Riots," as they had come to be known, and of the tense moments the missionaries had had before the rumor was quelled.

She was glad to have had this forewarning. Prudently she decided to conduct her demonstration of the human skeleton informally with her students, in the privacy of her own room, rather than risk alarming anyone by bringing the bones into the schoolroom.

One of the most sensitive issues with which the missionary to Korea was confronted was the Korean tradition of ancestor worship. It was over this issue that the early Catholics were persecuted, and for those Koreans who became Christians, giving up ancestor worship was often the most difficult struggle in the acceptance of Christianity.

When entering the homes of the *yangbans* (gentleman class), Dr. Sherwood would see the ancestor tablet house located in the courtyard. She learned that the tablet itself consisted of two strips of chestnut wood, a few inches long, and fastened together. This was set upright on a wooden base and the name of the dead man was written upon the tablet. A small hole left in the tablet allowed for the spirit to enter.

It was explained to Dr. Sherwood that the Korean belief was that every man has three souls. These separate at death, one entering the ancestral tablet, one remaining in the grave and one going to the lower world. For the *yangbans*, it was essential that the tablet be made of chestnut wood. The Korean believed that when a chestnut was planted, it did not rot until the tree growing from it bore fruit. Thus the chestnut symbolized the continuation of an unbroken family line. Ancestor worship was also practiced in the lower classes. However, only the *yangbans* were permitted to have ancestral tablets. The common people often used strips of paper to represent the abode of the spirit.

Only four generations were venerated at a tablet house. Thus, whenever the head of the house died, a new tablet was placed in the tablet house for his spirit and the oldest tablet was then removed and buried next to the grave of its owner. Other generations were worshipped at the grave site itself.

A three year mourning period was observed. At set times special services were held before the tablet of the departed. Sack cloth and large hats were worn during the mourning period and the anniversary of the death was observed by sacrificial offerings on eight special holidays. On one of these days, Dr. Sherwood witnessed such an offering first hand, as she describes in her diary:

> "October 5—A beautiful autumnal day; it is a Korean holiday—at least in the sense that most work stops, and the people go out to offer sacrifice at the graves of their ancestors.
>
> "As there were not likely to be any patients at the hospital, I decided to give my staff a holiday and take one myself. The Misses Paine and Lewis and I went in chairs quite a ways out in the country . . . Many graves cover the hills lying about this road, and we saw a great number of people, mostly men and children, but some women, all about, over these hills participating in the ceremonies of the day. We heard much 'howling' and some real weeping.
>
> "Thinking it would be interesting to watch at least one such rite from the beginning, we followed a closed chair carried by two coolies, with a woman servant behind bearing a load upon her head.
>
> "Some distance from the road over on a hillside, the chair stopped, and a lady got out. After searching about among the many round mounded graves, that look like hay-cocks in the distance, she evidently found the grave of her search. How they know or remember is more than I can tell, for there seems to be nothing marking the graves. We withdrew at a respectful distance and watched the proceedings.
>
> "First the servant went and brought some water, then the lady washed all the dishes, some of which were Japanese, and I noticed a foreign knife. Then she prepared all the food, carefully placing it in the dishes herself, the servant only

waiting upon her a little. There was the bowl of rice, something that looked like pancakes, dumplings, honey, wine, pears, persimmons and green prunes. After arranging everything in order upon a tray the lady covered it with an oiled paper, and gave it to the servant who placed it upon top of the grave, and then uncovered it. The lady then bowed herself at the side of the grave and began moaning and crying, and apparently praying. After some ten or fifteen minutes, she stopped, and then she and the servant began dividing the food, which she had just offered in sacrifice, between the chair-coolies and the men who cleaned off the dead grass from the grave, and some children (boys) who evidently go out this day in order to get these treats.

"Noticing me standing near, the lady politely asked me to come and sit down by her. I went. She offered me some of the food but I declined. I asked her if she did not eat any, and she said no, it would not be right for her to. I asked her if it was her husband who was dead, though I scarcely thought it could be as she wore a silver pin in her hair. She said no, it was her mother and father.

"She told me she had never seen an American woman before. I told her I was a doctor, and invited her to come to my dispensary sometime. She seemed like a nice earnest hearted woman, and how I longed to be able to talk more to her."

On December 15, 1891 Dr. Hall's ship touched at Fusan and here he was cordially welcomed by a fellow Canadian, Dr. R. A. Hardie, who had moved to Fusan that year as physician to the Custom's staff. Dr. Hardie also provided a medical mission to the fishermen of that port. From Fusan, Dr. Hall sent a telegram to the Reverend George Heber Jones that he expected to reach Chemulpo the following day.

Mr. Jones was there to greet the newly arrived missionary but had been able to obtain only one pony for the 27 mile overland trip from Chemulpo to Seoul. Mr. Jones later recalled that Dr. Hall, in action that was so characteristic of him, took in the situation at a glance, concluded that the pony was too small for his six-foot frame, and said he would be happy to walk the entire distance.

When Dr. Sherwood saw her fiancé that Thursday evening, December 17, at a prayer meeting at Dr. Vinton's, her heart was so full that she knew she would not be very successful at keeping the secret of their engagement from others much longer. Mrs. Scranton had assured her in a letter from New York that she would not divulge it until it seemed appropriate. Miss Bengel was the only one on the mission field who knew. Miss Bengel had confided to Dr. Sherwood that she and Mr. Jones were planning to be married the following year, and the two ladies had enjoyed sharing with each other their mutual secret and future wedding plans. Now Dr. Sherwood was worried that she had waited too long before telling Miss Rothweiler, for when Miss Bengel finally did speak about her own intention to marry, Miss Rothweiler was not pleased that the W.F.M.S. would be losing her.

No longer did Dr. Sherwood have to face decisions alone and she wrote a note to "her Doctor" that very evening to ask his advice in the matter. She did not wish to think only of herself and hesitated to add to Miss Rothweiler's discouragement so soon.

Dr. Hall wrote back that he did not think it would be selfish and as Miss Rothweiler was likely to hear of it at any time from other sources, he thought the news had better be broken directly. He wrote:

> "I wish I could assist you, as I feel for both of you. How I rejoiced to see you tonight, and how I longed to give expression to my feelings. I do praise God with all my heart that He has permitted us again to meet and that we are to labor for him in Korea."

Dr. Sherwood went at once to Miss Rothweiler, although it was after 10:00 P.M. She noted:

> "To say that Miss Rothweiler was *astounded* by my announcement does not half express her surprise. I don't understand it, but it seems to have been the general impression here that I would never look twice at a man. I am surprised myself at her great surprise; but oh, she was so lovely to me and she bade me 'Godspeed' with a kiss upon my brow and tears in her eyes."

Further, Miss Rothweiler penned the following note to Dr. Hall:

> "As far as you are concerned, I can offer my warmest congratulations for it is not the lot of all men to find as true and good a companion as Dr. Sherwood is, but when I think of the W.F.M.S. and its interests, which are also mine, I suppose I may be pardoned if my heart almost failed me. I am very thankful to be allowed to take the part of an 'older sister' and hope I may prove myself worthy the trust.
>
> "Wishing you God's best blessings, I am
>
> "Yours sincerely,
> "L. C. Rothweiler"

The next day Dr. Sherwood showed her fiancé around the hospital buildings. Her joy at being with him was so apparent in her features that even the Koreans could see that the lady doctor was a different woman.

Dr. Hall looked forward to setting a wedding date so that he could make definite plans as he began his new work. He learned that the Appenzellers intended to return to America on furlough in the summer and that this would mean their house would become available. He suggested to Rosetta that they avail themselves of this opportunity and get married in June. After a considerable struggle with trying to determine the right thing to do, Dr. Sherwood finally concluded that such a plan was not contrary to God's will.

She wrote a letter to Mrs. Skidmore at the New York office of the W.F.M.S. telling of her decision. In response, Mrs. Skidmore expressed considerable disappointment that Dr. Sherwood would think of breaking her five year contract and reminded her that in so doing she would be required to refund her passage money. Dr. Sherwood felt a little hurt that the W.F.M.S. seemed unable to see that she had not made her decision lightly, but had truly sought God's will in the matter. However, she hoped that in time they would come to understand. She certainly had every intention of refunding the passage money to enable them to send out another doctor in her place.

In the meantime, the Mission had decided to send Dr. Hall on exploratory trips into the interior to determine the best site for a new station. The outpost was to be established as soon as political conditions would allow.

On his arrival in Seoul, Dr. Hall had set up housekeeping with Mr. Jones. Since Mr. Jones was planning an extensive trip into the northern interior in the spring, it was decided that Dr. Hall should accompany him. Mr. Jones could thus initiate the new missionary into the rigors of country travel in Korea. They planned to journey together the 350 miles from Seoul north to the Manchurian border where, at Wiju, they would go their separate ways, with Dr. Hall returning to Seoul by way of Pyong Yang.

The missionaries left in the afternoon of a cold and windy day in early March, 1892. They planned to make the trip primarily on foot but so arranged the packs upon the horses that when tired, they could mount and ride. After a trek of seven miles, they found lodging at an inn with quarters so cramped that the doctor had to sit with his feet out the door. After another day of tramping through a drizzling rain and plunging along roads ankle deep in mud, they began their missionary work at Ko-Yang, fifteen miles north of Seoul. News of foreign medicine brought patients and the doctor began his first work in the interior. His companion later remarked:

> "It was then I discovered how real was my sainted companion's missionary spirit, for the simple administration of physical relief to these suffering country people gave him intense joy."[1]

Everywhere the two men stopped, people crowded around the doctor for treatment and medicine.

On one occasion, after a cold ride on a pack horse, he was offered a bowl of hot meat soup. Since it had been boiled, he had no compunction in taking it, and noted that it was quite tasty. Later, taking a short stroll, he noticed a fresh dog skin stretched on a roof to dry. His suspicions were immediately aroused. Upon inquiry, he found to his consternation that he had unwittingly partaken of dog soup! For a time after that he had no appetite for meat soups and, in fact, swore off native food for several days.

Mr. Jones described their journey northward:

---

[1] *The Life of W. J. Hall*, pp. 126-127.

"Passing Pong Son, we descended through the Tong-sol-ryong to the great plain which stretches to the banks of the Tai-dong [Taedong]. At this point we met the severest hardship of the entire trip. It turned bitter cold with a high wind. Against this wind we forced our way, finally reaching Whang-ju, where we put up for the Sabbath. Monday morning we started out with that terrible northwest gale still in our faces. At first we were light-hearted and courageous in spite of it, . . . but it kept on blowing, steady, keen, bitter cold, biting our faces and hands whenever exposed, forcing its way inside our wraps, numbing us so that we were driven to walk to keep from freezing, and unable, even with that exercise to keep warm . . . Both the doctor and myself suffered intensely. Our feet became sore with the walking, and yet we did not dare take to the horses for fear of freezing. Thus we struggled on over thirty miles, and finally reached the welcome banks of the Tai-dong. The river was frozen two feet thick, and on this carpet of ice we crossed into the great city of Pyong Yang, and Doctor Hall was for the first time on the field for which he was to give his life.

"We reached Pyong Yang March 14, 1892, and . . . from morn till night we were beseiged by visitors, and to one and all we preached the truth, cared for the sick, and spent a busy, happy week. Our Korean brethren had an exciting time. Opening a book counter in an accommodating store, in one day they sold eighty Christian books. This brought down an edict from the governor of the province prohibiting the sale. But this didn't worry us much, and we kept right on selling. We attempted to organize a class for instruction, but it proved abortive, for as soon as we left the men that joined disappeared. In the five days that we were there we accomplished our object . . .

"The following week was spent in busy work of a pioneer character on the road from Pyong Yang to Wiju. We reached the latter place Monday, March 28, 1892, after an absence from Seoul of twenty-six days. Here, for over one week, Dr. Hall remained with me, busy with medical work, and then he took the same road we had come, back to Seoul, while I plunged into the wild mountains . . . to the north . . ."[2]

---

[2] *The Life of W. J. Hall*, pp. 128-130.

For Dr. Hall, however, the greatest trial of his trip into the interior was not the physical hardships nor the potential dangers, but his long separation from his fiancée. He wrote on this occasion to Dr. Sherwood:

> "You know, Rosetta, how I long to be with you. My whole being yearns for you, and I have had to seek special grace from the Master. He has given me a heart to love. It costs me a great struggle to leave you so long, dear one, but now our wedding day will soon come, when we can be together at last."

Dr. Sherwood's work kept her busily occupied in Seoul. She found that the care of patients in the dispensary and the many outcalls requesting the lady doctor's visits helped to alleviate her fretfulness over the safety of her fiancé. She and Miss Bengel were ever watchful for a courier who might bring them letters from the two travelers. One can see from an entry in Dr. Sherwood's journal on Tuesday, April 12, 1892, that a wry sense of humor helped these pioneer missionaries bear the anxieties of such separations:

> "It is six weeks now since my Doctor went away. Last Thursday on my way to the classroom Rev. Appenzeller handed me a telegram which made me very happy. It said that the Doctor left Wiju Monday, the 4th, so we expect him in Seoul by the 18th—Saturday. Rev. Jones will stay a few weeks longer. Doctor comes back earlier so as to relieve Dr. McGill who wishes to make a country trip to the East of Korea, starting next week. It will seem so good to see the Doctor again . . .
>
> "Miss Bengel and I think that some of the letters must have been lost, as we never received any from Pyong Yang and they must surely have written from there. I asked Miss Bengel one day if she didn't think perhaps the Korean law had been executed upon them—decapitation for teaching Christianity, but she said I couldn't scare her that way.
>
> "She is expecting a nice long letter with Dr. Hall from Mr. Jones so is looking forward to the doctor's arrival quite as eagerly as I. We both promise when once married, to be like John Wesley's wife—to scold, and make home so uncom-

fortable that our respective husbands will be glad to get off upon long itinerating trips to the country; but as yet we are not quite equal to that sacrifice of self; and we feel we have been pretty brave to endure our separation with as much grace as we have."

Dr. Hall arrived on schedule and was much encouraged by his first country trip. He had had many interesting experiences and some hardships but reported that on the whole he was treated very kindly by the Korean people.

He prepared his detailed report for the Executive Committee of the Mission. In it he concluded that the city of Pyong Yang offered the best location for a new Mission station in the Korean interior. (His choice proved to be a good one, for in time, Pyong Yang became the banner Methodist and Presbyterian mission station of the world, boasting schools, colleges, hospitals and thousands of Christian converts.)

Dr. Hall quoted freely from what others like Samuel Moffett and Graham Lee of the Presbyterian Mission had said about Pyong Yang to support his choice. A number of facts pointed to the selection of Pyong Yang for the initial work of the Mission in the interior. First, it offered the greatest challenge. Pyong Yang had the reputation of being the wickedest and dirtiest city in Korea. It was also notorious for its violent mobs which took to stoning whatever people or institution incurred their displeasure. Furthermore, Pyong Yang had a population numbering over 100,000 and all the signs of becoming an enterprising, aggressive, and relatively prosperous city. In addition, it was located on the direct route from Seoul to Peking and had fair road and water connections.

It was indeed a city with a glorious history. An associate of Dr. Hall's, W. A. Noble, later described it in the following words:

"The city is located a little north and west of the central part of the kingdom. The natural basin in which the city is situated is boat-shaped, and the natives are superstitious in regard to its form. They think some genii of past ages prepared this for the present great city, and they fear to perforate the bottom in the digging of wells, believing that water would rush in and drown all the inhabitants. Beyond the prow of the boat is a high mountain from which a view can be had of the country for many miles in all directions; a view fascinating in beauty. At this point may be seen Ke-ja's [Kija] grave, the first King of Korea. On this mountainside for three thousand years the patriarch has rested undisturbed with the rise and fall of succeeding dynasties. Toward this well-tended mound ten millions of people turn their eyes in worshipful reverence.

"Around the city is built a massive stone wall running up the mountain ridge and culminating at its farthermost peak . . . Like the great mass of all Korea, the common people live in houses of mud walls and straw roofs. The life of the common people is representative of the nation, and emphatically so of those whom the missionary is called to serve. A view of one such home would introduce one into the Korean life and also transport him back to conditions that existed a thousand years ago."[3]

The Annual Meeting of the Methodist Mission was not scheduled to meet for action on Dr. Hall's report until August. With his initial assignment completed, he eagerly proceeded with his marriage plans.

It was no ordinary wedding that would take place that June. In fact, it was an international one, the first of its kind in Korea. The bride was a citizen of the United States of America, the groom was a Canadian, while the host country was Korea. All three flags would be in evidence at the wedding reception which was to be in Mrs. Scranton's lovely garden. The Scrantons had returned to Korea the previous month, much to Dr. Sherwood's special joy, for Mrs. M. F. Scranton, particularly, was beloved by missionaries and Koreans alike as the *Tai Pooeen* (Great Lady) and was a substitute mother to many.

Even the non-Christian Korean friends were jubilant about the wedding plans. They had long felt that Dr. Sherwood should be married, for practically no reputable Korean woman at that time would choose to remain single. They were glad that Dr. Sherwood's status would at last be normalized.

The Koreans were perplexed by the strange ways of Westerners as plans moved forward in preparation for the wedding. This Western bride not only had seen her betrothed before the wedding day, but

---

[3] *The Life of W. J. Hall*, pp. 343-344.

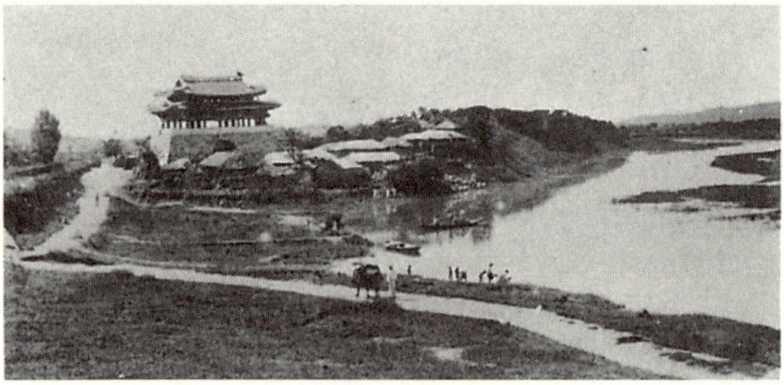

Futsu Gate, Pyong Yang

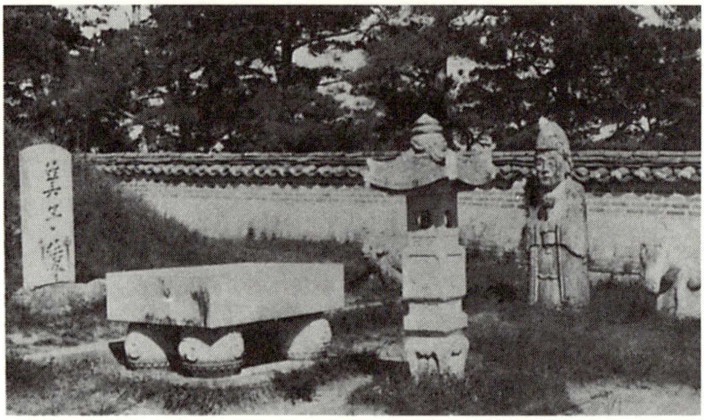

Kija's grave (first King of Korea)

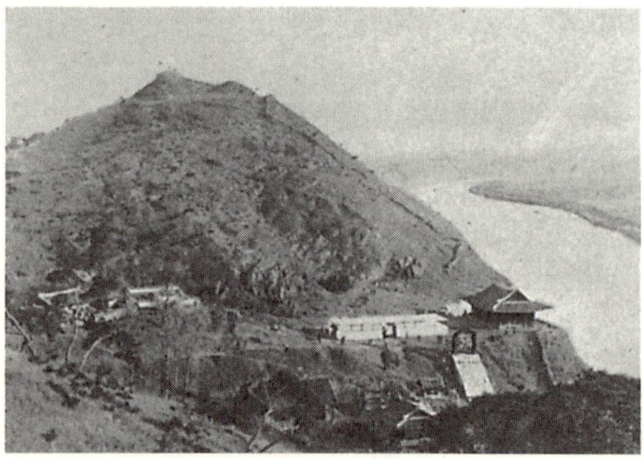

Peony Point ("Mo Ran Boong") outside of Pyong Yang

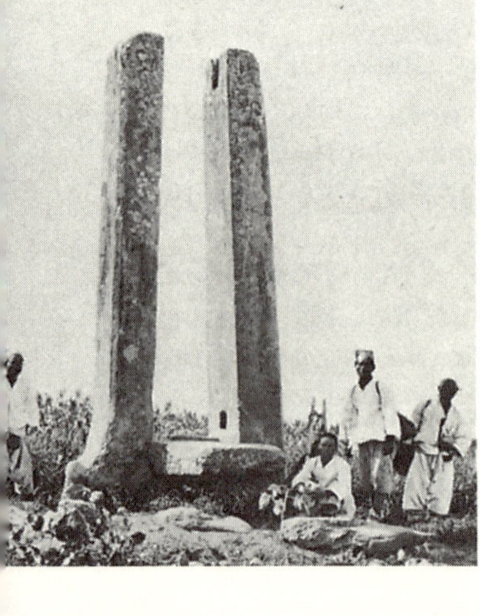

Mooring posts to which the boat-shaped city of Pyong Yang was believed to be fastened

was working by his side. The parents had not even arranged the wedding. Since Koreans viewed single adults as either deformed, sick or immoral, they would have been still more disbelieving had they been aware that Dr. Sherwood's mother was initially very much opposed to giving up her daughter to marriage, and that it was, in fact, only after a considerable struggle with her conscience that she had been able to write to her daughter:

> "The hardest thing I have ever written will be to answer Dr. Hall's letter. Now my dear child it is a hard job for me to give you away to another, for God knows I do love you . . . Your Pa and your sister of course consent to it. As far as I am concerned, if you are always going to do missionary work and you love Dr. Hall as you say you do, I will call it for the best . . . I have made up my mind to give you my consent to marry your doctor. Yesterday I didn't think I would or could ever do this, but somehow or other I couldn't get to sleep till I promised myself to put it down in black and white . . . I hope and pray that your marriage may prove a very happy one, a long and useful one."

In Korea the mother-in-law played a very significant role and had more control over the bride's life than even the husband. But in Dr. Sherwood's case the mother-in-law was far away. Who would guide and direct the bride?

With much consternation the Koreans learned that a white wedding gown was being made. Did the *wesa pooeen* (lady doctor) not realize that white is the color of mourning in Korea, and that a bride must wear bright colors? To be dressed in mourning would bring her bad luck.

The original plans for Dr. Sherwood's wedding gown had indeed encountered bad luck. She had sent three dollars to Mrs. Jenkins (the nurse at the New York Madison Street Dispensary) in America to purchase some silk lace for her gown, but the mail which contained her letter sunk with the Japanese steamer that carried it.

Instead, she was having a Korean tailor make up a gown from a piece of white silk she had purchased in Japan. But she could barely find time for the fittings, for two of the missionaries, Miss Bengel and Miss Lewis (a nurse), became dangerously ill. Both Dr. Sherwood and Dr. Hall gave them 'round the clock care, fearful for a period that they might lose them. However, both patients responded to treatment and had begun to recover when Dr. Sherwood wrote the following in her journal:

> "With all the other work, my tailor came last week and began my little bridal outfit. I verily believe I shall not have time to get married after all when the day comes. I could spend so little time in the fitting and supervision of the work as I'd like to. Well, I can be thankful that I have any at all. I think it will look pretty well, made up, with a full plain skirt and a basque with a bit of embroidered silk crepe in a point front and back—the silk laid in three folds on either side. I'd like a plainer basque but on account of my deformity [curvature of the spine] cannot well wear one."

Dr. Sherwood's fears that there would not be any time for a wedding did not materialize. In fact, she even had time for two weddings that beautiful June day! She wrote in her journal:

> "Between the Acts—At 9 o'clock Doctor and I, accompanied by Dr. and Mrs. Scranton, Rev. Jones, and Miss Bengel, went over to the British Legation and were married by Her British Majesty's Consul, W. C. Hillier. This marriage is legal anywhere within British rule, but to be legal in the U.S. it must be repeated before the American Consul, which will be done at 12 noon."

Some thirty guests were invited to the second wedding ritual which was held at the home of the Woman's Foreign Missionary Society, graciously presided over by Mrs. M. F. Scranton. On that perfect day, June 27, 1892, the noon wedding ceremony was performed by the Reverend F. Ohlinger, assisted by the Reverend D. Bunker, to unite in marriage Miss Rosetta Sherwood, M.D., of Liberty, New York, U.S.A. and the Reverend William James Hall, M.D., of Glen Buell, Ontario, Canada, in the presence of British Consul Hon. Walter C. Hillier and United States Deputy Consul-General Dr. Horace N. Allen. (This was the same Dr. Allen whose suturing skill in closing a Prince's wounds had helped to open up Korea to the Western World.)

The reception at the Scrantons which followed the ceremony continued to carry out the international theme. A Chinese chef, E. D. Steward, had baked and decorated the giant wedding cake. The "Royal Korean Palace Band" which had been trained by a German conductor provided music for the guests. Even the poor were not neglected, as a Korean custom of distributing money to them was followed. Korean coins (called *cash*), each worth about one tenth of a cent, were strung together through holes in their centers to form sets of 100 each. These strings of money were so heavy that they had to be brought on the backs of donkeys. The sets of *cash* were distributed to the poor outside the garden gate. Upon receiving the expected handout, the people beseeched the good spirits to bless the bride and groom.

Following the festivities, the newlyweds left for a honeymoon at the picturesque resort town of Chefoo, China, which was only a short trip from Korea across the Yellow Sea. They left for the port of Chemulpo at 2:00 P.M. Dr. Hall walked or rode a pony beside his bride's chair and entertained her with songs which brought back memories of her childhood. It was 11:00 P.M. when they reached Chemulpo, but their ship, the *Genkai* had been delayed by fog and was not yet in port. They took a room at Steward's Hotel where they stayed until their ship finally reached the harbor two days later.

Steward's Hotel was operated by the same Chinese gentleman who had baked their wedding cake. Originally he had been the steward of the ship that had brought to Korea the first U.S. Minister, General Lucius Foote. General Foote had persuaded the captain to let him have his steward, whose Chinese name was Eu Don. Ever since, he had been called E. D. Steward! In the early days of the Royal Hospital, he used to help administer the anaesthetic for Dr. Allen when the latter performed surgical operations. When Dr. Allen had left for a month to fetch his family to Korea for the first time, he had left E. D. Steward in charge of house repairs. An affable person of considerable enterprise, E. D. Steward had run the hotel in Chemulpo where for years missionaries stopped on their way to and from Korea. He also established a grocery store in Seoul known as E. D. Steward & Co. and for many years was the sole supplier of Western goods to the Seoul foreign community. He was always a warm and kindly friend to the missionaries and their children.

The young honeymooners found congenial fellowship with the other guests at the hotel at Chefoo. During the summer months the

Mission school there (operated by the China Inland Mission) was converted into an economical resort for vacationers from Korea and northern China. Chefoo boasted a lovely sandy beach with excellent swimming and boating facilities, and Dr. Hall promptly rented a rowboat for a month. He delighted in having the children of missionary families accompany Rosetta and him on their regular evening row. By the end of the honeymoon, Rosetta was beginning to master the technique of handling one of the oars while he rowed with the other.

The guests at the hotel took a special interest in the honeymooners, suggesting all kinds of different things to do and see. Perhaps one of the most intriguing suggestions was a ride through the town on a Chinese wheelbarrow, built especially to carry two passengers. It had a large central wheel and on either side were the passenger seats. One of the guests, an old timer with a merry twinkle in his eye, offered to make all the arrangements for this novel ride, which he assured them would be "something to write home about." The Halls cheerfully accepted his offer.

They found their seats on opposite sides of the contraption and after a little adjusting to get the right balance, were off to a merry start. The sturdy coolie behind, with a strap over his shoulders, grabbed the handles of the wheelbarrow; while two youths pulled it easily by ropes attached to the front. Since the strange vehicle moved comparatively slowly, there was no need to blow a horn. Anyway, the loud squeaks emanating from the poorly greased and complaining axle warned all pedestrians that a wheelbarrow was approaching. This was a common mode of conveyance in those days.

The Halls thoroughly enjoyed the experience and the chance it gave them to observe the bazaars at close range and in slow motion. At a distance the thoroughfares had appeared to be a dense blue, but as they drew closer, they saw that this effect was created by the blue garb of the people in the streets which were much more crowded than in Korea. There, of course, the women were kept in their homes. Here in Chefoo the women could be seen doing the marketing, but noting their hobbled gait, the Halls realized that they were witnessing first hand what they had before only read about—the bound feet of the Chinese ladies. It shocked them to see the pained shuffle of these women, and they began to wonder if perhaps the Korean system for keeping the women at home was not to be preferred.

They passed silk shops which displayed gorgeous Chinese brocades and pongee silk, woven from the thread of special silkworm cocoons. Chefoo was famous for its pongees, both the heavy suiting material for men and the thinner delicate fabrics for ladies. They priced some and learned that it sold for four dollars for a piece 18 yards long. They were told that what accounted for the peculiar quality of pongee silk was that the silkworms had been fed on oak leaves instead of the usual mulberry leaves.

The wheelbarrow squeaked its way past the coffin shops where they saw coffins built of thick wooden slabs which must have been very heavy. Their coolie explained that those who wanted to be sure of a decent burial made certain of this by purchasing their coffins in advance.

The Halls noted that the passers-by paid little heed to them, with the exception of amused glances from some of the obviously well-to-do men. Foreigners were evidently a much more familiar sight at the time in China than in Korea.

When the Halls returned, their genial friend who had made the arrangements asked them how they had enjoyed their strange ride. Mrs. Hall answered, "It was fun, but why did the better dressed men seem to be laughing at us?"

"Well, perhaps they were the only ones who could read," was the friend's quick response.

"Read what?" asked Mrs. Hall with a puzzled look.

Their friend smiled and with a wink at Dr. Hall, he replied, "Well, I must confess. There was a placard attached to the front of your vehicle which merely stated, 'Newly Married,' in Chinese characters."

On hearing this, Mrs. Hall blushed and everyone had a good laugh.

The China Inland Mission operated a sanatorium in Chefoo and the Halls enjoyed a visit to this work. It also served as a health center for people who worked in the interior of China. Dr. Hall knew a missionary of the China Inland Mission from his medical school days in New York, Dr. Randall, of Tong Shin nearby. Rosetta had visited the Randall family the previous summer when she was at Chefoo and they decided to visit Dr. Randall's dispensary and hospital. Here they were in for a unique experience which Rosetta recorded in her journal:

> "We saw a bound-footed woman remove her bandage for the doctor. She had walked four miles to get medicine for her husband on those poor little stumps of feet. The toes are all turned under except the great toe and at first sight, they look as if they had all grown to each other laterally and posteriorly

to the sole of the foot. But I found they could be lifted up. The great toe and heel are bent toward each other so as to shorten the foot as much as possible. Dr. Randall said the bones of the ankle are often dislocated this way. It is not very often one has the pleasure (?) of seeing such a foot. The Chinese women are very averse to showing them, but this poor woman had walked so far she complained of pain in feet and legs, and as we were very anxious to see such a foot, Dr. Randall succeeded in getting her to unbind them while he applied Iodine."

One of the things that impressed the Halls at Chefoo was the relaxed attitude of the China missionaries. They appeared less anxious than those who served in Korea. (Although as it later turned out, many of these very missionary acquaintances whom they met that summer would be liquidated in the "Boxer Rebellion" which occurred in China in 1900.) Basking in this cheerful tension-free atmosphere did the Halls a world of good and prepared them for what was to prove a "road of broken glass" ahead.

Their honeymoon at Chefoo was over, but still going strong in their hearts, when the Halls returned to Seoul. They set up housekeeping at the home of the Appenzellers who had just left on furlough as planned. The Halls enjoyed sharing their table with guests, especially the single ladies and the bachelors of the various missions in the capital. They both knew from personal experience how lonely one can feel in a strange land.

The Annual Meeting of the Methodist Mission met soon after their return from Chefoo. Dr. Hall had submitted his report in which he had strongly recommended opening work in Pyong Yang, and he offered to become responsible for half of the salary of a doctor sent to that field. His friend from New York days, Dr. John Bernard Busteed, was being considered for the Korean mission field by the Home Board and the Mission was hoping that he would be sent out at the earliest opportunity. Dr. Hall felt that, being single, Dr. Busteed might be the logical one to open Pyong Yang, and by helping to pay his salary, it might hasten the new doctor to Korea.

Bishop Willard Mallalieu concluded the meeting with the announcement of the appointments for the following year. Much to the Halls' surprise, Mrs. Hall was appointed to continue her work as physician in the Woman's Hospital at Seoul and Dr. Hall was appointed to open the mission work at Pyong Yang, and to be there most of the time except through the coldest months and the rainy season. The ban which prohibited foreigners from residing in the interior was still in effect and death was still the penalty for teaching Christianity. The mission that was being assigned to Dr. Hall was admittedly a dangerous one, but it was felt that a medical man could best perform it.

The Halls took the attitude, "It is all right, we feel sure, though it does look hard now. But surely the Lord is with us. He goes before." Only a few weeks after receiving his assignment, Dr. Hall set off for Pyong Yang making no specific plans as to when he would be able to return.

Four weeks after the doctor's departure, the Reverend and Mrs. W. A. Noble landed in Korea. Dr. Hall thought a great deal of Mr. Noble in their mission work together in New York and it was largely through the doctor's persuasion that the Nobles came to Korea. They, too, were newlyweds. The plan was that by the two couples sharing the Appenzeller home and taking turns with the meals, between them they could save enough money to pay the salary of another missionary to be sent to Korea for two years. When Mrs. Hall greeted her guests on October 18, 1892, she realized that they were not fully prepared for Dr. Hall's idea of combining households. Having some reservations herself, Mrs. Hall was sympathetic to their desire to begin housekeeping on their own and assured them they need not make the decision until the doctor's return from Pyong Yang. Meanwhile, they were welcome to be her guests.

Wondering in her diary whether she and the Nobles were selfish in their desire to each have their own household, she writes:

> "Finding that we were expecting them to live with us had great weight with them, especially as Mr. Noble knows and appreciates the Doctor so well, but I can see that they would both have to fight the same battle that I did before they could do it. Strange, but it seems to me that the Doctor did not have to do this. Is it pure selfishness with me and them? We are all very anxious to do what is right, and what will render us able to save the most to help others to come to the field, but somehow, it does seem unnatural for us to even think of trying to all live together in this way. But if it ever did to Doctor, he has kept it so well to himself that I can't

think it even . . . Both Mr. and Mrs. Noble have lovely Christian characters, and I am sure we can get on with each other all right should we deem it best to undertake it. I do wish the Doctor were here, and yet I don't know but that it is more fair to the Nobles that he is not, for he has a faculty of persuading people to do things quite against their wills often, and though as a rule, it is right and best, yet *perhaps* in this instance it may not be."

It turned out that the doctor's wish prevailed and the Nobles and the Halls found their shared households a very compatible arrangement. It proved to be a special comfort to the wives when their respective husbands were off on itinerating trips, for the loneliness of the long separations was not easy to bear.

On Monday, November 7, Mrs. Hall writes:

"Since I last wrote in my journal the Doctor has come and has gone again. He was home twelve days, but they went by like a dream and now the waiting time has come again . . . Oh, it was so hard to think of his going for so long again—even much harder than before. Day by day our love grows stronger and separation makes our hearts ache . . . I had to relieve a little of the heartache by crying, and all day Sunday, tears were bound to make their appearance above my strongest efforts to banish them; and I began to fear after the

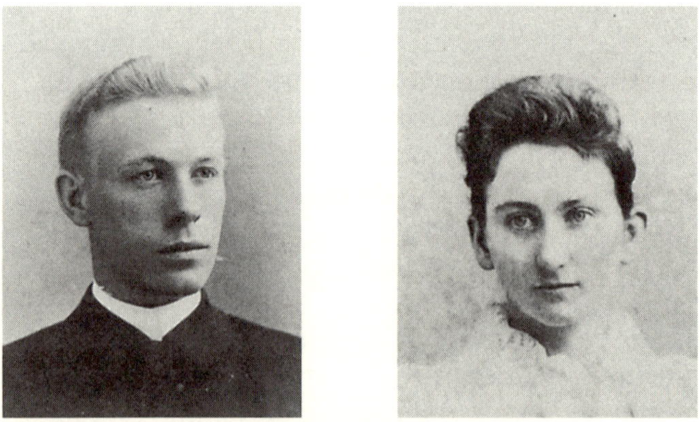

The Rev. W. Arthur Noble and Mrs. (Mattie Wilcox) Noble

Doctor had gone, no one could speak to me of him without my making a baby of myself. But now the day has passed and I have not shed a single tear, and I feel quite brave tonight. Surely God's grace *is* sufficient.

"Monday, December 5, 1892–My dear husband has been gone one whole month today, and not one word from him yet. When he was in America I heard from him oftener than this . . . 9:30 P.M.–A letter has just come from the Doctor, and though in one place he speaks of not returning till Christmas as he expected when he went away, of a later date he writes that he might leave in a week's time . . .

"Doctor feels that the way is opening up in a wonderful way for his work in Pyong Yang. Soon after he reached the city, he went to visit a little boy who was his patient there before, and who had quite recovered. His father is a man of means with a position with the Governor, and he was so delighted to see the Doctor again. He invited him to make his home there, gave him and Mr. Lee [Mr. Graham Lee of the Presbyterian Mission] the two best rooms in the house, and said he was more glad to see him than he would be to see his parents. It is a large 35 *Kang* house on a hill with a beautiful yard in front and to one side, though it is right in the midst of the city and in a good place for dispensary and evangelistic work. Later, Doctor asked the man if he knew where he could purchase a similar property, and the next evening he offered to sell his own house to him for $780, and that is Doctor's object in returning, to get permission to purchase the same and raise money for it.

"Doctor does hope our work will be together next year–separation is such a trial, but he says we don't want to sacrifice the Master's work to please ourselves and writes: 'I am glad after all, my darling, that God permits us to do hard things for Him. It is a special mark of favor. Let us not worry but be brave for Jesus' sake and get all the blessing from this trial that it is His will to bestow. God is training us and getting us ready for lives of great usefulness and it is all right.'"

When Dr. Hall left Pyong Yang to return to Seoul, he very nearly did not complete his journey. Along the road he came across a man who apparently had recently been killed by robbers. Another man lay beside him, severely wounded and certain not to survive in the freezing weather if left alone. It was the familiar Bible story all over again. Only the setting was different. For the first time, he fully realized how strong was the impulse of the passerby not to become involved. Although short of both time and money, he knew what he should do.

After giving the wounded victim first aid, he carefully lifted him onto his own pack pony and slowly returned with him to the inn from which he had started that morning. He was astonished and indignant to find that the innkeeper had no compassion for the wounded man and even refused to take him in. After considerable persuasion and hard bargaining, the innkeeper reluctantly agreed to provide the requested shelter. The doctor assured him that he would check on the situation when he returned.

Because most of his funds had been turned over to the innkeeper, Dr. Hall now had to ration himself to one meager meal per day. He comforted himself wryly with the thought that should the robbers attack *him*, they would not get much. The long daily treks without sufficient nourishment exhausted the doctor and he was on the verge of collapse when he chanced to meet a Japanese doctor friend who was on an exploratory trip to the North. His friend generously provided him with food and funds. This chance meeting was truly a "God-send" for his friend had originally planned to take another route off the main road, and had he done so, would have missed Dr. Hall entirely. The empty purse replenished, and refreshed in body and spirit, Dr. Hall resumed his journey. His arrival greatly relieved his wife who had been deeply concerned at the delay.

The Pyong Yang circuit to which Dr. Hall was appointed covered the territory from Seoul to Pyong Yang, a distance of some 180 miles. When Dr. Hall left on his fourth trip into the interior in February, 1893, he had Mission approval to make the Pyong Yang property purchases and to begin raising money for this undertaking. The Reverend Noble accompanied him, and he later wrote of his experiences on that trip with the Doctor:

> "The discomforts of traveling in Korea are multitudinous. There are peculiar trials that tend to bring out any sterling worth the missionary may possess.

"It was an inspiration to see Dr. Hall face these difficulties, even as joyously as if he had been traveling by the most luxurious railway coach. On leaving an inn one morning during our journey the coolies, as was their daily custom, began a general quarrel, each declaring that he had more than his share of the baggage to carry. At last they said they would not go another step. The doctor looked ruefully around upon his scattered baggage and upon the boisterous coolies and, without replying, sat down and, taking a paper from his pocket, he commenced to read. Such diplomacy on his part had the effect that entreaty or storming would not have had. They hastily placed the baggage on their ponies and were soon on their way. The doctor himself, seated on a pack astride of the strongest pony, would entertain with the brightest Gospel stories the coolie who trudged at his side . . .

"To the Korean mind the spirits around him have a great deal to do with his destiny. Every green tree, every bubbling stream, every green mound, the roof of his house, the walls, and the floor beneath are peopled with unseen beings, all to harass and none to cheer his weary life. On our journey at certain points we would pass small trees devoted to the spirit worship. At the foot of such a tree would be a pile of stones formed by the contribution of each passer-by; on the limbs were tied strips of paper and rags. The doctor would watch his coolies bow low to these places of worship, and at a convenient opportunity would, by question and suggestion, lead them to an acknowledgement that such worship brought them no satisfaction, and then he would offer Christ . . .

". . . If you tell the Koreans of the Western civilization, they marvel but little. If you tell them of the miracles of the Old Testament history, they will have something greater to tell. If you tell them of the great age of Methuselah, they will tell you of a man who lived two thousand years. Tell them of the waters of Eygpt that were turned into blood, they will tell you that the river of Pyong Yang, at a certain period, for three days ran blood. Tell them of the manna that fed the Israelites in the wilderness, and they will tell you of a clan that lived on the mountaintops fed with the dews of heaven; but tell them of the death and resurrection of Jesus Christ, and they are silent . . . and the great deep of the heart is moved, and they cry out, . . . 'What must we do?' . . .

"It was a great delight to have Dr. Hall back in his home after those trying journeys into the interior . . . The few days he would spend in Seoul . . . at the close of each trip from the interior would be in close application to the study of the language, looking after repairs upon mission buildings and frequently, also, the care of the hospital fell upon him . . . Yet he ever had time to give a helping hand to anyone in need and a word of cheer to those about him . . . That which he preached he lived, and to live in his presence was to know more of the Saviour he loved. . . .

"In his dispensary at Pyong Yang it was much the same. Seated on the floor like the Korean himself, the doctor would meet the people who thronged to see him, some coming from curiosity, others to be treated by the foreign doctor . . . none came under his care that did not leave . . . with the impress that they had been in the presence of a great and good man.

"At one time the people of Pyong Yang were aroused through the influence of an official with resentment against the foreigner. While sitting at an inn uncertain what would be the outcome of their animosity, Dr. Hall was asked how he felt over the prospects. He replied, 'If it is God's will to open up this city by the sacrifice of one life, I am not unwilling to be that one.'"[4]

Mrs. Hall was not idle during her husband's absence. An entry recorded in her journal on March 28, 1893 reports:

"I have just returned from the Great East Gate, where I began medical work the 15th of this month–going there every Tuesday and Friday. I do not have much work there yet, as the people have scarcely found it out, and the carpenters are still working at the buildings, but we have a nice site for work there, and I am sure it will grow."

---

[4] *The Life of W. J. Hall*, pp. 335-339.

This work did indeed grow and upon completion of the buildings, came to be known as the Baldwin Dispensary. Dr. Lillian Harris took charge of the Dispensary in 1897, but served only a few years when poor health cut short her service and she died in 1902. A hospital was built in her memory in 1912 which replaced the Baldwin Dispensary at the East Gate site and one day Dr. Rosetta Hall would serve as medical superintendent of that Lillian Harris Memorial Hospital.

In addition to this new clinic at the Great East Gate, and her regular hospital and dispensary duties, Mrs. Hall kept up her teaching in physiology and *materia medica* at the girls' school. Kim Chyom Tong continued to be an especially apt pupil and became a very decided help in putting up drugs in the dispensary and in caring for the sick. Her initial aversion to helping at the surgical operations changed after she had watched Mrs. Hall do an operation for harelip. Chyom Tong declared that she would like to be able to perform such an operation herself, and from that time on never gave up her determination to become a doctor some day should God open the way.

Chyom Tong was also developing the spiritual side of her life and when she was fifteen, asked to be baptized. In Korea, at that time, a woman lost her given name when she was married, usually around the age of fourteen. She then had no name of her own until she became a mother, at which time she was only known as such a one's mother. The missionaries, therefore, developed their own custom and gave women and girls "Christian names" when they were baptized.

When Kim Chyom Tong was baptized, she received the name, Esther. She was such a special help to Mrs. Hall that the latter hoped to be able to take Esther with her if ever she should go to the interior to work beside her husband.

In Mrs. Hall's March 28, 1893 journal entry she noted:

> "Doctor has been gone five weeks today on his fourth trip to Pyong Yang and his second to Wiju. It is just nine months ago, yesterday, we were married . . . and I know we love each other today more than we ever did. I want to quote from Doctor's last letter dated March 16th: 'Your precious letter reached me on Tuesday. Although it was as long as I could expect, yet while I was reading it, I was dreading that each page would be the last. Tonight my whole soul goes out to you in love. I have in you, my dear, the desire of my heart.

I praise God more and more each day for giving me such a precious treasure. You are my perfect ideal. I could not ask for more in a wife than I have in you my darling.'

"Doctor writes me that he has been able to purchase two very desirable pieces of property one of which will be just the place for medical and evangelistic work, and another farther back and higher up where it would be nice for us to live. He is hoping I may return with him in May when he comes back this time, and I want to very much. We are expecting our new lady Dr. Cutler this week, so probably I can be spared for a month or two.

"Doctor was having from 50 to 60 patients per day. The work has so grown in favor that the Governor (who hitherto has been difficult to deal with) replied to some who went to him to ask him to remove Dr. Hall: 'The foreigner is not a bad man, but a gentleman. He who cures the sick and helps the poor, is he not a good man? This same work is going on in Seoul, and you need not be afraid of him.' And he issued a proclamation stating this, and that these foreigners had permission from the King to travel in the interior, and anyone who interfered or made trouble with him, must be brought before the Governor.

"So Doctor thinks that already as much has been accomplished to remove prejudice as three years of ordinary work. Revs. Moffett, Lee and Swallen of the Presbyterian Church have gone up there now. They had not bought yet, but were going to move in Doctor's house when he and Rev. Noble went on to Wiju, for which they expected to start March 20th. They are working there now I suppose, and next Monday will start back for Seoul, reaching here about April 15th.

"God surely is wonderfully opening up the way for work in the northern interior, and I long to begin work for women there. When I asked Esther if she would be willing to go to Pyong Yang to work for Jesus, she replied: 'I will go wherever Lord open door for me. If He open door in Pyong Yang, I will go . . . I give up my life to teach my people about God even if people kill me.'

"Saturday, April 29, 1893– . . . Such a happy two weeks as the last have been. Doctor came home April 13th, two days before I expected him, and yet I thought of the possibility of his coming, and went and unlocked the door before I went to bed that night, and sure enough, about 11 P.M. he came, having traveled 140 *li* or 47 miles since morning. He is so glad to be home once more and we are so happy together . . .

"After the Doctor had worked nearly a month at Pyong Yang, and was gaining great favor among the people, he went with Mr. Noble to Wiju, and invited Revs. Moffett, Lee, and Swallen, who had come to Pyong Yang in the meantime, to live in one of his houses until they could buy for themselves. After Doctor and Mr. Noble left Pyong Yang, the Presbyterian brothers succeeded in purchasing property outside of the city, but they had not much more than done so before the people became alarmed at so many foreigners purchasing property, though of course, it had always been done in the name of their Korean helpers, as according to treaty, foreigners have no right to hold property outside of treaty ports.

"The Governor knew very well of Dr. Hall's relation to the purchase, and his plans for medical work there, and because they wanted the Doctor, he winked at it, and gave him his protection. But when so many more who were not doctors came in, he evidently changed his mind. At least he ordered Moffett to give back his deeds to the former owner, and them to give the money back. And also the people made it so hot for Moffett and Lee, that they had to leave the city. Swallen had already left upon an evangelistic tour through Whanghai Do.

"The former owners of Doctor's houses moved back, but as Doctor had the deeds with him at Wiju, he is still the owner in the name of Mr. You, his interpreter. When he came back, he was kindly received, and since he has been home, he has received letters from both of the former owners telling him not to be anxious; they will take good care of the property, and asking him to come back soon, that there are many sick people waiting for him.

"At the same time, we are having slightly serious times in Seoul. A politico-religious faction from the South, called Tonghak, came to the Palace and petitioned the King to send all foreigners to their own country. The King paid but little attention to them except to order them back. They went saying they'd return last Saturday 40,000 strong and they'd kill off the foreigners themselves.

"Some felt a great deal of anxiety as the day approached, especially the Japanese. The King sent guards to all of our compounds. By day they were disguised as farmers, but at night they were soldiers with musket and bayonet. They are still on guard, but everything has remained quiet. For a time it made a difference in the attendance of dispensary patients, especially at the East Gate. The people feared if they were seen going in and out of the foreigner's house, they too would be killed. But I think it is blowing over now, for day before yesterday I had 27 patients here, and yesterday had 13 at the East Gate.

"However, all things together, it hardly seems expedient for me to return with Doctor to Pyong Yang, as we had both been so much in hopes that I could do. I am very much disappointed and can scarcely give it up yet. I did so much want to see how they would receive me there before the Annual Meeting, so that if possible, we could make arrangements to move there soon after. But now Doctor thinks it the better policy to make haste slowly, and he will go back with Mr. You alone, and he feels sure he can get things in good shape again. And then, as it will probably be impossible for me to go with him next fall, he hopes that another year Dr. Busteed may be sent there (that is, if he comes out single), so that we may not be separated so much another year . . . We expect him now June 1st and from that time till after Annual Meeting I hope he can get a good start on the language, and Doctor can go up with him and establish him early next fall. Of course it will be best for him not to remain much more than two months at a time, perhaps, or three.

"This knocks a number of my calculations in the head. I had expected to take Esther with me there, and now I don't know just what is best to do with her. We think we have found the right husband in the person of Doctor's boy . . . He is 24 years old, tall, and good looking, very gentle and modest in manners . . . Mrs. Scranton is in a hurry for Esther to marry; she is such a great big girl and is sixteen now. The boy's name is Pak Yousan . . . Esther's mother was not pleased with the match when she heard that formerly Pak Yousan had been a hosteler, but after learning his father was a teacher whose death five years ago compelled Pak Yousan, his eldest son, to go to work, she has become reconciled . . . I have had such a nice letter from Esther about the proposed marriage, although no one could have blamed the girl if she too had felt badly about marrying a man from the lower class, as nearly every one of the school girls have married into the higher class. But this is the way this dear girl looks at it: . . .

"'My very precious sister . . . I was much pleased with your letter yesterday. You wrote to me very long and also say many strange words. Now I will tell you some strange words which I never tell. Do you know how my heart feel? Three nights I could not go to sleep and feel troubled, because I never like man, and also I do not know how to sew well; but Korean custom all girls have to marry—have to be wife and husband. I cannot help that, even if I do not like man. If our Heavenly Father send Mr. Pak here . . . to be my husband, then I shall be his wife though my mother do not like him. But my mother do not know him well. I tell my mother, what use to find he is low or high . . . I do not care rich or poor or high or low. You know I will not get married to one who do not like Jesus word. I think it will be very very queer if I get married. My heart will get very much different . . . From your sister, Esther Kim.'

"Dear Esther, what lessons of consecration she teaches me from day to day. I do love her."

Korean custom decreed that girls be married before they reached the age of 14. Because unmarried girls were easily recognized from the way they wore a long braid down the back, Esther, now 16, came in for considerable comment as she worked in the dispensary. Since her family did not wish to be disgraced (only dancing girls, the deformed, or the diseased remained unmarried in Korea), the missionaries either had to find a Christian husband for her, or the family would see to it that she married a non-Christian. That was when Pak Yousan, a young man converted in Dr. Hall's work, was selected as a possible groom. Dr. Sherwood's own happy marriage, though at first a great grief to Esther, later did much toward reconciling her to the idea of marrying. Subsequently Pak Yousan and Esther Kim were married in a Christian ceremony on May 24, 1893.

On June 27, 1893, Mrs. Hall wrote in her diary:

"This is the first anniversary of our wedding day. It seems so strange to each of us that we have been married a whole year—the time has flown so swiftly it is difficult to realize it. To each, it has been the happiest year by far of our lives. Doctor never tires of telling me how I have completed his happiness; he is so perfectly satisfied, and is ever expressing his great love both in words and in 'actions that speak louder than words' and yet he wishes he could tell me more. If a year ago it was impossible for me to put into words my love for my Doctor, it is still more so today, but I can put it into actions better than then. Dear Doctor understands me, and I him, and we are so happy.

"The future looks so bright before us, though we little know even where our work shall lie another year, but that is in God's hands, as are we, and we feel sure wherever He leads, is best. At present we are very comfortably situated in the house formerly occupied by Dr. McGill. We have our rooms upon one side, and the Nobles upon the other, with hall, dining room, storeroom and kitchen in common. We keep house together, just as before, Mrs. Noble housekeeper one month, and I the next. Dr. Busteed has been sent out upon Dr. Hall's and Mr. Noble's offers to pay his passage and support him the first year; so we are boarding him. We have been busy the last few days fixing up his rooms in the hospital building. They look quite cosy. We all like Dr. Busteed very much, and he is already quite one of the family.

"Mrs. Noble is housekeeper this month, and this evening she had a cake for supper beautifully frosted with the dates '1892, 1893' upon it, for us, and I had quite a large piece of the 'Bride's Cake' of my wedding that I gave to each. I have yet more to keep—think I can keep some for the 5th or 10th anniversary—perhaps the 50th."

The rainy season which begins in Korea in early July permitted the missionaries time for vacation and language study. Most of the

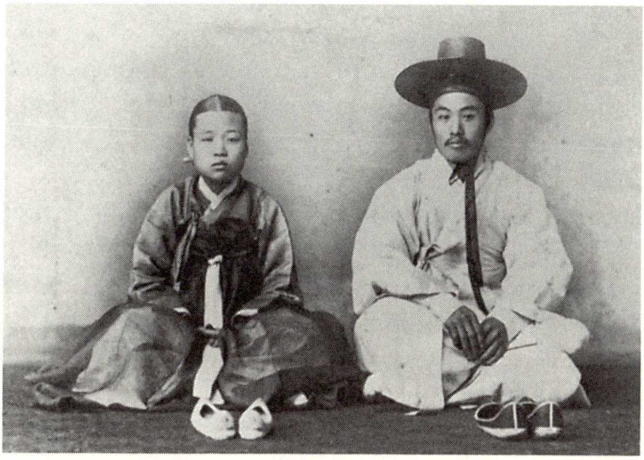

Esther Kim Pak and Yousan Pak

medical patients either could not make it in from the country over the flooded streams or were too busy with their farm work to come to the dispensary. With the medical work thus lighter, the Halls decided to camp out on a mountain near Seoul, Puk Han. It was Mrs. Hall's introduction to living in a tent and she declared she liked it. The tent in which they were camping had been used by Dr. Hall as a youth along the waters of his favorite Canadian lake, Charleston. It also was the same tent he had used when he had taken the 130 slum children to the lake during his New York Medical Mission days.

Mrs. Hall opened the July 26, 1893 entry in her journal with two quotations:

"'*Above all things have fervent love among yourselves.*' I Peter IV: 8.

"'The supreme happiness of life is the conviction that we are loved, –loved for ourselves, –say rather in spite of ourselves.' Victor Hugo

"Here we are living out of doors day and night upon top of Puk Han, the highest mountain near Seoul. Doctor put up his Canadian tent upon a bold promontory overlooking a beautiful valley, and here we sleep at night; but through the day it is too warm here, and we spend most of the time in our hammocks under some beautiful shade trees near. We have most of our meals served out here, but occasionally take our breakfast in the tent. We brought our cook with us, and

Doctor installed himself housekeeper, so I am relieved of all responsibility, and it is so nice. We are reading 'Peep of day' in Korean together through the day—one of the books in our course. Doctor generally studies it aloud while I sew.

"Every evening we take a mountain climb together. Often Doctor stops me saying, 'Give me a kiss my precious darling.' Indeed, this seems like another honeymoon even more sweet than the first. In short our whole wedded life has been but one continuous honeymoon, growing sweeter with each day. . . .

"Our daily routine here is generally about like this:

"We arise at 6:00 A.M., take our baths, dress, and are ready for breakfast at seven o'clock . . . Then we have our prayers, and later Korean prayers with the cook and Doctor's teacher; we then read a little from Frances Havergal's life if we have time before 9:00 A.M. when we begin studying Korean till noon when we dine . . . We read until 2:00 P.M. when we begin Korean again and study till five o'clock, then we meet with some other missionaries who are stopping in the Buddhist temple near us for the hot season, and we have a Bible study together . . . At six o'clock we have supper . . . take a walk . . . and retire by nine o'clock or before.

"So we are leading a very regular and orderly life even if we do live out of doors all the time like Gypsies and are becoming as brown as berries. We are just as happy as the days and nights are long. This morning after breakfast, Doctor said he had never felt so rested since he had been in Korea. I suppose we can have but one more week of this life, for then I must return to my work in Seoul—am engaged to officiate at the birth of Mrs. Moore's child which is expected somewhere between the first of August and the fifth, and then of Mrs. Swallen's about ten days later, and perhaps of Mrs. Reynolds another ten or fifteen days later. Also perhaps Dr. Cutler, who has been relieving me, will need a little vacation, and as Annual Meeting begins about the 23rd, it looks as if two weeks vacation is all I shall be able to get this year."

Bishop Foster presided at the Annual Meeting and appointed Dr. Busteed to work in Dr. Scranton's hospital. Dr. William James Hall and Dr. Rosetta Hall were appointed to work in Pyong Yang. The Halls were indeed thankful.

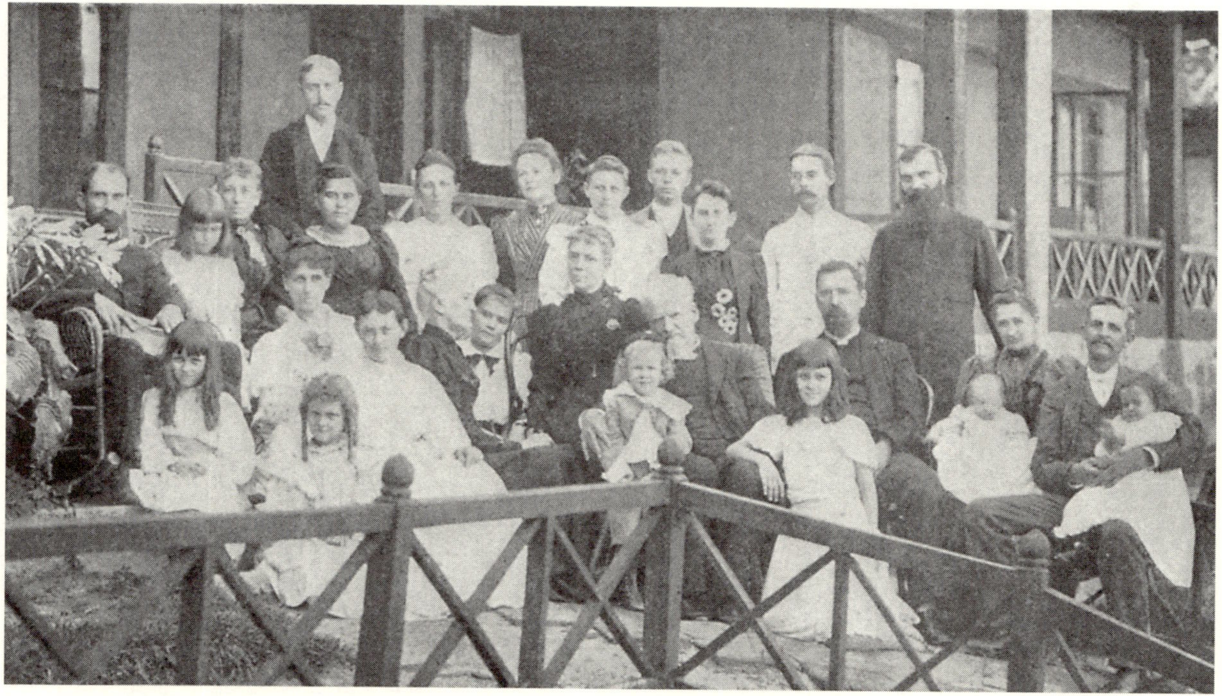

Methodist Mission in Korea, 1893, when visited by Mrs. Sarah Longacre Keen, Bishop Randolph Foster, and Corresponding Secretary of Foreign Missionary Society, Dr. Adna Bradway Leonard.

Seated, front row, l. to r.–Mrs. Keen (4th from left, profile view–see note, p. 120), Mrs. Margaret Bengel Jones, Mrs. D.A. Bunker, Bishop Foster, and Dr. Leonard. Seated, second row, 3rd from left–Mrs. M.F. Scranton. Standing, 1st and 2nd from left–Rev. George Heber Jones, and Mrs. Rosetta Hall, M.D. Standing, 1st, 3rd, and 4th from right–Dr. W.J. Hall, Mrs. Mattie W. Noble, Rev. W.A. Noble. (Others not identified)

As Dr. Hall gave his report about the status of the work in Pyong Yang, he noted that when he had returned to Seoul to raise money for the purchase of the houses and property there, his first encouragement had come from a meeting of missionary children that he had addressed. After he had told the youngsters of the need one of them had volunteered, "Dr. Hall, if that is the case, we shall ask God to give you a house."

Dr. Hall recalled:

> "I shall never forget those prayers; they went straight to the throne of God, and soon the answer came. After the meeting closed, Bertie Ohlinger came to my room with a bright silver dollar and said, 'Dr. Hall, here is a dollar to help buy a house in Pyong Yang. I wish I could give more, but it is all I have.' Next came Willa, his sister, a dear little girl of nine years, with ten cents. Following her came Augusta Scranton with fifty cents. It was only one dollar and sixty cents, and the prayers of God's little ones, but He who fed the five thousand with five loaves of bread and two fishes has multiplied the children's gifts until they have grown in eight months to $1,479.99. Today we have our property for hospital and dispensary well situated in Pyong Yang."

That fall, Dr. Hall had other cause for jubilation. He, who had always so loved children, was going to become a father!

N.B. At the time of her visit to Seoul in 1893, Mrs. Sarah Longacre Keen said that she always had her picture taken in profile, like the pose for the U.S. Indian Head penny, because she had served as the model for the figure on the coin when her father worked for the U.S. Mint Service. Dr. Rosetta Hall sought to verify the story in later years, and in 1945, received the following information, signed by Edwin H. Drench, Superintendent, United States Mint Service:

> "The legend is that during the administration of President Andrew Jackson, the Government held a competition to obtain the best design for the Indian Head cent; about 100 designs were submitted. Mr. James B. Longacre's design was selected. He was then Engraver of the Mint. His alleged inspiration was that in 1835 a delegation of Indian Chiefs traveled to Washington to visit the "Great Father," the President of the United States. They stopped off at Philadelphia to visit the Mint and Mr. Longacre entertained them at a dinner and reception at his home. His ten year old daughter, Sarah, made such friends with the guests that to please her, one of them took off his feathered helmet and put it on her head. An artist, who was present, made a sketch of her and handed it to her father, who was so delighted with it that he submitted it to the Government and it was accepted and used with some modifications. This is the story but we are in no position to vouch for its accuracy."

CHAPTER 5

Pyong Yang Legacy

The arrival of baby Sherwood at Seoul on November 10, 1893 created very little stir. In fact, life went on as usual in the capital except in the Hall household. Dr. Hall had wanted to be with his wife when their baby was born, but he was sure he would be useless as the attending physician. Therefore, Dr. Mary M. Cutler had been engaged for the delivery, and Miss Ella A. Lewis had agreed to be the nurse.

Mr. Noble records:

> "... The doctor's great heart was overjoyed with the birth of a son. This little fellow came November 10, 1893, the eighty-ninth anniversary of his Grandfather Sherwood's birthday, and he received the name of Sherwood Hall."[1]

Mrs. Hall's patients at the Seoul Woman's Hospital were also jubilant, for they felt that this birth event had at last made their doctor one of them. However, they continued to lament the absence of a mother-in-law to guide and advise the lady doctor.

One of the first things that Dr. Hall did after baby Sherwood's birth was to register the event at the British Legation in Seoul. A copy of the birth certificate was forwarded from there to the files at the Registry Office, Somerset House, London, England in case the original was ever destroyed (as it later proved to be).

While on the way home, Dr. Hall stopped off at the marketplace to see what he could find in the way of a crib for his new son. A large suit-case-like contraption made from woven reeds caught his eye. He was informed that Koreans called this type of basket-luggage a *cori*. It was equipped with a detachable lid, leather straps and a handle. Because the sides of the *cori* were fairly high, the doctor reasoned that it could be readily converted into a safe crib. Further-

---

[1] *The Life of W. J. Hall*, p. 341.

more, being lightweight, it would be just the thing to take with them when he and Rosetta traveled with their baby to Pyong Yang. This he hoped would be possible in the spring.

Sherwood was only three weeks old when his father had to return to the interior. This time it was doubly hard for Dr. Hall to leave. He wrote to Rosetta:

> "Our home is so happy; the only bitterness we have is our separation from each other."

However, he promised to be back for Christmas.

Dr. Hall was nearing the "City of the Beautiful Turf," as Pyong Yang was sometimes called, when he noticed a group of Korean men approaching him, all wildly waving and gesticulating.

"Am I to be their target?" Dr. Hall wondered, knowing the propensity for stone-throwing by the men of that city. It did not take him long to see that they were exceptionally friendly and had just come out to welcome him back and rejoice over the increase in his family.

Their first question was, "Are you now blessed with an *ahdul* (son)?"

Dr. Hall nodded yes with a smile that spread across his face from ear to ear. Then one of them stepped forward.

"You are indeed favored by the gods, for now you are assured of a son to worship at your grave."

The doctor then proceeded to the houses which had been purchased in Pyong Yang for the Mission. The deeds were registered in the name of Mr. You, the Korean interpreter, for foreigners were not yet permitted to own property outside of the treaty ports. Because of opposition from the Governor, the Christians had been unable to occupy this property for several months. One of the houses had formerly been used as a home for dancing girls and Dr. Hall found that it was again being used for that purpose. The men who had previously owned the houses had been forbidden by the Governor to let a foreigner stay in them. Rather than attempt to force the issue, Dr. Hall stayed at a local inn.

This "dancing school" was not simply a place where girls were taught to dance the "light fantastic." Rather, young and attractive girls were sold to these houses by their impoverished parents and became ordinary prostitutes. The more intelligent ones were trained to be entertainers, which included learning to play musical instruments, to sing and to dance at drinking parties.

After special training in Oriental arts, the best and most attractive girls were sold as concubines to the rich gentry for a fancy price. These women often reached positions of considerable importance, and through their masters, wielded real power in business or affairs of state. At times, the concubines would even be assigned the difficult and dangerous role of obtaining secrets or influencing government or business rivals by various and ingenious subtleties and coquetry.

Although they had no say in the matter, the girls, as a rule, did not seem to mind going to the "dancing school." They were well fed, gaily attired and lived an exciting life. However, those who served as mere prostitutes did not fare so well and usually had a short life span. Although the concubines lived much longer, they always faced the risk of a violent death as a result of the intrigues of their masters.

One evening, while Dr. Hall was sipping tea after his dinner, the other Korean guests at the inn became curious about his beverage. It certainly did not resemble the *sul* (liquor) which they were drinking. Being naturally curious, they inquired what it was and asked to try some. The doctor, glad for the opportunity to demonstrate his friend-

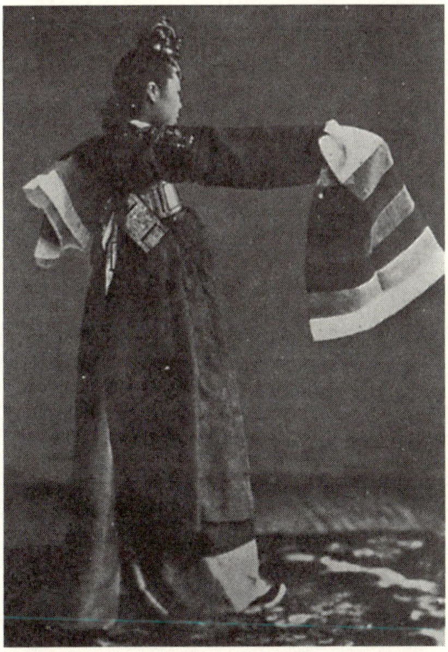

A Kisaeng *(dancing girl)*

FROM HULBERT, "THE PASSING OF KOREA" (DOUBLEDAY, PAGE)

ship toward them, poured them each some *cha* (tea). Tea-drinking had not yet caught on in Korea, even though the country was located between China and Japan where the practice was common.

Everyone was curious about the new drink. Besides tea, Dr. Hall had with him a quantity of white sugar and several tins of evaporated milk. The reaction of the Koreans to the milk, once they learned that it came from a cow, was one of repugnance.

"How dirty! It is unfit for humans. None of that in *our* tea!" came the unanimous voices of protest.

However, the Koreans consumed nearly his entire precious supply of tea and sugar. They expressed their appreciation by loudly sucking in the tea and smacking their lips, saying, "*Mat-is-so!*" (That does taste good!)

After some days, Dr. Hall finally succeeded in "dissolving the house of wickedness" and the dancing girls vacated the premises. He moved in with his Korean language instructor, Mr. P. S. No, who had accompanied the doctor to Pyong Yang to help him continue language study.

It soon became clear, however, that resentment for the Christians had not abated. They had not long been settled in the former dancing school when some twenty neighbors approached Mr. No.

They said, "Our Pyong Yang custom is that every year each house gives according to its wealth to the offering for the spirit of Pyong Yang. So you who are from Seoul, and especially that gentleman from the West," and they pointed to Dr. Hall, "can give us a lot of money to offer to our spirit. Then he will keep you and help you on your journey, and bless you all the year round."

Mr. No was asked to explain this matter to Dr. Hall but he objected, "People who serve God do not give money to this spirit."

"You do not have to give the money," they responded angrily. "Just simply tell that gentleman from the West as we told you."

Mr. No did so, and Dr. Hall said to tell them, "We have nothing to do with your spirit and we will not give it money, for we worship the true, living God who made us and you, and wants your worship too."

Mr. No described what happened next in a piece he later wrote called, "The Story of Saint Harak." Harak was the Korean name for Dr. Hall that appeared on his passport in Chinese characters.

"Then they were very angry, and they all went out; but a few minutes after, they rushed in, and they pulled me down, and also a young boy that believed, and they tore his clothes and hurt him. They beat me with their fists and kicked me with their feet and they said, 'This is not our work, but it is the spirit punishing you.'

"When they were through beating me and let me go, I went to Dr. Hall and told him what had happened, and my heart was very angry. He tried to comfort me, and asked me if I had not read how St. Paul was beaten. But I said I did not care; that if I continued to do this Jesus doctrine, my body would not last long, and I did not care about the good things I would get after I was dead. And I told him I would return to Seoul at once.

"Then he put his dear, loving arms around me and said, 'Let us pray, brother,' and we both knelt down, and he asked me to pray first.

"I could not pray with my angry heart, so he prayed for me. But I couldn't get over it yet; and he tried still to comfort me with such a loving, patient heart. After a little the young boy that also got hurt came in, and Dr. Hall bound up his wounded leg and paid him for his torn clothes, and he told us he was so sorry we were persecuted for doing right.

"After all this I became ashamed of myself, and got rid of my angry heart, and felt a good deal happier.

"After this, many people continued to crowd around Dr. Hall like flies around honey; yet at night, the stones would sometimes fly like rain pouring. We felt we were sitting out upon ice in the river . . .

"The doctor was always a friend to children. Wherever he went, many children followed him and bothered him, yet he loved them. Many times the children used to pull his whiskers, but he would only laugh and pet them. One day I asked him why he let the children bother him so much, and he turned to me and said:

"'Brother, what makes you so cold and hard? The Lord says in the Bible we are to have a child's faith and heart, for of such is the kingdom of heaven.'

"By this I perceived that his faith was like a child's. Many of the town people sometimes used to cry out, 'Good Saint Harak; he is one fit for the kingdom of God!' So when I went to write about him I called the heading of my story, 'Saint Harak.'"[2]

Unknown to the doctor, he had no sooner left Seoul, than baby Sherwood became quite ill with intestinal difficulties which did not seem to respond to any treatment. It was a new kind of anxiety for Mrs. Hall to learn to bear alone, and she added the following entry to her diary:

---

[2] *The Life of W. J. Hall*, pp. 396-398.

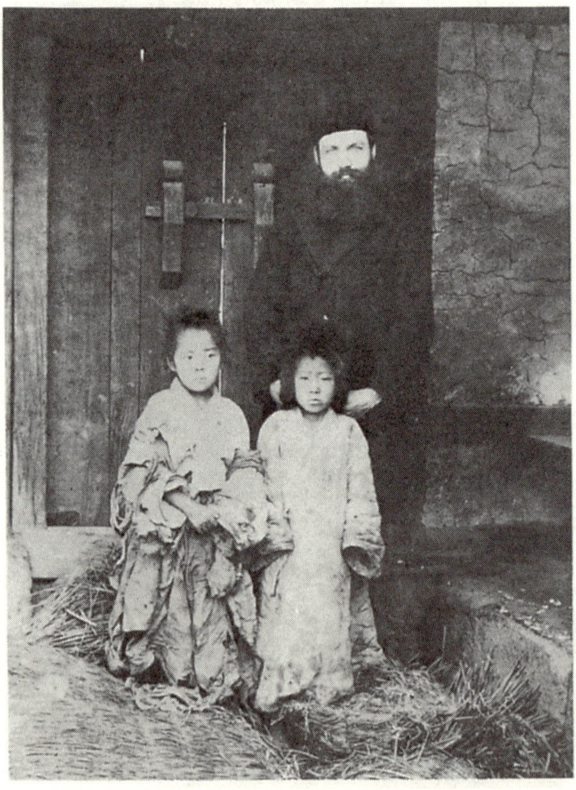

Dr. W. J. Hall and two Korean waifs

"Caring for Sherwood night and day those three weeks when I was not very strong, brought on my old backache again. It aches just as it used to when I was from twelve to fourteen years of age, and the curvature of the spine was taking place. It still continues. Sometimes it feels as if some of the bones must drop out, they hurt so. *Amah* gives it a good rubbing night and morning, and it is growing better now.

"Well, I am sure I can sympathize with mothers with sick babies as I never knew how to before. How many there are who have things much harder than I, and know much less what to do for the poor little suffering baby. I am sure, doctor and all as I am, I felt helpless enough often times. How I pity those who are yet more helpless."

When his father returned from Pyong Yang a few days before Christmas, Sherwood's health immediately improved. His mother began to suspect that it had been her own feelings of loneliness and anxiety that may have affected her baby when he nursed. She observed that she was more relaxed with someone there to share the responsibility of Sherwood's care and cure.

Dr. Hall felt that he had accomplished all that he could for a time at Pyong Yang, and it would be best not to stir up the anxiety of the non-Christians there by staying in the Mission houses too long at any one stretch. This way they could gradually get used to his comings and goings and build up a sense of trust in him as their friend.

In view of the circumstances, Dr. Hall concluded that he could profitably spend some of the winter weeks in Seoul studying the Korean language. He had been so busy since coming to Korea, that his language study had suffered. Yet he needed a minimum proficiency in the language to be fully effective in his work at Pyong Yang.

These carefully reasoned plans, however, were abruptly scrapped. Dr. Hall had scarcely been home a week when Dr. Scranton asked to see him. Dr. Hall was informed that he should return to Pyong Yang at once in order to begin construction of a Western style house, fitted out with Western style furniture, so that it would be in readiness to take his family there in the spring.

Dr. Hall was concerned that to move that rapidly into the appearance of Western permanence might alarm the Pyong Yang residents. His own idea had been to make the move very gradually and then to live in the Korean style house. This would give the residents of the city less cause for fear that the "Western barbarians" were taking over. He realized that until Dr. Scranton had experienced the situation first hand, such a notion undoubtedly appeared to evidence a lack of missionary zeal.

Despite his personal reservations, Dr. Hall promptly went to the British Legation to obtain his passport to travel back into the interior. The British Consul, Mr. Wilkinson, had had much experience with similar situations in China and so Dr. Hall asked his opinion of the suggested building plans. Mr. Wilkinson assured him that the treaty agreement at present would not allow such building, for Westerners were still not allowed to own property in the interior. He indicated that neither the British nor the American legations would be able to give him any protection if he so openly flaunted the treaty in that way. He did not rule out that such construction might be possible some day, but the time was not yet propitious.

Before Dr. Hall left for Pyong Yang, he shared with Dr. Scranton the Consul's opinion. Dr. Scranton agreed to hold the building matter in abeyance until he had a chance to visit Pyong Yang himself in early February.

On January 10, 1894, Dr. Hall again set out for Pyong Yang. He had never cared for solitude and so was very happy when a new missionary who had just recently arrived from Nova Scotia, the Rev. William John McKenzie, asked to accompany him. They proved to be very congenial companions. Even so, it was not easy for the doctor to leave his little family. He wrote to Rosetta hoping to reassure her:

> "Well, darling, I hope you have had a good night's rest, and that you and Sherwood are feeling well this morning. I have left you both with God and I am sure He will take good care of you. Lean heavily upon Him my darling. It is such a comfort to get where we can trust Him for everything. He is teaching us some good lessons now. We will cheerfully and patiently learn them for I am sure good will come out of them for us.
>
> "You are so precious to me darling. How dearly I love you. My love grows stronger for you every day, and for little Sherwood, dear little boy. He is getting very closely entwined around our hearts. I hope God may spare him to grow up to

be a good man, a comfort and a joy to us and a blessing to the world . . . When our home is so happy, we must not let the little things of life disturb us . . . God has promised to keep them in perfect peace whose mind is stayed on Him . . . I believe this trip will prove a blessing to each of us and let us cheerfully do hard things for Jesus."

Dr. Scranton journeyed to Pyong Yang in early February, 1894, and after being there awhile, agreed with Dr. Hall that any idea of building at Pyong Yang would have to be given up for the present. He acknowledged that it would be all they could do to hold onto what they had. It was readily apparent to him that the persecution of the Christians was still a grim reality and that progress could only be made in small steps.

It seemed wise to have some of the Korean converts from Seoul be the first to settle on the property that had been purchased by Mr. You for the Mission. Kim Chang Sik was formerly Mr. Ohlinger's cook and a very earnest Christian. Dr. Hall now employed him as his helper since Mr. Ohlinger's return to America. Kim Chang Sik and family were due to arrive in Pyong Yang in mid-March in company with another of Dr. Hall's helpers, Pak Yousan. When the doctor had seen them settled, he planned to return to Seoul. He wrote to his wife in February:

"It costs me a great struggle to leave you so long my darling, but I believe the blessings that will follow will be worth a thousand fold. We have started a boy's school and have an earnest Christian teacher and thirteen boys already. They study the catechism mornings and nights, and Unmun and Chinese the rest of the day . . . The light is beginning to dawn here for which I praise God . . . Several Koreans are to be baptized next Sunday . . . I have a meeting for boys every night before the regular service. About fifteen usually come and are very attentive. I questioned them last night upon what I had taught them before and was surprised to see how much they had learned.

"I am giving every morning to study and every afternoon to seeing patients . . . and the evenings to meetings. I treated sixteen patients today and three of these were outcalls.

Everything is going on smoothly and I am daily making friends and winning the confidence of the Koreans . . .

"Things were in such an unsettled state here for a time (we didn't know what the Governor or people would do with our being here) that it seemed unwise to lay any plans . . . But it seems to me now there will be no difficulty in your coming up as we had planned . . . I think we are in Pyong Yang to stay."

The overland trip took a week between Seoul and Pyong Yang, so on his return to Seoul, Dr. Hall investigated the possibilities of traveling by water. He found that although steamers ran very irregularly, going by boat would cut the travel time in half. He decided to take his family this way.

The Halls set sail on a small coastal steamer from Chemulpo on May 4, 1894. They were accompanied by Sherwood's *amah* (nursemaid), Sylvia, and by Yousan and Esther Pak.

How they were enjoying the scenery en route! The fishing boats with their orange sails added color and charm. Suddenly they noticed the small craft all heading for shore post-haste. Before they knew it, a typhoon was upon them with all its fury. Their ship had difficulty in reaching the shelter of one of the larger islands where it was obliged to anchor for thirty-three hours.

Finally the storm abated and they were able to start up the coast again. The boat entered the mouth of the *Taedong Kang* (Great East River) and they sailed up this majestic waterway to Posan, a point about twenty-five miles from Pyong Yang, which was as far as the steamer could safely go.

Dr. Hall recounted to his wife the story of the *General Sherman* which had met its fate on this river in 1866. It had been lured past Posan because floods and high tides made the river appear navigable. He noted that he had seen the anchor and chains of the American ship hanging upon the Great East Gate of Pyong Yang. They were displayed as trophies and served as vivid reminders of the fate of the gun boat. The Korean who had engineered its destruction had since become a Christian, Dr. Hall had been told.

The Halls were glad to get off the little steamer which had become filled with foul odors. They transferred to a rowboat for the rest of the journey, and were touched to see the native Christians waiting on the shore to greet them.

Many men and women crowded around Mrs. Hall and Sherwood. Not having seen a white woman or child before, they were full of curiosity. Dr. Hall assured them that on the afternoon of the following day, Mrs. Hall would be glad to let the women and children come for a *kugyang* ("look-see"). He said that they could come to her room in groups of ten for five minutes at a time, and that way they'd all have a fair chance to see her and the baby. They seemed pleased with the idea and did not seem to mind being sent away until the next day.

Mrs. Hall described her initial settling-in:

"We set to work and got our two little rooms cleaned, one of which I have for mine and the baby's bed, my trunk, a box, one chair, and a few shelves that do as dressing bureau for the present. In the other is our table, my steamer-chair and the two chairs Doctor brought up before. We swept the walls all down and bought new matting for the floors, and I adorned the walls with a few pictures. Doctor will put his cot up in this room every night and take it down in the morning for the present. After a time we will have one more room to use which will be our dining and sitting room. The Kims, the former owners of this house, are in there now. Yousan has the large Korean kitchen cleaned and we have put up the little cookstove and put in our boiler, like a Korean kettle, and two rice kettles for our Koreans. Although we are not all unpacked yet, we already feel quite at home. As I wrote to Mrs. M. F. Scranton last night: 'Perhaps you can imagine how happy I am and with what a sense of satisfaction I write "Pyong Yang" at the head of my letter.'

"The next day the sightseers began coming after lunch as arranged. Three sets of ten came in and went out on time and were very orderly, and many of those waiting in the packed court and outside the gate wished to continue the order. But later arrivals, who didn't well understand, would push in and soon the two rooms were packed so full that none could stir. The only way to get them to go out seemed for me to go myself upon the morrow and let them see by the courtyard full. This I did, and saw the courtyard packed full four different times, probably at least 1500 women and children . . .

"At about 4 P.M. Doctor started to go to the Magistrate to ask for a *Kuisyu* (soldier) to guard us on account of so many *kugyang* people (sightseers) and our walls and gates not being in a condition to keep order. Upon his way a messenger from the Governor met him and asked to see his passport etc. The Governor did not see him himself; said he was very busy, but had an underofficial see him. He asked Doctor about the houses. Doctor said they were bought by Mr. You, and he gave us permission to stop in them while we were here; that we could not stop in an inn as it was too small to see patients in. He wanted to know why I came. Doctor said I was also a doctor and came to see the sick women and children; that we were to return to Seoul after a little while. Kim was a young man in the employ of the Governor and one for whom Doctor got a broken watch fixed. Doctor brought it to Kim, without charge, from Seoul to show that he meant to be his friend. This young man was the son of the Captain of this district. He (the son) spoke up, before the doctor, and said to the underofficial that if they allowed me to stay here, one foreigner after another would come till Pyong Yang would all be taken by foreigners. The official said he thought the Governor would see Doctor in the morning.

"We had supper, prayers, and went to bed in peace and happiness to be awakened at 2 A.M. by two of the Pyong Yang Christians, Mr. O and Mr. Ni, coming to tell us that faithful Chang Sik, who has been living and teaching here ever since Doctor returned to Seoul, was cast into prison. Kim, the former owner of this house, and the former owner of Mr. Moffett's house, and Han, Mr. Moffett's preacher, were also in prison. It seems about 1 A.M. someone knocked at Chang Sik's window and said he was sent by Dr. Hall, so Chang Sik opened the door. He was taken by servants of the Captain of this district and beaten and put into stocks and was suffering very much. They said they would beat him again this morning. A little later Chang Sik's wife came. They said they did not dare beat Dr. Hall so they took Chang Sik in his stead.

"At 6:30 o'clock Doctor went to ask to see the Governor. He waited till 7:30 and they said the Governor was sleeping and wouldn't see him. While Doctor was gone, they sent word if we would give 100,000 *cash* it could save Chang Sik from a beating this morning. I did not have that much in the house, but told a man to go and tell Doctor. Doctor returned about 8 o'clock.

"He had been to the prison and saw them all. Chang Sik was suffering very much, the stocks being very tightly screwed on. Mr. O had accompanied the doctor, and just while the doctor was in the house a few moments, Mr. O was grabbed right in front of our ground and also carried to prison and put in with the others in the room for thieves.

"Doctor then started out again to send a telegram to Seoul. He telegraphed to Dr. Scranton: 'Chang Sik stocks. O, Moffett's Han beaten. Former owner of tree house all now prison. Ask protection family and servants.'

"He then went to demand an interview with the Governor. The English interpreter in the Chinese telegraph offfice has always been a friend to Dr. Hall and Doctor asked him as a favor if he would accompany him to see the Governor and he very kindly consented to do so. Doctor was gone this time from 11 A.M. to 2 P.M.

"*Kugyang* women and children kept coming in groups of ten and twelve all day. They were very orderly, the most of them cleanly dressed and very good faced people. I am sure I shall like the women of Pyong Yang very much. They scarcely noticed anything about the house, but spent all their time on the baby or me . . ."

While some thought that the baby was lovely, not all the remarks of the fascinated onlookers were flattering. Some commented on the protruding nose (Korean noses are somewhat flat) and others thought his ears were too large. Still others actually burst out laughing and exclaimed that he looked just like a dog. (Some Korean dogs have blue eyes.) Not able to pronounce the name, 'Sherwood,' they settled for calling him, 'Say-Oat.' Over the protestations of his *amah* (nursemaid), Sylvia, they tried to pinch him and soon discovered the little fellow had a good pair of lungs. His mother's story continues:

"I asked them if they were not afraid to come in this house as several of our friends had been cast into prison today, but they did not seem to be afraid. I had quite nice

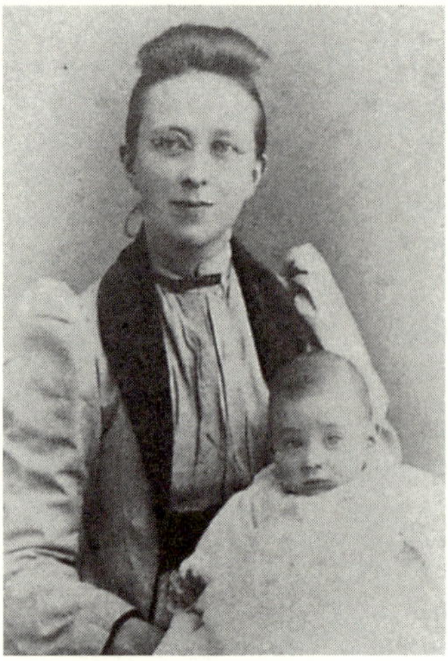

Dr. Rosetta Hall and son, Sherwood, age five months

talks with them; found out I could make them understand me well, and I understood them easily. It was of course very tiring for me (with the strain of the great disturbance all the time and our Korean helpers frightened) to keep a cheerful face and manner, but I did it.

"During this time poor Chang Sik came to this house under guard of his jailors, and they again demanded the 100,000 *cash* to save him from another beating. Later Mr. O came in the same way. He seemed very cheerful and said it was all right. He thought they would soon receive orders for their release. He didn't want me to give the money. I think Chang Sik did, but then he had been in prison much longer than Mr. O and had those terrible stocks pinching him, and it was enough to make his courage fail.

"About 1 P.M. a servant of the Magistrate came and asked to see me and gave me a paper written in Chinese. Esther said that they said we must get out of the house, so supposing it might be an order to that effect, I said I could not read it, and refused to receive it. They then posted it on the gate, and a friend of Doctor's afterward interpreted it as something like this:

"It was written by the Magistrate next to the Governor and addressed to Captain Kim of this district. It said that he must make the former owner of this house get it back; he had thus ordered a long time ago. Dr. Hall had now come with his wife which was a sign that he would live long here; therefore, right away the former owner must take the house back. Many *kugyang* people (sightseers) make a great disturbance; therefore, let only patients come. The other people he should tie up. No one must listen to preaching as both Catholicism and Protestantism were very bad.

"It had three official stamps upon it. From what afterward occurred, I do not know whether they gave it to me by mistake or whether the Captain, after reading it, sent it to scare us.

"At 2 P.M. Doctor returned saying this telegram had come from Dr. Scranton: 'Legations will act at once. Telegraph particulars of difficulty.'

"And he had telegraphed: 'All that can be found that have had anything to do with Moffett or self, in prison. No reason given. Governor refuses to see me, listen to appeals or give protection. We are ordered out of house.'

"Doctor again hastened off. The Governor still refused to see him even though the Chinese interpreter told him he had telegraphed to Seoul and would do so again.

"At 4 P.M. Doctor again returned with a telegram from Consul General Gardner saying: 'Will require Foreign Office to telegraph officials to release Korean servants and so forth at once and afford you and family adequate protection.'

"At this time servants came from the jail again demanding money or all would again be beaten. Also there came a servant from Captain Kim demanding the paper stuck upon our gate. Doctor had just previously received it, and we all thought it best to keep it, though we did not know at that time that it was addressed to Captain Kim. Doctor was about ready to eat when they first asked for it, so we told them to wait, and later, he told them to come in the morning; he was too tired to see them now (thought he would come across to them, Korean fashion). But they pleaded so much he finally went out, and they explained how they would be beaten if they went back to Captain Kim without that paper. He had been commanded by the Magistrate to secure it.

"I told the Doctor not to give it—that of course the Captain would tell them that, that they might use every means to secure it. Finally they went off. They had not much more than gone before I heard such a noise like a mad bull bellowing and pawing the ground in rage. It proved to be the Captain himself, the one that had Mr. No, Doctor's helper, whipped the last time he was here. Mr. No said he was no man, he was a pig . . .

"Doctor went out and tried to reason with him, but he would listen to nothing; went on blowing in the greatest rage I ever saw a man in. Little Sherwood had just gotten soundly asleep, and the noise made him wide awake in a few moments. Yousan happened to be out in the court. He had kept pretty close all day, and I only wish he might have been then.

"Captain Kim had him pointed out to him as one of Doctor's servants and he immediately set upon him, seized him by the top-knot, and beat and kicked him in white fury, and ordered him to be carried off. Doctor knew it was only to get hold of this paper, but under such circumstances, he could not withstand the appeals of Yousan to give it up. Then the satanic man went off satisfied.

"Eight P.M. Minister Sill's telegram came. It said: 'British Consul General and I have insisted that Foreign Office order the immediate release of Moffett's and your employees, and for facts and reasons laid before us together with your protection according to treaty.'

"At the same time a kind telegram from Mr. Moffett, saying: 'Joshua 1:9–Tell neighbors contents of telegram.' Joshua 1:9 reads: '*Have not I commanded thee? Be strong and of good courage; be not afraid, neither be dismayed; for the Lord thy God is with thee withersoever thou goest.*'

"We had prayer, and retired at 10 P.M. My bed crosses in front of a small paper covered window at the back of the room. Doctor had opened it to let in some fresh air. It was covered with a thin lawn curtain and I forgot it was open. I stood in front of it undressing, when suddenly there came a stone hurled evidently by someone who saw me standing there as there was a light in my room. It struck an earthen jar, breaking it, just in front of the window. It made such a crash, just like breaking a glass window, that it quite startled us all. Not knowing how many more would follow, I ran into Doctor's room and told Sylvia to bring the baby quickly.

Doctor got up and closed the window, and as no more seemed to be coming, I went to bed, taking the precaution, however, of placing my thick comforter between me and the window. We all had refreshing sleep.

"May 11–7 A.M.–The servant of the Governor (son of Captain Kim) came and said the telegram to the Governor had come (as we expected). But he said the message was that the British and American Minister had seen the King and had agreed that Pyong Yang was no place in which to preach the Gospel; that the King said Dr. Hall was a bad man, and ordered the Governor to behead all Christians today.

"Of course we think it must be a lie, but then they have changed Chang Sik from the cell of thieves to the death cell, and have put him in stocks again, and I don't understand that. Doctor went to see him, and he himself seems to have given up in discouragement. They beat him so much and threaten him with death all the time, so that I suppose the poor fellow dies a hundred deaths and at this slow rate of the Governor obeying the telegram, I am afraid he will die before he gets released. Doctor cries every time he goes to see him, it is so terrible. The reason he is treated so much worse than Mr. O and Mr. Han is because when they ask him to renounce the Jesus doctrine, he refuses to do so. When they ask him if he will preach anymore if he should be let out, he says he will. Praise the Lord for a Korean Paul!

"Doctor has gone to the telegraph office again to send word of Yousan's beating in his presence, and of what the Governor's servant says the telegram to the Governor said, and that instead of releasing them, they are put in the death cell.

"9 A.M.–The Captain of the district has ordered the water man to bring us no water under penalty of a beating. (There are no wells in Pyong Yang, and the water is brought from the river a half mile distant.) As we washed for baby yesterday, there is scarcely enough today for his food let alone ours. All continue to say that Chang Sik and Han will be beheaded today for having preached the Gospel. Our Koreans are all downcast, bewailing their coming to Pyong Yang. I am trying

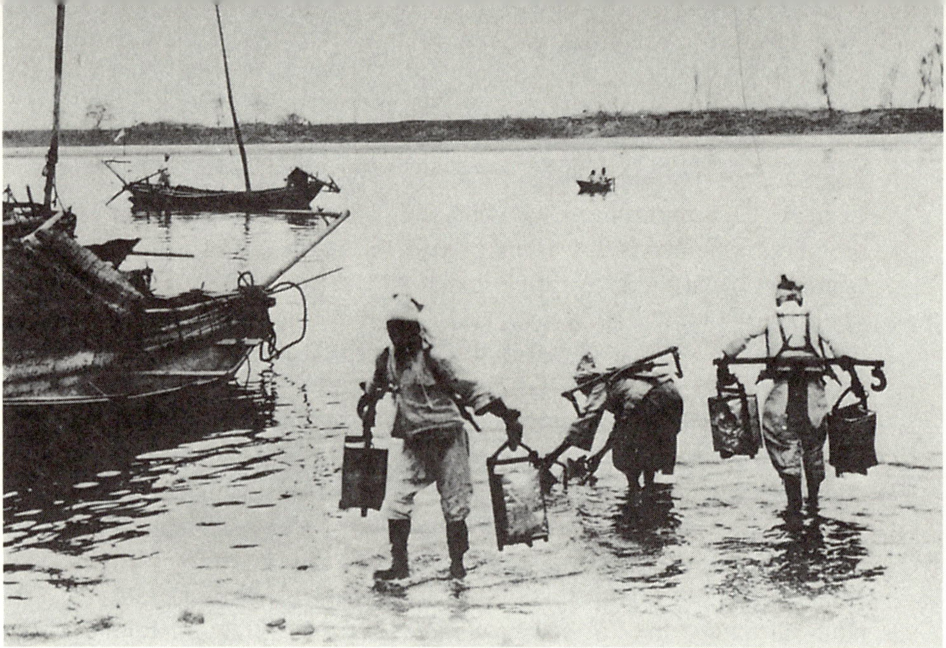

The Taedong River–water supply for Pyong Yang, 1894

my best to keep them cheerful and trustful, but Doctor himself seemed a bit discouraged this morning and they soon see that."

Dr. Hall wrote of his feelings at that time in a letter:

"We did not know the moment a mob might be upon us . . . We were the only foreigners in a city of one hundred thousand heathen, and you can imagine our situation when I had to leave Mrs. Hall and little Sherwood alone and unprotected, as much of the time I was away at the prison or the telegraph office. The Governor is a relative of the Queen, a powerful family here in Korea, and it began to look as though he were not going to pay any attention to the telegram from the Foreign Office. It seemed to us that the time had come for religious toleration for Korea, and God would require the lives of some of his children to secure it. We were ready to die for His cause. Grace had been given sufficient for every trial thus far, and we knew abundance would be given if it were required. My heart ached as I witnessed our faithful brothers in Christ suffering extreme torture, such as had not been experienced here by Christians for twenty-eight years, when thousands of Roman Catholics, including several priests, laid down their lives for their faith."

Mrs. Hall's journal resumes the narrative:

"At noon we received the following telegram from Consul Gardner in reply to that Doctor sent this morning: 'Telegram was sent last night at 11 P.M. to Pyong Yang by Foreign Office to release all Korean servants and Christians. Wire situation.'

"Doctor again visited prison. They yet continue to beat them and threaten them with death. They now tell us that the Governor says he doesn't understand his telegram, and that he will telegraph back to Seoul that our neighbors all tell him that we are Tonghak folks, and we and our helpers are building many houses all over Korea to help carry on that faction. Also they say he is a relative of the Queen and he does not fear punishment if he does not carry out the command of the telegram.

"So in answer to Consul Gardner's telegram, he sent word that they had cut off our water supply, had not released prisoners, and that they said we were all Tonghaks (a sort of political and religious faction that arose in the South a year ago, and threatened rebellion, and were put down by the Government). Also, that from every appearance, they might kill Chang Sik and Han soon if nothing further will be done.

"At 4 P.M. Dr. Scranton telegraphed: 'They will not dare kill them. Foreign Office has twice sent orders to release all. President of Foreign Office and English Consul now together. Shall see both at once. Telegraph three times daily or more.'

"Later another telegram came containing a copy of the order to the Governor. It demands 'immediate release of all imprisoned, asking if it has been done; if not, "other business" will follow,' and two such sent since. 'Moffett and McKenzie start north Friday. Arrive three days. Unless Governor defies America and England, you have nothing to fear.'

"Doctor was away at the telegraph office when news came at about 6 o'clock that the Magistrate had sent for all the men to appear before him. Esther and Sylvia were very much alarmed, and said now they would surely be killed. But I told them no. I thought it was good news, and that he would now release them. And about 7 P.M. poor Chang Sik came staggering in. He lay down on the floor, could scarcely speak, was limp and cold, and suffering extremely. Said he had been stoned all the way home by order of that Captain Kim's son, the servant of the Governor. I covered him up with a warm blanket, and gave him one-fourth grain of morphine in a little spirits of chloroform, and tried to keep the room quiet. Doctor returned very soon, and then went to telegraph that all had been released.

"About 9 P.M. Chang Sik began to feel somewhat relieved, and he ate some food, then he told us that the Magistrate wanted each of the Christians to promise they would not teach the Gospel anymore if they were released. Of course, poor fellows, after so much delay, and not knowing well the contents of the telegrams, they felt the only alternative was death, and being weakened by the cruel treatment they had received, and also the thought of their helpless families, Peter-like they promised—all except Chang Sik. He said though some might think it a bad doctrine, he knew it was good, and would live it and teach it. The Magistrate commanded him to deny Jesus and to blaspheme God. He said he couldn't do it. The Magistrate then told him to go, but sent no one with him, and this Kim at once ordered him to be stoned and killed, and boys and men pelted him all the way to our gate. Soon Mr. O also came. He had been home first. His wife is very sick. Twins were born to her but a short time ago, and she was not strong. This trouble was such a great shock it prostrated her entirely.

"Mr. Ni and a young man by the name of Kim, both of whom have courageously stood right by Doctor through it all, also came in and some little boys. Yousan, Sylvia, and Esther and I and Sherwood were in my little room, and we all had a short praise meeting together, Chang Sik himself reading Acts XVI and leading in prayer. The dear man that he is. Doctor said he felt like kneeling at his feet, such a faithful martyr for Jesus it is not the privilege of many to see."

An account by Mr. W. A. Noble tells of what happened on the "receiving end" of the cryptic telegrams from Dr. Hall:

"For once in the history of the Korea Mission all work was laid aside in the capital, and the missionaries of all denominations gathered for prayer. Each one seemed to feel that the crisis was of the deepest personal concern. Many were the prayers that went up in behalf of the two so well loved by all. It is a significant fact that at that hour, while the company was gathered in prayer, Dr. Hall wired these words, 'All released. Chang Sikey badly injured.'

"It was with deep, solemn gratitude that the missionaries returned to work, realizing that the epoch had changed and that the faithfulness of Dr. and Mrs. Hall had ushered in a new era. Never again could such opposition occur at these strategic points. The long-struggled-for opening was at last secured."[3]

Mrs. Hall recorded in her journal how the situation looked a week later:

"May 19, 1894–Saturday: Friday the 11th proved to be *the* dark day. Since then, no one has been injured and all have felt comparatively safe. All day Saturday those runners of the Governor continued to threaten and insult the Christians, but Sunday and Monday it lessened. Tuesday Mr. Moffett and Mr. McKenzie arrived. They came in eight-men chairs, but said it was a mistake. They could have gotten here sooner on horseback. We were very glad to welcome them. As Doctor said, he had had the care of both churches upon him and he was very glad to share the responsibility.

"Mr. McKenzie stays right with us, and Mr. Moffett takes tiffin and supper with us. Mr. Moffett's Han went out to meet him, and as he missed him on the way, and he had not returned yet by Thursday, Mr. Moffett sent for him. He came in during Mr. Moffett's absence and no more reached home than the Governor's servants were after him demanding more money, or he would get a beating. He gave them money. Mr. Moffett says he has had great agony of both mind and body,

---

[3] *The Life of W. J. Hall*, p. 345.

and will need Mr. Moffett's presence to cheer him up. So Mr. Moffett didn't come up here yesterday. He was afraid of more trouble if he should leave the place any length of time.

"Mr. Moffett sent a telegram to Minister Sill; Mr. McKenzie to Consul Gardner, and Dr. Hall to Dr. Scranton each giving a separate description of present affairs, but neither reporting what the other had said. Altogether it amounted to about this: 'Walls torn down. Stoned on street. Employees insulted. Former owner of house not removed. No adequate protection given. Can England give it?'

"Mr. Moffett tells us it is very fortunate that the trouble occurred with Dr. Hall and myself in the first place, for it is the U.S. policy to keep out of all religious and political trouble, and no doubt we should have at once been recalled to Seoul. U.S. Minister Sill could not give Dr. Underwood a passport to come up here, and would not give his official consent for Mr. Moffett to come.

"Of course, we are all very much in hopes that in the end, this trouble will bring religious toleration for Korea. If so, it must come mostly through England's demands. She may ask, instead, that Pyong Yang be made an open port. We would not like that as well, because it would mean that the Chinese and Japanese would all rush in, together with all sorts of business adventurers. Pyong Yang promises to prove the richest port in Korea, on account of coal mines, gold mines, farm products, etc. However, if that will be the only way we may legally be allowed to live here, it may be best. We are trusting God that in His own way it may all work together for the growth of His Kingdom.

"The idea of the three men sending the telegrams they did yesterday was that people in Seoul should do all in their power to push matters with officials to secure complete protection of Christian employees, and the occupation of our houses. But in addition to that, it did something they had not calculated upon. It alarmed them as to our safety in staying here, especially mine and baby's, and in reply Doctor got a telegram from Mr. Appenzeller that Dr. Scranton would start at once to take me home; for Doctor to stick to it if possible.

"As I am quite comfortable and happy here (as Doctor says, 'the most unmoved person of all through the whole trouble,') it seems like quite a needless expense for Dr. Scranton to come upon that purpose, and besides, we need him more at that end to push matters there. Also, if I should leave now, nothing would please these Pyong Yang officials more. They would feel they had gained the victory then, and we were scared out. Why, I wouldn't think of such a thing as going now. Doctor spoke to me about going that dark Friday, as the steamer was just about to leave and I could have made it, but I wouldn't listen to it then, and I am sure I would not like to now. So Doctor sent a telegram at once to tell him not to come; and this morning he sent another, fearing they might be anxious about me, saying I am happy and treating patients daily.

"We began Tuesday seeing patients down at the other property by the Gate. Doctor has one room, and I have two, one as a waiting room and one as dispensing room. Esther accompanied me. We went in our chairs. The first day we treated ten patients and took in 500 *cash*. The next day Esther had a headache and didn't go, and I treated thirteen patients, taking in 900 *cash*. Yesterday we again had thirteen patients and took in 1200 *cash*. Of course it is some trouble

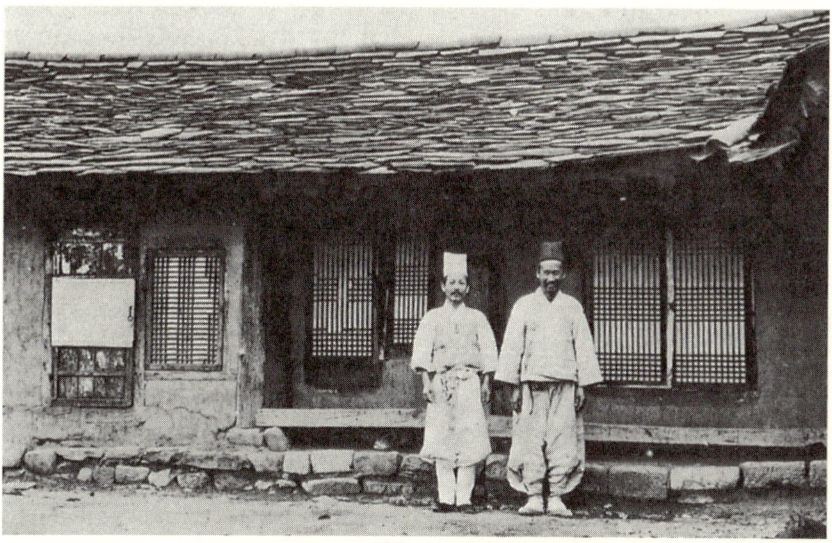

The building where the Drs. Hall began medical work in Pyong Yang, 1894

to make them observe order and to understand that I will only see one at a time, but it grows easier, as they learn if they will only wait, each will receive the same attention. There are many people who come only for a *kugyang*, but we keep them out pretty well until all the sick are treated and then I give them all a *kugyang* at me. We have not had any religious work as yet, but I think I will begin today after the dispensary and the *kugyanging*. I fear if we tried to do anything before, at this stage, we would not get much attention."

Dr. Hall's first Christian convert in Pyong Yang was Mr. O Syok-Hyong (who was among those cast into prison and later released during the recent persecutions). Mr. O had a little daughter who was blind. Mrs. Hall had encountered blind and deaf-mute patients in her medical work and longed to be able to do something to help them. However, the condition of both the blind and deaf-mutes in Korea at that time, Mrs. Hall discovered, was indeed pitiable. The deaf-mutes were considered imbeciles who survived by their animal instincts and the blind became fortune tellers or sorcerers (*mudongs*) if their parents were rich enough to have them thus trained. Otherwise, they were neglected and ignored, often poorly fed and clothed and allowed to sit in a corner until eventually they lost even the ability to walk.

Although Mrs. Hall had wanted to do something to help blind children, she had been cautioned that the Koreans might not understand her purpose. In time of any disturbances, they might point to the blind students as proof of the false tale that circulated during the Baby Riots of 1888 that doctors were taking out the children's eyes to make medicine.

When Mrs. Hall observed that Mr. O's eldest daughter was blind, she thought, "Here's my chance to begin. Her father is a Christian, and will not misinterpret my motive."

Mrs. Hall wrote:

"So I set about contriving a way to prick Korean oiled paper with a needle to teach little Pongnai."

Pongnai responded so eagerly and with such intelligence, that Mrs. Hall felt that she could be helped to learn to read if only Mrs. Hall had knowledge of the proper technique for teaching the blind. She resolved to learn more about it, for it could be a means of combating the superstition which prevented the blind from enjoying a life of usefulness.

The situation in Pyong Yang seemed to be settling down comfortably. Although both Sherwood and Mrs. Hall began to have some of the all too familiar intestinal problems that plagued foreigners in the Orient, the Halls tried to maintain their health by getting out of the city for walks. On one occasion they enjoyed a picnic on the scenic grounds above Kija's famous burial place nine miles north of the city. Other times, after dispensary hours, Mrs. Hall and Sherwood would ride out of the city in a chair to avoid the *kugyang* people and then get out and walk with Dr. Hall and their Korean friends. Sherwood seemed to especially enjoy riding on the shoulders of Kim Chang Sik.

Another health concern that prompted these daily outings was the persistent cough which had bothered Dr. Hall since his trip to Pyong Yang that winter. They greatly feared that the TB he had suffered as a boy might have returned as a result of the strenuousness and exposure of his winter trips.

To everyone's surprise, Dr. Scranton arrived on May 23 to take Mrs. Hall and Sherwood back to Seoul, on the explicit instructions of the British Consul General, Mr. Gardner. It seemed the telegrams sent by the three missionaries had not only been effective, but had given an erroneous impression that things were in a worse state than was the case. They thought that the Halls had been ordered out of their house and that the danger was too great to let Mrs. Hall and the baby remain.

What was actually the case was that the Magistrate had insisted that the former owner of the house resume his residence there. However, in response to the telegrams received from the Foreign Office and the additional pressures placed on the Magistrate by Dr. Hall, Mr. Moffett and Mr. McKenzie, the Magistrate had finally consented to tell the former owner to move out of the house.

Mrs. Hall felt that if Mr. Gardner knew this and that she was treating eight to nineteen patients a day, he would not feel her return was necessary. Dr. Scranton agreed that the situation did not seem to warrant sending her back to Seoul, but at the same time he thought Mr. Gardner's orders should be obeyed.

So it was that Mrs. Hall packed up her things and made ready to leave on the steamer the next day. Her intestinal difficulties had flared up again, but she thought she would be well enough to travel. However, when she found the tell-tale sign of dysentery, blood in her stool, her husband insisted she would have to go to bed instead of leaving on the steamer. Mrs. Hall rested for three days. She then felt well enough to return to work at the dispensary the following Monday.

It was beginning to look as though the illness had been Providential, when suddenly word came that another steamer had arrived at Posan. It had been sent up in haste as a transport for Pyong Yang soldiers who were needed to help quell a peasant rebellion that had arisen in the South. In view of that development, and not having any further word to the contrary from Mr. Gardner, Dr. Hall felt it his duty to take his wife and child back to Seoul at the first opportunity.

The Halls, the Paks and Sylvia reached the steamer at Posan on the afternoon of Wednesday, June 6. Waiting there was a good sized ship, the *Chong Riong*, but it had no accommodations for foreign passengers. However, the kindly German Captain Tessensohn insisted that they take his room. This time the trip from Posan to Chemulpo only took 27 hours, once they set sail Sunday, June 10. Mr. George Heber Jones met them at Chemulpo.

That afternoon the Jones and the Halls went out to visit the United States man-of-war ship, the *Baltimore*, which was to remain in Chemulpo harbor until the situation in Korea became more settled. Rear Admiral Joseph S. Skerrett invited them to his room for tea and told them all about his ship with considerable pride. There were thirteen warships in the harbor when the Halls arrived and rumors of thousands of both Japanese and Chinese soldiers landing on Korean soil.

It seemed that the Tonghaks had staged a revolt in the South, making good their threat of the previous year. The Tonghak rebels, reinforced by peasants who were disgruntled with governmental corruption, had marched toward Seoul with cries of, "Down with tyranny, Westerners and Japanese." They had succeeded in defeating the Yi government soldiers sent to repulse them. The Korean king had appealed to China for help. When China landed soldiers in Korea without letting Japan know, contrary to their treaty agreement, Japan also sent soldiers to Korea on the pretext of aiding the government against the insurgents.

The Halls traveled to Seoul by river boat this time, which proved a pleasant trip. At the landing they met Dr. Busteed on his way to America to be married. Mr. Noble was going with him to Chemulpo to see him off.

That evening it became apparent that Sherwood had developed a case of dysentery. It proved to be very slow in responding to treatment and caused Sherwood's parents considerable anxiety before it was finally brought under control, after several weeks.

On Wednesday night Mrs. Noble called Mrs. Hall to her room. Mr. Noble had not yet returned and she was unable to sleep because of recurring pains. She thought she might be in labor although she had not expected to be for another week. By 6:00 A.M. on Thursday, June 14, 1894, Mrs. Noble was delivered of a seven pound girl whom she named Ruth. The Halls and Mrs. Noble could hardly wait for Mr. Noble's surprised reaction when he walked into the room that evening at 6:00 P.M. to discover he was a father.

The Halls visited both the American and British Legations upon their return to Seoul. There they learned that word had gone from the Foreign Office to Pyong Yang ordering the punishment of the Governor's servant who had instigated most of the trouble in Pyong Yang and of the Magistrate who had helped him carry it out. The punishment was to take place before Mr. Moffett. They were also required to return the money extorted from Mr. Moffett's helper, Mr. Han, and then they were to be banished from the city. It appeared to the Halls that such news meant there should be little or no further trouble for the Pyong Yang Christians from then on.

The visit to the American Legation also apprised them of the fact that several American families were being recalled from outlying areas to come to the foreign settlement in Seoul. They could see for themselves that the Japanese soldiers were continuing to arrive daily and had established themselves at stations on all the surrounding hills. There were also rumors of thousands of Chinese soldiers landing along the coast.

Mrs. Hall noted in her journal:

> "Some say war has been declared between China and Japan. It is very difficult to forecast the outcome . . . I fear our people at home are pretty uneasy about us at this time, the papers filling with these rumors of war, so soon after hearing of our Pyong Yang trouble. I wrote home yesterday, and must try and write often. Dear people, they will mind it much more than we do no doubt. Poor Joe, he still worries about me."

Joe (Josiah) Wilson had been a black slave who escaped from the South by way of the underground railway before the Civil War. The Sherwood farm near Liberty, New York was one of the stops. Rosevelt Sherwood and Joe took an instant liking to each other and when the former invited Joe to make his home with the Sherwood family, he could see no reason for continuing on up to Canada. Joe, now 69, had virtually helped in the rearing of Rosetta from the time she was an infant and there was deep affection between them. Her diary account continues:

> "Mother writes: 'Joe says to tell you that he "doesn't want you to go to Pyong Yang . . . again. You have just escaped with your life, now keep away . . ."'"

The concern of the home folks was well founded. On July 23, 1894, the Halls were awakened in Seoul at five o'clock in the morning by the sound of gunfire. Japanese soldiers soon took control of the seven gates of the city and after twenty minutes of heavy and constant firing of guns, the palace fell into Japanese hands. The frightened Korean residents of Seoul streamed out of the city for days.

Dr. Hall and Dr. Scranton found that their formerly routine work at the Methodist Si Pyeng Won (Universal Relief Hospital) was suddenly exchanged for the work of a military hospital. Battle casualties began to pour in and the grim aspects of war became a reality. Dr. W. B. Scranton described his medical partner's efforts that summer:

> "Here Dr. Hall was called upon to be surgeon and nurse, druggist and steward, but he had a faculty for patient and tireless work without getting tangled in a complexity of duties as some of us do . . .
>
> "During these days in the Seoul hospital he was constantly at his post and tireless in his endeavors. One day when he had been most fully occupied and might well have remarked on his own weariness, I well remember how he said, and with what a genuine spirit, 'Doctor, how I enjoy this! I could spend my whole life in this way. It is so good to help people.' . . . Dr. Hall had learned the secret that the patient

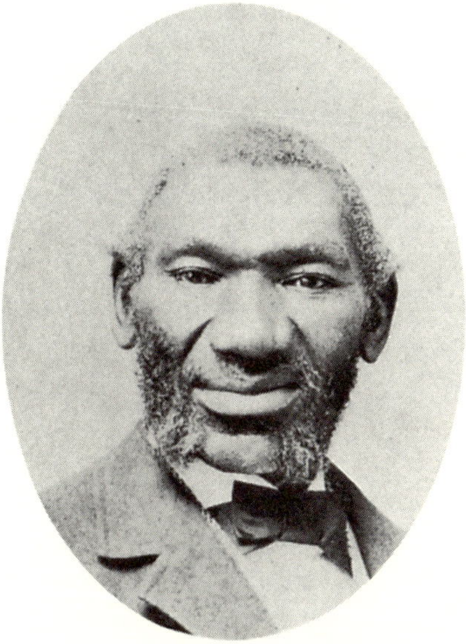

Josiah Wilson at age 65, 1890

and kindly touch of sympathy and love are the little things ordained of God to accomplish mightiest ends. They, and not the greater, are miracles in reality."[4]

The Tonghaks had set in motion forces over which they rapidly lost control. They could not withstand the confrontation with the two foreign armies that converged on them, the Chinese from the North and the Japanese from the South. The Tonghaks were crushed, the two leaders of their movement were executed, and thousands of their followers lost their lives. Furthermore, they had unwittingly provided the pretext by which China and Japan felt justified in declaring war on each other. It was a moment for which both countries had been waiting. They had been jealously vying for undisputed control of Korea.

On Saturday, September 15, 1894, the great battle of Pyong Yang was fought. It was the turning point of the Sino-Japanese war. The Japanese emerged victorious and the Chinese fled from the city, and were driven from Korea.

In the resultant peace treaty negotiated at Shimonoseki, Japan, the Chinese acquiesced to certain Japanese demands. China agreed to pay Japan a huge indemnity, enter into a special commerce treaty

---

[4] *The Life of W. J. Hall*, pp. 282-284.

which extended many favors to Japan, and open four new ports to Japanese trade. In addition, China ceded to Japan, Formosa and the Pescadores islands, as well as the Liaotung Peninsula in southern Manchuria. In response to later intervention by Russia, Germany and France, the Japanese reluctantly gave back the Liaotung Peninsula in return for increased indemnity payments.

The Treaty of Shimonoseki further recognized the independence of Korea, and removed Korea from its former vassal-suzerain role with China. Instead, Japan began to take an increasingly influential position in Korean affairs. Japan immediately assumed the role of advisor to the Korean government and began to restructure the Yi feudalistic system that had been so abhorrent to the Tonghaks. Postal, rail and telegraph systems came under Japanese control. New laws and regulations were rapidly introduced, often too abruptly to be greeted with anything but resentment by the Korean people.

Dr. Hall, in company with his Presbyterian colleagues, the Reverend Samuel A. Moffett and the Reverend Graham Lee, returned to his scattered flock in Pyong Yang in early October. Despite the hardships of war, Dr. Hall found the little Christian community had been able to maintain the Methodist Mission property intact. His Presbyterian brothers, however, found theirs had not fared so well and that their stores and things had been totally destroyed, so they stayed with Dr. Hall. The men met two foreign reporters in Pyong Yang who had been covering the war, Mr. Creelman from the New York *World* and Frederick Villiers from the London *Standard*, and both were invited to share in Dr. Hall's hospitality.

As late as October 8, Dr. Hall wrote of the scenes of war that remained around them:

> "We have partially visited the battlefield. It is strewn with Chinese bodies, some of which are still unburied, the rest have a few inches of dirt thrown over them. The stench is terrible and the sight indescribable. There were fourteen thousand Chinese and ten thousand Japanese in the armies."

The chair in which Governor Min was said to have fled from the city was lying overturned in a ditch. Dr. Hall and his companions had left Seoul on October 1 and reached Pyong Yang without too much difficulty. Dr. Hall's letter described that journey briefly:

"We saw a great many dead horses and cattle along the road, which had been used in conveying army supplies. Many villages were completely deserted, but the people were beginning to come back and settle down again. We had no difficulty in making our way through the army lines. We met the first large detachment of the Japanese army at Whoang Chu [Whang-ju], one hundred *ri*[5] south of Pyong Yang. They have four hundred and fifty prisoners there. At Chung Wha [Chunghwa], fifty *ri* south of Pyong Yang, we saw the graves of seven Japanese scouts, who had been killed by the Chinese. Between Chung Wha and ten *ri* south of Pyong Yang we saw one Chinese body partially covered. Ten *ri* from Pyong Yang we reached the river and were at once on the field of battle."

The Reverend Graham Lee recorded his impressions of the aftermath of that combat:

"The first few days we spent in viewing the battlefield, and truly it was a sight to one unused to scenes of war. That we may have some idea of this battlefield, which in future will be looked back upon as a crisis in the history of these nations of the Far East, let us present in general the plan of attack. Pyong Yang is a walled city, and it is most admirably situated for purposes of defense. In front runs the Tai Tong [Taedong] River, too wide and too deep to be crossed in the face of a determined foe. To the north, inside the city wall, is a hill, some hundreds of feet high, which commands the surrounding country for miles. No enemy could take Pyong Yang until its defenders had been driven out of this key position.

"The Chinese army had been in Pyong Yang some forty days, and had had ample time to entrench themselves most strongly in and about the city . . . The Chinese seemed to expect the main attack from across the river in their front, and here they were well prepared, but the Japanese did not

[5] One *ri* is about three miles.

see fit to give battle according as the Chinese had planned for it. For two days the Japanese kept up a cannon demonstration from across the river in front, and while the attention of the Chinese was turned that way, two divisions of the Japanese army marched around to the rear of the city and got in readiness to attack at a given time. On the morning of September 15 all was in readiness, and very early a combined attack was begun from three sides. The Chinese were driven out of position after position, and before night the Japanese were in possession of all the outer works. The Chinese still held the high hill at the north, and on this hung their fate. This was the key of the whole position, and once taken, the battle of Pyong Yang was over."[6]

After describing the disorganized flight of the Chinese army, Graham Lee continued:

"Were we, who saw that battlefield, asked why the Chinese made such a poor stand against a foe that from time immemorial they have despised as unworthy of their prowess, we would not be hard put to find the reason.

"Among other things thrown away by these fleeing Chinese were great numbers of fans and paper umbrellas. It is almost beyond the comprehension of a Westerner that a soldier should carry as part of his equipment a fan to cool his heated brow and a paper umbrella to shield his devoted head. The Chinese were armed with good guns, as the Krupp cannon and modern rifles among the trophies of war testify, but they were also loaded down with a lot of trumpery which was worse than useless in time of battle. As a trophy of this battlefield I picked up a large two-handed sword, which had a blade about two feet long and a handle about four. It was clumsy and awkward, and absolutely useless as a weapon in these days of the magazine rifle and Gatling gun. Also scattered about I saw many bamboo pikes with rough iron tips which were in perfect keeping with the big sword. Such things showed that the Chinese army was several hundred

[6] *The Life of W. J. Hall*, pp. 296-298.

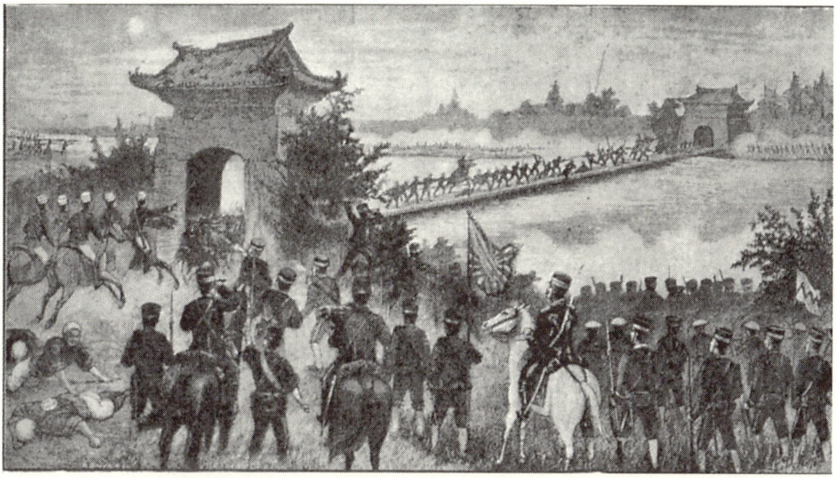

FROM "WAR IN THE EAST" (ZIEGLER) IN "THE LIFE OF W. J. HALL" (EATON AND MAINS)

Artist's rendering of the attack on Pyong Yang during the Sino-Japanese War of 1894 (Japanese crossing the Taedong River)

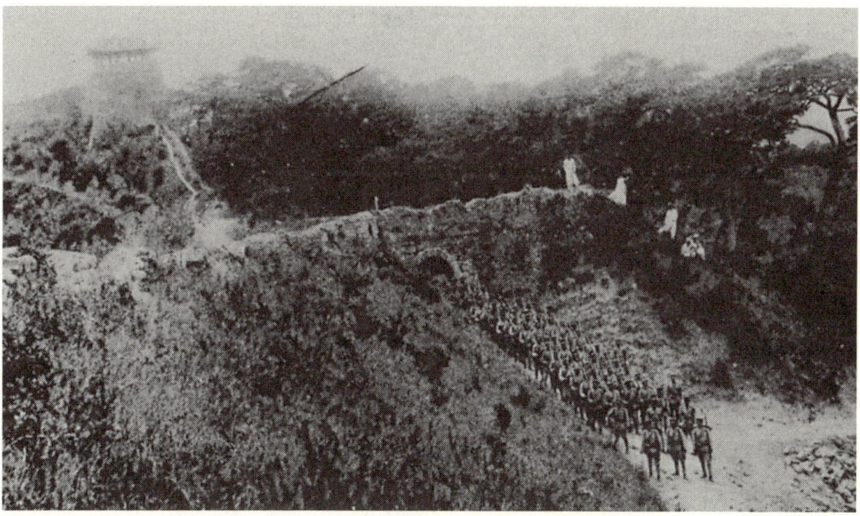

Japanese soldiers at Pyong Yang City wall

years behind the times. Is it any wonder that an army, unpatriotic, poorly drilled and badly equipped, could make no stand against an opposing force smaller in number, but patriotic to a man, drilled almost to perfection, and armed with the best of modern implements of warfare?

"Some of the sights to be seen on this battlefield were horrible in the extreme. The dead that fell near the city had mostly been covered, but those killed some distance away were lying all unburied. In one place I counted over twenty bodies literally piled one on top of another lying just as they had been shot down. In another place where a body of Manchurian cavalry ran into an ambush of Japanese infantry the carnage was frightful. Several hundred men and horses, lying as they had fallen, made a swarth of bodies nearly a quarter of a mile long and several yards wide. It was three weeks after the battle, and the bodies were all there unmolested even by the dogs."[7]

While his father busied himself working among the wounded in Pyong Yang, little Sherwood was about to celebrate his first birthday in Seoul. Ruefully, Mrs. Hall wrote in her journal on November 10, 1894:

"How much we miss dear papa today. In his last letter he wrote, 'How I long to see our darling little Sherwood. I will not be able to be down for his birthday after all.'"

Esther and Yousan Pak had become so close to the Halls that they seemed a part of the family. "Aunt Esther" penned a note to Sherwood in honor of his important first birthday:

"My dear darling Sherwood.

"It is your first birthday. I am very glad you came to this world and let me love you. I hope you grow very useful man and do many good things among the heathen like your father and mother, and honor to your parents and obey their teaching and be gentle and kind. I hope you grow up be best boy,

---

[7] *The Life of W. J. Hall*, pp. 299-300.

and love God keep His commandment. Will you dear child? I hope God may bless you on your sweet birthday and give you wisdom to understand many different things. Your father and mother and I love you so we want you to grow up to be a good man. O how much we love you. As you cannot read yet I will not write very much. With much love from Uncle Pak and Aunt Esther."

In Korea, the first natal day is very important for this is the auspicious time when the child is supposed to select his future career. Children and adults were invited to help Sherwood celebrate this special occasion and, observing Korean custom, to watch him select his life work.

Most of the parents looked on with amused skepticism while Sherwood was placed among the objects that would represent the direction of his future. He lurched forward with evident determination past the rag doll (beggar man), the attractively colored books (teacher), the Bible (preacher), toy hoe (farmer), right past a clutter of things to the most unlikely attraction of all—a stethoscope (doctor). Sherwood clutched one of the rubber tubes in his small fist while the audience laughed appreciatively. The Koreans nodded and said, "*Poya algeso*" (just wait and see), and his mother viewed the scene with ill concealed delight. Then, following Western custom, the guests sang "Happy Birthday" while Sherwood blew out the candle with assistance, and everyone enjoyed the simple party refreshments.

Dr. Hall worked day and night caring for the sick and wounded of Pyong Yang. He used his bamboo cot for a stretcher, and his fellow Christians served as an ambulance staff. He reestablished his school[8] and held a service every night with the Koreans. However, this strenuous schedule began to take its toll on the doctor's own health.

Samuel A. Moffett who was with Dr. Hall in Pyong Yang at that time described developments there:

"... The exposure of the past year in his numerous visits to Pyong Yang, had left him in poor condition to withstand

[8] The "Kwang Sung Academy," started by Dr. Hall with only 13 boys, continues to this day, although it has since been moved to the city of Seoul.

the dreadfully unhealthy condition of the atmosphere in and around this city, which had been the battlefield. The decaying bodies of men, horses, and cattle were so numerous that in whichever direction we went we came across them constantly, so that the atmosphere was foul beyond all expression. We all suffered from malaria, and as this seemed to have taken more serious hold upon the doctor we arranged to leave for Seoul by Japanese transport. Through the courtesy of the official we were able to do this, and after going down the Tai Tong [Taedong] River some forty miles we embarked on board a transport carrying some six hundred sick soldiers, who were suffering from dysentery and various fevers.

"We had a pleasant voyage, and when we reached Chemulpo all thought the doctor had almost recovered from his fever, but the sequel shows that he had probably contracted typhus fever . . . After a day in Chemulpo, in which he seemed fairly well again, his fever went up and continued to rise while we awaited the arrival of the small river steamer upon which we took passage for Seoul. Leaving in the afternoon, by dark we had reached a point opposite Kang-hoa [Kanghwa] Island, when we struck a rock and nearly capsized. All efforts to free the steamer were futile, so there was nothing for us to do but to get the doctor on shore, make him as comfortable as possible in a Korean hut, and seek for a junk. This we secured at daybreak, and after a slow journey reached Seoul the next morning. Here in the hands of his wife, and with all the care the doctors could give him, we hoped he would recover."[9]

Mrs. Hall recorded in a letter to a friend:

"Monday morning, November 19, just as I was getting some medicine ready to visit an out-patient, word came that Doctor had arrived. I hastily picked up our little boy and ran to meet him. He was too sick to stand alone even, and had to be carried to his bed. Nearly his first words were, 'I have

---

[9] *The Life of W. J. Hall*, pp. 305-306.

known what a joy wife and home are in health; now I am to experience what a comfort they are in sickness.'

"He seemed so bright and cheerful the first day after getting home that it was difficult to realize he was so dangerously ill; yet the fever thermometer would register one hundred and five degrees. He was able to help himself to water that stood close by him that night, but by the next night he was as helpless as a babe.

"Wednesday morning Doctor asked Mr. Noble to bring pencil and paper, and he gave him the items of expense in the trip he had just made; all his other accounts, he said, would be found in his books. He was ever thus careful about all business details. When he had finished he said, 'Now I am ready to live or to die; I would like to work longer for the Master if it be His will . . .'

"Already it was hard for him to talk, and it was beginning to be difficult to understand what he said. A gradual spreading paresis seemed to be involving the muscles of his throat. We had the best advice of five physicians, but it began to look as if he were going to leave us in spite of all that could be done.

"Now and then as I came near him, he would try to tell me how much he loved me, and that it was a love that would last through eternity. He asked after the little unborn one, and smiled when I replied, 'It seems so strong. It moves about so much more than Sherwood did.'

"Thursday morning Doctor asked for pencil and paper and attempted to write, but found that he was far too weak. His only trouble seemed to be because he could not tell all that was in his heart to say. His eyes would look sorrowfully into mine, but he could only stammer brokenly, 'I–love–you.' In the afternoon he asked for little Sherwood. He looked at him lovingly and longingly, but he who was known in both America and Korea as the 'children's friend' had to take a *silent* farewell of his only son. His last attempt to talk was to tell me not to regret his going to Pyong Yang, and he said, 'I did it for Jesus' sake, . . . He will reward me.'

"Dear Doctor, his faith was ever as simple as that of a child, and he never had any more fear of death than a babe of falling asleep in its mother's arms.

"Saturday, November 24, 1894, just at sunset, he fell 'asleep in Jesus,' to awake in the eternal Sabbath day.

"All that afternoon he kept his eyes fixed upon mine, and he seemed to want me to hold both his hands in mine, and that is how he left me. I closed those loving eyes, then, thinking how they could never look into mine again, I opened them for one long, last look; they were still so bright and so clear it seemed as if he must still see me. I then went to my room, took dear little Sherwood in my arms, and claimed God's promises for him and myself."

"The next day, Sunday," writes W. A. Noble, "we placed the form of our beloved brother in a huge Korean coffin, and bore it down to the banks of the beautiful Han. It is a peaceful place to rest, lying among those for whom he died."[10]

[10] *The Life of W. J. Hall*, p. 349.

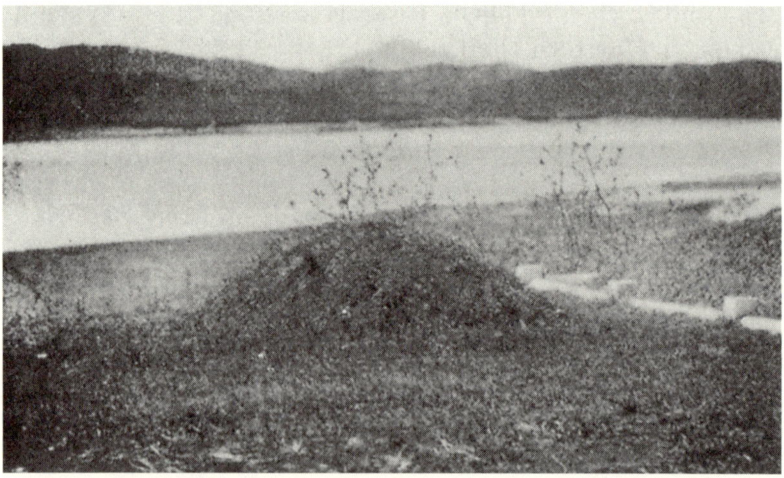

Dr. W. J. Hall's grave on the banks of the Han River, Seoul, Korea
Born Jan. 16, 1860–Died Nov. 24, 1894

CHAPTER 6

Edith Margaret

Soon after the beautiful memorial service at the Pai Chai School Chapel, Seoul, conducted by the Reverend W. A. Noble on November 27, 1894, Mrs. Hall began to make plans to return to her home at Liberty, New York with her year-old son. She was seven months pregnant with her second child.

Esther Kim Pak, who had been her faithful Korean assistant in hospital and Bible work, begged Mrs. Hall to take her along too. Mrs. Hall agreed that perhaps the time had come for Esther to pursue her long-cherished idea of studying medicine in America. The Mission approved and a little financial help was proffered by friends. Hesitating to separate Esther from her husband, Yousan, for so long a time, Mrs. Hall thought it best to take them both with her. All arrangements for leaving having at last been made, Mrs. Hall and the Paks bade good-by to their friends at Seoul.

The travelers reached the home of Mr. and Mrs. George Heber Jones in Chemulpo the evening of December 7. Several days before, they had feared that Sherwood might have contracted typhus fever from his father for his temperature had soared to 104.8°. However, he responded so well to medication that Mrs. Hall attributed the fever to teething and felt it was safe to continue with their plans. The next morning as they were preparing to board the boat that was to take them to Nagasaki, Japan, Mrs. Hall found Sherwood broken out with the measles. Because they could not expose the other passengers to Sherwood's illness, they delayed their departure, staying on with Mr. and Mrs. Jones. When finally they were able to resume their journey, they feared they had missed the connection with the *China*, the steamship that was to take them from Japan to the United States.

The crossing to Japan proved to be very rough and for fifty hours the adults were too seasick to eat anything. Sherwood did not seem to be bothered and was fortunate in being cared for much of the time by the Captain's wife. The night before they were due to arrive at Nagasaki, Mrs. Hall dreamed that the *China* was there, and would sail at 4 P.M. She mentioned this to the Captain and his wife, and they said they hoped it might be so, but the ship would have already sailed if the schedule had been followed.

When the pilot came on board at Nagasaki harbor, the Captain came running to find Mrs. Hall and said, "Your dream is true! The *China* is just in, and leaves this afternoon." The same storm that had made Mrs. Hall and the Paks so seasick had delayed the *China*. It set sail on Sunday, December 16, 1894 with the Halls and the Paks on board.

During the voyage, Mrs. Hall was befriended by a motherly stewardess who also became greatly attached to Sherwood. She was most solicitous of Mrs. Hall when she observed that she was carrying another child. Although the stewardess thought it would be wonderful to have a shipboard birth, Mrs. Hall prayed fervently that her baby would not arrive until she reached her home in Liberty. As it turned out, Mrs. Hall's prayer was answered.

Soon after they had all reached the old homestead, Sherwood woke up to find he was not "the only pebble on the beach." He had been joined on January 18, 1895 by a baby sister, Edith Margaret. Her name had been chosen long before in Korea by her parents—"Edith" because they both had liked it and "Margaret" for her paternal grandmother.

Mrs. Hall wrote in her diary:

> "Little Edith first opened her blue eyes in the home where her mama was born. In her papa's favorite chapter (Isa. 43) there is one verse that reads, '*Fear not; for I am with thee; I will bring thy seed from the East and gather thee from the West.*' And it seems strange to note that Sherwood was born in Korea in the 'Far East' while his little sister not fifteen months later was born ten thousand miles away in Liberty, New York."

Mrs. Hall found herself busy caring for her children, visiting with relatives in Liberty, and eventually taking up work in a medical clinic there. Rosevelt R. Sherwood, Mrs. Hall's father, delighted in his grandson and seemed to have a special affinity for him because of their shared birthdate. He proudly posed for a picture with little

Sherwood which the family labeled "Ninety and One," reflecting their respective ages.

In February, Mrs. Pak entered public school at Liberty, while her husband worked on Rosevelt Sherwood's farm. Different friends, believing in Esther's education as a practical form of mission work, boarded or paid for her board each month, and she made good progress in the schoolroom. In September of that same year, Mrs. Pak entered the "Nursery and Child's Hospital" of New York City where she was able to earn her way for over a year and at the same time receive tutoring in Latin, physics and mathematics. She entered the Women's Medical College of Baltimore (Johns Hopkins) on October 1, 1896–the first Korean to take up the study of Western medicine.

In July, 1895 Mrs. Hall took her children to visit their paternal grandparents, relatives and friends in Canada. The Paks accompanied them. Mr. Pak still wore his long hair rolled up in a top knot, concealed by a bowler hat! He created almost as big a sensation in the West as the "Western barbarians" had in the Far East.

A special service of welcome was held for Mrs. Hall at the Glen Buell Church in Ontario, Canada on July 31. Mrs. Hall listened to the warmth of that reception:

> "We welcome you to our community as one about whom we have oft conversed, and whose ways, for reasons well known, we have watched with keenest interest since we first heard of you.
>
> "We welcome you to our homes . . . and in our family midst–yourself and family and the foreign brother and sister, whom we are glad to greet as trophies of the power of Jesus to save in other tongues and lands than ours . . .
>
> "But we welcome you far from least of all for a reason that steals a little farther into our hearts as the beloved wife of one whose boyhood scenes and associations were these streets and farms and neighborhoods, and whose name is today far and near, 'as ointment poured forth.' . . .
>
> "Words are too feeble to express his genial manner, his kindness, his sympathy for all, and above all his unreserved consecration, anywhere and everywhere, to the work of the Master he loved. In all our hearts he has planted Korea, if for

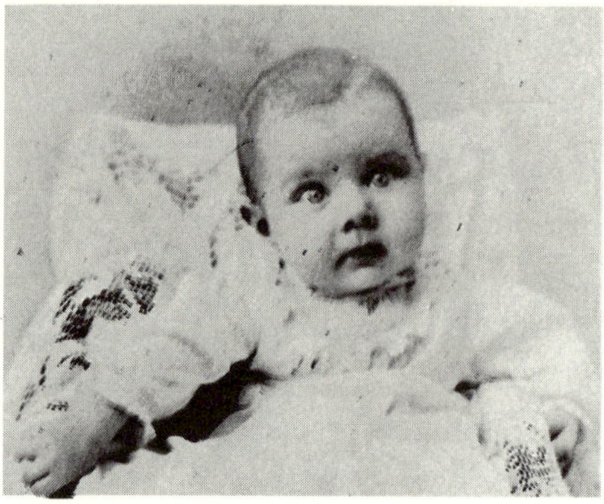

Edith Margaret Hall at five months, born Jan. 18, 1895

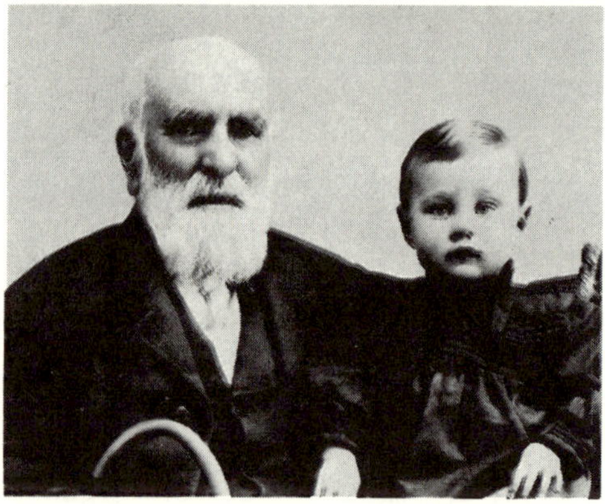

"Ninety and One"–Rosevelt Sherwood, born Nov. 10, 1804, with his grandson, Sherwood Hall, born Nov. 10, 1893.

no other reason, because it was dear to him . . . His letters breathed the same ardent spirit in yonder land, and for yonder distant people, as we had seen blossom into fragrance in our midst. . . ."[1]

It was evident from the many expressions of warmth and sympathy that Jimmy Hall had left his mark indelibly upon that Canadian community. A marble memorial plaque dedicated to him was installed in the front of the Glen Buell Church where it remains to this day.

At the time of her husband's death, Mrs. Hall had expressed the wish that the money remaining in the "Pyong Yang Fund" be used toward the erection of a hospital to his memory. The Reverend H. G.

---

[1] *The Life of W. J. Hall*, pp. 404-405.

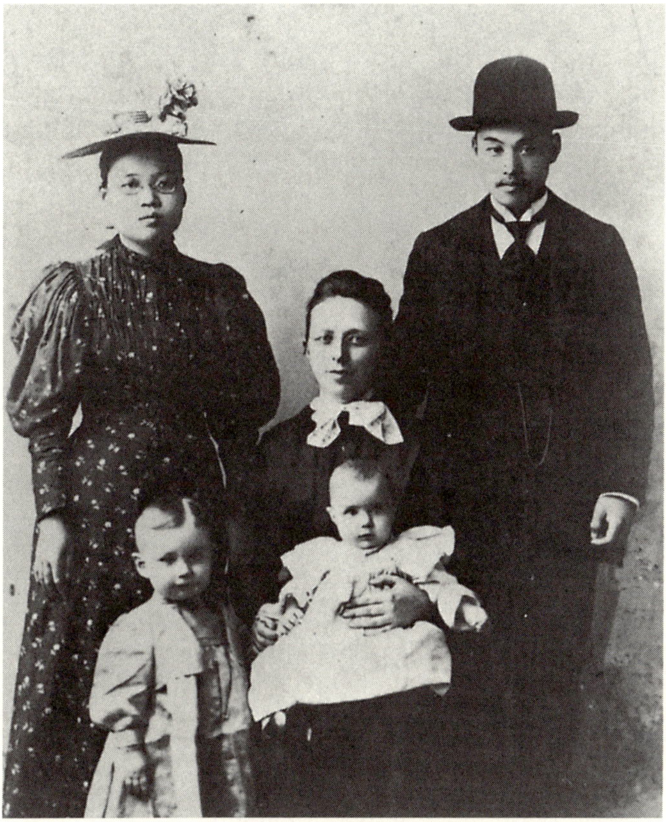

Esther and Yousan Pak, Dr. Rosetta Hall, Sherwood and Edith, Sept. 1895

Appenzeller, writing in the September, 1896 issue of *World-Wide Missions*, reported:

"Mrs. Hall feels that the true monument is not a cold, expensive shaft of marble or granite, but the foundation of some work for the uplifting of the race or the amelioration of suffering. Such a monument is alive, warm, and ever reproductive."[2]

In the *Korean Repository* for May, Mr. Appenzeller announced:

"Douglas Follwell, M.D., is the successor of Dr. Hall and to him is committed the pleasant, and we may say sacred,

---

[2] *The Life of W. J. Hall*, pp. 410-411.

work of erecting this memorial. It was our privilege to visit Pyong Yang, and with Dr. Follwell, on May 6, to begin this building by giving out the contract for the erection of a dispensary to a Korean carpenter, who agreed to finish it in five months.

"This dispensary is located inside of and adjoining the West Gate, on high ground, and but seven minutes walk from the commercial center of the city, which in Pyong Yang, as in Seoul, is marked by the big bell. This building will be 40 × 16 feet and in Korean style, containing a waiting room, clinic, drug room, and the doctor's office."[3]

In a report to Bishop Joyce and the Members of the Korea Mission, Dr. Follwell later wrote:

"Since February 1, 1897, the Hall Memorial Hospital has been opened to all comers. The building, without any expense whatever to the Missionary Society, has been erected through the self-denial of our late beloved Doctor Hall, his wife, also a physician, and their kind friends in Korea and the home land. . . .

"We are ready for all the work that comes to us if we only have the room to put the patients and sufficient funds to buy necessary instruments. I have repeatedly sent patients away either because I had no instruments suitable for operation or because of lack of ward room. A surgeon cannot work without proper instruments any more than a carpenter can build a house without saw, hammer, or nails. It is a great mistake for anyone to think that the medical missionary can get along with few instruments, and poor ones at best. We cannot afford to have poor results from our surgical work, that gives us the best success. I am hoping that the coming year will see these necessities to the carrying on of the medical work in Pyong Yang supplied. The results thus far have been most encouraging . . ."[4]

---

[3] *The Life of W. J. Hall*, p. 410.

[4] *The Life of W. J. Hall*, pp. 411-412.

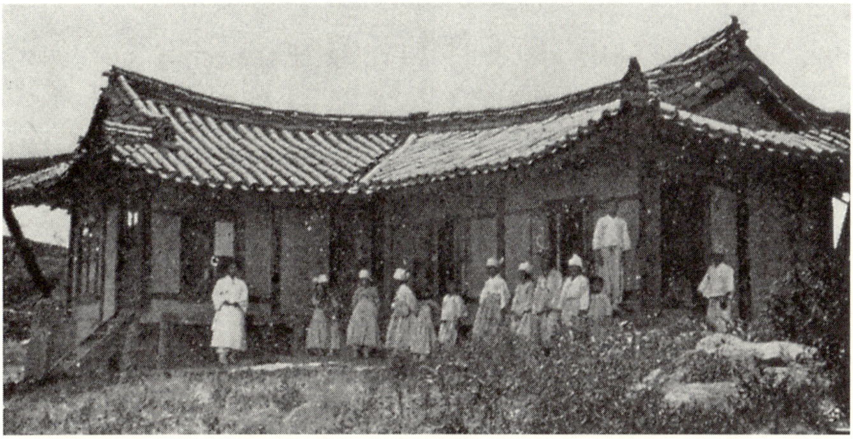

Hall Memorial Hospital, Pyong Yang

Dr. Follwell's report indicated that between February 1 and April 27, 1897, treatment had been given to 1,334 surgical cases and to 1,011 medical cases. The average in-patient attendance at the hospital had varied between 32 and 84 patients. The receipts in U.S. currency were $37.17.

Mrs. Hall had spent some of her time in the United States helping to raise money for the Hall Memorial Hospital in Pyong Yang. To this end, she also assembled material for a book on *The Life of Rev. William James Hall, M.D.* which was published in August, 1897 by the Press of Eaton and Mains, Publishing Agency of the Methodist Book Concern in New York. Mrs. Hall assigned her husband's youngest brother, Clifford Hall, to be the agent for the sale of the book in Canada. The proceeds from the book sales were added to the hospital fund.

Another matter that had remained in the forefront of Mrs. Hall's thinking was her concern for the plight of the blind in Korea. She began to look into the various systems then in vogue for teaching the blind. Louis Braille, a blind teacher in Paris, first published in 1829 the dot system he had developed. Superintendent William B. Wait of the New York Institute for the Education of the Blind developed another dot system in the 1860's which became known as New York point. Mrs. Hall had occasion to visit Superintendent Wait and from him learned his system. She concluded from her comparisons of the different systems that New York point best met the tests of correspondence and utility for adaptation to the Korean language.

By the Fall of 1897 Mrs. Hall could resist the call of Korea no longer. She decided to return there with her children and so help to bring to fruition her husband's work in that land. The Woman's Foreign Missionary Society of the Methodist Church, under whom she had served when she first went to Korea, offered her the opportunity to work at the *Po Ku Nyo Kwan* (Salvation for All Women Hospital) where she had first been assigned in 1890. She accepted. Mrs. Hall and her two children sailed for Korea on the *SS Empress of India* on October 11, 1897.

An entry in Mrs. Hall's journal for November 10, 1897 at Chemulpo records:

> "This is Sherwood's birthday—four years old today. It seems like quite a coincidence that he should have arrived in Korea, the land of his birth, upon the same day he first came, but such is the case as we just arrived per *SS Heigo Maru* at 9 A.M. and landed from the sampan at 10 o'clock—just the same hour Sherwood put in appearance four years ago today. But this time there was no loving papa to greet him. Mr. Jones was there to meet his wife and baby girl who traveled with us all the way from St. Paul, U.S.A., and Mrs. Follwell was down from Pyong Yang to meet her sister Dr. Lillian Harris, and Misses Paine and Frey from Seoul to meet Miss Nellie Pierce both of whom were also in our party from St. Paul and are W.F.M.S. missionaries to help in the work in Seoul."

Mrs. Hall was unable to leave for Seoul with the others, however, for both Sherwood and Edith became ill with whooping cough the day after the family arrived at Chemulpo, and then Edith developed pneumonia. By November 20th she was well enough to travel again and E. D. Steward carried her from his hotel to the boat landing. From here they traveled up the Han River to Seoul. They were to be housed there in the same quarters with the single missionary ladies of the W.F.M.S., who were making a special concession to Mrs. Hall to allow her to board with them along with her two children.

Mrs. Hall commented that her little patient:

> ". . . coughed but once going up the river. We started about 10 A.M. and landed about 4:30 P.M. It got quite dark before we reached the W.F.M.S. House. Mama carried her on her lap in a chair, and she was as warm and nice as possible

and was none the worse for the trip. We passed through rows of silk gauze lanterns in front of the Palace, ready for the Imperial funeral of the Queen on the morrow."

Ironically, when Mrs. Hall had arrived in Korea in 1890 for the first time, the country had also been in mourning for the passing of one of its queens—Queen Cho. Queen Cho was the Dowager Queen who had been responsible for appointing King Li H'oung to the throne, and for making his father Regent, with the title of *Tai Won Kun* (Prince of the Great House). The Regent and his daughter-in-law had long been engaged in a mutual power struggle. This ended for Queen Min on October 8, 1895 when she was brutally murdered by Japanese *soshi* (hired ruffian killers). Her body was soaked in kerosene and set ablaze in an attempt to destroy any evidence of how she died. A false edict, purportedly from the King, was circulated by the Japanese in an effort to discredit Queen Min by declaring that she was a prostitute.

In the months that followed, the King had lived in fear for his own life and refused to eat any food except that which was prepared in the homes of American missionaries. He distrusted the palace food, suspicious of a possible attempt to poison him. It was believed, although never proven, that the Japanese Resident Minister in Seoul at that time, Miura Goro, arranged with the Tai Won Kun for the murder of the Queen. The Tai Won Kun, it was said, was seeking revenge for past humiliations and defeats, while the Japanese were attempting to restructure the Korean government to suit Japanese ends. The Queen had been an unyielding obstacle to all their efforts at negotiation.

If the Japanese had hoped to thus increase their control of Korean affairs, the plan backfired when the King and the Crown Prince entered the Russian Legation on February 11, 1896 and were gladly given the asylum they requested. Here the King remained until February 20, 1897, still holding the seals of state and therefore the power to govern. The Russian influence with the Court successfully blocked Japanese expansionist plans for a few years, although it only postponed the inevitable confrontation between Japan and Russia.

On October 17, 1897 the King formally changed his title to Emperor and the official designation of his country to *Taehan Cheguk* (the Korean Empire). Queen Min received the posthumous title of Empress Myong Song.

Traditionally, Korean custom allowed for a mourning period of 100 days between the actual death and the formal state funeral, followed by a period of national mourning of one to three years. However, concrete evidence of Queen Min's death was destroyed when her body was burned. Because of this and the political upheaval which followed her assassination, her official state funeral had been delayed until November 21, 1897. So it was that the arrival of Mrs. Hall again coincided with a queen's funeral. The occasion reminded her of another funeral and made her return to Korea still more poignant.

On Thanksgiving Day, November 24, 1897 she entered in her diary:

> "Edith has improved right along—has scarcely coughed once—and is quite well. Sherwood does not cough either . . . We took chairs and rode down to papa's grave today. It is just three years ago November 24th that his body was placed there."

Mrs. Hall settled into the quarters provided for her and her children. An *amah* (nursemaid) was procured to care for Sherwood and Edith so that Mrs. Hall could attend to her medical duties at the hospital.

> "They have quite a good *amah*—a young widow. She is industrious and a very good worker . . . but she has not a very good knack for getting on smoothly with the children. She prefers to sit and sew to looking after them, and though mama tries to study faithfully every morning for three hours, it is often disturbed in looking after the children in one way or the other. Sometimes, mama wishes she had another room to study in, but it is probably better not—for no doubt a proper oversight over her babies is quite as much or more her duty than studying Korean, especially just now when they are so young, and among a strange people. How often mama, as well as they, has wished that Grandma might be here with us. It would be just lovely, if it were not for the terrible journey of getting here."

Feeling beholden to the single ladies for allowing her little family to live in the home, Mrs. Hall was sensitive to the strains inherent in such a situation. She wrote:

> "It is pretty hard living with two such little children in a family like this–none of them mothers, but each thinking, all the more, she knows how children ought to behave. However, there has been no real trouble. Only, mama has a feeling that most of the ladies think she doesn't make her children mind as well as they ought. Mama wishes they *did* do better, but they are such mere babes yet, with little or no pride for their reputations. In the dining room they sit in low chairs at a little table by themselves, and often have to wait until the whole eight ladies are waited upon, before they get anything, and it is so easy for them to get into disorder in that case. Being always alone, they don't advance any in table etiquette, but rather go backward. It will be good when we can get a little home of our own."

* * * * * * *

Although it is seldom easy to sort out fact from fancy of one's very earliest childhood memories, that winter of our return to Korea stands out in my mind as though it had happened just yesterday. It was December, 1897 and I had just turned four years old the previous month. Edith was two, going on three, and both of us were looking forward to Christmas with all the eager anticipation of childhood. Our requests to Santa had already been dictated. Edith wanted a doll almost as big as a real baby, so she could *ubba bai* (carry) it on her back the way young Korean girls strap on a baby brother or sister. I wished for a proper sled; not one of those crude homemade contraptions that my Korean playmates used, but one which could go as fast as the wind.

Mama had told us of the great difficulty our father had had in finding a suitable Christmas tree in this land of crooked pine trees. Paksabang, the gate keeper, had agreed to take us early for a long exciting trip of exploration to find just the right tree. Since there was no fireplace in our room, we were to hang up our stockings on the decorated tree. Little Edith was aglow with joy and anticipation and I confided to my mother, "I'll kie [cry] if Kismas [Christmas] day don't come again tomorrow." Was it a child's premonition?

Just the day before Christmas, an awful thing happened. Mama was away at the hospital, and we children were happily playing a game of tag around a desk in the ladies' home. Edith accidentally knocked to the floor a Korean ink well (*pyo roo*). The dark ink (*muk*) spilled out and all over the beautiful Oriental carpet.

We did not think too much about it at the time, for we were gleefully concentrating on chasing each other. However, just then, one of the single ladies of the home happened onto the scene and demanded to know who had spilled the ink. Edith freely confessed that she had done so. Since I had been chasing her at the time, I began to feel a bit guilty but said nothing. The lady then announced sternly, "Very well, we shall see about it when your mother returns from her work at the hospital."

We knew by her tone that the lady felt that Edith had done something terrible, but it had not yet percolated into our young minds the extent of the misdeed. To make matters worse, we innocently went on playing.

The ladies of the home had appointed themselves as a sort of "composite mother" to discipline us while our own mother was away at work. They apparently held a council about Edith's misdemeanor.

When my mother returned from the hospital, they called her before them. With serious expressions they told of the naughty thing Edith had done in spilling the ink and ruining the carpet. Moreover, they reported indignantly, Edith had shown no remorse but had gone on playing. This would never do. They then decided what punishment should be meted out to her, namely, that Santa was not to put anything in the children's stockings and Edith must receive no Christmas presents from anyone, not even from her mother. This would teach Edith a lesson she would not forget.

My mother, who felt that such a severe punishment for a child so young did not fit the crime, was about to protest. One of the ladies, sensing this, spoke up emphatically, "It would be no use to discuss the matter further. Our decision is final."

Mother realized, after all, that her children were in the home on sufferance, and it was only through the special favor of the ladies that they were allowed to live there at all. She felt helpless to oppose their decision or pursue the matter further. These same good ladies had come half way around the earth to help relieve suffering and pain, and would not have even thought of intentionally hurting any creature. Ironically, they had not the least conception of the great hurt they had inflicted on a young child in depriving her of Christmas joy, to say nothing of the mental anguish they had heaped on her mother and brother.

That Christmas morning Edith and I awoke to empty stockings. Perhaps for Edith the disappointment was not felt as keenly as it was felt by me, for she had really been too young to remember Christmas much from the previous year. However, as she observed the gift exchanges that excluded us, I thought of her bedtime prayer the night before for the W.F.M.S. missionaries: "God bless all them ladies." Added to my own consternation, it was almost more than I could bear to see Edith's eager anticipation now turn to bewilderment. My mother suggested that Edith and I accompany her to distribute gifts to the children in the hospital and this saved the day for us all.

My mother recorded in her journal:

> "How much interest Edith took in the sick folks, especially the children. After her afternoon nap she often came into the dispensary before mama got quite through with the patients. At night to her 'Now I lay me . . .' was often added such a petition as this, 'God bless all those Korean childrens. God bless the little babies at the hospital what's got the little bits of heads and one has sore eyes.' If a tooth had to be drawn or an abscess lanced, Sherwood was always quick enough to run away, but she stood her ground unless sent away. One afternoon she came in when mama was so busy with an operation she did not notice her. Some blood had spattered on mama's face. Edith saw Whey Whang sponging blood with some cotton, so procuring some, she placed a stool in position, and climbing up began to wipe the blood from mama's face! Mama felt sure she would make a physician herself some day."

Winter in Seoul that year had begun early. The Koreans had been forced to don their winter clothes sooner than usual. These consisted of quilt-like garments, so heavily padded with cotton that they ballooned out, making the Koreans seem nearly twice their size. To my child's eyes, they resembled the polar bears I had seen at the zoo.

Our *amah* decided one day in late January to take us with her to a Korean house where she wanted to get a beauty treatment. This consisted in having her hair pulled out evenly across her forehead. While there, Edith and I played with the Korean children in the courtyard, blissfully unaware that one of them had the measles. Both of us came down with measles soon after. Edith recovered fairly rapidly. My mother had not really expected me to get them at all, since I had already had the measles just as we were leaving Korea after my father died.

My mother wrote in the journal she kept for me:

> "Sherwood was ailing for a couple of weeks and one day, February 19th, was so severely ill that Drs. Cutler and Harris, as well as mama, considered him in grave danger, his temperature being 105½° in axilla, and continuing very high for nearly 24 hours. We of course thought it meant he was going to have some very serious disease like pneumonia, peritonitis or something, but it didn't turn out to be. In fact, the cause has never yet been discovered. But mama was very very anxious over her little boy, and prayed earnestly if it was God's will, to spare him to her, and no doubt others prayed too . . . and much to mama's relief and great joy, God spared Sherwood once more. . . . Mama does hope and pray that her little son may prove a great comfort and help not to her only, but to all who know him, as his dear papa was. Twice, now, God has given him back to mama, as it were from the very jaws of death, and this time it was almost more than mama felt she could expect. But God is merciful and good, so good."

Edith and I enjoyed playing with the other missionary children on occasion, but most of the time we had each other as companions. Edith had been given a large doll on her birthday by Gretchen Jones. This doll had brown eyes and flaxen hair and would often join us in our play. My mother described one such scene in her journal:

> "Edith says she will call her doll 'Mary' because it has hair like Mary Appenzeller, and her brother wanted her to

call it Mary . . . It is the finest doll Edith has yet possessed . . . Sherwood tried to persuade her that, 'mamas study,' and 'papas take care of the babies,' but he had to be put off with sitting down in his rocker beside the mama and her dolly Mary and reading the newspaper to them while dolly was rocked to sleep."

In such contented play, the winter months sped by. The snow and ice melted, as if overnight, and the Koreans, too, suddenly shrunk to almost normal size. We knew then that spring had come. It was the season when Korea was at its best. Cherry, peach and apricot trees flowered in regal splendor. The mountainsides appeared robed in purple garb, covered with exquisite Korean azaleas. It was indeed a glorious time of year to go to the interior. Fortunately, my mother had received her longed-for appointment to Pyong Yang.

We left Seoul on April 29, 1898 and sailed from Chemulpo the next day on the *Hai Riong*. We arrived in Pyong Yang on May 1, four years from the time (almost to the day) that my parents and I had arrived there to make our home before.

We were to stay with the Nobles, who were now working in Pyong Yang, until the house planned for us was completed. The next day we went to see our new home which needed only a few more

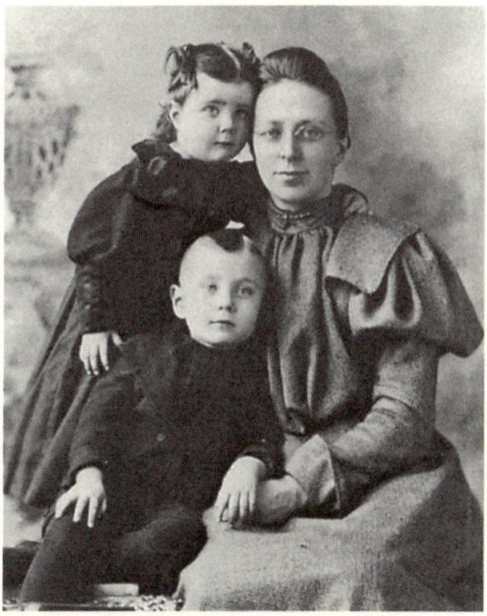

Dr. Rosetta Hall and children at time of her appointment to Pyong Yang

finishing touches. Edith gathered her hands full of white Korean dandelions in the yard and then flitted through the house like a little sunbeam. How happy we all were.

Our happiness, however, was short-lived. Soon after, all three of us were stricken with dysentery and Edith worst of all. My mother's journal detailed Edith's three weeks of nausea and pain which even opiates did not control:

"May 5 – Edith wanted to go to bed early, but didn't go to sleep before 2 A.M. Had a throat cough, vomited several times . . .

"May 6 – Complained of abdominal pain . . .

"May 7 – Seemed better . . . countenance looked bad–fretful, and no appetite.

"May 8 – . . . Has had only semi-solid food the last three days . . . Afternoon showed some symptoms of dysentery . . . Put on liquid diet.

"May 9 – Stools . . . all containing blood . . . Was restless and in pain . . . She got to sleep 4 A.M. and slept well until about 6:30 A.M. . . .

"May 10 – Complains bitterly of stomach-ache after eating . . . Consultation with Drs. Wells and Follwell . . .

"May 11 – Complained bitterly of pain . . . dropped off to sleep on bed pan . . . 10 P.M.–Absolutely refuses ice, milk or anything in the mouth; took a little ice water . . .

"May 12 – 2:30 A.M.–Refuses anything by mouth . . . Face anxious, and appears to be in much pain often. Asked, 'Is this our house?' . . . 12:30 P.M.–Unusually restless, tossing and turning . . . Talked in her sleep–said, 'Goodbye,' . . . 'Sherwood, don't you want some of my medicine?' . . . 'I want to go to my house and play with Sherwood and Mary [Mary Appenzeller].' . . .

"May 13 – Has been restless all day . . . Her lips are drawn upon her teeth almost like a dead child's–eyes somewhat sunken–dark lids . . .

"May 14 – Vomited 14 times during this 24 hours–Pain before and during stools much increased . . .

"May 15 – . . . Stools . . . contain more bright blood and tissue again . . . and it would seem as if a new portion of the bowel were becoming involved . . . had 30 stools during 24 hours and vomited 7 times . . .

"May 16 – It would seem there has been a complication of malaria . . . Respiration has increased . . . some catarrhal involvement of lungs also . . .

"May 17 – It has been her best night and mama feels encouraged again, and so thankful if God's will be to spare the comfort He so kindly sent her, when He took Papa away . . .

"May 18 – Lies on her back altogether now, except when turned, and then at first has to cough and has some difficult breathing before she can get adjusted to the change. Is getting pretty thin . . .

"May 19 – Seemed decidedly weaker tonight.

"May 20 – Her temp. kept down but stomach began to give out again . . . will not eat . . .

"May 21 – . . . Temp. kept down to 100° nearly all day . . . symptoms of local peritonitis . . . Breathing much more oppressed . . . She seems so weak–difficult to understand her . . .

"May 22 – When given food would insist, . . . 'Keep it for tomorrow days.' At noon, moved her to Mr. Lee's guest house and she liked the change and seemed rather better for a time . . .

"May 23 – . . . At 3:30 in the morning seemed to be suffering much again . . . Asked to be rocked almost for the first since she was sick . . . Seemed to be suffering, with such an anxious look upon her dear little face–her brow so troubled and perplexed. She begged mama to hold her–but as long as there was any hope at all, mama feared to do it, for her heart was so very weak, and any change of position was likely to make her vomit or have difficult respiration . . .

About 10 A.M. mama placed some white dandelions in her hand which she enjoyed and held for a long time. Mama then went to lie down–

> and Grandma Webb [Rev. Graham Lee's mother] nursed Edith; Drs. Wells and Follwell, one or the other, being present most of the time.
>
> . . . At 3 P.M. her hands and feet were cold–face and body hot–temp. 103.2° . . .
>
> 6:45 – Restless and sighing–Nauseated
>
> 7:15 – Temp. 105°
>
> 7:30 – Hypodermic
>
> 8:00 – Sucked with relish a little ice-cream from brother's little spoon . . .
>
> 8:25 – Temp. 106° – Resp. 52 – Difficult. Mama took her in her arms and rocked her like she used to when going to take her afternoon nap–She breathed much more quietly–seemed content. Her face became peaceful, her breaths farther and farther apart, and with wide-open eyes looking into mama's her little spirit wended its way, back to the God who gave it, at 8:40 P.M. Monday–May 23, 1898. . . .

> ". . . Another great sorrow has come to us . . . and our precious one, the 'little comforter' God sent us in our first great sorrow, was removed from our loving arms before we ever got settled in our new home in Pyong Yang. Sherwood said when he first heard that God took her, that he thought it was 'because papa wanted her so much.' . . .
>
> "After she was dressed for the last time in her dainty white clothes, he went with mama to see her. He seemed to realize that it was only her body and that her spirit had gone. He picked some white clover blossoms and placed them in her hands. He seemed a bit chary of touching her, but he kissed her forehead then, and again when we saw her for the last time in the pretty white casket after the beautiful service. He made no remark about it at the time, but later, several times when describing anything very cold he would say, 'It was as cold–as cold as Edith's forehead.'"

That final memory stayed with me many years and was perhaps a greater shock to me than my mother realized. For a long time I suffered from nightmares and often woke up sobbing.

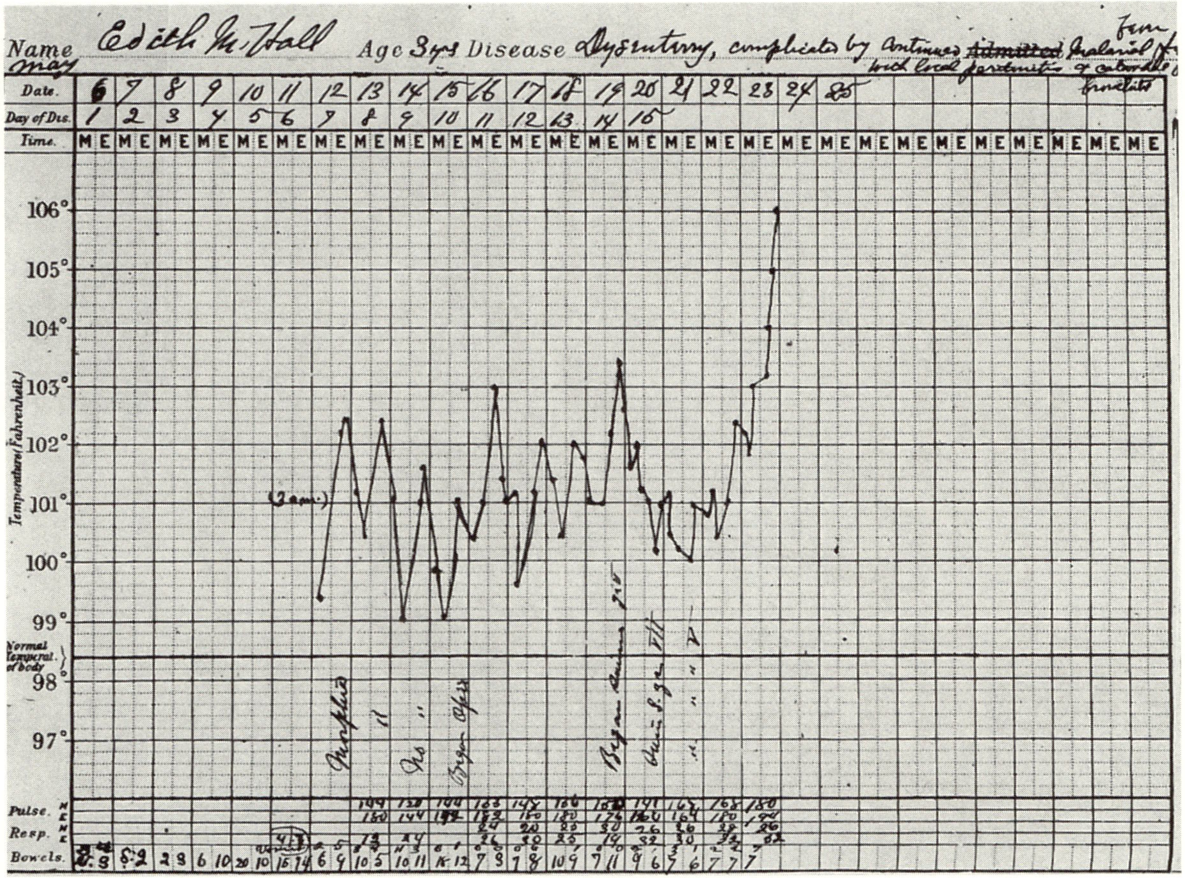

Edith Margaret's temperature chart May 16 to May 23, 1898

A final entry in the journal my mother kept for Edith notes:

"It was mama's wish that the precious body of her baby daughter might be laid at rest by papa's. Mr. Lee kindly soldered of tin an airtight box, and accompanied by faithful Kim Chang Sik the little body of the dear child her papa never saw in this life made the long overland journey to Seoul that he had so often made, leaving Pyong Yang May 26th and reaching there June 1st."

The following extract from Rev. H. G. Appenzeller's letter tells the rest:

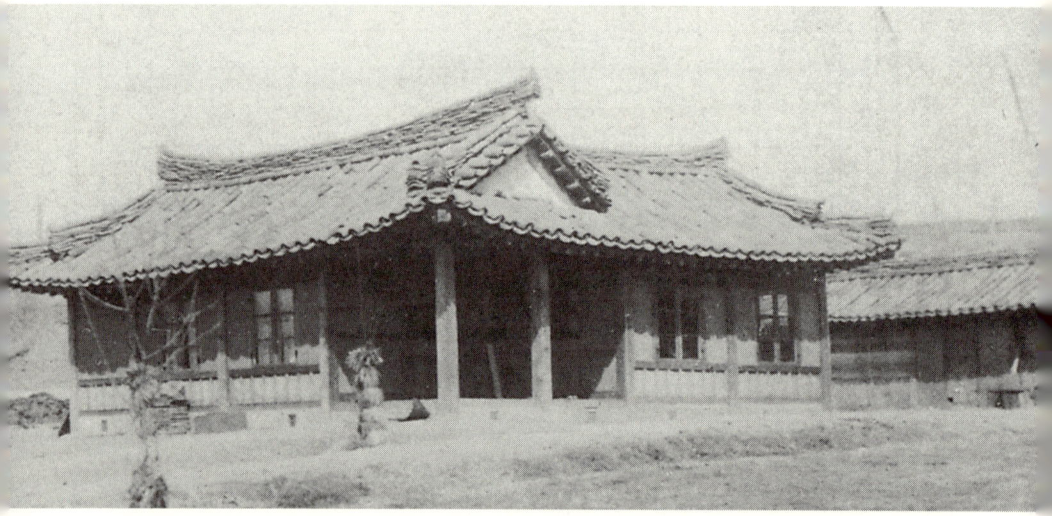

Graham Lee guest house where Edith was moved during last days of illness

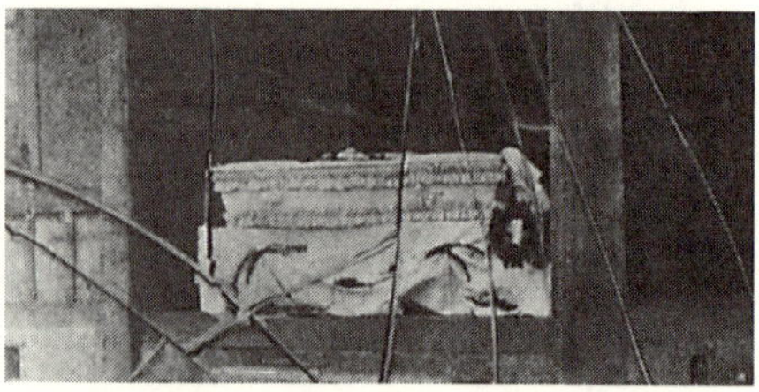

Edith's coffin on porch of guest house

"'At noon yesterday, as I came down from school, I found Brother Kim at my door. I was prepared to see him as I had learned that you proposed as was quite natural and eminently proper to have little Edith buried by her papa in our cemetery here . . . Miss Pierce bought a bunch of white peonies, my wife sent a wreath of white roses, and Alice made a cross of white roses. These we laid upon the coffin as it rested over the open grave. I read the words, 'I am the resurrection and the life' and we sang in Korean, 'Asleep in Jesus, blessed sleep.' The flowers were then removed and Brothers Bunker, Swearer, Kim and myself lowered the coffin, after which I read our beautiful burial service, and called on Brother Kim to lead in prayer followed by the Lord's prayer in concert. The whole was a beautiful, simple impressive service, such as I know you would have liked. The mound was heaped up, and the flowers placed on top. Your dear little girl sleeps now by her father's bosom, and the two will rise again at the call of the last trumpet. Half of your family is in Heaven.'"

CHAPTER 7

Picking up the Pieces

"Time passes so quickly and mama is so busy that she can only touch upon some of the changes that came to Sherwood."

So began the journal entry recorded in May, 1899, a year after Edith's death. It continued:

> "Last December mama took a little country trip of a week, leaving Sherwood with Ruth Noble. He didn't like it very well when he found mama was really gone . . . but he got on very well and was a pretty good boy, and most delighted to receive mama back home. He petitioned next time, however, that mama should take him along; so in March of this year, when mama went again, Sherwood went too.
>
> "We went by boat to a point near where Kim Chang Sik lives; then went overland, Sherwood riding the pack-pony. He enjoyed it . . . The first place we stopped, and where we finally spent the night after leaving the boat, there were two 'setting-hens' in the room with us. At this place Sherwood picked the first 'grandmother flowers' of the season.
>
> "At Sam Wha he enjoyed himself playing with Mr. Kim's children. At 'Nampo (Chinnampo) he got some small black pigs that were just across the way, and played with them. We spent Easter Sunday here, and had a nice service. The first 'collection' ever taken up in 'Nampo was taken by Sherwood this day in his cap. It amounted to 131 Pyong Yang *cash*, an average of half a cent apiece for those present. Kim Chang Sik told them about the first collection papa ever took in Pyong Yang, and how though not so much as this, they were in time able to build their own church. And he suggested that this money form the nucleus of a fund for such a building in 'Nampo.

"We returned home overland–taking three days for the trip–spent one night at Sam Wha, and one at Kang Syo–held an interesting meeting at each place. Altogether we visited six different villages traveling 450 *li* or about 150 miles. We taught in 11 different houses, holding two and three, sometimes four women's meetings daily. Of course, Sherwood was a great sight of all the places, being the first foreign boy the people ever saw; but he was rather a help than a hindrance. The fact that I am a married woman and have a son gives me a standing with the people who don't know foreign ways and can't understand our unmarried missionaries."

The house that was being finished for us when we first arrived in Pyong Yang shared the same roof with the woman's dispensary. The dispensary work opened on June 18, 1898. A day or two before the opening, my mother had received a call from the Governor of Pyong Yang to visit his wife. After several house calls, his wife was relieved of her suffering and Governor Chyo, in gratitude, sent my mother a present of 100 eggs and three spring chickens. A little later when the Governor was asked to name the newly opened dispensary, he chose to call it the "Women's Dispensary of Extended Grace" and predicted that multitudes of people would be helped as his wife had been, through the grace of the workers there. My mother observed:

"So we are beginning our work under quite a different relationship with the present governor than with the former who favored our persecution in '94."

In addition to her routine medical work in Pyong Yang, my mother was actively engaged in several other projects dear to her heart. She began to implement her dream of establishing some wards for Korean children as a memorial to Edith. The W.F.M.S. was at the same time trying to secure funds to build a Woman's Hospital and my mother hoped to have the "Edith Margaret Children's Wards" form a wing of the new hospital. Gifts from relatives and friends, added to the nucleus of Edith's small savings, provided enough funds to actually begin building the children's wards by the summer of 1899.

My mother reported to those who had helped to make her dream possible:

> "Last August we began building. So far all the buildings in Pyong Yang, including those occupied by missionaries, are of the native style–one-storied, mud-walled, tile-roofed structures. The Children's Wing is the first two-storied building in the city, the first to be clap-boarded and to have a galvanized iron roof. It is also the first to have a brick chimney. When you know there are no sawmills in Korea, and that all the material has to be prepared by hand here, and that even the 'boss' carpenter had never seen such a building, you may understand something of the undertaking. Our funds grew low and the cold weather came on before we were able to complete it; but one ward and the kitchen and helper's room is finished enough for use this winter, and we hope to be able to finish all, to paint and to paper in the spring."

Another unique feature of the Edith Margaret Memorial was its large cement cistern, which gave the city its first pure water supply. Contaminated water was a major cause of dysentery, the disease which had claimed Edith's life, so my mother was particularly eager to provide another source of water than the Taedong River.

However, she ran into immediate difficulty when she tried to obtain the necessary building permit. You will recall that Pyong Yang was believed to be a boat. The officials argued, therefore, that if my mother made a hole for the cistern, it would cause the boat to sink. They did not wish to lose their fair city in this manner. So my mother had to convince them that by lining the "hole" with brick and cement, Pyong Yang would not sink. They finally agreed this was the case and allowed her to proceed with her plans.

Special metal pipes led from the galvanized iron roof (which had been imported from America) into the cistern. My assigned chore during each good rainstorm was to turn a special lever in the pipe to drain off the first dusty water, and only when the water became clear, was it allowed to flow directly into the cistern, which resembled a reservoir. It was large enough that before a cover was finally placed over it, I was able to try out the raft I had made.

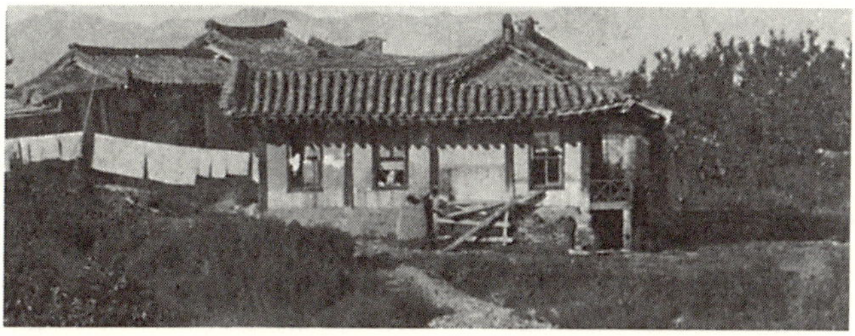

Woman's dispensary opened in 1898

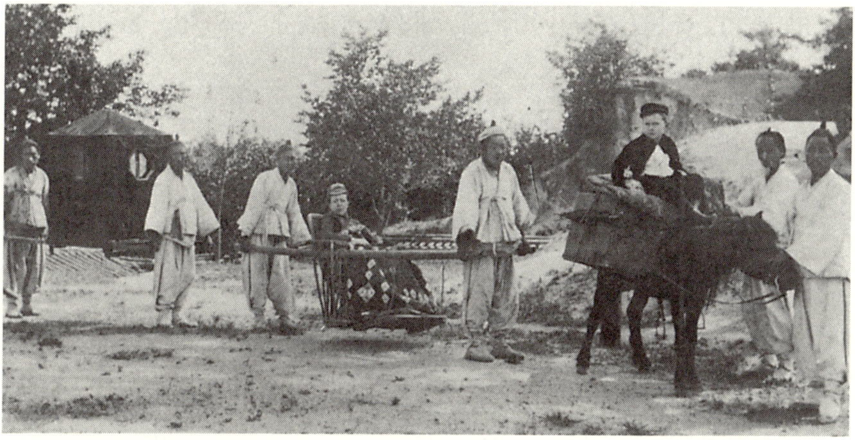

Dr. Rosetta Hall with Sherwood leaving for work in the country

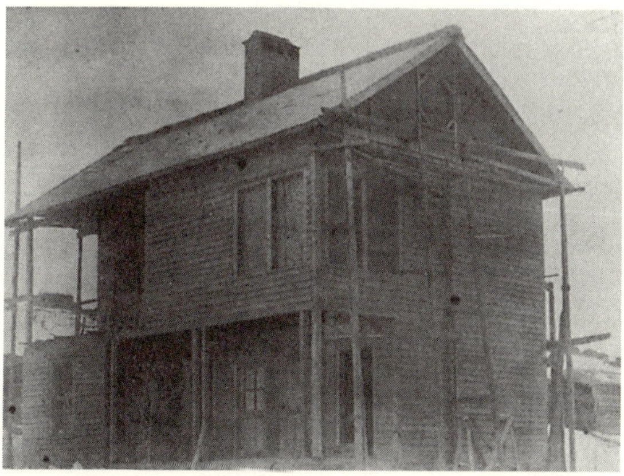

Edith Margaret Children's Ward, January 1900

When the Edith Margaret Memorial was near completion, my mother invited some little Korean girls to celebrate by giving a party for them on the fifth anniversary of Edith's birth. The reason for the celebration was explained to the children and their mothers. They were told how Edith's maternal grandmother always sent a silver dollar to her grandchildren on their birthday and how the last one sent to Edith was providing for this treat. My mother said that the memorial building in which they were meeting was God's wonderful answer to prayer.

The following year, 1901, my mother wrote sadly in her diary:

> "Dearest Grandma, we can't see her again in this world—God took her home May 5th, while we were in China, just about the time Sherwood was writing her. It is a great grief. . . . The night we received the news Sherwood did all he could to comfort mama . . . He seemed to realize what it meant to us both."

Although I remember my mother's weeping when she received this news, it was not until years later that I understood the battle with grief that lay beneath my mother's courageous exterior. I was reading the journal which my mother kept for Edith and came upon the following entry recorded on May 23, 1900, the second anniversary of Edith's death:

> "'*A voice was heard in Ramah, lamentation, and bitter weeping; Rahel weeping for her children refused to be comforted for her children, because they were not.*'
>
> Jeremiah 31:15"

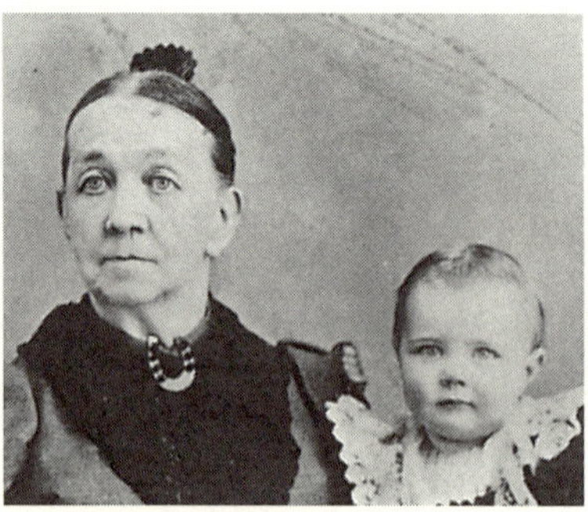

Phoebe Gildersleeve Sherwood and granddaughter, Edith Margaret, May 1896

"'The's a good many different sorts an' kinds o' sorro' that's in some ways kind o' kin to each other, but I guess losin' a child's a specie by itself. . . . The's some sorro's that the happenin' o' things helps ye to fergit, I guess the's some that the happenin' o' things keeps ye rememberin', an' losin' a child's one o' 'em.'

From *David Harum*"

"This day finds mama and Sherwood at Shanghai, China. Our darling Edith has been gone two long years, and as we see Ruth [Noble] and Gretchen [Jones] and Mary [Appenzeller], we can't help but to wonder what she would have been like now. . . . Perhaps it is because mama is not feeling well, but somehow the loss of her little daughter grows harder and harder to bear . . .

"Not long after writing this mama had such a nice talk with dear Mrs. Fitch of Shanghai. She seems to have gotten into perfect harmony with God and his plans, and it makes mama long to do likewise. But so many times mama has earnestly tried to get in closer relations with God, and even with dear papa's help never quite succeeded, that she finally thought it could not be for her, and that she must not covet such experiences. At least they were not for her yet. Mama is so material, and these experiences seem to be for the more spiritual. Our natures are not alike and we can't expect like experiences. Yet, mama can't help longing for a *happier* experience, and she has tried to lay her Isaac on the altar, and to let God do with her the best he can. And even where she may have succeeded in this, it seems as if God himself *has taken* her most precious things . . .

"She has tried to learn the lessons he would have her [learn], and not be rebellious. But somehow, as time goes on, even the faint outlines that at first she thought she could discern of these lessons, have grown dim, and more dim, and there has been no result. . . . Of late, rebellious feelings do arise sometimes, and she feels farther away than before these great losses came into her life. Something is wrong no doubt.

"Mrs. Fitch said that mama couldn't help feeling the heaviness of her losses. And neither could she expect to understand just how it could be better for her and Sherwood that papa and Edith should be removed, but she must just give her feelings over to Jesus and trust him implicitly. Mama has surely tried to do this. But as she told Mrs. Fitch, it has been more because there seemed nothing else to do, in sort of a stoical way; not counting it a privilege so to do, in this particular loss, and secretly feeling that she could have trusted him better if he had not taken her precious ones away.

"Now this is a plain fact we fear, though very unbecoming of a Christian and a missionary to say. Mama has been trying to examine her heart. It is hard to diagnose one's own case, but one trouble seems to be that she can't quite bring herself to where she *wants* to feel that these losses were best . . . Somehow as yet she can't *will* to have these wounds closed. It would seem like forgetting her dear ones. So, foolish as it may seem, and short-sighted as no doubt later it will look even to her, she goes on hugging those wounds, really refusing to have them healed! Though, up to the present, she has never quite realized it. Putting it into words makes it seem worse. If God were to heal those wounds in spite of herself, . . . she realizes it would be blessed. But for herself to *will* it seems, somehow, she knows not how to express the *feeling*, but in cold words something like sacrilege!

"This is a queer state of feeling to be in. The more she thinks of it, the more foolish it seems, for she knows those very loved ones would not have it for a moment. As much as papa loved mama he desired her soul's good above all. Poor stupid mama, she knows she has grown very dull of late. It has been all work and no play, and promises to continue to be. Something must be done. May God continue to have mercy on her. May his Holy Spirit teach her and bring her out of this low spiritual state. '*Thou has chastised me, and I was chastised, as a bullock unaccustomed to the yoke; turn thou me, and I shall be turned; for thou art the Lord my God.*'"

The "promise of more work" certainly came to pass, and judging by all she accomplished, it would seem her prayer for guidance also came to be. My mother's work with the blind claimed her attention soon after her return from that vacation in China.

One of the initial uses of the newly completed Children's Wards was to temporarily house four blind girls whom my mother had begun to teach. Her teaching aids were those she had prepared and adapted to the Korean language from the New York Point system. During the winter of her return to Korea, she had spent her spare moments transcribing Korean teaching materials to the system. These included the Korean alphabet, syllabary, *A Korean Primer* written by Mrs. George Heber Jones, and the Ten Commandments. She did this by pricking the appropriate dots with a pin in stiff Korean oiled paper which resembled cardboard.

After moving to Pyong Yang, my mother had started working again with Mr. O's blind daughter, Pongnai. Teaching Pongnai with these new resources was at first slow and tedious work, but once she had mastered the alphabet and the syllabary, it was plain sailing. In a year, Pongnai could read all that my mother had been able to prepare and she learned to write in point and to make her own lessons from dictation. My mother also taught her to knit.

Patients, seeing Pongnai so happy and industrious, would ask my mother if other blind girls they knew might join her. Thus began the first school for the blind in Korea, and after the Pyong Yang Girls' School was built, a classroom for blind girls was added. My mother's belief was that the blind girls should be taught together with the seeing girls and should participate in their games. All that was necessary was to add a special teacher to the school staff for the beginners. Pongnai eventually became such a teacher as the work for the blind and deaf expanded.

The week following my sixth birthday, my mother had planned another country trip. This time she had been invited to visit the thirty-nine churches which were the outgrowth of the church my father had started in Pyong Yang. Susan No, Mother's capable Korean assistant in the dispensary, was to accompany us. Susan also served in the role of "Bible Woman," reading to the patients from the Scriptures.

Our caravan was made up of three pack ponies and their *mapoos* (drivers). The packs were arranged so that the medicines and supplies were carried in boxes hung on each side of the pony. The bedding on which we sat was spread out on top of it all. A small guard rail supported our backs or, in case of need, could be grabbed to keep one's balance. Everything was strapped on quite firmly. When we needed to give some relief to the ponies and wanted a chance to stretch our legs, we drew alongside some roadside bank and easily jumped off. It was a lot of fun, especially for a young boy.

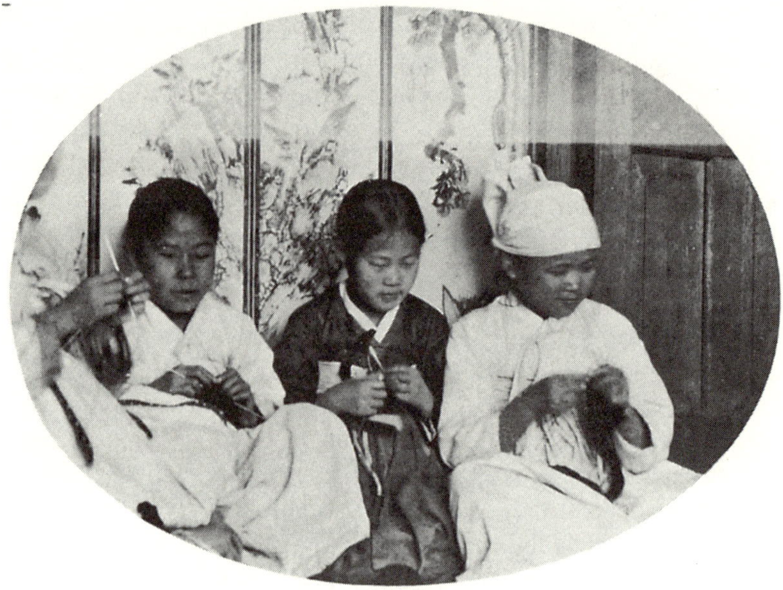

Knitting class in the school for the blind begun by Dr. Rosetta Hall in Pyong Yang

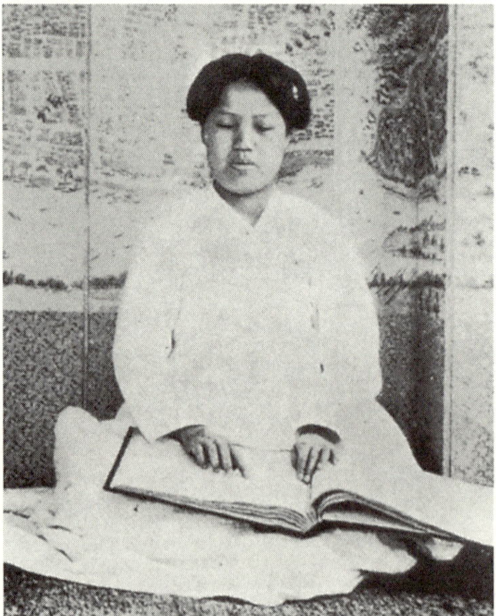

Pongnai, the first blind Korean to study by means of embossed books

The ponies had bells slung around their necks which made quite a "jingle-jangle." We created no small sensation as we passed through the towns and villages, bringing forth such exclamations as, "*Po ra! Po Ra!*" (See! See!) from the curious onlookers. The people, for the most part, received us gladly, and clamored for treatment and medicine. Our nights were spent in the local inns where only the liberal use of kerosene and insect powder kept us free of the bedbugs and lice which were always a part of the "company" at the inns.

After passing through the walled city of An Chu (Anju), we had to cross the Chyong-chyong (Chongchon) River to Unsan. We dismounted, and pack ponies and all were ferried across the river in a flat-bottomed boat. The Oriental Consolidated Mining Company, known more familiarly to us as "the American gold mines," operated a shipping point here for the gold ore mined at Cheraepalpe six miles to the north.

On the night of November 18 we reached Unsan and the home of Mr. O and his wife, Susanna. Both were Korean Bible workers who had been established in this area by the Reverend D. A. Bunker in order to bring the Christian message to that mining community. Mr. Bunker had been one of the ministers who had officiated at my parents' wedding.

Because the custom of female seclusion was stricter here than in Pyong Yang, Susanna had found Bible work among the women to be especially difficult. Susanna had a daughter, Lucy, with whom I enjoyed playing. Although Lucy was older than I, she was smaller in size. She had attended the mission school and was proving quite helpful to her parents' efforts because she was able to teach the women to read.

I had been looking forward to visiting the American gold mines ever since I had met Mr. and Mrs. D. A. Bunker in Pyong Yang the previous summer. The Bunkers were then missionaries in the Unsan area and had told me all about the processing of gold and the other operations of the mines. They were especially kind to me and had patiently answered my endless questions. Their descriptions had made me very eager to visit the mines.

The mining operation at Cheraepalpe was a pleasant walk of five or six miles beyond Unsan. As we came over the last hill, we saw spread out below a little piece of America. There were wooden houses, two and three stories high, with shingled roofs and glass windows and brick chimneys. The sounds of the push and bustle

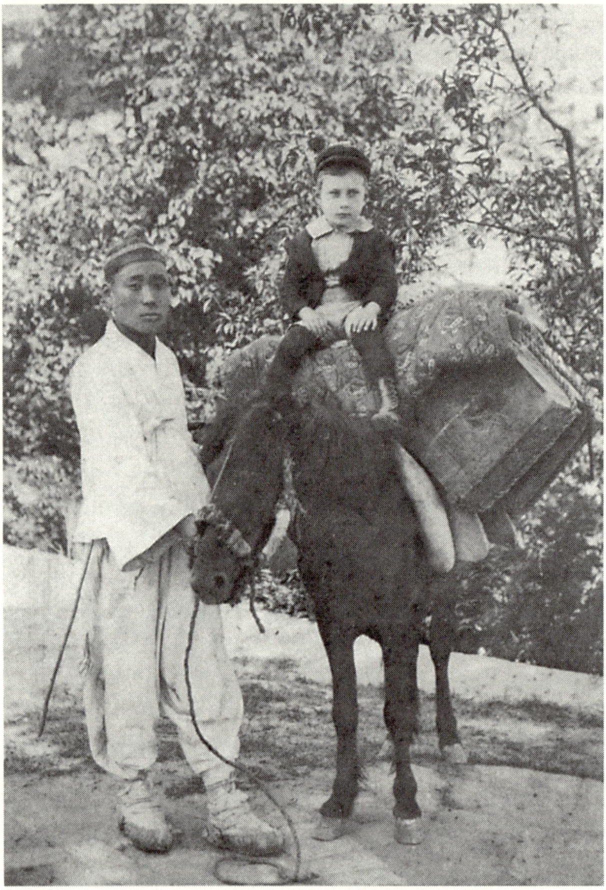

Sherwood, age six, on second country trip with his mother, 1899

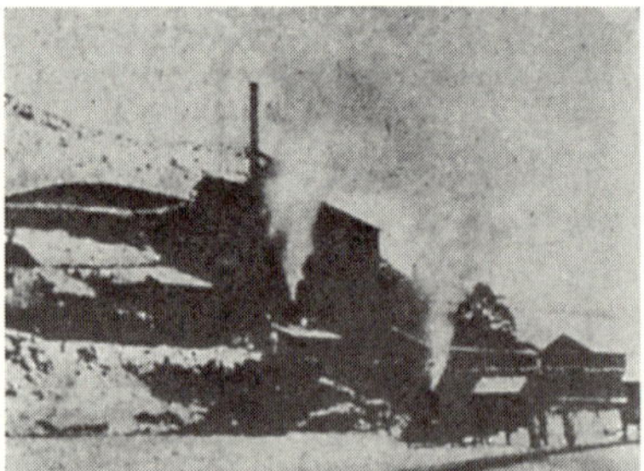

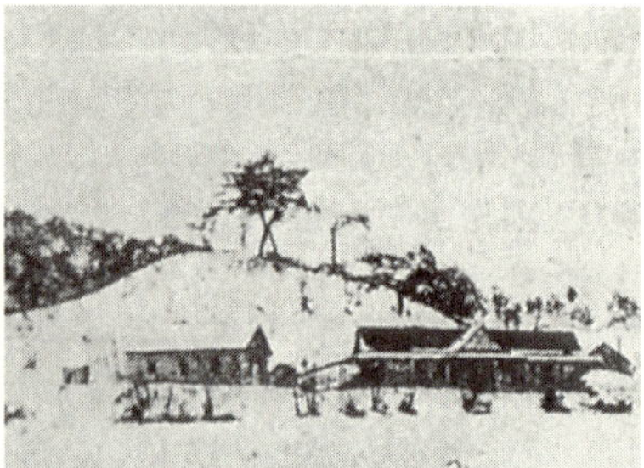

American Consolidated Gold Mining Works and homes of American employees at Cheraepalpe, six miles north of Unsan

of American enterprise greeted our ears as a noon whistle sounded and machines, wheelbarrows, carts and wagons were everywhere in motion.

I was thrilled to be taken down a mine shaft, holding a lighted candle and marching in single file. There, many feet beneath the ground, we watched the miners at work and saw the huge buckets of ore sent up from the shafts still deeper below. The processing of the ore was patiently explained to me, and for years I treasured the small fragment of gold ore given to me as a souvenir. To the untrained eye the ore looked like mere stone, although we were shown some pure gold at the office which had a yellow-brassy color. It was explained that most of the gold was exported in the form of amalgum.

Most of the Americans at the mines were away from mothers, wives or sisters and they told us it was a red-letter day to be visited by a woman and a little boy. My pockets were stuffed with all the candy and nuts they could hold.

Our host, Mr. Taylor, Superintendent of the Mines, insisted on furnishing us with an armed escort on our way back through the mountains, which were reputed to be infested by robbers and tigers. My mother protested, but I thought it was a capital idea and hoped that a tiger might be shot en route. I was not quite so enthusiastic about the robbers. We returned to Pyong Yang without mishap from either.

Our nearest white neighbors were the Nobles, who were also my parents' dearest friends during those early days in Korea. This friendship had continued and served to double our joy in times of happiness and to halve our sorrow in times of grief. Frequently, I would go to the Nobles to play with Ruth and her younger brothers. They, in turn, would play at our house. Ruth had a real flair for dramatics. She had written a charming, vividly imaginative play which she called "Power Woman," in which she had the boys dress up in the strangest costumes. Ruth patiently drilled us to play our respective roles and although it was great fun, I found out early that I had no talent for the stage.

Our fun often included Mr. Noble's young Korean secretary who wanted to learn conversational English by associating with us in his spare time. He had a young wife who also worked at the Nobles and had the same ambition. These two Korean friends introduced us, in turn, to the joys and skills of Korean games.

The boys were taught how to fly "fighting kites" which was a popular sport in Korea then. The goal was to down your opponent's kite and keep your own flying high. Small bits of broken glass were glued to the string near the kite, and the object was to cut the other fellow's kite before he cut yours. This required considerable skill and the secretary proved a patient and able instructor. The girls of our group learned how to play see-saw standing up, the art being to see how high one could jump without falling off the see-saw.

In the winter months the Korean children would join us and show us how to make a Korean type of snowman with a long stick for a pipe. They also enjoyed whipping their hand-carved wooden tops on a cleared area of ice, making them spin merrily. They would then invite us to try it and would laugh at our frantic attempts. Our tops merely balked. However, Mr. Noble's secretary taught us the technique and we persisted in our efforts. By the time winter was over, we could keep our tops spinning almost as long as those of our Korean playmates.

We children grew fond of these sports and our enthusiastic teachers. Sometimes our games were interrupted by the arrival of a pack-pony caravan on its way to the American gold mines at Unsan. One pony always bore two heavily guarded mysterious wooden boxes which were carried into the missionary bungalow.

We later learned that they contained Korean silver dollars called *won*, for the salary of the Korean workers at the mines. They preferred to be paid in silver coins rather than in paper money. Because there were no banks in Pyong Yang at the time, it was thought safer to keep the wooden boxes in the missionary bungalow. The other equipment was deposited at a Korean inn nearby.

This arrangement worked well at first, but one time it was noted by the American officer in charge of the caravan that the boxes seemed lighter when reloading them onto the pony. Sure enough, on counting the silver coins, it was discovered that some of the coins were missing, even though they had been guarded and the inner closet door had been carefully locked.

Since no thief could be found, the question was, "What to do?" Someone remarked that he had seen several steel spring bear traps in the equipment in the storage room at the mine. He suggested that these traps might be used to catch the thief.

On the next trip the plan was put into effect. Some protested strongly, especially Mr. Noble; but finally his objections were overruled. Openings were cut in the lids of the wooden boxes only big enough to insert a hand. The traps were then placed on top of the silver coins in the boxes and the lids closed back.

Since the closet was dark, the thief would not be able to see the trap, and would probably thrust in his hand and literally be caught red handed. It was predicted that some dangerous criminal would be found in this way.

However, to the surprise of all, especially to Mr. Noble, the criminal trapped was his beloved secretary. In fact, the unlikely thief had been able to drag the heavy wooden box some distance before the armed guards found him in a faint from loss of blood.

The guards opened the box and unsprung the trap, but his hand had been badly mutilated. Since he was still bleeding profusely, he was rushed to the nearest hospital which happened to be where my mother was working. She checked the bleeding and dressed the wounded hand. But what hurt the patient most was the disgrace that he felt he had brought to his parents and the missionaries. He begged to be forgiven. I also put in a plea to forgive him, for I had grown to love him.

The officer of the gold mines agreed not to turn him over to the authorities, and instead, assigned him to the custody of the missionaries. At the time, Korean laborers were being recruited to go to work in the sugar cane and pineapple plantations of Hawaii. It was decided that the secretary had suffered enough punishment and justice would best be served by sending him and his young wife to Hawaii. This plan was promptly carried out.

Spring was the time of year for traditional stone throwing contests in Korea. Two teams competed, each chosen for their ability to throw stones the farthest. The older boys would spend hours polishing and rounding stones for their favorite team. These competitions drew large crowds, as boxing matches do in the West. The arena was just outside the city wall, and the wide top of that wall near our house served as the viewing stand. It was thus a very great temptation for me to go over and join the crowds watching this dangerous sport. Sometimes, the contestants' stones fell into the crowd, making it really quite a hazardous sport both for participants and onlookers. My mother, therefore, discouraged me from watching it.

Sometimes the excitement grew so intense, however, and the stone throwing yells (*Oo-you-ya! Oo-you-ya! Ka-ja! Ka-ja!*) so compelling, that I too would be carried away in the fervor of it all, and would run to join the mad crowds to see which side was winning. I took my just punishment without resentment, for I knew I deserved it.

Another thing for which we children were severely reprimanded was playing hide-and-seek under the huge hats of the Korean ladies. These were too large to be brought into church and so were stacked outside. In the South, ladies used light green cloaks to hide their faces when on the streets, but in the North, the ladies wore very large basket-like contraptions. These covered up their heads, but were supported by their hands. If a man came into view, all the lady had to do to hide her face was to tilt the hat forward over her head.

What excellent devices these hats provided for a good game of hide-and-seek! While their owners were at a meeting, we would hide under the headgear and the person who was "it" would have to guess under which hats his playmates might be concealed.

But life could not continue to be all play and the question arose of what to do about my "three R's." In Chefoo, China, where my parents had enjoyed their honeymoon, there was an English-type school operated by the China Inland Mission. However, that school was 300 miles from Pyong Yang across the Yellow Sea. My mother was not keen on sending me so far away to school, for I was only six years old.

Another Pyong Yang family, the W. L. Swallens, were faced with the same problem. (The Reverend Swallen was one of the original group of Presbyterian missionaries who had come to Pyong Yang to purchase property for the Presbyterian Church shortly after my father had been successful in opening his mission in the city.) Mrs. Swallen had been giving lessons to her own children and had allowed me to join them, but both my mother and the Swallens realized that soon this would be inadequate. They felt a growing urgency to procure a teacher who could meet the educational needs of the children of missionaries without having to resort to sending them to Chefoo.

Thus it came about that my mother and the Swallens decided to establish a school for missionary children. Other families soon joined the effort. Dr. and Mrs. William M. Baird, Sr., Presbyterian missionaries also in Pyong Yang, had three boys who were nearing school age. Since the Bairds were about to set out for America on furlough, they agreed to assume the task of trying to secure a teacher for the school. It eventually became known as the "Pyong Yang Foreign

School." Later it was to attract students from all over Korea and even from China, Japan and other parts of Asia. Olivette and Gertrude Swallen, John Baird and I were among the first scholars at its inception in June, 1900 but very soon others joined us.

Qualified teachers were brought out from America. They were mostly single ladies who often married on the mission field. The school was patterned after those in the United States. My mother had proposed that the courses prescribed by the New York Board of Regents be followed in order that the students would have no difficulty when transferring to American schools. This proved to be the case. The Pyong Yang Foreign School had no dropouts and most of the students went on to higher learning.

Our first teacher was Miss Louise Ogilvy who had been recruited at a missionary meeting which the Bairds were conducting in Topeka, Kansas while on furlough. Miss Ogilvy and her mother had attended the meeting, and upon hearing of the need for a teacher to teach the children of the missionary families, she told her mother that she was moved to respond. Since she was only 18 years old, both the Bairds and her mother demurred. However, by the time the Bairds were

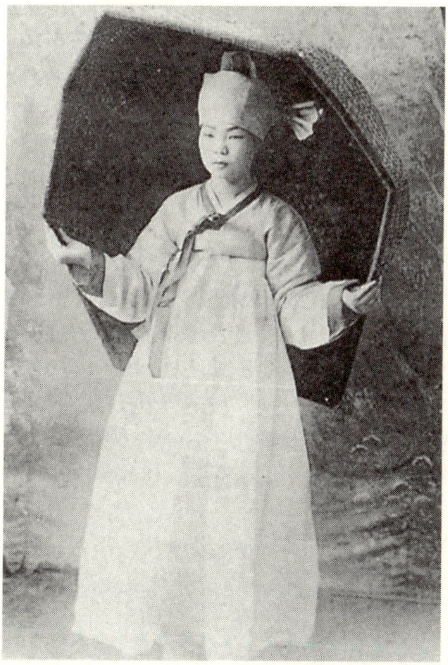

A lady of Pyong Yang with a basket hat

ready to return to Korea, no one else had volunteered. They contacted Miss Ogilvy and agreed with her that God must have intended her for the job. She later married the Reverend Charles D. Morris, a Methodist missionary then stationed in Pyong Yang. I remember that while she and Mr. Morris were courting, they caught me spying on them through the window of the schoolroom. For my snooping I received a well deserved spanking.

The school was located outside the city wall in the Presbyterian compound, where most of the scholars lived. We children of the Methodist Mission, who lived inside the city, had to walk or ride a donkey about a mile to reach the school. Although I tried to train our large calf to take me, she had little interest in the trip, preferring the grass along the roadside. Finally, a relative in New York sent me out a bicycle. However, as it was the first one in the city, it attracted too much attention. Pedestrians, like chickens, often would change their minds without warning and after starting across my path, would suddenly retrace their steps. I would frequently land among a wriggling heap of humanity. Some were good natured, but others heaped invectives on my already bruised head and made me wonder if walking might be less painful.

Esther Pak had returned to Korea from the United States with her M.D. degree in 1900. She was a great help to my mother in her expanding medical work. In her first ten months of practice, Esther treated over 3,000 patients. We were all very proud of her, for she was the first Korean to study Western medicine. Her husband, Yousan, who had remained in the United States to help support Esther through medical school, became a victim of tuberculosis while working in a Baltimore restaurant. Esther nursed him through his illness until his death which occurred during her final year at the Women's Medical College of Baltimore (Johns Hopkins University).

I had grown very fond of Esther. She lived with us and seemed like one of the family. She had a sweet melodious voice and used to read to me in the evenings from such books as *The Last Days of Pompeii*, by Edward Bulwer-Lytton; *The Spy*, and other novels by James Fenimore Cooper; and the stories and poems of Sir Walter Scott.

In a letter begun on November 23, 1900 while on a country trip, my mother wrote:

> "Soon after Esther returned, when I was talking about the great need of work among the country women, and that

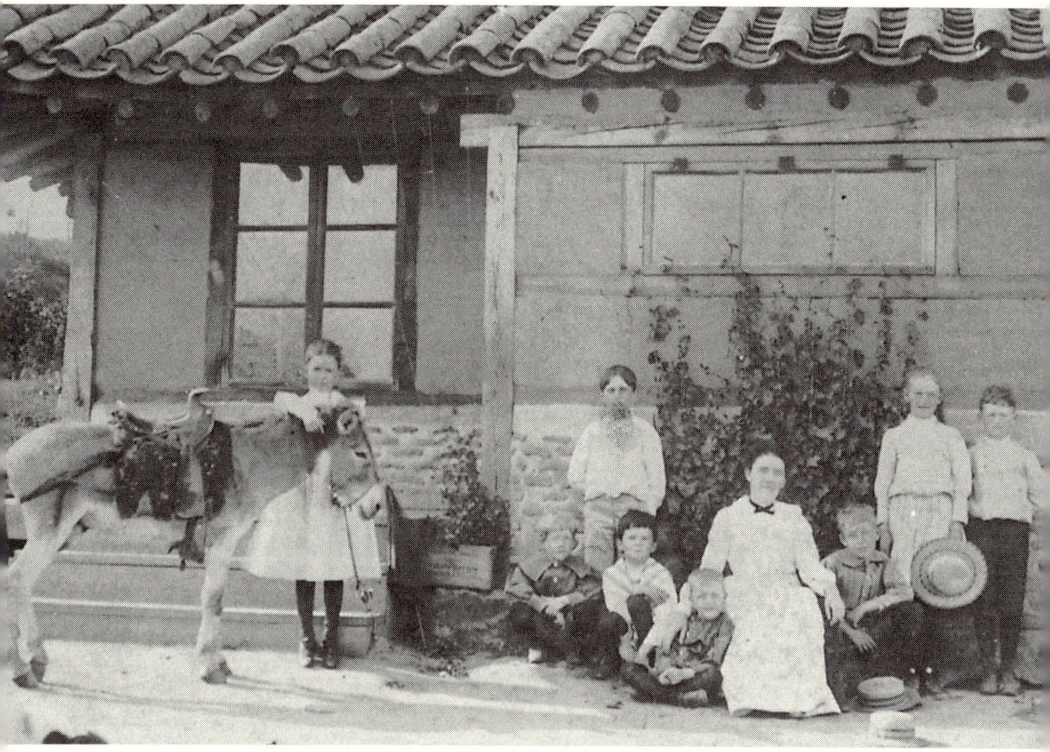

Pyong Yang Foreign School for the children of missionaries (Ruth Noble, left; Sherwood, 3rd from left; Miss Armstrong, the school's second teacher, center)

now I hoped we could do more of it, she asked to be excused from it this year. So I left Sherwood and the dispensary and children's wards in her charge, shut up my house and brought my cook . . . and Susan, and came myself.

"Sherwood goes to school now mornings and afternoons too, so these short days he is gone from prayer-time to dark. He loves Korean food, and Esther will of course see he doesn't get anything he shouldn't have. He will sleep in Susan's room with Pongnai, my blind pupil-teacher, and his *Amah* will look after washing and dressing him, taking him to school, putting to bed, etc., so I feel he will be all right. At first he felt badly about my not taking him, but then he loves his school; and when he found he could have Korean food just the same as if he went to the country, he was comforted. . . .

"On Saturday preceding the Tuesday I planned to leave . . . Sherwood was taken sick and the next day his temperature arose to 104.5°. . . . Monday it went down through the day without again rising. . . . However, I deferred my trip a day. On Tuesday Sherwood was quite well again and Wednesday morning he went to school, and we started on our trip in spite of another discouraging thing that I learned the day before.

"Mr. Noble came in upon Tuesday with a copy of a telegram from Dr. Underwood at HaiChu [Haeju] for Mr. Moffett in Latin as follows: '*Omnibus praefactis mandatum secrets mittus est in mensis decimi idibus mones chretians occident*,' which means that there have been secret orders to all the magistrates to kill all the Christians 15 days from that time–*à la* Boxers. We had heard rumors of such placards being up in the northern districts before, and we don't know whether it really means anything or not; but Mrs. Noble thought I ought not to take the trip now. She was so opposed to it, that I began to feel that if others too felt that way, that I might have to give it up. However, after talking to Dr. Follwell, Mr. Lee and Mr. Morris, I decided to go, only to cut the trip a little short. You see everyone feels so long as we have had no word from our Consuls, who must be on the alert for these things now after the lesson in China, that we better not disturb our Christian natives with such reports, and not needlessly scare them half to death as it would. As my horse and all were engaged, time set, and boxes packed, to suddenly stop now after surmounting all the other difficulties, and stay at home without giving a good reason, they would surely suspect something. And if there should be nothing in the report, it would cause needless anxiety, and the work of my country trip would remain undone. I had calculated anyhow to get back before the prescribed time for the killing to take place, and now I will go a day or two sooner, and I feel all will be well. I do hope it will prove a false alarm, and that we may not have to go through what they have in China."

After describing her visits to several villages, my mother's letter continued:

"Sunday afternoon we visited two other villages nearby where work has been begun from here; had one room full of women and one of men in each place. At one place they implored me to go in and see an insane woman.

"Poor soul, she is a bright good-looking woman of 34, a widow for three years, with two children—taken crazy, they claim, only four months ago upon a visit to Pyong Yang. For three and a half months now they have kept her shut in a tight room with but one door—no window—just unpapered mud walls and floor—no mats—no nothing—a gourd shell contained a little pigs feed. The odor of the room was worse than any pig pen.

"When she was first taken sick, they had *mudangs* to dance and make their racket about her for 20 days—they also pounded her to drive the spirits out, and burned her in various places so deeply she still has the scabs over the ulcers thus made. After this treatment, she was so demented that they had to shut her up the way I found her, filthy and lousy.

"She would answer questions intelligently as long as you could hold her attention, but her mind seemed constantly wandering, and she would try to catch the devils she kept seeing, and would sing much like a *mudang*. She is certainly insane, but I believe if she could have proper medicine, food and treatment she might be well again. I would like to try it and see. As I told them, a well person would be driven insane to be shut up in a cell like that and be treated like a pig. (They'd not have a pig pounded and burned that way.) Why, they burned her vulva every night for six nights, as well as back and top of head.

"We had one insane patient already in the children's wards—she tried to drown herself when she first came—jumped in the cistern I was digging and had stopped on account of the rainy season. We rescued her, but she got so much water in her lungs, that she had a light pneumonia. And during the time she was really sick, she obeyed so well, eating her food and medicine (she had refused to eat for four days before she came to us), that she was really better after she got over the pneumonia than before.

"I set her to piecing some of the bright calicoes that came in a box from East Orange, and she pieced a whole quilt, becoming very interested in it. She went to church, and desired to be taken on probation—said grace before meals and was fond of her children again—in fact, was practically well when I discharged her.

"But before she jumped in the cistern, she was a great care to Susan. She climbed out of the window one night when Susan was sleeping alone with her with the doors locked. It was a dark rainy night and we had a great time to find her when Susan missed her. I decided then to take no more such cases until I had a proper place and more help. But now I have Esther and her sister extra, if I can fix up one of our wards for it, I would like to take in these pitiable cases. . . . If I only get money enough appropriated, I'd like to build two more wards than I have planned for—one for contagious cases and one for the insane."

The letter described the remainder of the country trip and then concluded with a final comment written on December 1:

"Reached home Wednesday, November 28 in time for Thanksgiving Day this year. A year ago we spent Thanksgiving on the road I remember. . . .

"Had a pretty hard journey home, it was so muddy. It would be better to make this trip when the ground is frozen again. Got home 3:30 P.M. in time for me to go and bring Sherwood home from school. It seemed good to see my brave little boy again. He had gotten on nicely during my eight days' absence. I left him in Esther's care you remember. She had carried on the dispensary during my absence and also saw to the two patients in the children's ward, and made the necessary outcalls—so she was busy and happy.

"I feel it a great privilege, indeed, to have the work thus skillfully cared for during my absence, and I mean to have her continue while I get caught up a little in my accounts, reports and building plans. Also hope to make some advancement in work for the blind. Have four nice girls now in this department of our day school, but I need to get out more work for the pupil-teacher.

"As you can imagine, it was with some anxiety that I asked the first missionary I met for 'news' [of the plan to slay all the Christians]. I soon learned that the warning was well founded—and that shortly after I left, a letter came from the U.S. Minister saying that no women could be allowed to visit the country, and that even the men better not—and all were to have a care. He thought the present trouble averted. But such orders as I wrote of in the early part of this letter (including not only Christians, but *all foreigners*, to be killed) . . . were actually sent out through Confucian schools to all the magistrates. And one magistrate favorable to Christians (in fact himself a Christian), at the risk of his life should it be found out, took a copy of the order and sent it to the U.S. Minister Allen."

After missionaries have served a number of years on the mission field, it is customary for them to return to the homeland for a furlough. During this time they may undertake postgraduate studies to keep them current in their area of specialization. My mother's furlough had come due and we left for America in June, 1901.

CHAPTER 8

White Boy in the Hermit Kingdom

Toward the close of my mother's furlough in the late summer of 1902 I was given a pair of Belgian hares to take back to Korea. The hares accompanied us to London, our first "port o' call." Here we found that our steamship reservations had been unexpectedly cancelled, and due to the Coronation of Edward VII, all passenger lines were booked full for weeks ahead. It looked as if we might be marooned in London indefinitely. As it happened, we were there for six weeks.

I found London to be most interesting, but Mother was vexed by the delay and left no stone unturned to find passage for us to the Orient. During this time I would take my rabbits out for a hop in a small park near our boarding place. One day they encountered an organ grinder's monkey who seemed to have it in for bunnies. When the monkey attacked my pets, I jumped to their rescue and, in the process, was scratched and bitten until the organ grinder called off his animal.

One evening after Mother had been trudging around all day to various steamship offices, she returned smiling. She announced, "I have been able to book our passage to Kobe, Japan on a freighter, the *Glen Logan*, and though it sails via the Black Sea, we shall be able to get to Korea sooner than waiting for a passenger ship."

Our freighter was to load tin from Swansea, Wales and exchange it for kerosene at the Port of Batum (Batumi), Georgia which is at the "toe" end of the Black Sea. This shipment of kerosene was to be distributed at Shanghai and Kobe where oil products were in great demand.

I eagerly looked forward to the trip. Because the ship was a freighter, I would be able to roam wherever I wished. In addition, I would be allowed to care for my pets. By this time a tom turkey and two hen turkeys had been added to the menagerie. I had purchased them in Swansea.

The captain warned me, however, that if the ship was delayed, they might have to serve up the birds for some special occasion, such as a Christmas dinner. But Christmas was a long way off and I felt confident that he was just kidding, so I did not allow the remark to worry me. During the voyage the care and feeding of my animals kept me well occupied. The only other passengers were W.F.M.S. missionaries, Dr. Mary M. Cutler of Seoul, and Miss Margaret J. Edmunds, a nurse appointed to my mother's hospital in Pyong Yang.

From the Mediterranean, we entered the Aegean Sea with its fabulous isles. We then passed through the Dardanelles (which the ancients called the Hellespont), separating Europe from Asia Minor, into the Sea of Marmara. When we approached Constantinople, as Istanbul was then known, we saw an unusual sight. The numerous mosques and minarets were lighted up in a snow storm through which the sun was shining. This gave the city the appearance of an enormous sparkling jewel.

The voyage so far had been quite smooth sailing, but when we left the short Bosporous Straits, we encountered a raging storm in the Black Sea. Waves seemingly mountain high broke upon us with great fury and swept unchecked over our decks. No passengers were allowed on deck and I was concerned about my pets. I found out later that one of the crew had taken pity on them and had fed them. How relieved we were to reach the haven of Batum.

This was indeed a strange city. It was inhabited by people of various races, especially the fierce looking Georgian men who wore cartridge belts criss-crossed from shoulder to waist in which were tucked a pistol and a dagger. The Russian Cossacks, armed to the hilt and riding on fiery chargers, policed the turbulent area. Here one did not have to go West to see "Westerns," for actual shootings often occurred in the streets when the Cossacks rode rough shod through the crowd, madly discharging their guns or wildly waving their big curved swords.

When there was no unloading of our cargo of tin week after week, our usually jovial Captain James McGregor turned into a dour Scotsman. The delay was first due to the rainy season, which was then in progress, and after that, to strikes, and then to race riots, and finally, to holidays.

At times we ventured forth on land for a stroll, or for a ride to the attractive countryside in a picturesque Russian *drosky* with quaint wooden arches over the shoulders of the horses. The bearded drivers looked so fierce that it was easy to imagine they were driving us directly to a den of thieves.

Eventually, we were able to communicate to a driver that we wanted to visit the U.S.A. consulate. Here we were most warmly welcomed by the James C. Chambers and were urged to come back to a Thanksgiving dinner in several days. I was relieved to know that my turkeys would now be spared their traditional role. When we were on the point of leaving after a wonderful dinner, the consul's family invited us to have Christmas dinner with them, for in this out-of-the-way place they too were lonesome for fellowship with those of their own kind. We thanked them for the cordial invitation, but as it would take only a few days to unload and then reload another cargo, we declined. We assured them that in all likelihood our ship would be sailing long before then. They gave us a knowing smile and said, "We shall be expecting you for Christmas."

Sure enough we were back for a delicious Christmas dinner at the consulate, and my turkeys escaped another potential hazard. It was explained to us that although the strikes were over, there were now prolonged Christmas holidays. It seemed that because of the various religious groups in this area, there were *three* different dates for

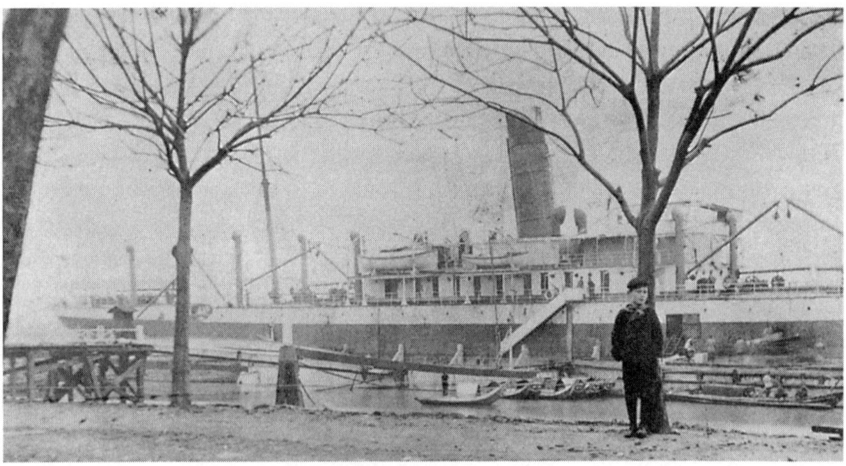

Sherwood in front of freighter SS Glen Logan

Christmas. Furthermore, no one group would allow other groups to work while the former was celebrating its own Christmas holidays.

Other ships which also were being delayed anchored near us. A few of these had children about my own age on board and we used to take turns visiting each other's vessels and comparing them. Each, of course, claimed his own ship was the best.

The reputed Garden of Eden was not far away. We also could see in the distance a view of Mount Ararat, the traditional resting place of Noah's Ark. Although these trips beckoned us, Mother decided against yielding to such temptations. She did not wish to risk being stranded here for any more months.

One day when we returned from a short excursion into town, we were delighted to see the longshoremen unloading our cargo. They swarmed like bees all over the ship and worked in shifts night and day under arc lights. Before we knew it, the old cargo had been discharged and the new cargo of kerosene loaded. The whistle blew a deafening blast. The workers swarmed down the sides of the ship, the crew closed the hatches, and the anchor was raised amid great rejoicing.

Captain McGregor came out of his cabin where he had secluded himself for three months and greeted us with a smile that stretched from ear to ear. He ordered the ship's siren blown again and again as we passed the other waiting vessels whose passengers and crew must have been green with envy.

After our return to Pyong Yang in March, 1903, my mother's medical duties kept her ever busy. In addition, she had again become a builder. Sufficient donations had been received to build the women's hospital onto the wing that formed the Edith Margaret Memorial Children's Wards. The main building was to be of the same frame construction, two storied, along with staircases and galvanized iron roof and brick chimneys. These features were still a curiosity to the Korean residents of Pyong Yang and people came for miles to see the kind of structures the Western barbarians had designed.

Some exclaimed, "*Howlung howo!*" (wonderful). Others, rightly, thought that their Korean type of tiled roof with curved up corners was more artistic. But these were far more costly than galvanized iron roofing and required heavier timbers to support them. Not everyone liked the two-story idea, but here also the overruling factor was economy. In any event, the modern buildings were neat and functional, and they served to greatly enlarge and improve the hospital facilities. The new building retained the name that Governor Chyo had given to the Dispensary and was known as "*Koanghyoe Nyo Won*" or, "The Women's Hospital of Extended Grace."

The political situation in Korea during these years was tense as foreign nations attempted to establish their areas of power and influence at the expense of Korea. It was a familiar story and by February of 1904 the ominous rumblings of the Russo-Japanese War could be heard in the land. As it turned out, the war, ironically, may have saved us from fighting for our own lives.

A report reached us that we could expect an attack from the Tonghaks. Previously we had heard rumors to this effect and had taken the precaution to lay in supplies, store water, and to fill sand bags to barricade the windows. In fact, our hospital staff had been supplied with firearms and ammunition, but most of them were innocent as to how to use these weapons.

Following the Tonghak defeat of 1894, a new leader had emerged, Son Pyonghui. He had gone to Japan and sent for many young Koreans to come there to study. In 1904 when Russian-Japanese relations appeared strained, Son Pyonghui instructed the Tonghak followers in Korea to form a political party. Under the name of the Progressive Society, the political organization set about to pursue its former goals of ridding the government of corruption and paving the way, by popular force if necessary, for the political independence of Korea.

Unknown to those of us who were expecting the anti-Western attack, the leader whom Son Pyonghui had assigned to carry out the political aspects of the movement sold out the Progressive Party to the Iljinhoe, a notorious pro-Japanese group. Son Pyonghui, angered by the news, decided to divorce religion from politics, and changed the name Tonghak to Chondogyo. He returned to Korea and established more than 30 schools and over 100 preaching stations, hoping to achieve his aims of national independence through education and training. In later years the Chondogyo was to work in cooperation with Christian organizations in the cause of Korean independence. But that was later. In 1904, we were preparing for an unfriendly assault by the Tonghaks, mindful of the fate of Westerners during the Boxer rebellion in China only four years before.

Our home was situated on a hill with a large clear space in front, so we were in a good position to spot any approaching intruders. We could have withstood a siege for some time. My assignment was simply to raise a flag if attacked by day, or put a red cloth around a kerosene lamp if attacked by night. This was to serve as a signal to the Nobles, who were then to come over for refuge in our improvised fortress.

I was all keyed up for the attack and was frankly disappointed when it did not materialize. I felt that we could have given a good account of ourselves. The next day we began to surmise why the Tonghaks had not made an appearance when we looked through our binoculars.

We could see far in the distance a thin black line approaching, which turned out to be the vanguard of the Japanese army. The army engineers soon started to throw pontoon bridges across the river and the few Japanese civilians in Pyong Yang were busy repairing the breaches in the city wall near our house. Russian Cossacks had been seen just north of the city. These were reported to be huge bearded giants mounted on beautiful swift chargers.

The people were fleeing the city in droves and all shops were closed. We realized how very fortunate we were to have laid in a good reserve of supplies. To distinguish the white missionaries from the Russians, the Japanese had issued us small red, white and blue badges. These were to be concealed in our clothing and displayed only when we were challenged.

As there had been no fighting, I had gone that morning as usual to our school outside the city wall. However, on my return, I found Japanese sentries guarding the city gate. One of these soldiers roughly grabbed me. I was not worried and I proudly displayed my badge. I could soon see that he had never heard of it, and evidently thought I might be a Russian spy sent to find out the Japanese strength and positions. I knew then I might be in for real trouble.

They spoke neither Korean nor English and several so-called spies had already been shot on the merest suspicion. So I gesticulated frantically, trying to communicate by using sign language. I pointed in the direction of our house. By chance, a passing officer, who spoke some Korean, noticed my arms wildly waving and stopped just long enough to find out what all the fuss was about. He at once sent one of his subordinates to check, and upon verification, I was released.

The fighting this time was not at Pyong Yang, but north of it, although near enough so that the Japanese brought their war dead to the bank of our river for cremation (they do not bury their dead). This was indeed a ghoulish sight for a young boy to witness as they heaped up hundreds of bodies on the funeral pyres. When the pyres started to burn, the bodies seemed to twist and turn, and some even appeared to sit upright as if they were alive.

After the war, I visited "203 meter hill" at Port Arthur where one of the crucial battles was fought. Here I was shown the wide, deep trench which the Russians had dug to defend the hill, and which had been filled instantly with live Japanese volunteers so their comrades could walk over their bodies to victory. I picked up a shell fragment from the hill as a souvenir.

The turkeys I had introduced to Korea were still thriving. Some Japanese soldiers returning from fighting the Russians were very curious about these birds and stopped to look at them. My two gobblers seemed to have it in for anyone in uniform and boldly attacked these men, who then retreated in great haste. Perhaps my turkeys were just showing their resentment for my previous capture at the city gate.

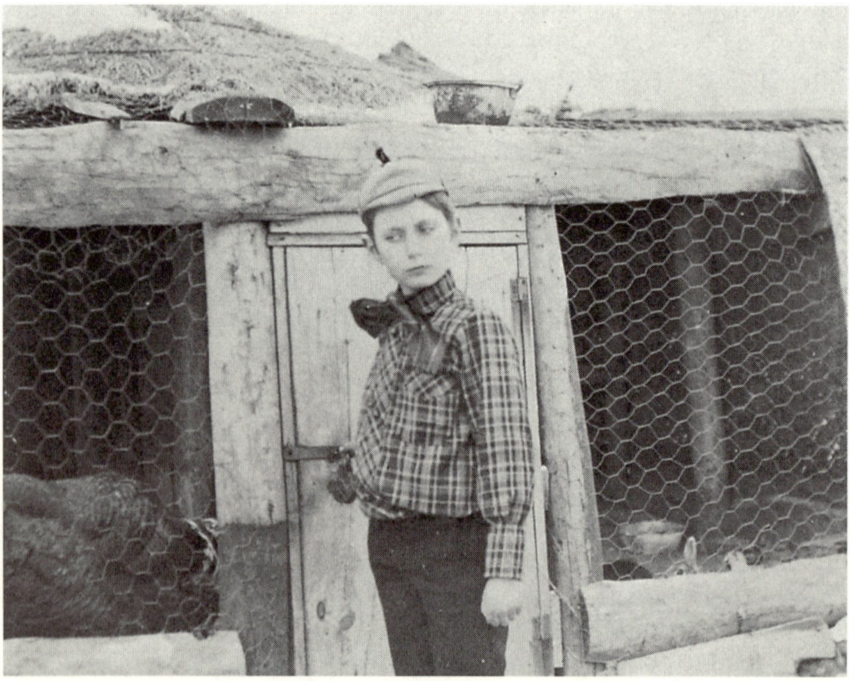

Sherwood with his turkeys and Belgian hares

The war finally ended with Japan as the victor. Following the Treaty of Peace signed at Portsmouth, New Hampshire on September 5, 1905 and mediated by President Theodore Roosevelt, Russia acknowledged Japanese primacy in Korea. On November 17 of that year, Japan secured control of Korean foreign relations by treaty. Thus in 1905, Korea became an official protectorate of Japan. This led to the eventual abdication of the Korean Emperor on July 19, 1907 in favor of his son, who served as a mere figurehead until the formal Annexation of Korea by the Japanese on August 22, 1910.

Many of the missionaries felt the need for some relaxation after the tensions of the preceding months. My mother chose for us a houseboat trip up the river that flowed past the city. The Korean riverboats were long and flat bottomed, of very shallow draft, and were used primarily to bring rice to the city from the hinterland.

In preparation for our journey, a temporary superstructure was built on one of these boats. It consisted of a thatched roof and matting sides, mounted on frames. Hinges were attached to the frames which could then be opened up in the day. The structure had three rooms, each separated by matting screens: a large living room in front, which we furnished with a table and chairs; a small room in the center which we used for our bedroom; and a large room in the rear which served as our kitchen and the quarters for the crew. A narrow catwalk on the sides made it possible for the crew to go either to the prow or stern without disturbing us. I owned a very small, light, flat bottomed boat, which I sculled when fishing. This was attached to the houseboat.

The crew consisted of a so-called captain, who steered the boat by a rudder which resembled a long oar; two men who poled, one in front and one in the back; and three who towed the boat by walking along the bank. These three would help in rowing when we traveled downstream.

Progress up some of the rapids seemed by inches only. We often questioned whether the crew would make it, and I would get out and add my little might, to the amusement of everyone. At least my presence seemed to lend encouragement.

As we went farther and farther up the river, the mountains increased in height and the scenery became more spectacular. The other missionaries, in similar houseboats, left us at the fork of the river. We preferred to explore the smaller east branch where the scenery was yet wilder and where there were huge river caves which

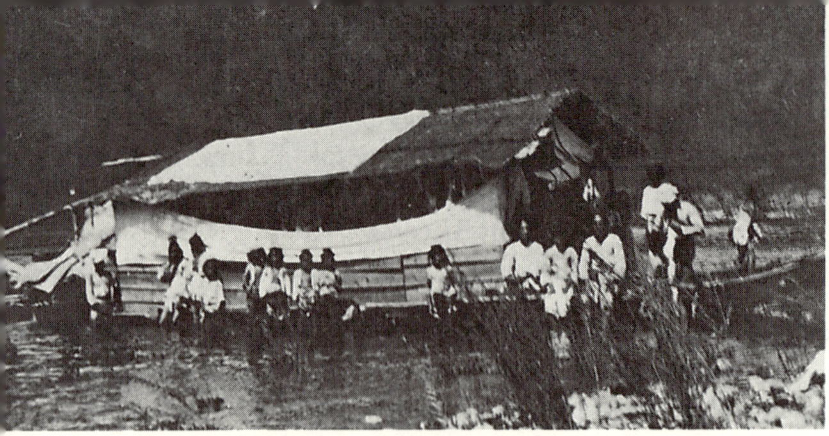

Houseboat on the Taedong River

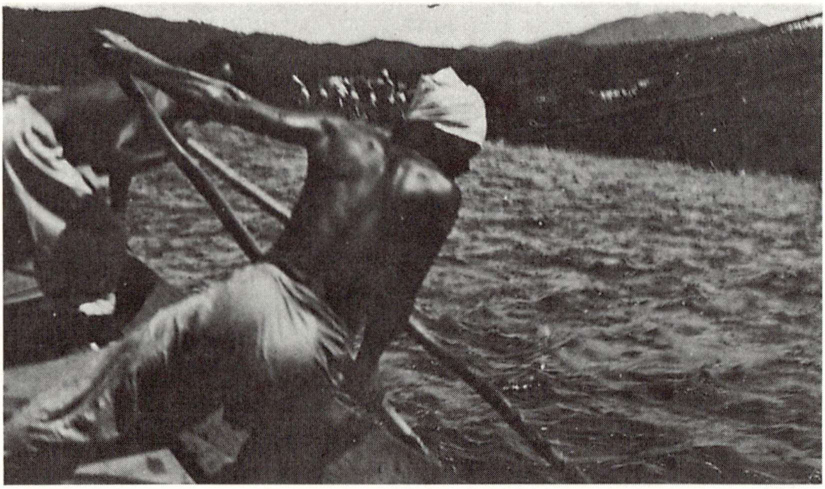

Poling upstream

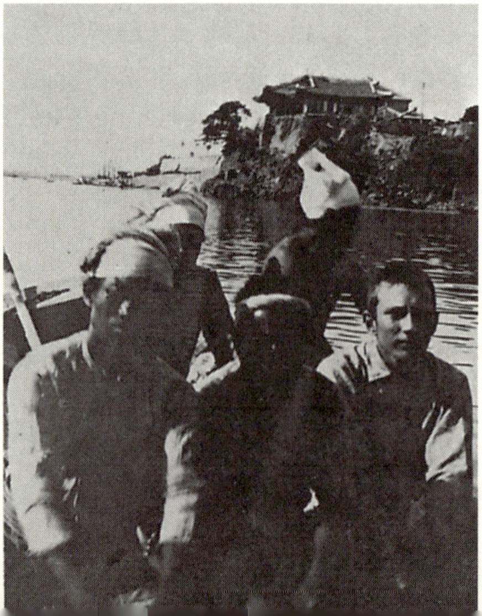

Sherwood and crew rowing downstream

our entire houseboat could enter. Here we found that we could keep cool even in the middle of the day. I especially enjoyed exploring the caves which contained lovely stalagmites and stalactites. However, after a near slip down one of the yawning chasms, my mother put a stop to this. Then we went over to one of the beautiful sandy beaches for a swim.

As fishing was supposed to be especially good here, I thought I would try my luck. In Korea, one did not use earthworms for bait, but went upstream a bit and scattered handfuls of fly maggots. Then quickly one sculled downstream a ways. As the wiggling maggots slowly floated down, the fish would swarm after them. All that remained for the fisherman to do was to haul in his catch by hooks or nets. This really made it all too easy and took away much of the sport.

Somehow in this particular area, my catch seemed to consist mostly of eels, which were considered a great delicacy. We had more eels than we could eat, and since in those days there was no refrigeration, I thought the best way to keep them was by letting them swim around in a little water at the bottom of my skiff. How little I knew about the tricks of eels. That night we had a rain shower and my whole catch slithered out over the wet sides of the boat.

On another occasion, we moored our houseboat to the trunks of the trees along the riverbank. In the morning we found that our houseboat had risen to the branches of the trees. Evidently a storm higher up had caused the river to rise suddenly during the night.

Every day there was a change of grand scenery and always a new area to explore or a new beach where one could bathe. It was an ideal way to spend a vacation. However, word came by courier that my mother was urgently needed at the hospital. Reluctantly, we had to ask our captain to head our boat downstream.

Shooting the rapids anywhere is exciting, but doing so with a rather unwieldly houseboat is even more so. One has to work hard and expertly to avoid the sharp rocks that seem to speed past. Also we had to take care that the boat did not turn sideways or the waves of the rapids would have swamped it. We maneuvered the rapids with much excitement, but without mishap. Soon we were home.

I, too, had what I considered to be urgent work. In reading about the early history of our city, I had noted a small paragraph about a secret passageway in the extreme northern part of the city that the ancient kings had used to escape in times of peril. It was supposed to lead under the river to a large island in its center. There might possibly be some hidden treasure in it. Although I knew I could not aspire to the wealth of Captain Kidd, I talked the matter over with my chum, John Baird. It had to be a "hush-hush" affair, for it would diminish our gain to have to share it with too many, and others who heard of our plans might even beat us to it. John waxed as enthusiastic as I, and we set out on our secret mission. We were well aware that it might prove impossible to discover the opening of the passage. We made discrete inquiries but no one in that area seemed to have even heard of any such opening. In a way, this was all to the good.

We systematically started to comb the entire area, keeping in mind where a king on the run might flee. We knew it would have to be near the river in some remote and secluded spot. Luck was with us, for just about where we had figured it ought to be, there was a heavy clump of overgrowth and a deep trench-like depression which slanted down finally to a dark and forbidding opening in the side of the hill. We both exclaimed at the same time, "This is it!"

Who wanted to go in first? John looked at me and I looked at John. We both hesitated. Then we decided it would be foolish to attempt to enter such a dark place without matches and candle, as well as defensive weapons, in case of attack by snakes or some wild animal.

After carefully covering up our tracks and looking around to see that no one was observing us, we hastened to our homes to try our luck the next day when we would be better prepared. That night we dreamt about what we would do with all the treasure we might find.

We returned to the site the following day equipped with shovels, candles and matches. We entered the hole and found a stone walled passage which we followed for some 30 yards. Here it was blocked by another wall constructed of heavy stones. We began to dig in the earth at the base of the wall but found nothing but some old bones. We dug further, thinking at first to burrow beneath the obstructing wall, but wisdom prevailed. We decided that to dig under the wall would be too risky, for it would very likely cave in on top of us. Reluctantly we gave up our expedition.

From toy pistols and rifles, I graduated to a twenty-two caliber rifle. The campanile, with its large bell, made an excellent target within rifle range from our house. Every time I hit the bell, it gave forth a ring, which was a pleasant sound to my ears but a puzzlement to any passerby. When I became a reasonably good shot, I asked my

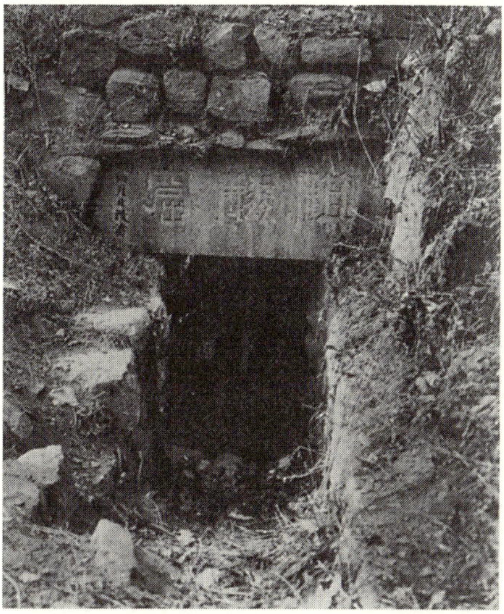

Escape route of ancient kings in Pyong Yang explored by John Baird and Sherwood

mother for permission to go on a ten-day hunting trip on my next winter vacation. My request was granted, with the usual admonitions. I felt, at last, quite grown up, for now I was really on my own.

In those days, geese and ducks often literally darkened the sky, so I had no trouble in bagging a large quantity of them near home. But I was after bigger and more exciting game, and had to go farther afield. Some Korean farmers wanted me to shoot a Siberian tiger that was killing their livestock. I politely informed them that this time I had only my small rifle with me so could not oblige, but if they told me where I might find deer, I would be glad to share some venison with them.

This offer seemed to satisfy them. One youth agreed to accompany me to help carry the game back to the village. The first few days I did not have any luck, although we did a lot of tramping through the snow without spotting anything worthwhile. We did stir up a few pheasants, which were often so close that they startled me as they flew up from right near my feet with a noisy flutter of wings. Then, one day, we saw some tracks in the snow that suggested a sizeable herd of deer. Sure enough, just across the valley we sighted a beautiful herd of spotted deer.

How to steal up on them before they might see us was the problem. I had taken the precaution of wearing a white Korean *turamagie* (coat) so the deer would think I was just a harmless Korean. (Koreans then were not allowed to carry firearms.) Well, the ruse seemed to work and I was able to get within fair rifle range for a shot at the leader.

The deer were all off like a flash and I thought in the excitement I must have missed. But when we reached the place where the deer had been, we found the snow quite red, and I knew I had wounded one. I then decided to track it down to put it out of its misery and to bring back some venison. I was to be disappointed on both counts. We soon found the wounded animal and just as I was about to shoot it again, my companion put his hand on my rifle and yelled, "Stop!" in no uncertain terms. I demanded to know the reason.

He surprisingly responded, "My brother has TB and the village doctor says if he sucks the blood from a live deer, he will recover."

I was not in a position to dispute him, but as I looked into the doleful eyes of the wounded deer, I vowed never to shoot another. I have kept that vow.

We had quite a few mulberry trees in our yard. This gave me the idea of raising silkworms. It would be nice to give my mother a dress spun from the silk of cocoons my silkworms had made.

Since this required about six yards of woven silk fabric, it would mean supplying the weaver with some 4,000 coccoons. My responsibility in the total process would be to feed the larva from the time they hatched until they reached the pupa stage and had spun coccoons on the pine branch framework which I would provide for them. The silkworm eats about fifty times its own weight. The feeding period extends over some 42 days with the worm having four twenty-four hour rest periods. After each of these sleeping periods, the worm sheds its old skin and with a new skin proceeds to continue its voracious eating.

At first, feeding the silkworms was easy; but when they grew larger, I had to be gathering the leaves from the mulberry trees almost night and day to satisfy their ravenous appetites. At last, all was in readiness, and a Korean friend undertook the remaining tasks of plunging the coccoons into cauldrons of boiling water and then unwinding the silk filament from the coccoons onto reels, and weaving this into fabric. This gift I then proudly presented to my mother.

In August, 1906, the Pyong Yang missionaries invited a Canadian medical missionary stationed at Wonsan, Dr. R. A. Hardie, to lead them in a series of meetings. It was Dr. Hardie who had first welcomed my father to Korea when the latter's ship had touched at

Fusan. To pay my respects to Dr. Hardie, I attended a special Korean language service that he was conducting in the church that my father had founded in Pyong Yang.

Dr. Hardie did not speak eloquently, nor even emotionally, but directly and sincerely from his heart to the hearts of his listeners. Somehow, that day, I was ready to receive his message. My recollection of it was essentially as follows:

"The heart of the Christian gospel is the message of God's grace. To strive for heavenly rewards or to struggle to avoid dire eternal punishment is to miss this message. Attempts to be good by our own efforts usually stem from human pride and a lack of faith which only serve to harden our hearts.

"The lesson of faith for the Christian is the power of God to save His people from their sins, not just in the hereafter but in the here and now. Christ gave the most amazing statement of the ages, considering the circumstances under which it was uttered, when he said, '*Father, forgive them, for they know not what they do.*' This simply means that God wants also to forgive and abundantly pardon us, no matter what our mistakes have been.

"Once we have acknowledged to God that the energy of human flesh is not adequate to empower our ideals, aspirations, and resolutions, we are open to receive His promised gift of the Holy Spirit to be our ever present teacher and comforter. By our obedience to the promptings of the Holy Spirit we are able to respond to God's unconditional love on the one hand and to offer that love to our fellow men on the other. Not only does belief in Jesus Christ as the Son of God offer us the assurance of unearned eternal life, but we are enabled by the Holy Spirit working in us to make our resolves come to fruition in our temporal life. Our resolves, too, take on a different focus as we change from wanting to bring glory to ourselves to a desire to glorify God.

"High ideals and lofty motivations are not enough without the necessary spiritual power to carry them out. Remember, this power can only be realized through constant prayer. Just as our bodily strength can only be sustained through daily food, so our spiritual strength can only be maintained through daily prayer."

I had heard similar statements before and have since, but somehow, Dr. Hardie's message was etched indelibly on my boyish mind and heart. At this particular time and place, my heart had need of it and I gratefully responded to it. Although I had planned to go to the Western World and train for a business career, I resolved, instead, to become a medical missionary and return to Korea.

In the past, I had made New Year resolutions and had broken them. I well knew, left to my own strength, I might also break my resolution of returning to Korea. But because Dr. Hardie had given me the simple guidelines of how best to realize the spiritual power that my heart craved, I was confident in my new resolve. The details I would have to fill in myself, according to my own individual needs and temperament and guidance of the Holy Spirit.

Dr. Hardie delivered his message throughout Korea. It resulted in the "Great Korean Revival" of 1907. During that time thousands were brought into God's Kingdom, including a young white boy in the "Hermit Kingdom."

The medical and educational work in Pyong Yang continued to expand. Periodically the home-based Mission Board would send representatives to visit the work on the mission field in order to better keep in touch with the needs there. My mother was especially delighted, therefore, when the J. Sumner Stones came to Pyong Yang in the fall of 1906. My father had lived with the Stones while he was working in New York City. Showing the mission work to these visitors had special meaning, therefore, for my mother.

It was when she was seeing the Stones off on the train at the conclusion of their visit that my mother had an accident. She had remained on the train too long when saying her farewell. Suddenly, she became aware that the train had started. Without thinking, she jumped impulsively to the platform from the moving train. All too late, she painfully realized that she had been foolhardy. Her leg was broken. My mother now became a patient in her own hospital on the second floor.

On November 2, 1906 I was attending classes at the Pyong Yang Foreign School when someone nearby had noticed a billowing dark cloud in the direction of the Women's Hospital. He rushed into the schoolroom yelling to me, "Your hospital is on fire!"

Knowing that my mother was confined to a room in the upper story of the hospital, I frantically raced all the way to the conflagration. By the time I reached the scene, flames and smoke were pouring from the windows of the very room where I thought my mother to be. I was desperate and tried to push my way through the crowd, but was roughly thrown back as I shouted, "My mother is up there. Do rescue her!" My frantic pleas seemed to go unheeded and it was only some time later that I learned that my mother had already been taken out by means of a ladder thrown up against the building just in time. She was resting comfortably in a nearby native hut.

Both the women's hospital and the Edith Margaret Memorial Children's Wards burned to the ground. All that remained standing was the main brick chimney. Later, this posed a problem, for should it collapse in a high wind, it might cause injury. Fortunately, one of the miners from the American gold mines at Unsan offered to dynamite it under proper precautions and this potential hazard was safely eliminated.

My mother was then faced with the problem of finding quarters for the medical work while waiting for a new hospital to be constructed. The General Board of the Mission had negotiated for the purchase of some native buildings in a downtown area of the city known as Ku Kole. My mother was able to reopen her work there and the funds which the W.F.M.S. hospital paid in rental eventually paid for the Ku Kole buildings. The mud floors and paper windows and minimal equipment recalled the pioneer days of medical work in Pyong Yang.

Mother also began regular religious services there and eventually a church was established at Ku Kole. That church remembered its founder every Christmas by sending my mother a bolt of white homespun material for hospital uniforms.

After the experience of the fire, Mother decided that the new hospital buildings should be made of brick and granite. As soon as possible she began rebuilding. This time the site was changed back to near where she and my father first began their medical work in Pyong Yang and across the street from the Hall Memorial Hospital.

Largely through the efforts of personal friends, funds were secured for a larger, better hospital and dispensary which would include a hot water heating plant and plumbing. The type of building my mother envisaged was also quite an innovation at that time in Pyong Yang. My mother assigned me to the job of supervising the work and my Korean friend, Ko Syo Bong, to be my right-hand man.

My first task was to take the head carpenter, Mr. Kim, to Seoul to help him get the idea of what a brick building looked like. He had never seen one, for up to this point the mission buildings had been built close to Korean style.

The job of "boy foreman" was a considerable responsibility to assign a lad of fourteen, and Mr. Kim and I often felt that we were in the position of the blind leading the blind. Nevertheless, experience

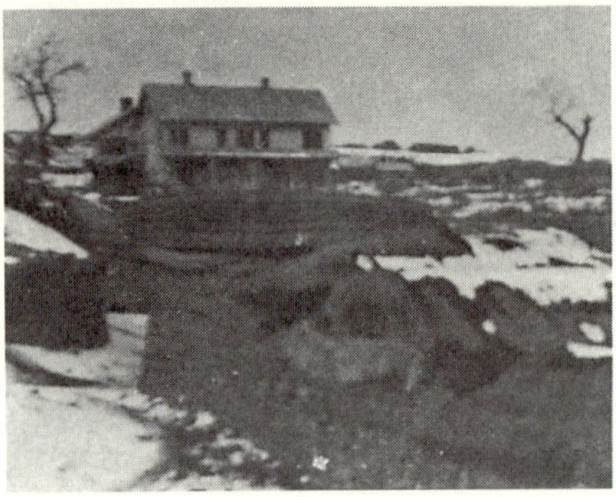

Original Woman's Hospital in Pyong Yang–built 1903, burned 1906 Edith Margaret Children's Wards at left of main building

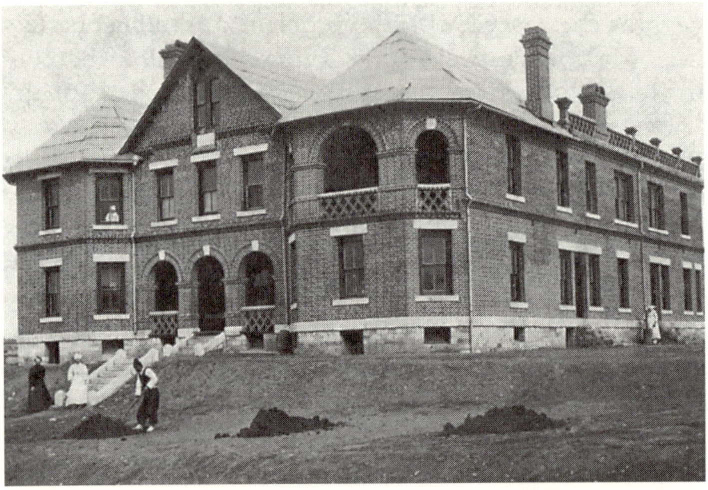

New Woman's Hospital of Extended Grace, completed 1908

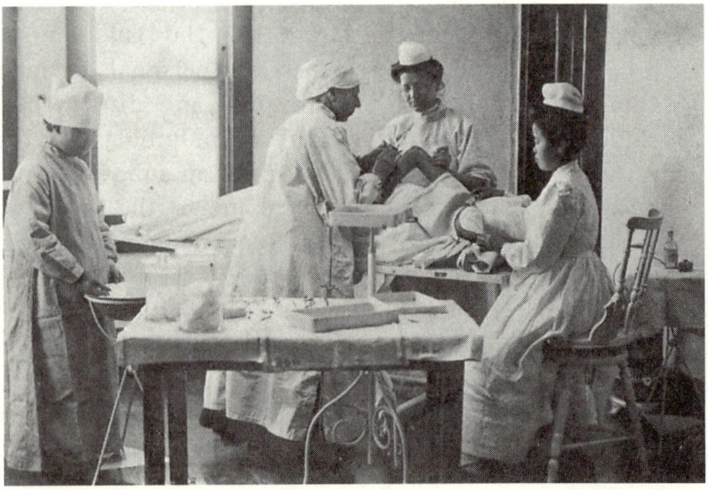

Dr. Rosetta Hall in operating room of new hospital

proved to be an excellent teacher, and by 1908, the building was sufficiently completed for the medical work to be moved from Ku Kole to the new location. It only lacked the heating plant and the plumbing which were installed later. The following year, the educational work for the blind was also expanded to include deaf-mutes.

The Pyong Yang Foreign School, at that time, did not continue past the eighth grade. By the fall my mother had decided to send me for my high school work to the British school run by the China Inland Mission in Chefoo, China. Two later famous Americans, Henry Luce and Thornton Wilder, also attended this school. It was run along strict disciplinary lines and I was not very happy. My mother did not care for the long separation and decided to withdraw me after one term and tutor me at home as time allowed. In another two years we would be returning to the United States on furlough and Mother had plans to enroll me then in the Mount Hermon School in Massachusetts.

I had turned fifteen. Mother realized that I needed to have some lessons in managing my own funds responsibly and that I must start earning toward the expense of my future education. The year before, my efforts to earn money had not been notably successful. In fact, I had only broken even from a project of collecting butterflies and insects for a Russian naturalist. This was because I had not counted on shipping delays, and many of the specimens had arrived in Moscow in a moldy condition due to the extreme humidity of the Korean rainy season. My mother hoped that I had learned from this to plan more carefully and to invest my money more wisely.

Mother decided to let me have some of the funds which my father had left me from his life insurance. Since I had just had the practical experience of helping my mother rebuild the Women's Hospital, building construction seemed a logical place to begin. Two new missionary families were coming out to Korea, but if housing could not be found for them in Pyong Yang, they would likely be assigned elsewhere. This seemed a practical way for both helping out the Mission and my educational future.

I decided to invest my funds in building a duplex which could house both families at less cost than a single unit dwelling. It was to be three stories tall, a true "Pyong Yang skyscraper." From previous experience, I had found that the millwork took a long time for it had to be all done by hand from unseasoned timber. After making inquiries hither and yon, I decided to order the woodwork (floors,

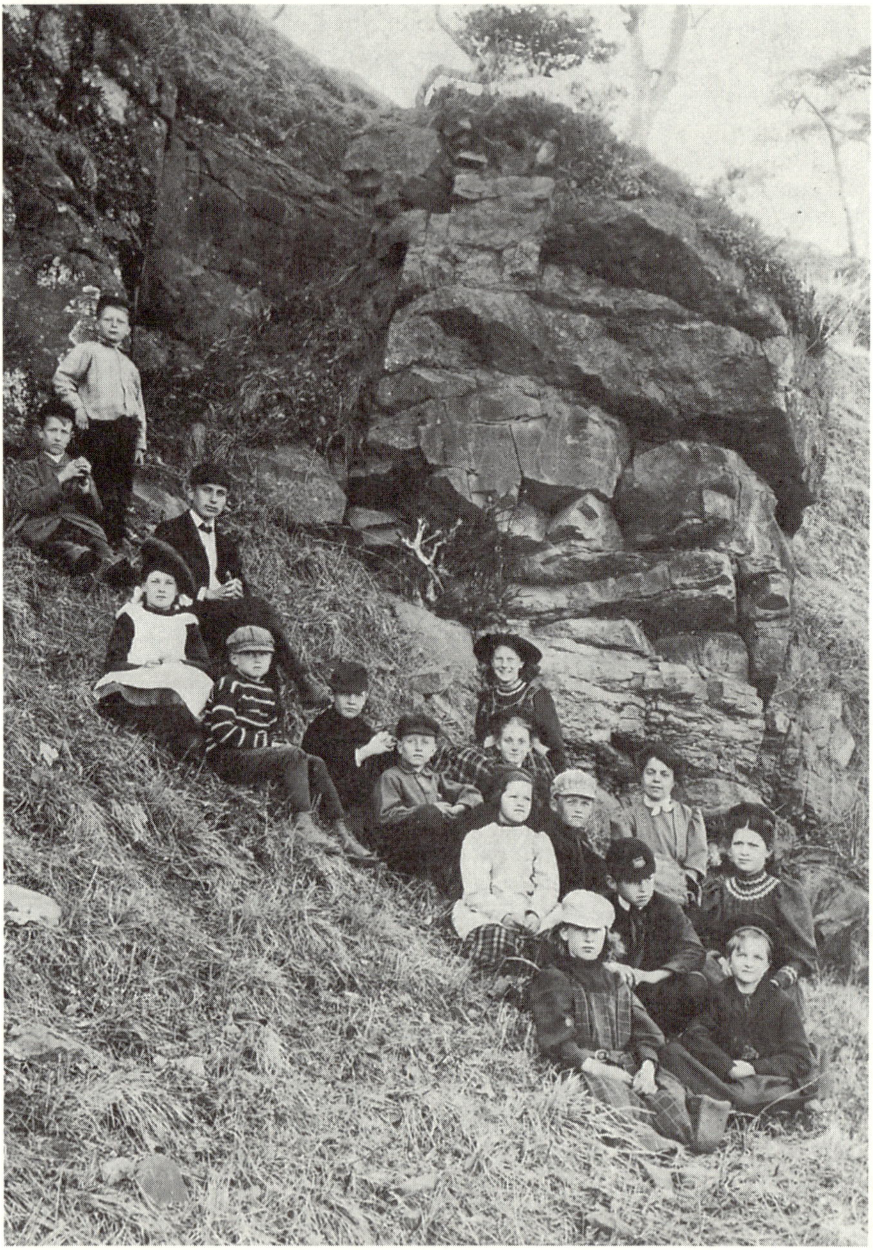

Students of the Pyong Yang Foreign School on outing at Peony Point

l. to r.–William Baird, Alden Noble, Florence Follwell, Sherwood Hall, Graham Lee, Richard Baird, Scott Wells, Ruth Noble (large hat), Gretchen Jones, Gertrude Swallen (white smock), Mylo Lee (plaid cap), Virginia Wells (white hat), Miss Strang, teacher, Wilbur Swallen (school hat), Olivette Swallen, Margaret Lee (front)

doors, window frames) and hardware, premanufactured, from Tacoma, Washington. This would save much time and money and prevent complaints which were bound to arise when using unseasoned materials.

The only major snag I ran into in this project was the digging of the cellar. Here we struck solid rock. As time was of the essence, it meant we would have to blast it out with dynamite. But we were within the city limits and my Korean contractor had no permit for blasting. However, I, being a foreigner, would be allowed if I did the blasting myself. The Koreans could drill the holes for me.

At that time a railway was being built from Seoul to the Manchurian border via Pyong Yang. We used to ride flat cars as far as the rails had been laid. Much blasting was in progress, so I went to get a little know-how and to procure caps, fuses and dynamite. In testing the fuse, I found that it tasted sweet but that I would be well advised not to bite on it. Mother had gone to Shanghai, China for a medical conference, so I was completely on my own to do foolish things as well as wise ones.

Dynamite was almost as costly on the black market as sticks of gold. I discovered that a number of people had their eyes on my precious supply of dynamite which I had bought with considerable difficulty. I felt that the safest place to store it was in my own bedroom closet under lock and key. No thief would think of looking for it there. But I did not consider the possibility of being blown to "kingdom come" in case of fire.

The blasting went well at first until one time a charge failed to go off. What to do? It would be risky to try to dig it out. So it seemed best to just add another stick of dynamite, and put on extra dampened rice straw mats as covering, to prevent fragments of stone from the blast from scattering. However, I evidently had not accurately figured the terrific force of the explosion, for it was like a small volcano erupting, scattering fragments far and wide.

I said to myself, "Now I have had it." Although frightened people came running up from all directions, providentially, no one was hurt. It did not take long to pacify them. The police, however, admonished me not to make such a "big noise" next time, as it terrified the "ignorant people." I felt like telling them how much it had also terrified me.

The house was finally completed in July 1909 after six months of labor. The missionary families thus were enabled to accept assign-

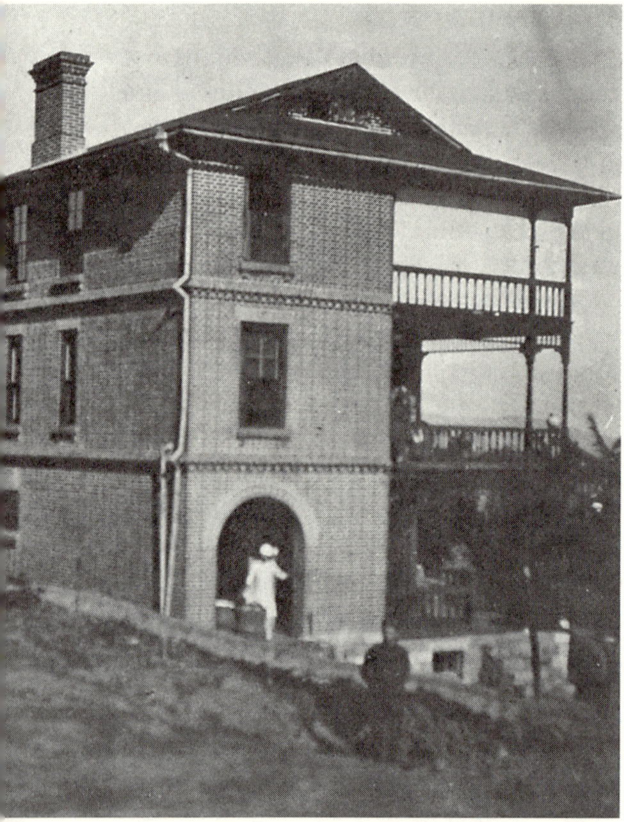

The three-story duplex "investment" house

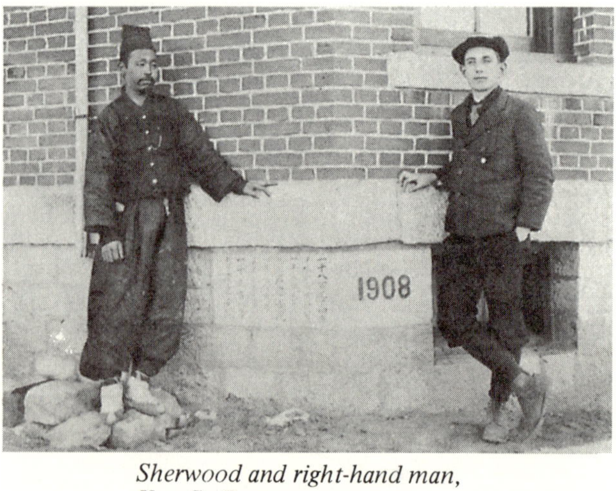

Sherwood and right-hand man, Kyo So Bang, at cornerstone

ment to Pyong Yang. At the same time, I was helped in funding my future education.

May 28, 1909 was a very special day for "our doctor," Esther Kim Pak. She was invited to the capital where the Woman's Educational and Woman's Enterprise Societies were combining to honor Korea's first women college graduates, Mrs. N. K. Ha, B.A., and Mrs. Esther Kim Pak, M.D. Carriages conveyed them in grand style to the grounds of the old Mulberry Palace where the ceremonies took place. Following the addresses they were each awarded a gold medal. How proud Esther was of hers. However, she would have less than a year in which to bask in the sunshine of this recognition, for she was fighting a losing battle with tuberculosis. I was heartbroken when I learned that she had contracted the disease, and in those days there was no sanatorium or proper treatment facility where she could be sent in Korea. After only ten years of practicing medicine and teaching in the Mission Bible Institutes, Esther died on April 13, 1910.

Esther's death came as a shock. I resolved to do all in my power to help prevent the disease that had snatched her away in her prime and wasted the lives of so many of her fellow Koreans. I vowed that I would return to Korea as a TB specialist and would establish a tuberculosis sanatorium.

To that vow I harnessed the words etched on my memory four years ago by Dr. Hardie:

"High ideals and lofty motivations are not enough without the necessary spiritual power to carry them out."

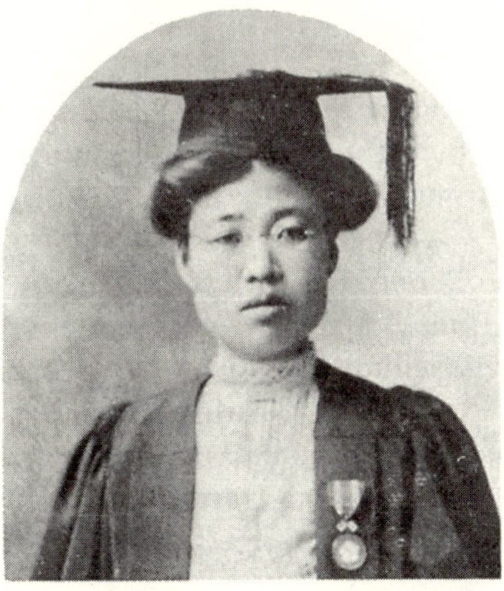

Esther Kim Pak, M.D.

CHAPTER 9

Western Exposure

Mother had been appointed the official delegate from Korea to the World Missionary Conference in Edinburgh, Scotland in 1910. She was a great believer in travel as part of my education, and in this I was not a reluctant pupil. I was sixteen and ready to start a new world of adventure.

The journey we had planned through Manchuria and Siberia was rather ambitious for those days. The Manchurian portion of the primitive railway on which we were to travel had been completed by the Russians shortly before the Russo-Japanese war. Its construction was considered a remarkable engineering feat because of the mountain ridges and unstable soils that had to be traversed. The railroad was used extensively during the 1904 conflict to rush troops and supplies to the front.

Our trip through the mountains offered the excitement and thrills of a breathtaking roller coaster ride. The train seemed to precariously hug the steep mountainside. When we looked out of the window, we became uncomfortably aware that it would take only one small mishap to plunge us into the deep gorges below. The train travelled only during daylight hours and at night we sought shelter in crude mountain inns.

On the second day of our journey, I noticed my mother looking methodically through all her travel documents instead of admiring the wild scenery which so fascinated me. Then she came up with a surprising proposition.

"You seem to be enjoying this 'roller coaster' trip so much, how would you like a repeat journey? I find that I must have somehow left our Trans-Siberian Railway tickets behind at Pyong Yang. I shall telegraph Miss Emily Haynes to meet you at the Korean-Manchurian border. You will have to make the trip there and back here to Mukden by yourself, for we do not have enough travel funds here for both of us."

That was a little more excitement than I had bargained for, but there was no alternative. The part I did not particularly relish was being alone overnight in a Manchurian inn, which I had heard were often attacked by bandits. Then, too, there was the uncertainty of whether Miss Haynes would, in fact, be at the border to meet me. These possibilities raced through my mind.

At the inn that evening, I decided to familiarize myself with exit routes in the event I needed to escape in a hurry. I had not walked far before I encountered not bandits, but ferocious Manchurian dogs. These canines, I soon discovered, were quite different in temperament from Korean dogs. As soon as a man stooped to pick up a stone, a Korean dog would run away. When I tried this ruse now, it seemed to only serve as a signal for the Manchurian beasts to close in on me. I was saved in the nick of time by a passer-by, who with some difficulty was able to call them off. The dogs growled and bared their savage looking teeth at me as I made a hasty retreat. After this experience, I decided it was safer to return to the inn and face the possibility of a bandit attack.

I was so relieved to see Miss Haynes with our tickets at the border that I surprised her with an impulsive kiss. She laughingly said that she now felt repaid for her special trip. Miss Haynes was involved in the educational work of our Mission in Pyong Yang and I had always found her to be delightful.

Now all I had to do was to deliver the precious tickets safely to Mother. That night at the stop-over, the innkeeper offered to have a fire built under me for it had turned quite cold. In his broken English, he made it sound much worse than it actually was. In this way, he introduced me to a Manchurian winter bed, which is really ideal for cold weather. The Koreans heat their floors, but the Manchurians heat just that part of the floor that forms their bed. This is simply a raised stone and mortar platform. Under this, smoke flues are extended from a small fireplace in the kitchen to the chimney at the far end of the bedroom. In other words, one sleeps on a prostrate chimney and thus can keep warm even in the coldest weather. The fact that the bed is above the floor level makes it more convenient.

These Manchurians were a different breed of men than their fellow Chinese. They were taller, many over six feet. They gave women more freedom and did not engage in the practice of binding their women's feet. The Manchurians seemed to prefer a diet chiefly of soya beans (from which a milk powder substitute is made) and millet. Their excellent diet may have accounted, in part, for their superior strength. Anyway, they quite impressed me because of their physical fitness.

Mother, though not usually demonstrative, received me back with a warm hug and kiss. I could see that she was greatly relieved to see both me and our precious tickets. We resumed our journey and finally reached the Manchurian-Siberian border. The border town looked bleak and dismal, and we were doubly glad that our passports, visas and tickets were all found to be in order so that we would not have to be stranded at this forlorn outpost.

It was certainly good to be on a big train again, even though we were traveling "Russian hard," which was an apt name. Seating consisted of two long, narrow wooden benches with no padding provided. Although we had brought along our own cushions, the seats seemed to grow harder as the trip progressed.

Our fellow passengers were very curious about us. We were less curious about them for they were perfectly innocent of soap and deodorants. To while away the hours, they spent much of their time in de-lousing one another. One was so kindly disposed that she even offered to de-louse us, but Mother expressed an emphatic "no" in the universal sign language.

The scenery at first was just rolling plains, which stretched to the horizon with hardly a village in sight. The locomotive here burned coal. Later, when we passed through an area rich in oil, an oil burner would be attached, and still later, when we went through the dark forests, we would have a wood burner. I kept a sharp lookout for game. We soon had passed the area where the Siberian tigers abound, without seeing one, although we saw several varieties of deer and an occasional bear. At night when we stopped at some isolated station, we would hear the blood curdling howls of the Siberian wolves and were glad they could not get at us.

We made rather infrequent stops, but when we did, they were of sufficient duration that we could get off, stretch our legs and get boiling water for our cocoa. The heated water was provided free at every station or from the boiler of the engine. I soon learned the Russian word for boiling water, *keepertock*. We could also buy milk, butter, eggs and black bread at most stations at fantastically low prices, which nicely supplemented what food we had brought with us. In fact, every day of the trip, which normally took ten days, was a picnic for us.

THE GREAT

TRANS-SIBERIAN

ROUTE

SPEED & ECONOMY

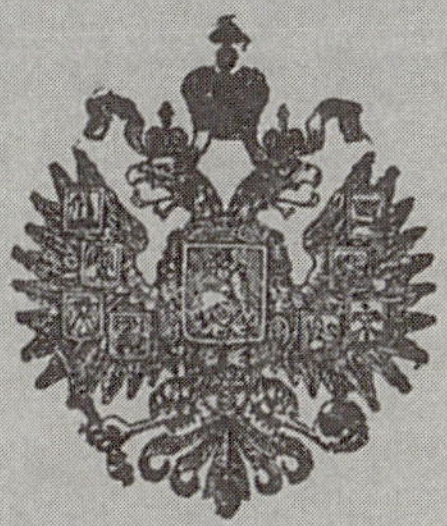

COMFORT & EASE.

QUICKEST & CHEAPEST ROUTE BETWEEN THE FAR EAST & EUROPE

This Route has opened up a New Era in World Travel, annihilating distances & bringing the Occident & Orient within easy reach.

LOCAL CONNECTIONS FROM THE FAR EAST

Passengers have the choice of various interesting routes from all parts of the Orient in connection with the

TRANS-SIBERIAN RAILWAY

Three Express Trains, each week, from Wladivostok to Moscow & St. Petersbourg, connecting directly with the Daily Express Trains thence

TO ALL PARTS OF EUROPE

and with the Trans-Atlantic Steamship Lines from European Ports

TO AMERICA

The great variety of interests in the new territories opened up; the spacious & Luxurious Compartment Sleeping Cars, with vestibuled Corridors the entire length of the train, well heated in Winter and ventilated in Summer; Private Lavatories; Bathrooms; Fans, Electric Light; handsomely appointed Dining, Smoking & Library Car; Excellent Cuisine & Service; Broad Guage & Easy Motion; all combine to dispel the fatigue of ordinary train travel and to make this

THE IDEAL ROUTE AT ALL SEASONS OF THE YEAR

For Tickets, Rates, Hand Books, Maps & General Information, Address, or Apply to

INTERNATIONAL SLEEPING CAR COMPANY

(See Official List of Agents page 7.)

1

Train schedule of the Trans-Siberian Railway Circa *1900*

(Route map is shown on inside cover)

(See Official List of Agents page 7).

SPECIAL NOTICE.

THROUGH TICKETS

Issued for the ENTIRE journey from any principal points in the FAR EAST, to any principal points in EUROPE and to AMERICA.

BAGGAGE

Each Adult passenger holding "INTERNATIONAL" Ticket, I or II class, through to points in EUROPE &c., is entitled to 110 lbs. of personal luggage registered FREE in the Baggage Car; which may be checked through to ticket destination, with Customs examination ONLY at the FRONTIER of the country of destination.

Each Adult passenger holding Ticket, I or II class, to points in RUSSIA only, is entitled to 50 lbs. of personal luggage Registered FREE in the Baggage Car; subject to examination at the various frontier Customs Houses en route.

In addition to the above, each I or II class passenger is entitled to carry FREE, such portable hand luggage as may be accommodated in the Sleeping Car Compartment without inconvenience to the other passengers; subject to examination at the various frontier Customs Houses en route.

The Co.'s Agents will arrange for Storing, Insuring & Forwarding to destination, by sea routes, such luggage as passengers may not wish to take with them via the Trans-Siberian Line.

PASSPORTS

All travellers in RUSSIA are required to have a PASSPORT, which will be issued at their respective Consulates and must be viséd at a Russian Consulate before leaving the Far East.

These passports will be viséd when entering and leaving RUSSIA, and when staying over night in Hotels, or Houses.

CHILDREN

RAILWAY.—Between 10 and 4 years—pay SPECIAL CHILD'S FARE.
Under 4 years—FREE for one child accompanying each Adult Passenger; each additional child pays SPECIAL CHILD'S FARE.

SLEEPING CAR.—Over 4 years—pays Adult berth fare.
Under 4 years—FREE (if no separate berth is required).
Any child occupying separate berth, pays Adult berth fare.

DOGS

If properly muzzled and on a leash, will be carried in a section of the Baggage Car, fare between WLADIVOSTOK & MOSCOW, Roubles 10.55.

The Company assumes no responsibility for the Dog, and its food and care must be arranged for by its owner accompanying it.

INTERNATIONAL TRAINS DE LUXE

DIRECT THROUGH SERVICES from WLADIVOSTOK & HARBIN To MOSCOW, WARSAW, BERLIN, PARIS, LONDON, VIENNA, VENICE, GENOA, BORDEAUX, LISBON, RIVIERA, &c.

SPECIAL COUPON TICKET BOOKS

issued, containing Coupon Tickets covering each separate section of entire journey by any of the various routes, either in connection with the

TRANS-SIBERIAN LINE

or for Single Trips, or Local Circular Tours including all the principal places of interest in

JAPAN, CHINA, KOREA, MANCHURIA, SIBERIA, PHILIPPINES. JAVA, SIAM, INDO-CHINA, BURMA, CEYLON, INDIA, AUSTRALIA, &c.

(This is a distinctly new feature and of great convenience for all Residents and Tourists in the Far East).

Train schedule (cont.)

SUMMER SCHEDULE
(From May 1st to Oct. 1st.)

THE G

VIA WLADIVOSTOK.

ROUTE I.

Lv. Shanghai......	Ac. to tide	—	Sat.	—	RUSSIAN VOLUNTEER FLEET.
Lv. Nagasaki......	6.00 p.m.	—	Mon.	—	——
Ar. Wladivostok ..	9.00 a.m.	—	Thur.	—	Weekly Steamer.

ROUTE II.

Lv. Nagasaki......	5.48 a.m.	Fri.	Mon.	Wed.	IMPERIAL JAPANESE RYS.
Lv. Tokyo	11.00 p.m.	,,	,,	,,	——
Lv. Yokohama ...	11.52 p.m.	,,	,,	,,	
Lv. Kobe............	8.18 a.m.	Sat.	Tues.	Thur.	Sleeping and Dining Cars.
Ar. Maibara	1.20 p.m.	,,	,,	,,	——
Lv. Maibara	1.35 p.m.	,,	,,	,,	Daily.
Ar. Tsuruga	3.20 p.m.	,,	,,	,,	
Lv. Tsuruga ...	5.00 p.m.	—	Tues.	—	Tri-Weekly Steamers.
	8.00 p.m.	Sat.	—	Thur.	
Ar. Wladivostok ..	11.00 a.m.	Mon.	Thur.	Sat.	

Passengers have the choice of various other Local Routes from the Far East in connection with the Trans-Siberian Line. Special Coupon Tickets are issued for Single Trips and Circular Tours covering the principal places of interest in CHINA, JAPAN, KOREA, MANCHURIA, SIBERIA, PHILIPPINES, INDIA, AUSTRALIA and all parts of the FAR EAST.

For Tickets, Rates, and Detailed Information, Address, or Apply to the

INTERNATIONAL SLEEPING CAR COMPANY

(as per our official List of Agents at all principal places in the Far East.)

(See Page 7.)

WLADIVOSTOK & HARBIN TO MOSCOW & ST. PETERSBOURG.

Lv. Wladivostok...	3.00 p.m.	Tues.	Fri.	Sun.	TRANS-SIBERIAN RAILWAY.
Ar. Harbin	3.10 p.m.	Wed.	Sat.	Mon.	——
Lv. Harbin	4.00 p.m.	,,	,,	,,	Three Express Trains Every Week.
Ar. Irkoutsk	8.30 a.m.	Sat.	Tues.	Thur.	——
Lv. Irkoutsk	10.10 a.m.	,,	,,	,,	Compartment Sleeping and Dining Cars.
Ar. Moscow	7.45 a.m.	Fri.	—	Wed.	——
Ar. St. Petersbourg	5.45 p.m.	—	Mon.	—	International Train-de-Luxe Days shewn in RED.

Through Tickets are issued for the entire journey from any
Registered Baggage is checked through to Ticket Destinatio
Passenger; and children proportionately. Passengers n
Through Services "International Trains de Luxe" from Wla
Trans-Siberian passengers arriving at Moscow on Friday m

OUS ROUTES FROM THE FAR EAST TO EUROPE &

in connection with

REAT TRANS-SIBERIAN

VIA PEKING & HARBIN.

ROUTE III.

Lv. Nagasaki ... Lv. Shimonoseki .. Ar. Kobe	5.48 a.m. 2.40 p.m. 6.27 a.m.	} 24½ Hours.	IMPERIAL JAPANESE. RAILWAYS.
Lv. Tokyo .... Lv. Yokohama ... Ar. Kobe	6.30 p.m. 7.08 p.m. 9.00 a.m.	} 14½ Hours.	Sleeping and Dining Cars. Daily.
Lv. Kobe .... Lv. Moji .... Ar. Tientsin	10.00 a.m. 1.00 p.m. — a.m.	} 5 Days.	OSAKA SHOSEN KAISHA. NIPPON YUSEN KAISHA. Two Steamers Weekly.

ROUTE IV.

Lv. Shanghai ...... Lv. Tsingtau ...... Lv. Chefoo .... Ar. Tientsin	Ac. to tide „ „ „	} 3½ Days.	VARIOUS LOCAL STEAMERS. Every few days.

Lv. Tientsin ...... Ar. PEKING	8.50 a.m. 11.39 p.m.	3.48 p.m. 6.55 p.m.	4.37 p.m. 8.15 p.m.	IMPERIAL CHINESE RAILWAYS. Daily.

ROUTE V.

Lv. Shanghai ...... Ar. Hankow	Midnight Noon	Sun. Thur.			YANGTSZE RIVER STEAMERS. Daily.
Lv. Hankow ...... Ar. PEKING	10.45 a.m. 5.00 p.m.	Fri. Sat.	— —	— —	IMPERIAL CHINESE RAILWAYS. Sleeping and Dining Cars. Weekly.

Lv. PEKING ... Lv. Tientsin ...... Ar. Shanhaikuan..	7.20 p.m. 11.25 p.m. 7.50 a.m.	Mon. „ Tues.	8.30 a.m. 11.47 a.m. 6.22 p.m.	ORDINARY TRAIN.	Daily. Sleeping over night at the Railway Hotel Shanhaikuan.	IMPERIAL CHINESE RAILWAYS. Day & Dining Cars. Express Train Weekly. Ordinary Train Daily.
Lv. Shanhaikuan. Ar. Mukden	8.00 a.m. 6.45 p.m.	„ „	8.00 a.m. 6.45 p.m.			
Lv. Mukden ...... Ar. Changchun ...	9.15 p.m. 5.00 a.m.	Tues. Wed.	Fri. Sat.	Sun. Mon.		SOUTH MANCHURIA RAILWAY. Sleeping & Dining Cars Tri-Weekly.
Lv. Changchun ... Ar. HARBIN	6.32 a.m. 3.00 p.m.	„ Wed.	„ Sat.	„ Mon.		CHINESE EASTERN RAILWAY. Daily.

MOSCOW TO EUROPE.

Lv. Moscow	9.45 a.m.	Fri.	"NORD-EXPRESS" (Train de Luxe.) Sleeping and Dining Cars. Weekly.	9.30 p.m.	Wed.	"STATE" EXPRESS. Sleeping and Dining Cars. Daily.
Ar. Warsaw	11.00 a.m.	Sat.		9.05 a.m.	Fri.	
Lv. Warsaw	12.22 p.m.	„		5.02 p.m.	„	
Ar. Alexandrovo..	4.10 p.m.	„		9.52 p.m.	„	
Ar. Berlin	10.53 p.m.	„		6.38 a.m.	Sat.	
Lv. Berlin	10.59 p.m.	„		1.00 p.m.	„	
Ar. Paris	4.00 p.m.	Sun.		7.30 a.m.	Sun.	
Ar. London via Ostend	10.00 p.m.	„		7.50 a.m.	„	

chedule Days of the "INTERNATIONAL TRAINS DE LUXE" are shown ir

principal point in the Far Fast to any principal point in Europe, and to Ame
, with Customs examination only at the Frontier of the country of Destinatio
ost be provided with Passports, which most be viséd by a Russian Consul, before
ivostok & Harbin to Moscow, St. Petersbourg, Warsaw, Vienna, Berlin, Paris
nings, by the "International Train de Luxe," may transfer directly to the "N

Train schedule (cont.)

ROUTE.

This Schedule is subject to change after Oct. 1st.

VIA DAIREN & HARBIN.

ROUTE VI.

Lv. Tokyo .... Lv. Yokohama ... Lv. Kobe	3.30 p.m. 4.11 p.m. 7.25 p.m.	30 Hours.	IMPERIAL JAPANESE R'WAYS. — Sleeping and Dining Cars. — Daily.
Lv. Nagasaki	1.10 p.m.		
Lv. Shimonoseki	10.00 p.m.		
Ar. Fusan	8.30 a.m.	11 Hours.	Steamer—Daily.
Lv. Fusan .... Ar. Seoul	10.40 a.m. 10.23 p.m.	10½ Hours.	KOREAN STATE RAILWAYS. — Day and Dining Cars. — Daily.
Ar. Chemulpo......	9.08 p.m.		
Lv. Chemulpo ... Ar. DAIREN	— —	36 Hours.	OSAKA SHOSEN KAISHA. NIPPON YUSEN KAISHA. Frequent Steamers.

ROUTE VII.

Lv. Nagasaki ...... Lv. Shimonoseki.. Ar. Kobe	5.48 a.m. 2.40 p.m. 6.27 a.m.	24½ Hours.	IMPERIAL JAPANESE R'WAYS. — Sleeping and Dining Cars. — Daily.
Lv. Tokyo .... Lv. Yokohama ... Ar. Kobe	6.30 p.m. 7.08 p.m. 9.00 a.m.	15½ Hours.	
Lv. Kobe .... Lv. Moji .... Ar. DAIREN	10.00 a.m. 1.00 p.m. — a.m.	3 Days.	OSAKA SHOSEN KAISHA. — 2 Steamers—Weekly.

ROUTE VIII.

		A		B	
Lv. Shanghai	Ac. to tide.	Sat. or Sun.	—	Thur.	A.—S.S. "Saikio Maru" B.—S.S. "Kobe Maru" Bi-Weekly.
Ar. DAIREN	„	Mon. or Tues.	—	Sat.	

Lv. DAIREN...... Ar. Changchun ...	11.00 a.m. 5.00 a.m.	Tues. Wed.	Fri. Sat.	Sun. Mon.	SOUTH MANCHURIA R'WAY. Sleeping and Dining Cars. Tri-Weekly.
Lv. Changchun ... Ar. HARBIN	6.32 a.m. 3.00 p.m.	„ „	„ „	„ „	CHINESE EASTERN R'WAY. — Daily.

ST. PETERSBOURG TO EUROPE.

	RUSSIAN "STATE" EXPRESS.—DAILY.					
Lv. Moscow ...... Ar. St. Petersbourg	9.30 p.m. 9.30 a.m.	Fri. Sat.	7.05 a.m. 6.30 p.m.	6.30 p.m. 8.30 a.m.	8.00 p.m. 9.00 a.m.	11.30 p.m. 11.00 a.m.
Lv. St. Petersbourg Ar. Wirballen...... Ar. Berlin .... Lv. Berlin .... Ar. Paris .... Ar. London via Ostend	6.00 p.m. 10.30 a.m. 10.55 p.m. 10.59 p.m. 4.00 p.m. 10.00 p.m.	Sat. Sun. „ „ Mon „	Wed. Thur. „ „ Fri. „	"NORD-EXPRESS." (Train de Luxe.) — Compartment Sleeping & Dining Cars. Bi-Weekly—Petersbourg to Berlin. Daily—Berlin to Paris and Ostend.		

RED LETTERS.

ica.

110 lbs. of Registered Baggage are carried FREE for each Adult I & II class arriving in Russia.

Ostend (London) &c.

ord-Express" Train de Luxe for Warsaw, Berlin, Paris, London, &c.

Each station presented a curious group of onlookers, who gave the impression that they had nothing to do but to watch the infrequent trains go by. We often wondered how they ever got any work done. This apparent leisure stood out in marked contrast to the "bee like" activity of the congested Oriental lands that were now fast receding from us. I marveled at how the Russians had been able to get as many troops, horses and supplies to the front as they did over the long single-track railway. No wonder their soldiers were dispirited and no match for the numerous and almost fanatical Japanese soldiers who fought so loyally for their "Sun god" Emperor.

When we were nearly half way across Siberia, I developed a high fever. Once I had almost passed out with malaria while visiting China and now Mother grew quite alarmed. She decided, against my protests, to get off at Irkutsk, 3,000 miles east of Moscow, near beautiful Lake Baikal. This was, at that time, only a rough pioneer town with few paved streets. Our *drosky* sank in mud nearly to the axles.

Mother found a place for us to stay at a log cabin, something like the one in which my father had been born in Canada, although this was more primitive. She also had succeeded in finding a Russian doctor, a big bearded man who at first glance looked as if he had escaped from a convict camp. However, he proved to be very kind and capable, and with the aid of Latin medical terms, confirmed that I had a severe attack of malaria. Fortunately this was one of the few diseases of that day for which there was an excellent specific medicine in the form of quinine.

I responded so well to treatment that we were able to board the Trans-Siberian train of the following week, and so our time schedule had not been too badly disrupted. It had also been interesting to experience what life was like in a pioneer Siberian town. We had found the living rather drab and had no desire to return. By contrast, however, it made the places that we were yet to see all the more attractive.

We were not sorry when we reached Moscow and had to part with our lice-hunting fellow passengers. However, the trip through the Ural Mountains, which separate Asia from Europe, had been very scenic and enjoyable. Perhaps one of the things we welcomed most in Moscow was the chance to get a bath and remove soot from our hair (fortunately, we found no lice).

Moscow impressed us as being a city of domed churches. These were often filled with devout worshippers either standing or kneeling before their favorite icons that were bedecked with precious jewels. One of the domes stood out from all the rest, due to its special spiral markings. We were told that "Ivan the Terrible" had had its architect blinded, lest he design a more beautiful dome.

One could not have imagined that only seven years hence, many of the devout now in these churches would declare themselves atheists and denounce all would-be worshippers. It would also have been hard to believe what was to be the fate of the handsome Czar of all the Russians. He was to be shot down, together with his beautiful family, by some of the very same individuals who now cheered him as he rode in state through the "Red Square" to the Kremlin, the walled citadel. It was with much difficulty that we were able to peer through the madly cheering crowds to even get a glimpse of the Czar. When we succeeded, we were struck with his close resemblance to Edward VII, whom we had seen in London at the time of his coronation.

We were frequently told by our guides about that fateful winter march of Napoleon to Moscow. We were even shown the bed where he had slept, before he was turned back by the brave Russians and the rigors of a severe Russian winter.

St. Petersburg proved to be a more modern city than the Moscow we had just left. In a comparatively short time (1924), this city would be renamed Leningrad after Vladimir Lenin. It would have been difficult to have predicted that the people would dismiss the many historical ties the city had with its founder, Peter the Great, in favor of one who was not generally known and who had made no contribution to the establishment of the city.

Soon after our arrival in St. Petersburg, we were startled by earthquake-like tremors which seemed to alarm no one but ourselves. When we remarked about it, we were merely reminded that Peter the Great had built his city on a spongy bog, and we would soon get used to such vibrations every time a tram car went by, and think nothing of it!

However, I soon had in store a more frightening experience than mere earth tremors. We had gone to see the "Winter Palace," by far the largest palace in the world. The innumerable rooms soon began to all look alike. While Mother was particularly interested in viewing the lovely paintings and works of art, I was far more interested in exploring. I promised that I would be rejoining her after I had had a look around.

Evidently the palace guard on duty had temporarily left his post, which marked the limits where visitors were permitted, and before I realized it, I had strayed beyond bounds. I was having the time of my life peering into the countless chambers which seemed to lure me on and on.

Finally I decided that I had better return and tell Mother about my explorations. However, as it turned out, I was just going around in circles and was lost in the maze. What was worse, it was growing dim, and I realized it would not be long before it would be pitch dark. Yelling did no good for I only heard the faint echoes of my own voice. I knew the Russians to be a very suspicious people, and when I was found, they might think I had been up to some mischief and punish me accordingly.

In the meantime, Mother was beginning to become concerned, especially since it was growing dark and all visitors were being asked to leave. She had tried in vain to get the guard on duty to initiate a search but he stoutly maintained that no one ever got by him. Probably he did not want to admit to his superiors that he had left his post. With difficulty, Mother finally located the head palace guard. At last she was able to convince him that I might still be inside the palace. So with the aid of lanterns, they started the search.

In due course I saw a shaft of lantern light through a corridor and began to shout. The guards were not in a friendly mood when they reached me. They first searched me, evidently looking for weapons. When they were satisfied I was not armed and had not stolen anything, they sullenly led me through the maze of rooms to where my mother was anxiously waiting. She then thought we could leave without further delay. Little did she know of Russian mentality. It was not as simple as that.

The officer in charge said, "Does the young man not know that he has committed a very serious offense by breaking into a royal palace?"

I tried to explain but he refused to listen and demanded to see our passports and visas. Mother, therefore, had to leave me to their tender mercies while she went back to the hotel to get the necessary documents.

Mother, fortunately, had been able to persuade our hotel proprietor to accompany her on her return, for the guards' knowledge of English left much to be desired. After much haggling and the payment of an unofficial fine, I was finally released. I vowed that the next time I would confine my explorations to caves and not to Russian palaces.

Our travels took us to Bavaria, where we were deeply moved by the Passion Play at Oberammergau; then on to Paris and London. We reached Edinburgh, Scotland in time for the official opening of the "World Missionary Conference" to which Mother was a delegate from Korea. It was the first conference of its kind on such a large scale, and the delegates came from many lands. The huge auditorium was filled with people from all parts of the missionary world.

Dr. John R. Mott, world famous for his Y.M.C.A. and missionary activities, presided over the conference. He was the one who, in 1897, had advised my mother to return to Korea with her two small children. He had visited us in our home there. It was, therefore, a special joy to meet this personal friend again. The conference proved to be a real inspiration, and when it was over, we sailed from Glasgow to Montreal, and thence, to the United States.

I was to complete my high school education at the Mount Hermon School in Mount Hermon, Massachusetts, fulfilling a dream of my father's. Dwight L. Moody had founded the school, and when my father had attended the D. L. Moody Summer School at nearby Northfield, he had been much impressed by the caliber of Mount Hermon. It was at that time that my father had decided to prepare for a medical missionary career by training in New York. He later told my mother that should they ever have a son, he would hope that he could attend this school which had given birth to the Student Volunteer Movement. Thus, the paths of destiny led me to Mount Hermon. Before me lay the prospects for growth, study and adjustment. Little did I realize the extent of that adjustment nor how very different life in America would be from my boyhood in Korea.

When my mother returned to Korea at the completion of her furlough in 1911, I stayed on at Mount Hermon. Perhaps I had gone more native in Korea than most missionary children. I was a lone child, and my mother was away at the hospital all day. Many of my playmates were Korean children. I had learned to play, think, and often act as a Korean. During those early weeks of becoming acclimated to a new life style, I would often think back nostalgically to a more carefree time.

Somehow, I never acquired the Westerner's sense of urgency and timing. The Koreans, for the most part, had no timepieces and adopted an easy-going philosophy of life which seemed to appeal to my nature. "There will always be tomorrow," they would say. So it was hard for me to have to keep my eyes glued to the clock, and to work as if "tomorrow never comes."

Then, too, there had always been someone at my beck and call, and I easily acquired the habit of saying, "Let the *amah* do it." So there was indeed much adjustment and a great deal for me to learn at Mount Hermon.

The school had a unique feature called the "work hour" where students could contribute toward tuition expenses by working two hours each weekday. Since work was not done on Sunday, one could put in extra time on Monday by working an additional hour and a half. Overtime pay was only twelve and one-half cents per hour. I was, practically speaking, financially on my own, so I had to put in considerable overtime.

They started me off working on the school farm, and of all places, in the silo. As the cut green cornstalks were blown in from above, I was told that all I had to do was to simply spread them out evenly in the interior pit of the silo. The farm foreman, with a twinkle in his eye asked me, "Do you think you can do it?"

In my ignorance, I replied, "Sure."

In the first place, it was very dusty and hot as Hades in the silo. Even before the work started, I felt certain that I was suffocating. Then the green cut fodder started to descend on me, and suddenly I acquired a sense of dire urgency, for had I stopped even for a minute I could see that I would be buried alive in the deluge. So there was nothing to do but to work as if, in truth, there would be no tomorrow.

Finally the farm foreman could see that I was all done in and he assigned me the job of milking, which I was certain would be much easier. Alas, those who have never milked by hand do not know what is in store for them. First, the cow objected to my gentle touch and simply kicked me off my stool. It was here that I discovered her hoofs were not padded. Next, she put one of her dirty hoofs in my milk pail, which did nothing for the purity of the milk nor for the serenity of my disposition. After some time when I thought that I had acquired the hang of it, the one in charge came along and found that I had not stripped the bags enough. In no uncertain terms, he informed me that at the rate I was going I would have all these prize cows dried up in no time.

My next assignment was to pick tomatoes. Except for backache, which at first was considerable, it really was not too bad. By this time, however, I was beginning to feel the work hour was a cruel invention of the devil. I decided I was definitely not cut out to be a farmer, though previously I had dreamt of one day owning a farm of my own.

Just as I was becoming adjusted to some of the more interesting types of farm work, I was transferred to janitor duty at one of the dormitories. I found myself inwardly protesting, but soon I was promoted to work at West Hall, which housed the kitchen and large dining area. After a brief kitchen apprenticeship, I was assigned to waiting on tables. This job had a pattern of promotion already established. One graduated from waiting on the students, then the farm supervisors, to, finally, the most coveted of all the jobs—waiting on the teachers. The rewards, in addition to the status, were reaped in the superior food which we could also enjoy. In the kitchens of Mount Hermon I learned the Western value of time and punctuality.

The school had an enviable scholastic achievement record and I found much of the teaching to be inspiring. I attended the compulsory Bible classes taught by a much loved teacher from Australia, Dr. M. C. Harrison. These were held in the very room where the great Student Volunteer Movement had its birth. A classmate was the son of the Reverend John Forman, missionary to India. It was the Reverend Forman who had brought my father into the Student Volunteer Movement back in 1887 which ultimately resulted in my father going to Korea. I, naturally, joined the Student Volunteers and did some deputation speaking in the surrounding churches.

Soon after I had come to Mount Hermon, other students from Korea arrived, including my chum, John Baird. Indeed, some of the "Korea girls" at Northfield (the companion school across the river) had preceded me. I would often trudge the nearly two-hour walk there and back to have the privilege of a half-hour chat with them. We would compare notes concerning our respective schools. We agreed that D. L. Moody would be remembered by later generations more for these two schools and the Bible Institute at Chicago than for being the flaming evangelist of his day, although that fame was deservedly considerable.

In 1912 I had the privilege of meeting Fanny Crosby, the renowned and beloved blind hymn writer. She had been a great friend of my father's during their association at the Madison Street Mission in New York, and had written a farewell hymn in honor of his departure for the mission field.

Fanny Crosby received me most kindly at her home in Hartford, Connecticut. She entertained me with stories of my father and her work with him at the Medical Mission. Even now, I can see her happy face, as she told me how she had composed "Saved by Grace," and some other beautiful hymns. I could not help but fall in love with the winsome personality of this saint of God.

She was humorous at times and asked me with a smile, "Do you believe I have ever been in prison?"

I replied, "I could hardly think so."

Then she answered, "Well, I go to prison every Sunday, for I have a Sunday School class composed of some of the worst convicts there. I love it, and I love them."

My apprenticeship at Mount Hermon drew to a close with my graduation in June, 1915. I felt that it had not only prepared me academically for my future, but had given me the needed tools to bridge two very different cultures. I was ready for college.

On a brief visit to the dear friends of my parents, the J. Sumner Stones of New Rochelle, I met their son-in-law, Mr. Wilson, a minister. He waxed eloquent over the advantages of a small college where one was not just a number. He had graduated from such an institution, Mount Union College in Alliance, Ohio. Although I had originally planned to attend a large university, he so convinced me that I allowed him to make the arrangements for my enrollment at his alma mater. I have never regretted it, for it led to my meeting the most important person in my life—Marian. But that is a later story.

At Mount Union College, I was fortunate to have a remarkable roommate, Fred G. Bratton, who had quite a flair for writing. He later published a booklet entitled, "Friends Unique." I was one of those whom he described and here I quote in part from his essay:

> "It was my first day in college, and I was engaged in the process, common to all 'Freshies,' of seeking a rooming place. I found a front room in a house overlooking the campus, but was informed by the landlady that it had already been engaged. . . . I saw another dejected looking individual in the hallway who had also been disappointed. We looked at each

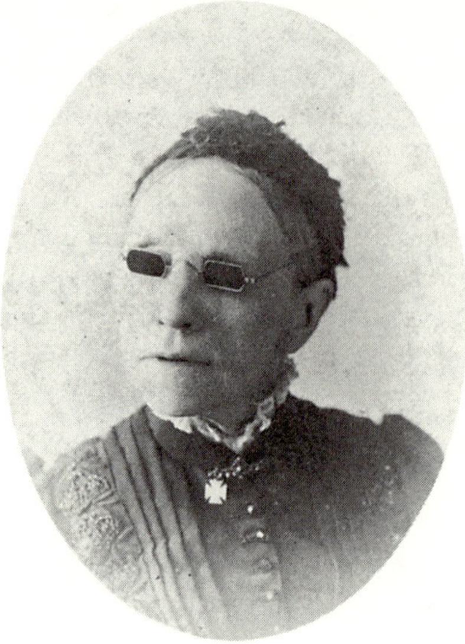

Fanny Crosby

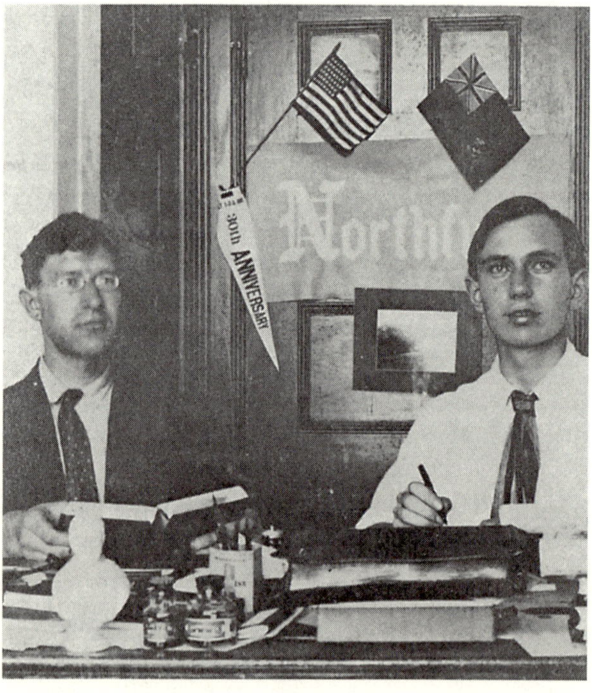

Harry Studwell and Sherwood at Mt. Hermon

other and were about to depart when the landlady spoke, 'See here, I have a room in the back part of the house which is in good condition and big enough for two. Take a look at it.'

"A common cause always makes friends of strangers. We looked at each other, this time in a more scrutinizing manner as if each were reading the character of the other, then at the room, which suited us.

"'Well, what do you say?' I ventured.

"'I am game if you are,' my new acquaintance shot back.

"'We'll stay,' I told the landlady. . . .

"Through such a circumstance, or shall I say, Act of Providence, was I thrown in with Sherwood Hall of Korea . . .

"I have found Hall to be an ideal companion, and one of the most interesting characters I have met. Many a pleasant evening have we spent in our den, where I would listen eagerly to the remarkable experiences which Hall, perched on the bed opposite me, would relate. . . . I had asked Hall to tell the story of the scar on the back of his head. He had just had a close haircut, so the scar was very much in evidence.

"'Well, that represents a mighty close call for me. It was this way. My mother had been on one of her furloughs and we had been out on the Pacific ten days. Suddenly the captain awakened to the fact that it was July 4th, and as there was no other ship in sight, determined to celebrate by letting loose the signal gun in salute. In my boyish curiosity, instead of keeping at a safe distance in the rear, I edged toward the front to see just how a cannon is fired. With a loud crack, the cannon burst into a thousand pieces. One of the pieces whizzed past me, grazing my head and struck a Chinaman next to me, who was killed instantly. I first thought I must have been killed, too, when I saw the blood spurting from my head, but on second thought, as I felt pain, I realized I must still be alive. For once, I appreciated the value of pain. Had my head been tilted back even a little, I would not be here to tell the tale.'

"I congratulated Hall on 'keeping his head,' and myself for being privileged to live with such a 'Hair's Breadth Harry.' . . ."

Bratton in his essay referred to a Dr. Isaac T. Headland who was Professor of Missions at the college. He had served in China and his wife, also a Dr. Headland, had been physician to the Empress Dowager of China. When I shook hands with Dr. Headland the first day I was at college, he told me that he had sailed to China in 1890 on the same ship with my mother whose destination was Korea. He had never dreamed then that he would return to the U.S.A. twenty-five years later and teach her son.

Bratton's essay continued:

> "Hall's uniqueness was soon recognized, and while at college, he has lectured on Korea in churches, missionary societies, and kindred gatherings. His lectures concern Korea, the work of his parents, and personal experiences in Korea and elsewhere. One of the reasons for the popularity of his lectures is that he accompanies his talks with curios, illustrating Korean customs and uses.
>
> "Then he always entertains the children with tiger stories, for the Koreans are not without their folklore . . . Often, articles ornamenting the room are . . . fans, human hair rope, Korean articles of clothing, embroidery, paintings, and photographs of Korean life.
>
> "Needless to say, Hall is a member of the Student Volunteer Band, in fact, he is its President. He is also Chairman of the Deputation Work Committee of the Student Volunteer Union of Ohio Colleges. Hall is a Brother and fellow member of the Phi Kappa Tau Fraternity. He is a conscientious student and also supports various other college activities . . .
>
> "Hall is not talkative, that is, not superfluously so, but his opinion is respected and he usually says something worthwhile. . . . Our friendship has been of mutual inspiration and blessing. . . . The influence of this versatile character on my life has been of lasting benefit. I thank Providence, that it is my privilege to number among my friends, my college roommate, Sherwood Hall!"

I heartily reciprocated Bratton's sentiments. He told much about my life in his booklet, but for some reason, omitted one of the most important aspects—my romance. Perhaps this was because he thought it too personal; or maybe it was still too young when he first took up his pen to compose his essay. At any rate, that romance has run through my entire subsequent life like a golden thread.

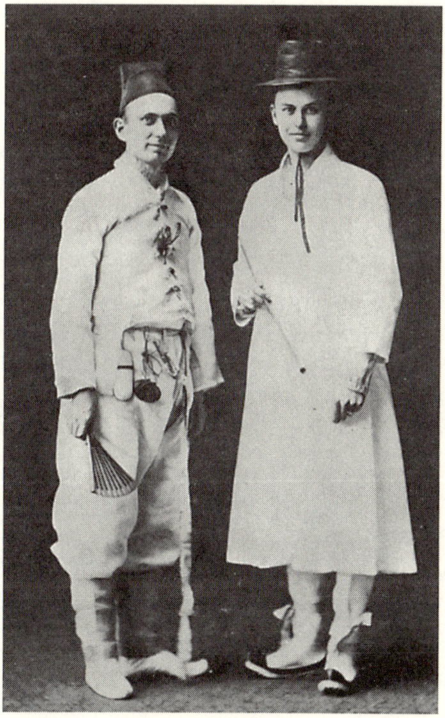

Sherwood Hall and Fred Bratton dressed in Korean garb

CHAPTER 10

Search for Tomorrow

The Dundons, who were fraternity brothers of mine, had made arrangements for me to speak at their home church in Rootstown. This was about twenty miles from the college. These speaking assignments had become quite frequent so I anticipated nothing particularly special about this one.

In my talk at the church, I alluded briefly to the fact that my father had been a member of a church in Athens, Ontario, Canada, similar to their church in Rootstown, and had gone out to Korea as a medical missionary. After the meeting, a number of people came around to shake my hand and exchange pleasantries.

Among those who introduced themselves to me was a young lady, Miss Marian Bottomley, and her mother, Mrs. Mary Bottomley. The minister of the church, the Reverend Norris Lineweaver, was unable to be present because he was attending Annual Ministerial Conference with his wife, Emma, Marian's sister. The Bottomleys were officiating at the parsonage in their behalf and expressed regret that the Lineweavers had not heard me speak.

Miss Bottomley then startled me with her query, "Is that your father's picture which hangs on the wall of the Sunday School room of the Athens Methodist Church?"

My amazement was ill concealed. How was it possible that someone in this remote country village in the United States should happen to know that a picture of my father hung in the church of another remote country village in Canada?

"Yes it is!" I responded wonderingly.

Arthur Dundon's mother met Emma Lineweaver later that week when she had returned from the Ministerial Conference and reported, "When Mr. Hall came back to our house after the church meeting, he appeared to be in a daze. He told me, 'Mrs. Dundon, I have just met a young woman who knows about my father. You don't know what that means to me!'"

Marian and her mother had told the Lineweavers about my talk. They were very much interested and felt that more people should hear my story. Through Arthur Dundon they arranged for me to return for an evening meeting and church social and be their guest to dinner at the parsonage before the gathering. When Marian did not appear before the meal was served, my heart sank. I was afraid she had already returned to Canada. Just then she emerged from the kitchen where she had been helping her sister. I felt an immense sense of relief.

Following the church social, Mrs. Lineweaver realized that in all the preparations for the evening she had neglected to fetch the milk from a nearby farm as was their daily custom. When I heard her ask Marian to get the milk, I eagerly offered to accompany her. We crossed the street from the church to the parsonage for the milk pail and proceeded down the road.

During the brief walk to the dairy farm that evening, I heard from the lovely girl who had walked by my side that she was a school teacher at Bishop's Mills, a town near Athens, and would be returning soon to Canada. Marian knew many of the friends and relatives on my father's side of the family. I suggested that I would appreciate it if she would kindly take a small gift to my grandmother, to which she readily agreed. For me to deliver the gift would necessitate another visit to Rootstown on the following weekend.

When Arthur Dundon had failed to find me at the parsonage, he decided that I must have returned to his home ahead of him. The headlights of his car illuminated a young couple carrying a milk pail between them. Arthur later confessed to me his disbelief at the sight. He had said to himself, "That can't be Hall! He never takes out a college girl on a date. He even refused to escort anyone to the college prom, so he would hardly be taking a country girl from up North on a walk at this hour! But it must be Hall. No one in Rootstown would be dressed in a light pongee suit but that importer of Oriental silks himself. It *is* Hall!"

I had the unexpected privilege of hearing Marian sing a solo at the regular church service in Rootstown that next Sunday. Although I had heard the same hymn many times before, somehow, as Marian sang "In the Garden," its real loveliness was borne in on me as never before. I had never heard it sung as beautifully nor heard a voice so melodious to my ear.

I was received back kindly at the parsonage. I welcomed the opportunity to get better acquainted with this girl from Canada whose beautiful voice and vibrant personality had already had such a moving effect on my heart. It had for me been love at first sight.

I could see that I had allies in Marian's mother and sister but I was not sure about Mr. Lineweaver. I later learned that he had someone else in mind whom he felt might become interested in Marian. But he failed to get to first base, for as it turned out, Marian had become interested in me.

Marian's family felt that she should plan to return to the United States, and perhaps later, enter Mount Union College. That too was my fervent wish and I was delighted when Marian concurred. Time passed all too swiftly and I had to leave, but not before I had received a promise from Marian that she would write to me regularly, and of course I would want to hear all about my grandmother's reaction to the small gift.

It is true that notes between Marian and me were, at first, rather brief and were concerned chiefly with happenings and events of more general interest rather than personal. However, through our correspondence, the story of Marian's life began to unfold.

She was born in England on June 21, 1896 in the small village of Epworth, famous for being the birthplace of John Wesley, the founder of Methodism. Marian and her elder sister, Emma, often served as self-appointed guides to show visiting tourists the historic town. (This was how Emma happened to first become acquainted with Mr. Lineweaver, a Methodist minister. He had been a tourist visiting Epworth from the U.S.A. When Emma moved to Canada, he pursued her, and the romance eventually led to their wedding in the Athens Methodist Church. Mr. Lineweaver was then assigned to the Methodist Church in Rootstown, Ohio.)

The girls' parents were the first to be married in the new Wesley Memorial Chapel at Epworth. Their mother was the church organist and their father served as a Methodist "lay preacher" on Sundays. He was a photographer by profession and Marian as a child was much interested in his work and often assisted him.

Following the death of her husband, Joseph Bottomley, Mary Keightley Bottomley took the venturesome and courageous step of moving to Canada in 1911 with her two daughters, then of high school age. It was on the suggestion of one of her former Sunday

School students who had moved to Canada that Mrs. Bottomley chose to settle in the village of Athens, Ontario.

Here Mrs. Bottomley set up an attractive photography studio and Marian attended Athens High School, completing the four-year curriculum in three years much to the amazement of the local townspeople.

Marian finished her teacher's training at normal school in Kingston, Ontario, and was soon teaching Canadian youngsters their "three R's." She had many exciting experiences as a school marm in the rural schools. One morning when she arrived at school some of her students, whom she thought to be devoted to her, unceremoniously began to pound on her and rub her nose vigorously with snow. Shocked by such behavior, she had demanded an explanation.

They replied in a shrill chorus, "But teacher! Your nose was frozen!" This, evidently, was the locally accepted treatment for frostbite.

From the farmhouse where she was boarding, Marian made the trip to the school during the winter months on snowshoes. She had become quite proficient at maneuvering on them. Once, while traveling to another school by sleigh, it overturned in a snowdrift and both she and the horse had to be extricated. Marian decided then that snowshoes were a surer way.

All the various wheels that had been set in motion finally succeeded in bringing Marian to the United States in the summer of 1917. She was to teach at the Rootstown School in the fall, but she also needed to earn as much money as possible for her future college education. She took an interim job in the next town at a factory which had big war orders for wool yarn and wool products. The other factory girls looked on the newcomer with condescension and pitying smiles. Some said, "Poor thing, she does not know how long it takes to learn how to handle these complicated machines before piecework is profitable. Besides, the foreman is a rough sort. She will soon be in tears and fleeing from here. This is no place for a school marm."

Marian went to work on the new spinning machine assigned to her which the foreman had briefly explained how to use. Almost at once it had jammed and the other factory girls gave each other sly knowing smiles. Under their breaths they whispered, "Now she will get it from the foreman. She can't last much longer."

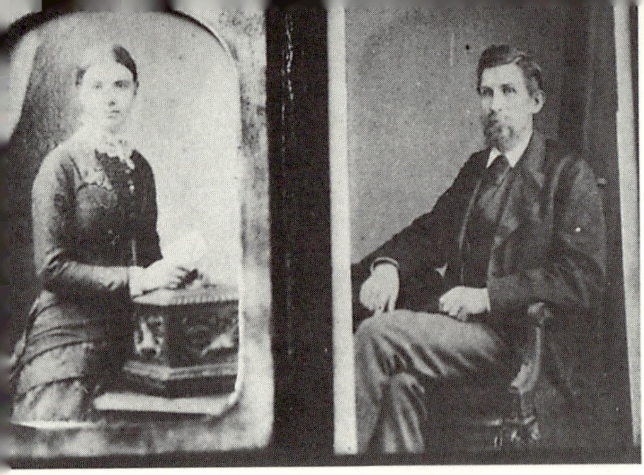

Mary Keightley Bottomley and Joseph Bottomley, Marian's parents

Marian in England with village of Epworth and spire of Wesley Memorial Chapel in right background

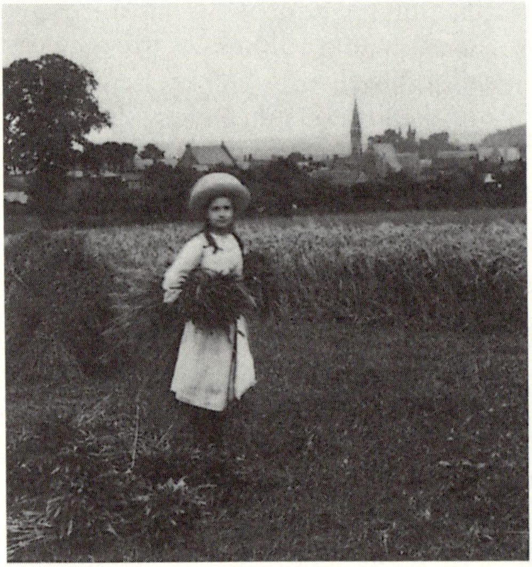

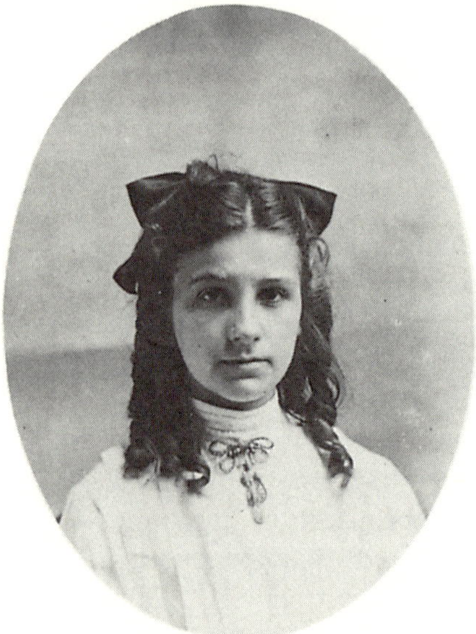

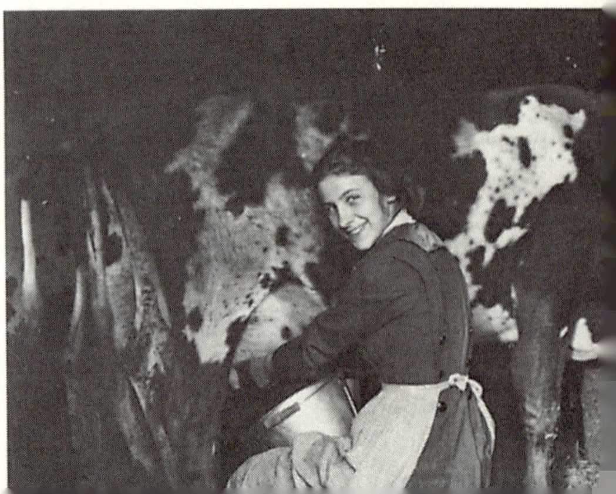

Marian in Athens, Ontario, Canada

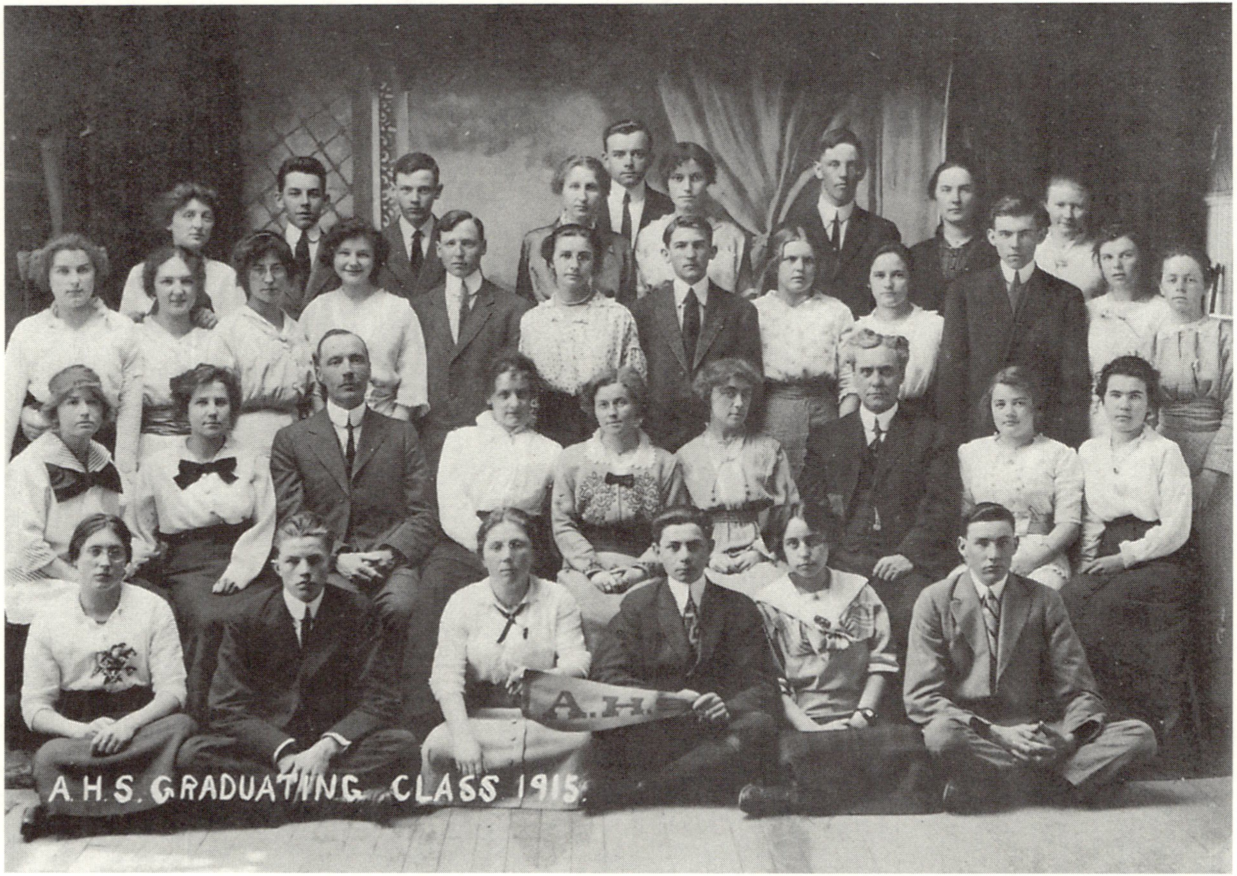

Marian's Athens High School graduating class, 1915

Marian did not hesitate to go up to the foreman, but what she asked him nearly toppled him off the high stool on which he was perched. She ignored his sneer and demanded to see a diagram and printed instructions of the machine, for she wanted to figure out for herself just how this machine worked.

He said rudely, "You never would be able to understand it, even if I did show it to you."

She stuck to her guns until, to get rid of her, he reluctantly turned over the diagram and instruction sheet. In no time at all, Marian had it figured out and was operating the machine like an old hand.

All were taken aback, especially the foreman, who soon assigned her a more complicated machine which usually took considerable time to master. This time, however, he had given her the diagram from the beginning.

Marian was soon turning out piecework at a much faster rate than the old timers. The foreman really did not want her to leave when school opened but some of the girls, who felt Marian had set them too fast a pace, were frankly relieved when she departed to resume her role as school teacher.

The consolidated school was much larger and the classes more difficult to manage than the one-room schoolhouse Marian had been accustomed to in Canada. Discipline was a particularly difficult problem. One day a mischievous pupil started to disrupt the class by noisily snapping his fingers. Marian detained the boy after school.

"You seem to enjoy snapping your fingers," Marian observed. "Very well, Wilbur, you may snap them all you want for the next fifteen minutes when you will not be diverting your classmates."

A delighted grin crossed Wilbur's face and he started snapping his fingers loudly with both hands. It was not long before his smile vanished and he was soon having difficulty in snapping the fingers of even one hand. Marian reminded him to keep up his pace. At the end of fifteen minutes, she dismissed the offender.

"I'll do it again tomorrow!" Wilbur called back, still unrepentant.

"Fine!" replied his teacher. "If you do, you may stay after school and snap your fingers for me for thirty minutes."

"Oh, I couldn't do it any longer," Wilbur responded with feeling.

After that Miss Bottomley did not encounter any more behavior problems and her class became known as the best disciplined in the school. She did not mind the riddle the children asked each other: "Why is Miss Bottomley's class like a Ford car?"

The answer: "It is run by a crank."

She knew that both the children and the music teacher, in particular, appreciated the order that she was able to maintain in contrast to the unruliness of the other classrooms.

Although Marian was now relatively close, we found that we had little time for dating. Marian had her teaching assignment, and when I was not studying, I was helping to support myself through college by selling silks and laces from Chefoo, China. Later, I added kitchenware and cutlery to my line.

I did find time to remain active in our Student Volunteer Band, and Marian shared this interest with me. She confided that she, too, had aspirations to become a missionary. It seemed especially appropriate, therefore, that she should attend the Student Volunteer Convention that was scheduled in March, 1918 at Baldwin Wallace College in Berea, Ohio. I was to be a delegate from Mount Union College, and I invited Marian to accompany me as my guest.

The convention was an inspiration to us both. On the way home we discussed its meaning for us. In the predawn hours, we sat over breakfast in the restaurant of the Cleveland railroad station. Whiling away the long wait for our train connection back to Alliance, we talked about Marian's future. Marian seemed responsive to my suggestion that she become a medical doctor and in that capacity fulfill her aspiration to become a missionary. I leaned forward eagerly and asked her, "Marian, will you accompany me to Korea?"

I was totally uprepared for her facetious unhesitating reply, "It would hardly be proper, would it?"

I was so taken aback that I missed the twinkle in her eye. I fell into an awkward silence for most of the remainder of the trip. I, who generally tried to be so careful with my words, had fallen down badly on my most important speech. I realized, too late, that a public location like a railway station, at such an early hour, was hardly the romantic time or place for such a serious proposal.

I was even greener than I had realized. My fraternity brothers later instructed me that the correct way for a college "Greek letter man" was to back up his proposal with a jeweled fraternity pin, which he should pin on his beloved as soon as she gave him her maidenly nod. I would not leave the matter to chance the next time.

Fortunately for me, Marian was a great lover of wildlife and had much to teach me about the various species of birds to be found in the woods near Rootstown. A pleasant excursion into the woods would afford the ideal mood and setting.

The first suitable weekend, I invited Marian to accompany me, not to Korea, but just to the woods to study bird life. Marian accepted my invitation. It was a perfect day in April for our excursion. It was good to be alive.

At the propitious moment, I made my proposal. This time I assured Marian that it was as my *wife* that I wished her to accompany me to Korea. She rewarded my proposal with the coveted "yes," and received my fraternity pin graciously and lovingly. Momentarily, our rapture in each other eclipsed our mutual interest in wildlife.

Somehow news of our engagement spread like wildfire among my special college friends, who now felt they had discovered a new Hall, or at least a new side to my character. Each one seemed to have different unsolicited advice for me, but I felt that this was my own personal business. I soon learned to live with a lot of good natured

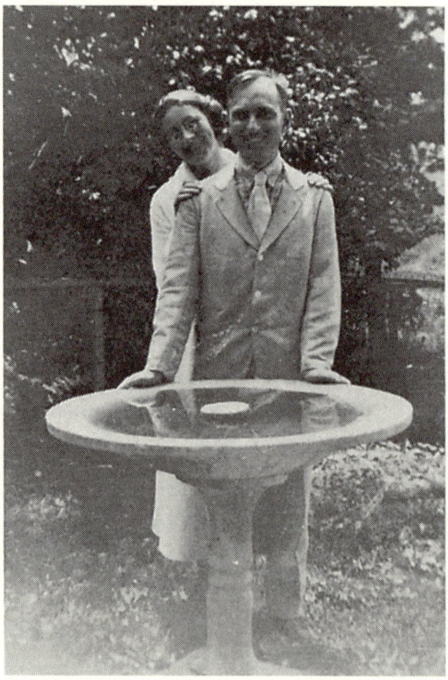

Marian and Sherwood at Mt. Union College, Alliance, Ohio

kidding. One individual, however, seriously thought I was making a great mistake and that it was his duty to caution me, for he feared my plans for the study of medicine would never be realized. Another wanted to know why one of the college girls was not my choice and named off a few possibilities. Still another suggested that I should go out with different girls before settling down with a relatively unknown girl from another country.

While these suggestions may have had merit, they came too late. I had already fallen in love. Marian and I were floating on a cloud of happiness.

All too soon we had to come down to earth. The reality of the Great World War was getting closer to us since America had become formally involved the previous spring. I had attended a British recruiting meeting in Canton, Ohio, where no pains were spared to secure volunteers for the British Army. However, I was reluctant to volunteer, for my mother was scheduled to return to the United States on furlough in May. If I were to join the British Army, I would have been sent overseas immediately.

The other alternative was to volunteer for the United States Medical Reserve Corps where my premedical courses at Mount Union would serve me well. There was some question of my losing my Canadian citizenship if I took this step, but it would mean that I would be stationed at Pittsburgh for the training period and my mother would be able to stay at YWCA quarters nearby.

After consulting with President W.H. McMaster of Mount Union College and with Bishop Herbert Welch, Methodist Bishop of Korea, I decided to apply for United States citizenship and volunteer for the U.S. Medical Reserve Corps. All males of military age who were not enemy aliens were subject to the draft. By enlisting in the Medical Corps I would at least be in the service area of my choice.

My application was accepted and I was ordered to report to the Alliance Draft Board for my physical examination in the late spring of 1918. Marian and her family had invited me to Rootstown for the preceding weekend. I had planned to leave by the interurban electric train on its last trip on Sunday night in order to be back at Alliance in good time for the induction on Monday. One thing I had not reckoned with was that in the world of love there is no sense of time. Before we knew it, I had missed the interurban. Hitchhiking at that hour was out of the question. I had no option but to walk the twenty-odd miles. I made it, though tired and footsore. The blisters on my feet made even that "one step forward" command a painful ordeal. Apparently I passed the physical despite the blisters and was ordered to report to the Army Training Center at the University of Pittsburgh Medical College on September 30, 1918.

On June 18 I went to meet my mother's train at the Alliance railroad station. I was especially pleased when later, after meeting Marian, Mother said she was favorably impressed by my fiancée.

I was enrolled in the Summer School at Mount Union College and Mother decided it would be fun to take some courses along with me. Although Marian had originally felt that she should go back to the factory to earn some extra funds for the college year ahead, Dr. Headland thought otherwise. He had been instrumental in helping to secure a scholarship for her and she was thus enabled to enroll in Summer School with us.

The Lineweavers had invited my mother to visit them before Summer School opened. They had now been assigned to a church in nearby Middlefield, Ohio. Marian and I traveled to the Lineweavers with my mother and on June 21 we all celebrated Marian's 22nd birthday. Mother stayed on to speak to some of the ladies' groups in the church about Korea and then the three of us enrolled for the summer session. We enjoyed Dr. Headland's Bible course immensely, which featured the Book of Job. All too swiftly summer was over.

The Army Medical Training Center was located in Pittsburgh on the campus of the Medical College of the University of Pittsburgh. Here we newly enlisted recruits were to receive our special training. Crude barracks had already been erected adjacent to the Medical School and a playing field nearby had been converted for our drilling ground. So it was drill, drill, drill and intensified medical study. We were so bone weary when we turned in for the night that we hardly had energy enough to remove our clothes or even complain about the hard bunks.

Then came the fateful "Spanish Influenza" Epidemic of 1918. Because medical personnel were in short supply, the Department of Health and Charities in Philadelphia requisitioned my mother to help as a temporary physician. All church conferences planned by the Mission Board had been cancelled, for city health departments were placing a ban on large public gatherings because of the epidemic.

The Anatomy Department at the University of Pittsburgh Medical College had no difficulty in obtaining cadavers because of the many fatalities from influenza. Each of us was allowed one corpse apiece, instead of two people having to work on the upper extremities, while another pair were working on the lower extremities. This experience in dissecting was not usually available to first-year medical students.

However, the flu came even closer and was no longer impersonal when it hit our barracks. It seemed that every morning one or more of our buddies would be carried out on a stretcher to the infirmary. Some were taken directly to the morgue. Each of us began to wonder whether he would be next. We began to feel that this place was even more dangerous than the field of battle.

I wrote to Marian that I, too, had contracted the disease. She realized that because of the crowded conditions throughout the training center, it would be impossible to get proper nursing care. She paid me a surprise visit and accomplished the almost impossible, by getting permission from the authorities for my immediate transfer to a private rooming house where a motherly landlady could help to look after me. I was in the early stages of fever, aches and pains. I am sure that this bold and timely deed of Marian's was responsible for my recovery.

The wonderful news of the Armistice reached us on November 11, 1918. This was an occasion for real jubilation. However, it would still take some time before my formal discharge papers from the Army came through. The medical training was continued, but without the early morning military drills, which thus gave us more time for our studies. We were also permitted to live outside the barracks.

My mother's emergency assignment as a physician in Philadelphia had terminated. At the end of November she was able to arrange for us both to have rooms in the private home of Mrs. Cassidy, sister of a wealthy friend of my mother's, Mrs. Woolverton. The latter friend was to play a significant role in our lives at a future time. My job at Mrs. Cassidy's was to wind her huge collection of rare clocks and see that they all chimed in unison, a task that proved quite challenging.

Marian seemed to be getting along beautifully in her college work at Mount Union. She was able to join us in Pittsburgh for a week at Christmas, and we talked much about the future. Through summer school work, Marian planned to speed her undergraduate training so that she would have sufficient credits to enter medical school by the fall of 1920. That way we could be married in seven years after the completion of her internship.

Meanwhile, Marian had been pledged by the Tri-Delta sorority. She was continuing to help support herself through school by working in the kitchen and dining room of Elliott Hall. We had little time to see each other but made up for it through correspondence.

By the end of the college year, I finally received my honorable discharge from the army. My studies at Pittsburgh, and the previous summer work at Alliance, had earned me enough credits to graduate with my class in June 1919 from Mount Union College.

My guardian, and my father's great friend, Dr. Omar Kilborn, as well as his talented son, Dr. Leslie Kilborn, felt strongly that it would be best for me to take my medical training at the University of Toronto. After due consideration I agreed. With their help I had no difficulty in transferring my credits. The American Methodist Mission Board and the Pennsylvania Medical Missionary Society agreed to assist with my expenses. With this substantial aid plus what I was able to earn during vacations, I was able to carry through financially.

Because I would now be living in Canada, I would be unable to complete the residence requirements for U.S. citizenship. The application expired, and I remained a Canadian. My future career as a missionary made it doubtful I would live in the United States ever long enough to meet the residency requirements.

I was attending Toronto University at a very exciting period. Dr. Frederick Grant Banting and Dr. Charles Herbert Best were doing their research work on insulin in the treatment of diabetes. My good friend, Dr. Leslie Kilborn, was also on this research staff and was able to get me into the exclusive laboratory to watch this wonderful team at work. It was a thrill to see such dedication and enthusiasm, though it was then still some years before their great breakthrough and subsequent worldwide fame.

Marian had shown greater faith than I when she began her medical course at the Women's Medical College, Philadelphia, Pennsylvania in September 1920, and I could not help but be in awe of her pluck and determination. Her three summer sessions had speeded her undergraduate work as planned and earned her enough credits for admission to medical school. She would complete her undergraduate credits the following summer, and could then formally receive her B.S. degree at the Mount Union College graduation exercises in June, 1922.

Marian greeted her future with only a few dollars in her pocket, the assurance of a scholarship for tuition, and the promise of a free room. However, her faith was rewarded almost from the first, for the kind lady who had offered her a free room, Mrs. Isabelle West, said soon after her arrival, "Marian, I shall of course expect you to board with us too. My mother is frail and I do not like to leave her alone. However, I often have to go out in the evenings, so if you will plan to stay home when I am out, this service will pay for your room and board."

This indeed was an answer to one of Marian's prayers. In various providential ways, other channels always seemed to open as a need developed.

After Marian had finished her final Mount Union College course work in the summer of 1921, we were able to spend a few weeks together in Battle Creek, Michigan. We both had been hired by the Laboratory of the famous Kellogg Sanatorium there. It proved to be a congenial place for gaining some practical experience while at the same time earning money toward our medical school expenses. We were grateful to have a little time together for the separations necessitated by our education were becoming harder and harder to endure.

Long engagements may have been ideal in Bible times. That was hardly so for Marian and me, especially since we were in different countries. This was long before the day when colleges and universities built dormitories for married couples. Marriage for college girls was severely frowned upon at that time, and it was generally assumed that any girl foolish enough to marry would not be able to finish her academic training. The chances were also considered quite dubious for the married college man, especially if he did not have a large bank account.

Thus, it was very difficult to buck the trend of that day, especially against the advice of our well meaning elders and relatives. We felt, nonetheless, we must be true to ourselves and cast aside our plans for a seven-year engagement. We would be wed on June 21, 1922. This date had special significance to Marian, for it was her natal day as well as the date on which she was to receive her Bachelor of Science degree. It would thus mark a triple anniversary. I laughingly told her that it would also be advantageous for me, for it would only involve one present for the triple event.

Hairsplitting timing was required that day. I had to first complete an important final examination the day before, then catch an overnight train from Toronto, soon after, for the close connection to the train for Alliance. The first part went off like clockwork, and I was beginning to feel quite elated when unexpectedly, we encountered a freight train wreck ahead.

Marian had already arrived in Alliance earlier from Philadelphia. Her anxious eyes were rapidly scanning the large audience at the commencement exercises but her bridegroom was not in evidence. Even the unusual and glowing tribute that Dean Bowman had handed Marian, saying how much influence for good to her fellow students she had been while at college, did not divert her concern for her absent lover.

Hair disheveled and completely out of breath, I entered the auditorium just at the conclusion of the ceremonies and waved to my relieved bride-to-be. Immediately following the graduation exercises, Marian, clutching the coveted sheepskin, slipped out by the nearest exit, not waiting for the congratulations of friends. She fell into my eager arms. We rushed to a waiting car, which was to speed us the some 50 miles to East Liverpool, Ohio, where our wedding was to take place.

Marian's sorority sister and very close friend, Phyllis Crook, and Phyllis's dear parents had made all the beautiful arrangements for the church wedding and a reception. Marian's brother-in-law, the Reverend Norris A. Lineweaver, together with the Reverend Isaac Wood, were to conduct the marriage ceremony. Marian's sister, nephew, and mother had arrived ahead to welcome us and give us their blessing. My mother had returned to Korea in 1920 and regretted very much that she could not be present with us.

After enjoying the wonderful hospitality of Phyllis and her parents, we were off the next day to Canada. We stayed a brief while in Toronto and then left by steamer down the St. Lawrence River through the fabulous Thousand Islands to Brockville, Ontario. We traveled by car the 25 miles to Charleston Lake, the place where my father went camping many years before. For us Charleston Lake remains to this day the most beautiful lake in the world. Here we spent our honeymoon on a remote and uninhabited island.

We were totally unprepared for the announcement that awaited Marian upon her return to medical school from our honeymoon. The Woman's Foreign Missionary Society announced that they were

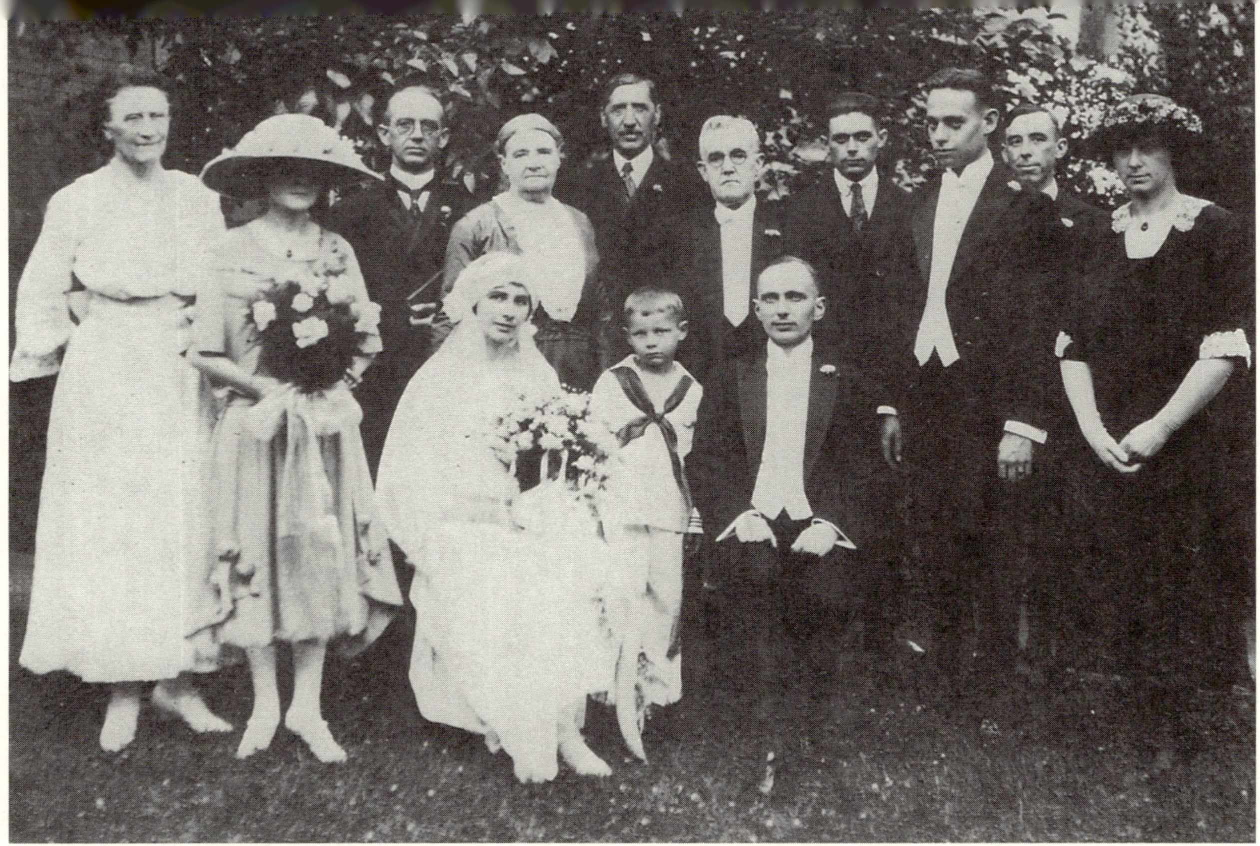

Wedding day–June 21, 1922
Front: Miss Phyllis Crook, Marian, Norris E. Lineweaver (Marian's nephew), Sherwood, Walter Ashbaugh (best man), Mrs. Emma Lineweaver,
Back: Mrs. Agnes Crook, the Rev. Norris A. Lineweaver, Mrs. Mary Bottomley, the Rev. Isaac Wood, Mr. Frank Crook, Paul Binsley, Sanford Almy

immediately discontinuing their scholarship aid to Marian because of her marriage while yet a student. This really hurt. The Society, of course, had the perfect right to stop their help, for which Marian had been most grateful, but we felt they should have given us sufficient warning at least to allow us to make alternate arrangements. We had kept our marriage no secret. It had been understood that Marian would give free medical care for the women of the Society when we reached the mission field, which she was glad to do anyway. However, the college proved understanding and gave Marian a partial scholarship. The Pennsylvania Medical Missionary Society came to the rescue with the remaining needed financial assistance. Marian was thus able to pursue her medical studies uninterrupted.

After obtaining my degree from the Medical School of the University of Toronto in 1923, I was naturally drawn to Philadelphia for my internship. Marian was in her senior year at Women's Medical College. My internship at the Stetson Hospital in Philadelphia began in June, 1923. Many of the patients at the hospital were connected with the famous Stetson hat factory.

Soon after beginning my work there, I received an urgent telephone message to the effect that Marian, while out attending a patient, had fainted and had been admitted to a hospital as an emergency. After I obtained permission from Dr. Tracy, the Medical Superintendent, I rushed to the hospital where she had been taken. I found to my consternation that the young intern there was about to do a lumbar puncture, which could be a rather serious procedure, especially in unskilled hands. Upon my quick examination of my wife, I believed she was not suffering from meningitis (there was no rigidity in her neck muscles) but from a severe case of heat stroke. It had been unusually hot that day. I told the young intern that I strongly felt that a lumbar puncture was not indicated, which did not please him. My diagnosis proved correct.

However, I later made another diagnosis on a patient at Stetson Hospital which did not prove to be correct. The patient was attending our maternity clinic, and on listening with my stethoscope over her abdomen, I thought I could discern two heartbeats. I proudly informed her that she was carrying twins, which immensely pleased the parents-to-be. When she came in for delivery, everything seemed to work out as previously diagnosed, and the young mother was delighted with her newborn twins. Since the mother and babes were o.k., I left the nurse in charge and stepped out for a brief coffee break.

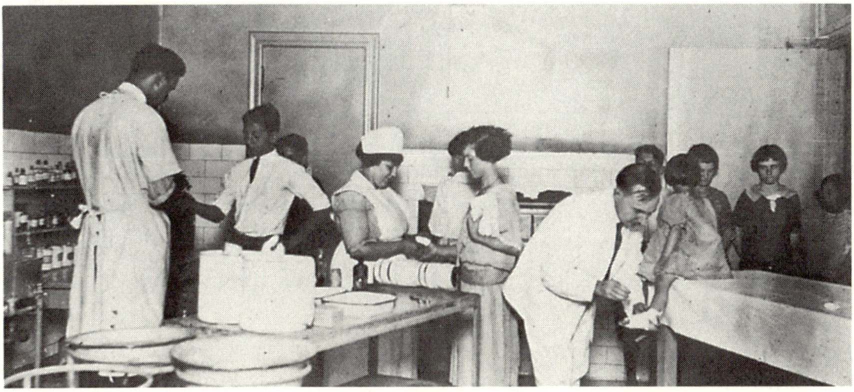

Sherwood in emergency room of Stetson Hospital, Philadelphia

I had not been out long before the nurse rushed in and said, "Oh, Doctor, come quickly."

Thinking that perhaps the mother was having a hemorrhage, I was immediately at her side.

"Sorry, Doctor, but I feel as if I am having another baby."

I tried to assure her not to worry, for that would not be until her next pregnancy.

Then she exclaimed, "I can't wait! Here it comes now!"

How right she was. With chagrin I had to admit, "You now have triplets!"

Time sped by busily and happily. Marian received her M.D. degree in June, 1924, and appointment to an internship at South Side Hospital, Pittsburgh for a year, while I was to specialize in tuberculosis at Suffolk Sanatorium and Clinic in Holtsville, Long Island, New York. I enjoyed splendid training in tuberculosis under Dr. Edwin Kolb and his staff.

I now had my Ontario License and we both had the U.S.A. National Board License, so we were at last both qualified to practice medicine. It looked as if this long, long trail of preparation for our life's work was about over. We applied confidently to the Methodist Mission Board for appointment to the mission field in Korea.

Marian had had superior training and experience in surgery under Dr. Hugh McGuire and other outstanding members of the South Side Hospital staff. We were conceited enough to believe we made a fine team. I would tease Marian and tell her she could cut up the patients and I would make them better. Imagine our dismay, therefore, when we were told by the Mission Board that they simply could not send us out to the mission field because of the financial recession of 1925. Lack of funds prevented the Board from even returning missionaries who had completed their furlough. This news was indeed a stunning blow to us.

When I had been in Toronto, Dr. Wilfred Grenfell (later knighted "Sir") addressed our Student Volunteer group and told the medical students of the great need for doctors in his Labrador Mission. After the meeting, I had spoken to Dr. Grenfell personally. He had become especially interested when I told him that my wife was soon to be a doctor, too.

He had said, "You two are just the kind of medical team we are looking for. If you accepted service with us, we would see to it that your wife received a full salary also."

I told him about our commitment to Korea.

He then said, "If you should ever decide not to go to Korea, please give us the first chance."

This I had promised to do. Thus, after receiving the disappointing news from the Mission Board, I wrote to Dr. Grenfell to inquire if his offer was still open. I received an immediate reply saying that it was. Although we were reluctant to have to give up the idea of going to Korea, it seemed that another door was opening. Dr. Grenfell's offer, besides the wonderful challenge it suggested, would enable us to get on our feet financially. So, all in all, it was very attractive.

We were on the verge of writing to accept it, when we received an urgent letter from Mrs. Edith Beaver Woolverton of New York City requesting us not to make any plans about our future work until we have first seen her. She invited us to meet with her and her sister, Mrs. Miriam Tilge, at their New York City apartment as soon as possible, which we did. I knew them to be good friends of my mother, but I had never met them, although I had roomed at a third sister's home, Mrs. Margaret Cassidy's, when in Pittsburgh.

It seemed that when my mother heard the news about the Mission Board not being able to send us out to Korea, she immediately apprised these wealthy ladies (who had helped her so much in her own work) of our situation to see if they might be interested in sending us to Korea. After our meeting with these generous people, who were not even of our church, we found that they were willing to guarantee our financial support. This way the Methodist Mission Board could send us to Korea.

I suggested that they contact Bishop Herbert Welch, the Methodist Bishop of Korea, who at that time was on a visit to New York. With him they could work out the details.

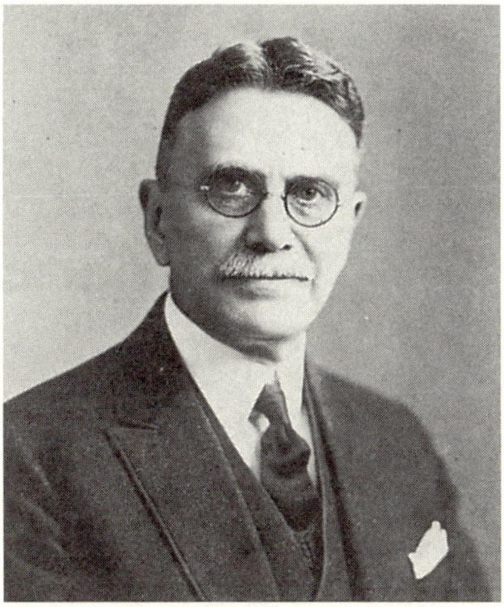

Herbert Welch,
Methodist Bishop of Korea

After I had introduced Bishop Welch to the ladies, they at once started working out the financial arrangement. We were to receive from them, through the Mission Board, the same salary as other missionaries of the Board. It was hoped that the Board could assume responsibility for our support after a three-year period. This arrangement included not only travel expenses, but something additional for which we had hardly dared to hope. The surprise package was in the form of an intensive six-month course in Oriental diseases at the famous London School of Tropical Medicine. From there we would proceed to our mission appointment at the Norton Memorial Hospital in Haiju (Haeju), Korea.

This happy turn of events after the dark moment of our recent discouragement seemed to us like a miracle. We breathed a heartfelt prayer of gratitude to God, and to all who had helped to make it possible. Many had told us that it simply could not be done that year. We remembered, however, that "*with God, all things are possible*." With the zest of youth, we looked forward eagerly to exciting new experiences and high adventure in our life mission across the seas.

CHAPTER 11

Korea Bound

Our sailing date of August 15, 1925 had arrived. We were to travel from New York to Glasgow on the one class passenger liner, *SS Cameronia*. Marian had put the last finishing touches on her packing and had carefully listed everything. My methodical bride, who liked order and system, did not think much of my masculine tendency to stuff things in suitcases every which way. (To this day, she remains the "packer" of the family.)

By the time we reached the ship, there was already a small but very important group of relatives and friends waiting on board to wish us "Bon Voyage." Some had rather special significance to this departure. Mrs. Woolverton was there, accompanied by the widow of the late Dr. George Heber Jones. Mrs. Jones was now working at the New York office of the Mission Board, and had come, not only as their official representative, but as a personal friend. It seemed especially fitting that Mrs. Jones should see us off, for she had traveled to Korea with my mother in 1890 when they were both new missionaries and single. It was the Reverend G. H. Jones who had been the first to officially welcome my father on his arrival in Chemulpo, Korea in 1891 and escort him to Seoul. Mrs. Jessie T. Skidmore and Dr. Simonson, friends from my days at Suffolk Sanatorium on Long Island, had been busy decorating our stateroom with the flowers that had been sent to us, so that it looked like a bridal bower. Indeed, we were known as "the honeymoon couple" all the way to Glasgow.

The usual rolls of colored ribbon were tossed to us as the ship weighed anchor. While our relatives and friends held on to the other ends of the unwinding balls, the ship pulled away and one by one these ties of friendship parted, but not the love they symbolized. It meant a final parting here on earth from some dear ones, like Marian's wonderful mother, the Stones, Mrs. Skidmore and Dr. Simonson. Farewells such as this would now be a part of the life we had chosen. They would always contain that peculiar mixture of sadness at leaving and joy in anticipation which is the lot of a missionary's life. This initial departure was harder on Marian than for me, for she was going "from," while I was going "to," which stirred different emotions in us. However, she brightened at the prospect immediately ahead, which was to be a visit to her birthplace en route to our studies in London.

After touring Scotland and the English Lake District, we journeyed on to the quaint old town of Epworth. Here John Wesley shook all England with his vibrant message and proclaimed "the world as his parish." What was more personal and pertinent to us at that moment was that Epworth was Marian's birthplace and childhood home. This was, indeed, to be a happy day for her, when she could introduce her man to her relatives, old friends, and former classmates. Furthermore, she was now the proud possessor of an M.D. degree, rare for a woman from this area.

When we arrived at the Epworth station, all travel-stained, clothes wrinkled and sooty from the smoke and cinders of the train, we decided to change and freshen up a bit at the rest rooms. We were eager to make an acceptable appearance when we met the folks in town. But to our consternation, when we went to claim our suitcases, we were informed that they had not arrived. The Station Master assured us that they could not have been lost or stolen, but probably had been only held up somewhere at one of the transfer stations. After a session of frantic telephoning, we discovered that they had

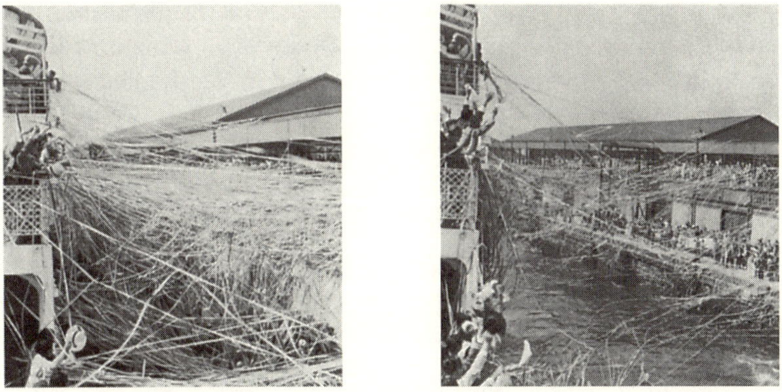

Departure–parting ties of friendship

been sent back to Lake Windermere, for we had not removed the Windermere labels. This would have been done by more experienced travelers as a matter of course. It was with due chagrin we had to admit our ignorance.

Marian was now doubly glad that she had not previously informed her Epworth friends of the date and time of our arrival. After a rather tiresome wait, our baggage finally caught up with us, and we were able to change into something more presentable. We then located an old fashioned trap, a two-wheeled vehicle pulled by a rather spirited young horse, to take us the four miles from the station into Epworth, the Mecca of Methodism.

We were hardly settled in the home of one of Marian's relatives before Marian pulled me out for a quick tour of her beloved home town. The first place to see would be the old Bottomley homestead. Somehow it appeared to Marian that the house had shrunk with the years. She had remembered it as large and spacious. Strangers now occupied the home, but they were friendly and invited us in. Marian pointed out the room where she first saw the light of day, and the courtyard where her father had captured the photograph of her as a child, giving a tea party for her cat.

Then we entered the parlor which was rather dark. In vain, she looked on the walls for the beautiful painting which had been auctioned off regularly once a year by the tax collector, and as regularly bought back by her father. This was because her father, in protest as a Methodist, refused to pay a tax that supported the "established church," and thus he registered his view.

We visited the place where John Wesley used to preach so eloquently and effectively, using the tombstone of his father, Samuel Wesley, as his pulpit. Marian reminisced, "As children, we used to come here and in our play try to imitate John Wesley's preaching from the tombstone."

I was shown the bell tower where Marian used to watch the bell ringers toll out Christmas carols. Then there was the window in the rectory where it was alleged John Wesley had been rescued from fire. However, Marian pointed out that she could never figure out how this could be the very window when the old rectory had burned to the ground.

A special reception to welcome us was held on the beautiful lawn of the Wesley Memorial Chapel. Marian's parents had been the first couple married in the church where her mother had been the organist and her father had conducted services as a lay preacher. I spoke first

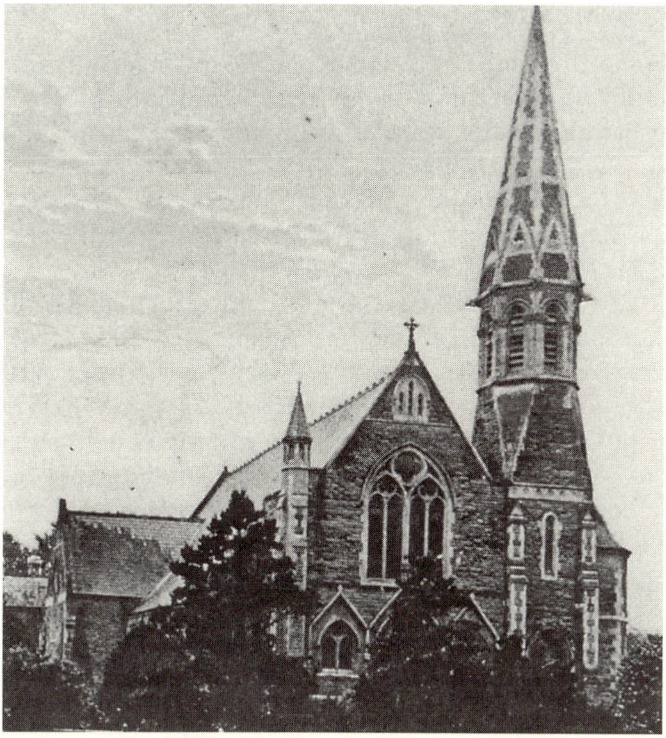

Wesley Memorial Chapel, Epworth, England

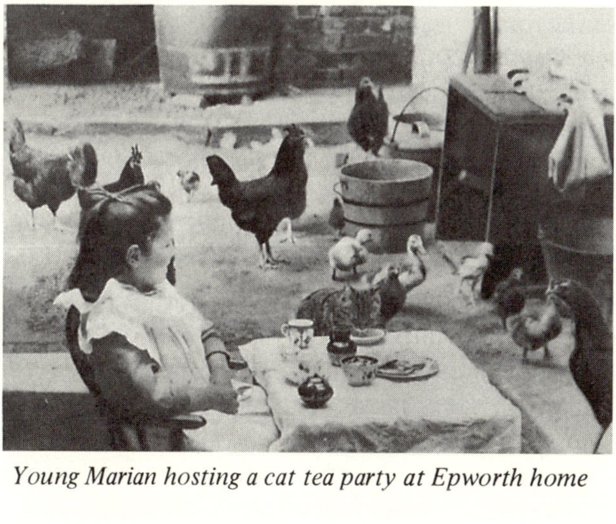

Young Marian hosting a cat tea party at Epworth home

at the Sunday School, where I recounted one of my Korean tiger stories. But I could see that the story fell flat. Later, I discovered that the children here had never been to a zoo or circus, and had no conception at all of a tiger or its nature!

It was apparent to me that the people of Epworth had been very fond of Marian's family. They now had reason to be immensely proud of her.

In London, we were able to locate a place providing board and room near the London School of Tropical Medicine. It was here I learned to eat cabbage or cauliflower every day, and could well understand why some called the "cauliflower" the national flower of England. The tiny gas heater in our room operated in response to pennies deposited in a slot, and by perching on a rotating stool in front of it, one could warm various cold parts of the body by turn. After a winter in London with no central heating in our lodgings, we could well appreciate why the English had been such wonderful colonizers. It must have been in order to escape the winter chill.

The students at the school were from all parts of the Orient, including those British doctors who held responsible government medical posts in the colonies. In all, it was a varied and stimulating group. Here too we became known as "the honeymoon couple," or the "American tourists," for on weekends we often visited some historic place in the environs of London, and at the tea break, the doctors would cluster around us to hear about our adventures.

The staff of the London School of Tropical Medicine were all prominent authorities on tropical diseases and had written extensively in the medical journals. Several had been knighted for some special achievement, such as Sir Leonard Rogers for his pioneer work in the treatment of malaria and for his special and successful treatment of liver abscess.

We also were most fortunate in having ready access to clinical material from the four corners of the earth. In the quarantine and isolation hospitals of the Port of London were many sailors and passengers who had acquired a variety of tropical diseases. Thus we had the rare opportunity to see actual cases of diseases that were normally encountered only in the tropics or the Orient. We observed the skilled treatment accorded the patients and the method of taking their histories. This experience later proved of immense value to us when we reached the mission field. It enabled us to make more accurate diagnoses and give appropriate treatment without going through a long trial and error learning period.

We learned that we would be dealing with many diseases not generally covered by our medical courses in the West. Take, for example, liver abscess, which is so often met with in the Orient but is rarely seen in the Occident. Besides the specific emetine treatment, some doctors recommended surgery, which often proved fatal. Sir Leonard Rogers, however, had worked out a simple aspiration technique which nearly always saved the patient.

In the case of dysentery, successful treatment depended much on proper diet. The usual one prescribed was a bland milk diet, but in this instance, milk was found to act as a "foreign protein" poison which could cause the patient's death. Thus, intravenous feeding was advocated initially, to be followed by barley water and gruel. At a later time, and soon after arriving in Korea, I was able to help save the lives of two children of missionaries who had been going steadily downhill on their previous milk diet regimen. While all this seemed so simple, it could mean the difference between life and death.

We learned to do some rather unusual things too. I had had considerable experience in doing dissection on earthworms, frogs, dogs and human anatomy. But I had never even heard of dissecting a mosquito, or killing one in a test tube, although I had swatted them with a heavy hand many a time while they were extracting blood from me. In this instance, however, the mosquito had to be tenderly preserved, intact. It was amazing how a comparatively light tap of one in a test tube would knock it out. After it had thus been stilled, with a delicate touch and still more delicate instruments, we were shown how to pull out its entrails and press them between two slides. We could then easily examine the contents under the microscope. Here was revealed to us the amazing world of malarial parasites.

These malarial mosquitos are not usually seen in the Occident. The females of the species are the offenders and "more deadly than the males." When biting they almost stand on their heads, which is one of their distinguishing features, for the ordinary mosquito rests in a horizontal position. The malarial mosquito injects parasites into the victim's bloodstream which results in malarial fever (from which I had suffered so as a boy).

With the enrichment of our training at the London School of Tropical Medicine behind us, we were eager to reach Korea and begin the work for which we had so long prepared. Our route to the Orient allowed time in Europe for a "second honeymoon."

Marian, as president of her class at Women's Medical College, had once had the privilege of introducing Madame Marie Curie when the latter was lecturing at the college. Famous for her work in the discovery of radium and its use in the treatment of cancer, Madame Curie had extended a warm invitation to the students to visit her Institute if they ever came to Paris. We were eager to take advantage of her invitation. When we reached Paris, we found to our great disappointment that we had missed Madame Curie, but her daughter, Eve, a scientist in her own right, received us most graciously and showed us her parents' remarkable laboratory.

We also visited the renowned Pasteur Institute which had been instrumental in saving many lives. The research work they were doing on rabies fascinated us. Little did I realize that in due course the Pasteur treatment for rabies would play such an important role in our own lives.

Somehow the usual tourist attractions of Paris seemed mundane to us in comparison to what we had just seen. After a cursory round of the conventional sights, we were impatient to be on our way. While at the School of Tropical Medicine, we had learned of the remarkable cures achieved by the Rollier Medical Clinic at Lausanne, Switzerland on so-called "surgical tuberculosis" patients by the natural means of heliotherapy. I felt that we should visit this renowned clinic in view of the fact that my specialty lay in the area of chest diseases and tuberculosis and that we were going to a land stricken with TB.

The trip up the mountains to Lausanne was certainly breathtaking. The Rollier Clinic was situated high in the Alps on a plateau surrounded by snow-clad peaks. Thus it was well protected from dust and winds. We were amazed to see the patients walking in the snow, clad in nothing but a loincloth, and enjoying the healing ultraviolet rays and warmth of the sun in genuine comfort. We were introduced to Dr. Rollier who received us kindly and took great pains to explain his technique. He showed us many x-ray plates and photographs of "before" and "after" treatment. Later he took us on ward rounds where we saw some of the actual patients whose pictures we had seen. Large, ugly, swollen TB glands had disappeared without surgery. Hunch-backs had become straight, and abdomens bloated with intestinal tuberculosis had been restored to normal. All this was long before the advent of the so-called "miracle drugs," and certainly some of his cases seemed like miracles.

The secret, as we saw it, was the ideal location of the clinic, where the healing ultraviolet rays could easily penetrate the dust-free atmosphere. Besides this, we observed that the clinic staff were strict disciplinarians and insisted that each patient have the correct dosage or exposure to the ultraviolet rays. Temperature and pulse were recorded before and after each treatment, and if there was the slightest rise, the period of exposure was reduced for the next treatment. Any patient not obeying the strict rules was immediately dismissed and forfeited his chance for further treatment. In due course I was able to introduce a modified form of the Rollier Clinic on a much smaller scale in Korea, with moderate success.

From Lausanne, it was not a long run to Marseilles, the port of our embarkation. Here we were joined by Drs. Tay, Khoo, and Li, our Chinese friends who had also attended the London School. We boarded the British owned liner, *SS Macedonia*, for the Orient. Enjoying the companionship and conversation of our Chinese friends, the voyage passed pleasantly for us. Traveling by way of the Suez Canal and Aden, we soon found ourselves at the port of Bombay, India. Here we had time to disembark briefly to do some sightseeing and I recalled that my father had also touched at this port on his way to Korea.

We were appalled by the sights of poverty in our tour of the *chawls* of Bombay, the notorious slums of the city. Here several families were crowded into a single room and the moral and sanitary conditions were indescribable. One area, where the Methodist Mission had its work, stood out in marked contrast to the scene we had just passed. Here people were working with new hope, incentives, and above all, the Spirit of Christ.

A more attractive part of Bombay housed the Haffekin Institute, the place where anti-venom serum was made from the snakes of the four poisonous species found in India. We were told that these snakes annually claimed hundreds of victims who were not able to have this serum. Fascinated, we watched the technicians extract the venom. The snakes were firmly held, and then prodded so that they bit a stretched rubber diaphragm, dispensing their venom into a bottle. From the venom thus collected, the anti-venom serum was prepared after a rather complicated process. We were fortunate in being there at feeding time. One snake looked particularly lethargic, and we were not prepared for the lightning speed with which it devoured a live rat the moment it was thrown into the snake cage. We had studied about these poisonous snakes at the London School and had heard of the fine work of this Institute, so it held a special interest for us.

We had just time enough left to visit the "Towers of Silence," the place where followers of the Parsee religion (a Zoroastrian sect descended from Persians) brought their dead for the vultures to consume the flesh. A Parsee gentleman we met on the site engaged us in conversation. He considered the custom of burial of the dead more revolting than his religion's custom, for he declared that in our case worms devoured the body. However, he did admit that occasionally the vultures might inadvertently drop a piece of flesh on a lawn tea party, which could prove upsetting to the guests. Well, it all lay in one's point of view.

Our ship next touched at Columbo, Ceylon (Sri Lanka). A short inland trip through real tropical jungles brought us to Kandy. It was here we saw displayed the teeth of Buddha, visited the botanical gardens, and had our first introduction to peppery hot curry. A Ceylonese acquaintance, seeing our dire distress at the first mouthfuls of the hot dish, reached quickly for a nearby plate of bananas and urged one on us.

"These are the fire extinguishers," he assured us.

Sure enough, the terrible burning in our mouths was at once relieved.

As we touched at the respective ports that were home to our Chinese doctor friends, there was great excitement. Dr. Tay lived in Penang, situated just over 300 miles north of Singapore, Malaya (Malaysia). Dr. Tay wanted us to meet his parents and to show us a bit of his fair city. His home was particularly beautiful.

After delicious refreshments, Dr. Tay took us to see the famous Snake Temple, for he knew of our keen interest. Here we saw many species of live, poisonous snakes entwined around pillars and candlesticks in the temple. At first we kept a respectful distance from them. But when we were told that the reptiles were quite harmless, for they had been doped, we moved closer, although not to the point of stroking them. The king cobra, however, was kept in the temple yard for he had not proved so docile and had to be caged. We might respect these snakes at a distance, but it was hard to see how anyone could come there to worship them.

Later it was Dr. Khoo's turn to welcome us to his home in Singapore. We were surprised to find that this home was truly palatial. It appeared that his father was one of the rubber plantation kings at a time when rubber had no rival. They received us most cordially and invited us to see one of their plantations. The rubber plantation

Sherwood, Dr. Tay and Dr. Li at Snake Temple in Penang

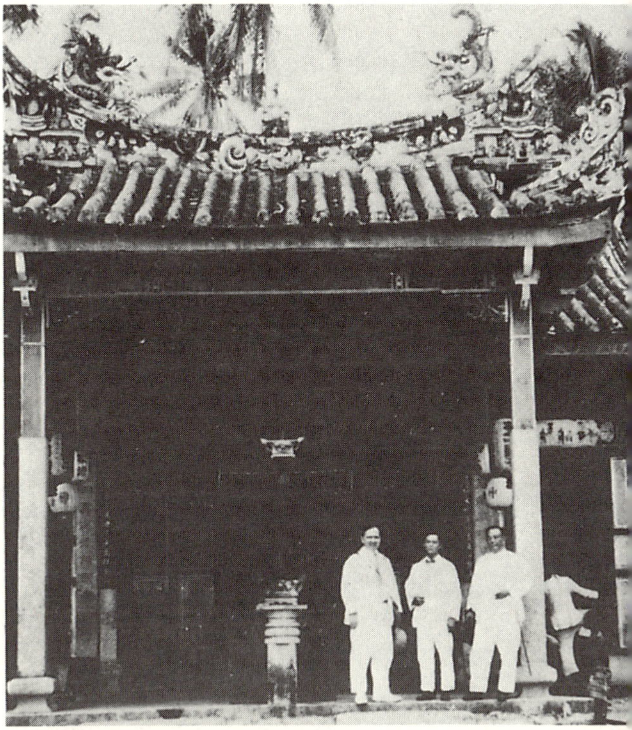

"Residents" of Snake Temple

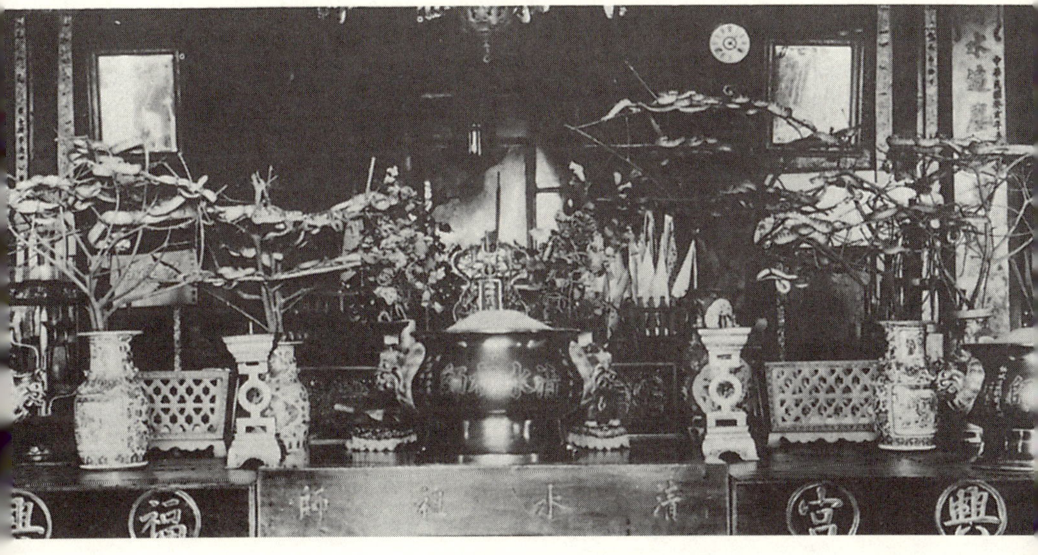

reminded me, in a way, of a maple sugar grove in Canada, and the process of taking sap from the trees was similar. We visited various points of interest, and took a drive to Jahore, a neighboring native state.

Dr. Li, having noted our surprise at seeing the large homes of the other two doctors, cautioned us ahead of time not to expect an even grander home when we visited him in Hong Kong, for he had come from more humble circumstances. However, he now had a very responsible medical post. Dr. Li showed us some of the sights and modern hospitals of Hong Kong and introduced us to some of his colleagues. Since he had to keep a special appointment, he was unable to accompany us to the Matilda Hospital which gave discounted rates to missionaries. The hospital, though not large, was very well staffed and equipped. Beautifully situated on The Peak, it had a spectacular view of Hong Kong harbor.

The ride down the hill proved a hair-raising experience in a jinrickshaw, from which we were nearly dumped off The Peak on two occasions. We figured that we might not be so lucky the third time, so we politely conveyed to our rickshaw coolie that we no longer needed his services. We dismounted from the vehicle and paid him. We then returned via the "Peak Railway." Our cable car seemed to drop down as vertically as any elevator, only this descent was more exciting, for one could see into just which portion of the harbor one would fall if the cable should break.

The final stop of our ship was Kobe, Japan, where we eagerly disembarked on April 10, 1926. Japan seemed like a picture-book fairyland. This was in early spring when the numerous cherry blossom trees were at their best. Of course we had to see the famous cherry blossom dance, "Osaka Odori," at Osaka. This was indeed enchanting, and more attractive to the eye than the accompanying music was to our Western ear. We did not have the patience to sit through the four-hour long "tea ceremony," knowing there were so many other exciting things to see as we passed through Japan.

Prior to our departure for Korea, we visited one of the lovely gardens for which Japan is famous. This was not the usual type of garden or park. There were no boisterous children or noisy picnics. They were really special places for meditation. Everything contained in the garden had a symbolic meaning, and each garden contained prescribed minimum features: a small waterfall, two small lakes with an artistic arched connecting bridge, a tiny grassy plain, and a miniature mountain. Rustic benches were placed at convenient intervals and in a quiet corner stood an attractive tea house where one could brew a pot of tea and sip it from handleless cups, as one contemplated life.

The birds twittered in the crooked pine trees, and the carp jumped after some invisible insect. There were not many people in the garden in the early morning, so we had brought a bundle of welcome letters with us. They had been there to greet us when we landed in Kobe and we had not stopped long enough to read them properly.

Many of the letters cheered us and offered us real encouragement. It was good to know we had so many friends on whom we could rely. A letter from Miss Pearl Lund, R.N., the American Superintendent of Nurses in the Mission hospital at Haiju, conveyed heartwarming assurances of how needed we were and the eagerness with which our arrival was anticipated.

But some of the letters troubled us. These had been written, we were sure, with the intention of being helpful, although they proved rather disconcerting. One was from my own dear mother. She frankly told us that she thought we were making a serious mistake by not going to work at the Pyong Yang Union Christian Hospital[1] at Pyong Yang where I "rightly belonged." I realized that there was considerable logic to my mother's statement. However, we had not been appointed to Pyong Yang. There was already an excellent missionary doctor in charge, and I suppose, in the back of my mind, there was the feeling that I was inadequate to follow in the footsteps of my sainted father. Besides, from Haiju, as from Macedonia, came the persistent cry, "*Come over and help us*." At Haiju, which was some 70 miles south of Pyong Yang, we were desperately needed. Furthermore, there we could make a fresh start on our own.

The work in Haiju had been the exclusive responsibility of the Methodist Episcopal Church since 1909. Up until that time the Presbyterians had been active in this provincial capital, but a mutual agreement between the two denominations had assigned this territory to the Methodists to avoid duplication of effort. Dr. Arthur H.

---

[1] In 1920 the Hall Memorial Hospital and the Pyong Yang Presbyterian Hospital joined under the name of the Hall Memorial Union Hospital. In 1923 the Women's Hospital of Extended Grace joined the union and the whole institution was renamed the Pyong Yang Union Christian Hospital.

Norton had operated from a simple dispensary until he had been able to construct a two-story brick hospital building in 1913, the Louisa Holmes Norton Memorial Hospital. The hospital served the Haiju District, which comprised one-third of the area of the entire province of Whanghai (Yellow Sea Province). The thirty-bed capacity soon proved inadequate to the opportunities there for service. Even when occupancy could be tripled under emergency circumstances by putting patients on the floor (Koreans were accustomed to sleeping on the floor in their own homes), the staff was inadequate to handle the increased patient load.

In addition to the medical needs at Haiju, the educational facilities were being pressed. The Methodists operated a girls' school and a boys' school there, each with a staff of four teachers and an approximate enrollment of 100 students in the girls' school and 280 in the boys' school. The girls were housed in a comfortable brick building, but the boys' school was described by an American visitor as "unfit to house a Ford." Nevertheless, the institutions were providing valuable services. With the need for medical and educational staff so great, we felt that we could make a contribution by accepting our assignment to Haiju.

We reviewed the letters. One was from Dr. Y. J. Kim who was trying to hold the fort at the Norton Hospital as best he could. Dr. A. H. Norton had been transferred to Severance Hospital in Seoul in 1922. He had then had to return to the U.S.A. for health reasons. Dr. K. W. Hidy had followed Dr. Norton at Haiju, but had remained only two years.

In his letter Dr. Kim told us how glad he was that the son of Dr. William James Hall and the son of the Reverend Kim, Chang Sik would now be working as a team in Haiju, as their parents had once worked to help overcome superstition and prejudice through the healing ministry of Christ. Our parents had together endured the persecution of the Christians in Pyong Yang in 1894. In the unfathomable ways of Providence the sons of this pioneer team now found their paths uniting.

Kim, Chang Sik had been licensed to preach in 1901 and was ordained a deacon. He was thus the first minister to be ordained in the Protestant Church in Korea. In 1904 he became the first Korean District Superintendent of the Methodist Church, appointed to the Yeng Byen (Yongbyon) District for six years. His final appointment was to Haiju where he retired and was now living with his son, Dr. Y. J. Kim.

In contrast to the letters of welcome, the remaining letters contained words of admonition and advice. One wanted to know why we chose the isolation of the country when the larger centers needed us so much and where we could render greater service. We could augment the teaching staff of one of the mission medical schools, we were told. Others were even more personal and wanted to know what right I had to take a young wife to a remote area where she would languish in loneliness, or drag me back to the States before I could even complete my first term. Obviously this one did not know Marian!

Another writer wondered if we had never contemplated having a family. If so, how cruel it would be to bring up children where they could have no playmates of their own kind and could not attend school with children of their own race. Such children would be bound to grow up misfits in any society.

The tranquility of the garden helped us to sort over these well meaning suggestions and put them in perspective. Some of the points may have been well taken, but we had already made our decision and nothing convinced us to change our plan to go to Haiju. We never had cause to regret it.

CHAPTER 12

Return

To reach Korea no longer required the long trip on a crude coastal steamer that my father had taken in his day. We had only to cross the Korea Strait on a night ferry and then take the train to Seoul. A railway had been built from Fusan at the southern end of the Korean peninsula all the way to the Manchurian border in the North. The engines that hauled the trains had a familiar look, for they had been built just outside of Philadelphia at the Baldwin Locomotive Works.

Usually Marian was up first, but on this auspicious spring morning, I was up with the crack of dawn. In the light of the rising sun I beheld the distant Korean Coastal Range in all its glory. I had sometimes wondered why Korea, so often war torn, had ever been called the "Land of the Morning Calm." Now I understood. We approached the coastal mountains in a perfectly calm sea, without so much as a ripple to disturb its tranquility. To the East was the golden path caused by the rising sun. Mountains covered with twisted pines outlined the rugged coast and were this day perfectly reflected in the sea mirror. Against this green background, on a point of land that projected into the sea, was the pink bloom of the cherry trees. Their reflection turned the sea into a delicate pink which merged with the golden path of the sun. The peace and beauty overwhelmed me.

By the time Marian had joined me on deck much of the early splendor had vanished and I realized that I must have been seeing things through "rose tinted glasses." In part I was living over some of my boyhood experiences, and those associations that might arouse my feelings and render the scene so especially appealing to me would not be present in another without that early background.

However, Marian became enthusiastic and excited as we drew nearer and could clearly see the quaint thatched huts at Fusan with gourd vines growing over the roofs. The men wore white baggy trousers and black laquered "fly-trap" hats (made of silk and the hair from horses' tails). The women were clad in pea green cloaks which also covered their heads. One could see naked children peeking from behind their mother's cloak, proclaiming to the world that spring had come. These sights proved refreshingly different for Marian and drew from her exclamations of surprise and delight. Marian's happy reactions added to my own joy.

Marian said to me, "You will be jabbering away in Korean as soon as we land at Fusan, and I shall feel out of it for I can't even say a word of greeting. Please teach me at least one sentence, so I can join in the excitement."

Perhaps it was the elation of the moment—the intoxication of happy feelings that had gone to my head—which caused me to toss sobriety and good sense to the winds. I responded mischievously, "There is a very simple sentence you might use which is bound to create a sensation. Just say, '*Nai ga cham nab-e-o!*'"

Marian kept repeating over and over the sentence I had taught her. She proved a perfect mimic.

My mother, who had come down from Seoul, was the first to greet us. She was accompanied by Korean friends who lived in Fusan. After sixteen years of absence I wondered whether I might have forgotten how to talk in Korean. However, just as the swimmer who has been away from water for some time discovers he can still swim, I found that I was easily conversing in my boyhood-style Korean, as Marian had foreseen.

From the corner of my eye I could see that Marian was not entirely left out in the cold for there was also a cluster of Koreans about her. At first I could see on their faces expressions of incredulity, thinking that she might be addressing them in English. Then as Marian slowly articulated and repeated her carefully memorized sentence, I could see comprehension dawning on them, then broad smiles.

All would have been well if it had stopped there. However, a dignified Korean gentleman, who finally caught the full impact of Marian's carefully rehearsed sentence, spoiled everything with a loud guffaw. I was forced to come to the rescue at this point, but my interpretation of the sentence to Marian did not help matters much and I made a hasty retreat.

The translation of "*Nai ga cham nab-e-o!*" is, "I am a monkey!" It was the last Korean sentence Marian ever allowed me to teach her.

My mother scolded me roundly for my juvenile and tasteless joke and I received her rebuke meekly, knowing it was well deserved. She then taught Marian a more socially acceptable phrase, "*Mai-o-pong op simneda!*" meaning, "I am happy to meet you!"

We were naturally eager to be on our way but Fusan friends insisted that we accept their invitation to a welcome party at the Fusan Cherry Tree Garden. They claimed that the blossoms were now at their best and the cherry trees in the North would not yet be in bloom. When Marian began to politely demur by saying we had to get to our work, an older Australian missionary volunteered a word of advice.

"Young lady," he said, "remember you are now in the Orient where time does not count. You will no longer be using your watch, except to count the heartbeats of your patients. If you are to last in the Orient, you will have to learn to take things at a more leisurely pace or you will find yourself being sent home as an invalid."

Marian graciously thanked him for his admonition and we accepted the invitation. In doing so, Marian looked at her watch and with a roguish smile added, "We shall try to be there on time so that we do not keep you waiting."

He chuckled.

The cherry blossom trees provided an idyllic setting for the informal gathering. Since so many of the missionaries stationed in Fusan came from Australia, the kangaroo was mentioned as an inevitable topic of conversation. Marian asked if anyone knew how large a kangaroo was when it was first born. Various sizes were estimated but none proved correct. Then Marian surprised them all with her knowledge.

"It is just a little nubbin, not much larger than one's thumb, which the mother places in her pouch after its birth. She helps it to attach to her nipple there where it further develops. I saw one once at an autopsy in a zoo."

A breeze stirred the waters as the party began to break up. I noted that where I had seen two cherry blossom gardens that morning, now there was only one, for the wind had wiped out the mirror image of the other in the sea. As we thanked our hosts, the gentle breeze showered us with pink petals, a beautiful conclusion to the welcome given us on our arrival in Korea.

The train sped us swiftly northward. At first the scenery was filled with fields of young rice plants which rippled like an ocean in the breeze. As we neared Seoul, the train was flanked by rugged

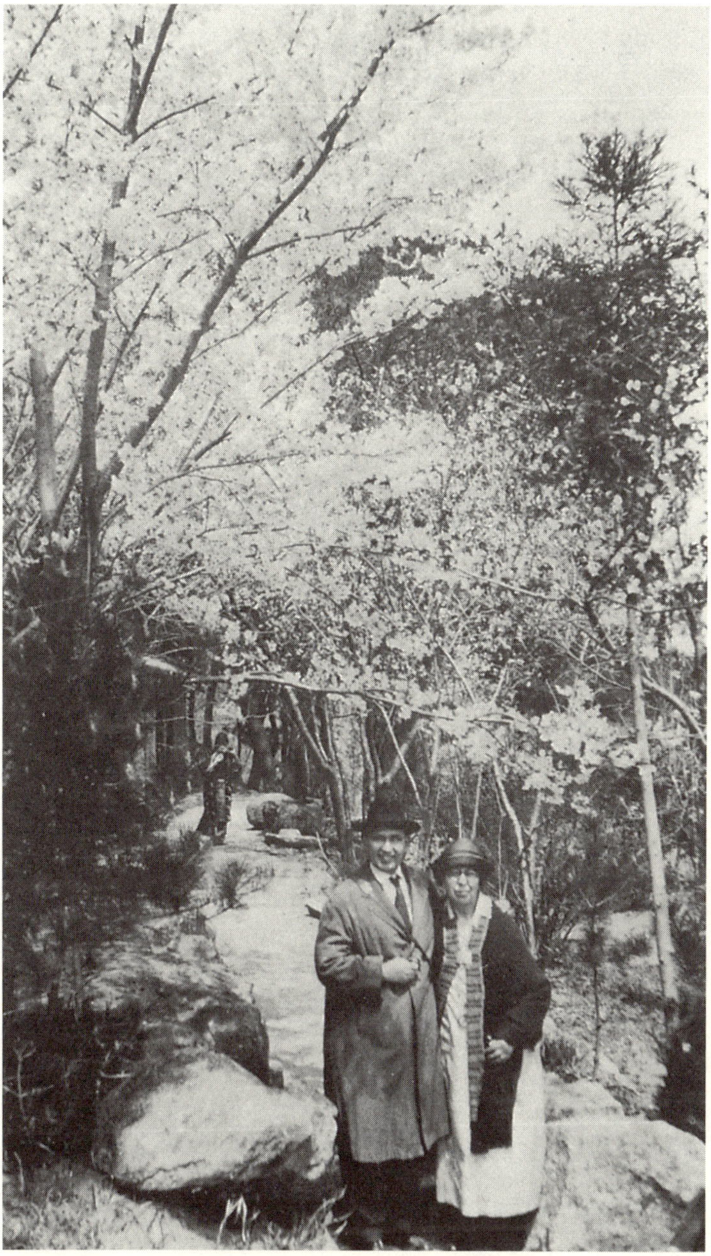

Sherwood and Dr. Rosetta Hall under the cherry blossoms at Fusan Garden

mountains covered with the ever picturesque crooked pine trees. At last we pulled in to Seoul, the city of my birth and scene of my childhood. I was deeply stirred with joy and gratitude to God. I had returned.

I could find no words to adequately portray my emotions to my lovely bride beside me, but somehow I felt that she understood. The gentle pressure of her hand on mine let me know that she was sharing in my inner excitement and happiness.

At the Seoul station, hands from all directions reached out to greet us. The sea of faces around us was like a kaleidoscope. My poor mother was frantically trying to make introductions but names became a blur to us, especially to Marian. We had hardly focused on the faces in front of us before new faces appeared. We were relieved to be gently led to my mother's special two-passenger rickshaw. (Mother had imported it especially for use in her medical work. Unlike the more typical Korean one-passenger rickshaw, both doctor and nurse could travel to the scene of an emergency in this one, and be assured of arriving together without the risk of getting separated in a crowd.) There was a "puller" coolie in front, and a "pusher" coolie in the rear.

Soon we were speeding at dog-trot rate through *Nam Dai Moon*, the Great South Gate of Seoul which now was no longer closed at night. Thus we entered the city proper. Marian was all eyes now and amazed that buildings in this area looked quite modern and the street so wide.

We then took a short cut to the *Tong Dai Moon*, or Great East Gate. The streets were narrow and crooked here and crowded with Koreans from all walks of life. Coolies with their *jiggies* (pack boards) mingled with children carrying a baby brother or sister strapped to their backs, while merchants hawked their wares. Housewives crowded around the open food stalls, no longer kept at home by a rigid curfew as in the days when my parents first arrived in Korea. The changing variety of the Korean street scenes completely intrigued Marian.

The constant clang of the bicycle bell attached to the shaft of our rickshaw noisily heralded our approach, but with little effect. Indifferent pedestrians apparently wondering at our urgency, slowly moved aside to let us pass.

Eventually we emerged onto another broad street. A tram car passed us. It was packed full like a sardine can. Passengers spilled onto the steps where they clung perilously to anything that offered them a place to grasp. Some boys were even attempting to climb onto the roof.

This was not the same sight that would have greeted a traveler almost three decades ago, when trams were first introduced to Korea. I could remember back to a time when the tram car had not always been so popular. In fact it was once an anathema to the Koreans, who called it "an invention of the foreign devil."

The arrival of the tram car in Korea unfortunately coincided with a long period of drought. When geomancers placed the blame on the tram cars for the lack of rain, the natural suspicion of the Koreans toward this strange contraption was further aroused. Only the fortuitous onset of the rainy season averted certain trouble–but not for long.

To understand the incident that followed shortly thereafter it should be explained that the summer period of the Korean rainy season means months of sweltering heat and high humidity. It was not uncommon for the Koreans to seek relief from their stuffy, airless huts on hot summer evenings by choosing, instead, to sleep right out in the middle of the street. Unlike the Occidental, who prefers a soft downy pillow, the Oriental likes nothing better than a smooth block of hard wood on which to rest his head. The street sleepers soon discovered that the tram car tracks served admirably for this purpose.

The incident that was now brought back to my mind occurred on a misty morning in the summer of 1899. My mother was scheduled to attend some missionary meetings, and I was to have an appointment with a dentist, so we had come to Seoul from Pyong Yang.

The first tram car of the day began its run. The dense fog of the early morning hour had obscured the conductor's view and the wheels of the tram car ran over a number of Koreans who had been sleeping in its pathway, using the tracks for pillows. They were decapitated.

When the fog lifted as the sun came out, the gruesome tragedy became apparent to horrified onlookers. Pandemonium broke out and a mob of frenzied coolies attacked the hapless conductor and overturned the tram car, setting it ablaze.

It was one of the vivid recollections from my childhood. The over-loaded tram car that I saw today was ample evidence that in the course of time the Koreans had overcome their initial distrust and

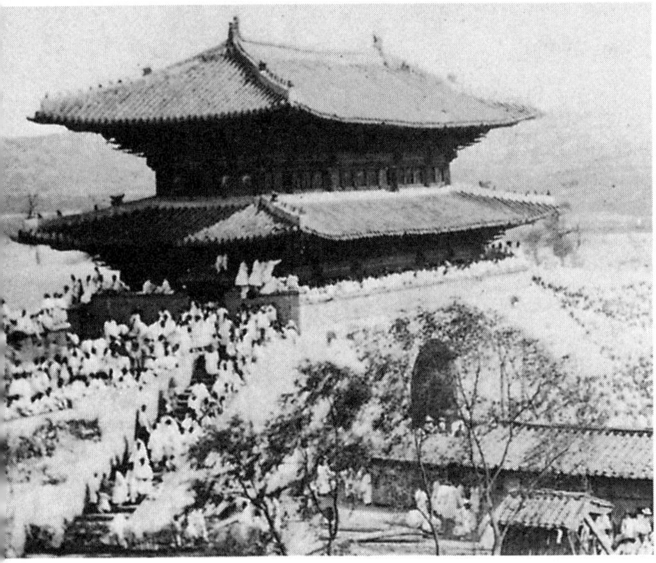

Great East Gate in Seoul at introduction of electric streetcar–May 20, 1899

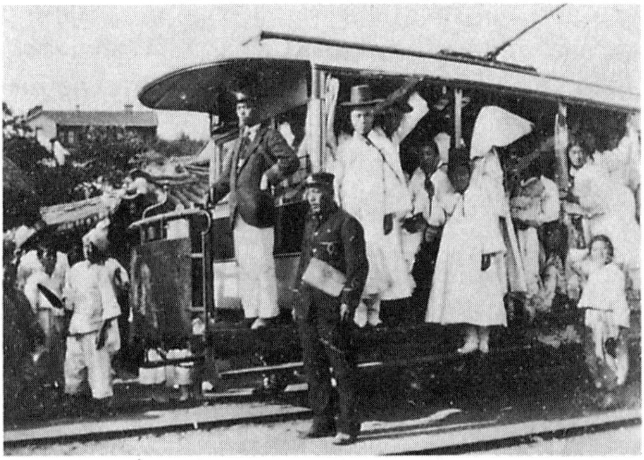

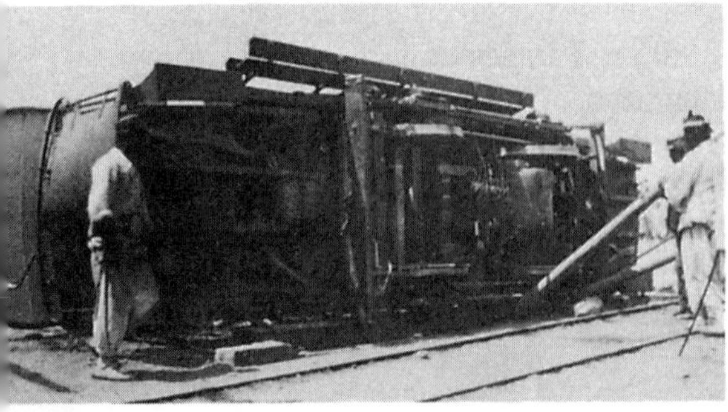

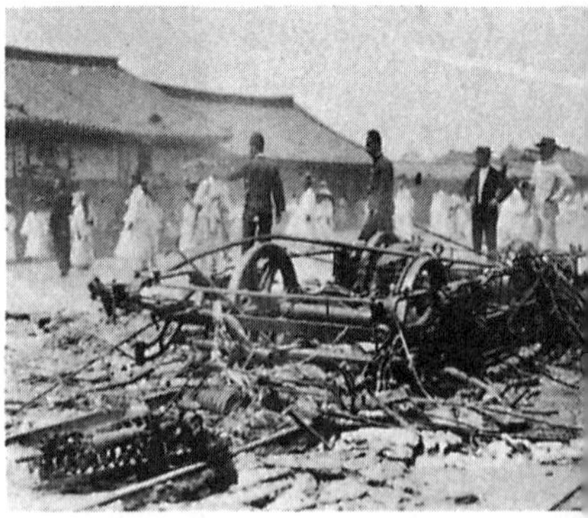

Overturned and burned streetcars

fear of this "foreign devil invention." Indeed it was but one of many signs that pointed to the evolution of a broader acceptance of more modern ways.

Marian broke into my reverie as she nudged me, asking if the gate we were now approaching was the Great East Gate. It was. This *Tong Dai Moon* was not as large as the *Nam Dai Moon* (Great South Gate) but was to me more picturesque, situated in an artistic curve of the city wall against a background of quaint straw-roofed and tile-roofed houses. From this location, a rather steep hill ascended to the Lillian Harris Memorial Hospital where my mother was the Medical Superintendent, and to her residence adjacent to it.

Marian exclaimed, "We can't allow these poor coolies to pull and push our rickshaw up this steep place! Let's get out and climb up the hill ourselves."

This I was perfectly willing to do, but not for the reason Marian gave. I knew from my boyhood days that these "poor coolies" had the strength of oxen and were capable of carrying a four-hundred-pound load on their backs over much longer and steeper mountain passes. They considered this to be all in the day's work and did not mind it as long as they could take time out to smoke their long-stemmed, small-bowled pipes. Thus the coolies made no protest as we dismounted from the rickshaw. They smilingly watched us puff up the steep grade.

When we reached Mother's home, we had hardly had a chance to get a bite to eat and unpack our suitcases when there were Korean callers at the door to greet us. After they had left, Mother wanted to discuss plans before we became too deeply involved, and she briefly outlined the crowded agenda. We were scheduled to make a number of official calls, such as seeing the British Consul-General, Mr. A. Hyde Lay, and registering at the consulate. Of course we should call on Bishop Herbert Welch and his wife. He was now our bishop and we had been appreciative of all he had done to help us in New York.

Mother knew we would want to call on her distinguished Korean Christian friend, Baron Yun, Tchi Ho. We had known his daughter, Helen, when she was a student in the United States. Baron Yun was a Korean nobleman who had served as interpreter for the first American Minister to Korea, General Lucius Foote, in 1884. He had left Korea following the December émeute of 1884 and had gone to Shanghai. There he became a Christian while studying at a college run by the Southern Methodist Church. He went on to earn distinction for himself as a student at Vanderbilt University in the United States. He returned to Korea to serve in educational and diplomatic posts for the Korean government and still later in religious and educational work for the church. When we went to call on him, he had been retired some six years from serving as General Secretary of the Korean Y.M.C.A.

Mother especially wanted us to pay our respects to Viscount Makoto Saito, Governor-General of Korea, and his wife. (The Viscount later became Premier of Japan and was assassinated in 1936 for his peace activities. His wife was wounded when she bravely tried to defend her husband from the assassin.) Korea, you recall, was under Japanese domination at this time, having been formally annexed to Japan on August 22, 1910. Under the Japanese, Korea was referred to officially as Chosen.

The Japanese officials on my mother's list were not simply government officers to her, but warm personal friends who had already expressed to her a wish to meet us. Mr. Yasuma Oda of the Foreign Affairs Department was a Japanese official loved by all. It had been said that he was so tall for a Japanese that the Emperor of Korea had taken him to be a Korean. Since the Emperor could not be wrong, his verdict was allowed to stand. We were also to meet Mr. I. Yamagata, Editor of the *Seoul Press*, a paper printed in English. He was a champion for the training of Korean women doctors, so Mother felt a special kinship toward him. The list seemed never-ending.

Mother finally concluded, "There is to be a big reception for new missionaries at the time of the Annual Conference of the Methodist Church in June. That will give you the opportunity to meet missionaries from other Korean mission stations. Since Language School begins on Monday, you will need to plan your time so that you can fit in some of these official visits in the early weeks. The Welches are not due back in Seoul until June 15, so that visit can be postponed, but the others can be made in the near future. Miss Lund is coming to Seoul for the Nurses' Association Meeting on Monday and has written that she would be glad to escort you to Haiju when she returns there at the end of that week."

I sensed that Marian could not help but feel more than a little overwhelmed by such a list of obligations on top of the day's new experiences and sensations. I interrupted Mother, therefore, to

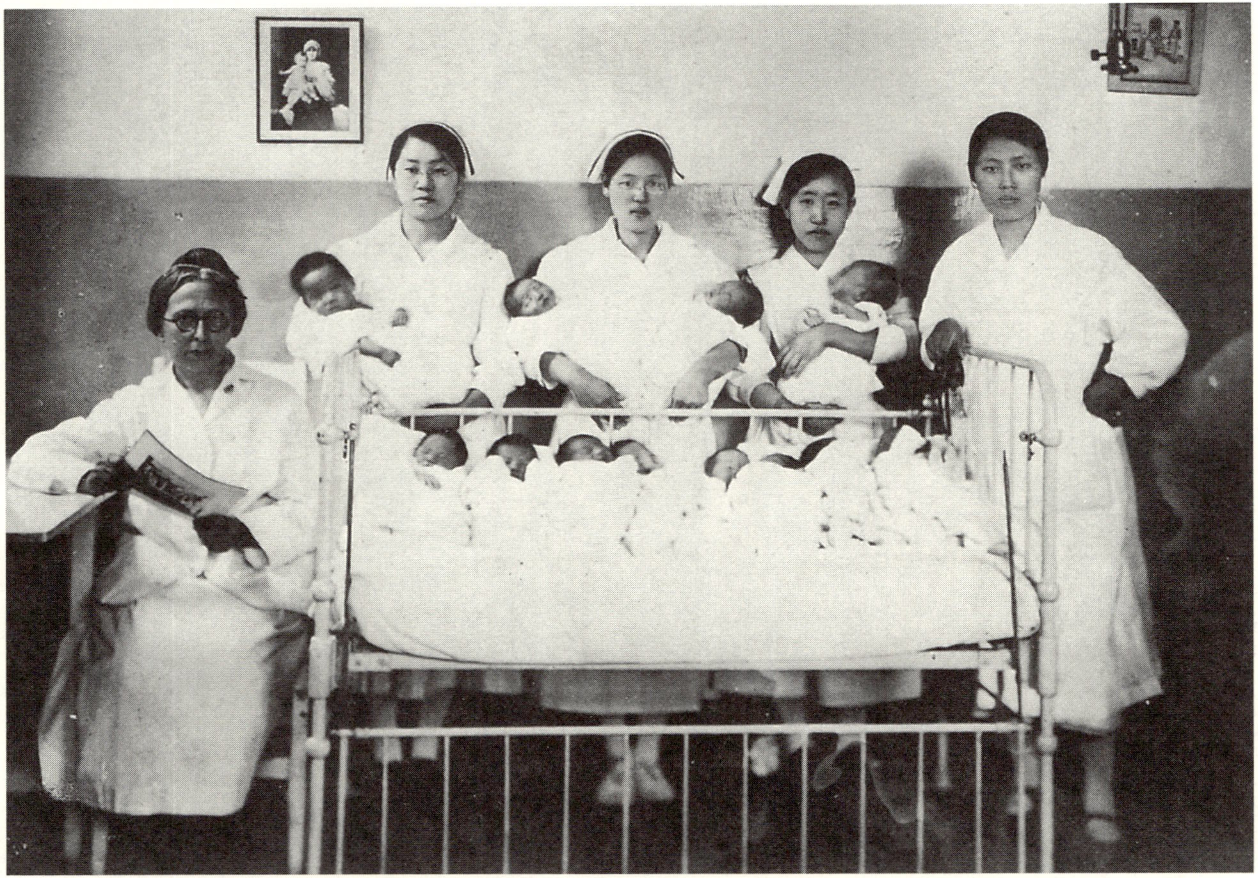

Dr. Rosetta Hall and nurses with "a week of babies" delivered at Lillian Harris Memorial Hospital, Seoul

announce that we had decided to get an introductory look at our mission station before language school opened. It would probably be easier to do it before we became involved in our studies, and by leaving on Friday, the following day, we could return to Seoul on Monday with Miss Lund.

Mother seemed startled that we would want to crowd that trip in so soon after our long voyage, but she could appreciate our eagerness to see where we would be located after so many months of anticipation.

We boarded the 8:05 train Friday morning which would take us to the railroad station nearest Haiju, known to the Koreans as Sariwon and to the Japanese as Shariin. At that time the railway did not extend to Haiju but traveling northwest through Songdo, we could reach Sariwon which was about 30 miles due north of our destination. The remainder of the journey would be by jitney. It was estimated that the entire 128 mile trip would take about five hours.

The jitney of those days was a remarkable contraption consisting of a converted Model T Ford, which "Henry" would hardly have acknowledged as one of his vehicles. The seats had been removed and were replaced by three narrow wooden benches. These left practically no leg room and were calculated to give even men "housemaid's knee," for the knees were forced to knock and bump against the seat in front. The vehicle was redesigned to seat nine, but the Korean jitney resembled the proverbial circus car in that the number of passengers was unlimited.

We had been forewarned to limit our intake of fluids before the trip, for there were no comfort stations on the jitney route. It was presumed we would not care to use the side of the road in the customary manner of the Korean. Later, some of the passengers became car sick, which added further to the discomforts of this mode of travel.

We soon came to a ferry crossing that proved rather tricky to negotiate. This provided some excitement and gave us an opportunity to stretch our legs. We were also required to give a mighty shove to the jitney, when it sank down to its hubcaps in the sand. After we all joined in the unison chant, "*Oo-ya-cha, oo-ya-cha!*" we finally succeeded in getting the jitney pushed onto the ferry. On the boat we were crowded between two stalwart oxen. We were reassured that as long as we did not maneuver too near either their front or hind ends, we would be comparatively safe. Furthermore, if the ferry wobbled too severely during the crossing, we would have a ready-made support.

The river was in its spring flood and the current was quite swift and turbulent. Thus it was necessary to tow the ferry a considerable distance upstream before crossing if we were to land on the opposite bank above the rapids. I remembered the fun I had experienced as a boy in shooting the rapids, but I would not have cared to repeat the experience with so many on board and the water still so cold. There was really no worry for our oarsmen were strong and sturdy. They utilized the current to help land us at just the right spot. Then with more huffing and puffing, we all succeeded in pushing the jitney up a steep bank and onto the road. Seated in the jitney once again, our knees continued to knock against the hard wooden benches in front as we were bumped and jolted over the potholes in the dirt road which led to our longed-for destination. We all heaved a sigh of relief at journey's end.

The hospital staff and a flock of Christians had turned out to welcome us led by Miss Pearl Lund. The students of the Christian Boys' School were all lined up and saluted us smartly. As I acknowledged their salute, I was politely informed that the School Board had chosen me to be the new principal, for the Reverend V. H. Wachs was leaving soon and for health reasons would not be returning. Marian suggested that we should see how my hospital schedule worked out before accepting the honor.

We were promptly assured that the position would really take very little of my time, and besides, there was no one else available. I realized that this was hardly the time or place to pursue the matter further.

We were introduced in quick succession to those with whom we soon would be closely associated, both in the immediate future and down through the years. Dr. Y. J. Kim was one of the first to clasp my hand. He said warmly, "I am so glad that at last you have come. I felt that I would not be able to hold out on my own much longer. Some difficult cases have long been lined up for you both."

"We consider it a privilege to be associated with you in building up this medical work," I responded, "but I hope that you have also left us some easy cases."

He smiled. "No doubt you will consider them all easy ones."

The next person to be introduced was a prim and proper lady, who fit the typical stereotype of the old maid, Miss Jane Barlow. I

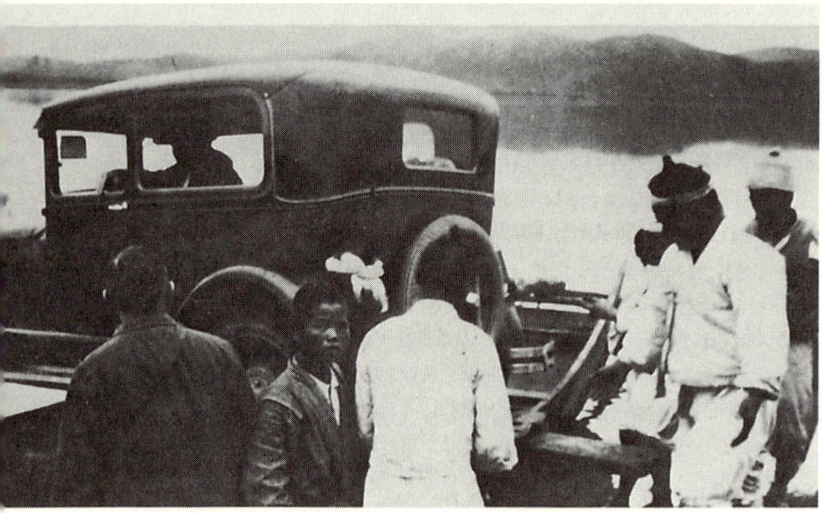

Loading car onto ferry between Haiju and Seoul

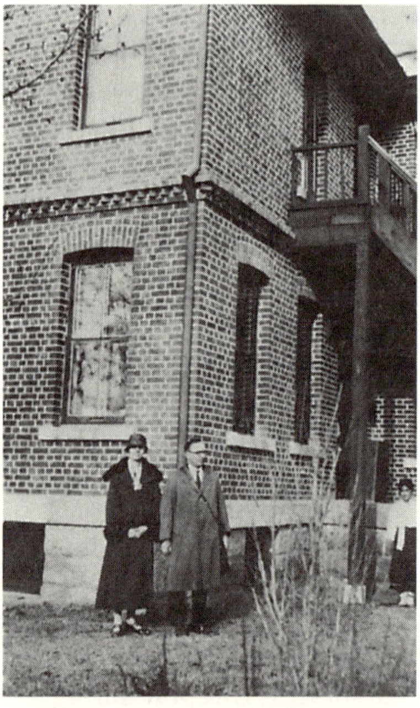

Sherwood and Marian in front of Norton Memorial Hospital in Haiju

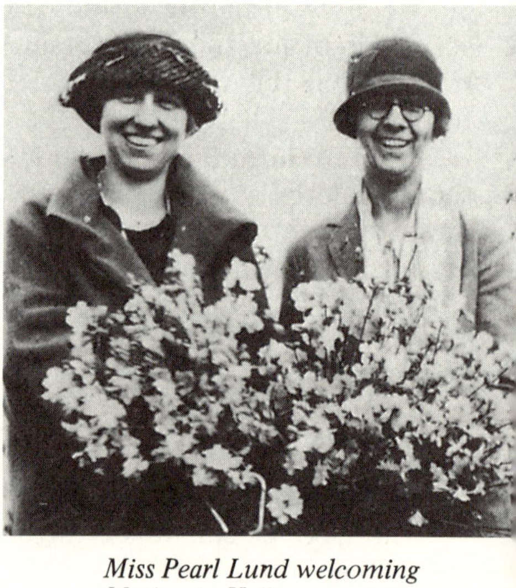

Miss Pearl Lund welcoming Marian to Haiju

had an intuition at once that she would never be one to let us call her "Jane," nor would we particularly want to. Her first remark to us was, "I am glad that you have no children so that you both can better concentrate on the Lord's work."

I am not quick at repartee, especially when I am taken off my guard. Marian, however, promptly responded, "Miss Barlow, we may disappoint you in that regard one of these days."

Later we became more accustomed to Miss Barlow's blunt manner and grew to be very fond of her. One could not help but admire her sincere dedication to the evangelistic work of the Mission.

Miss Belle Overman was standing in the background and I could see by the knowing smile on her face that she had overheard some of our conversation and approved of Marian's forthright reply. Belle was Principal of the Lucy Scott Memorial School for Girls. She was to prove very helpful to me in school matters, and to be to us both, an understanding friend. We were then introduced to the various Korean Christians for whom we would acquire a true affection.

The Reverend Victor Wachs and his wife, the missionaries we were to replace, extended their hands in greeting. We would soon be bidding them farewell. Mr. Wachs was known by the Koreans as the "motorcycle missionary" for he visited his large circuit on a "putt-putt" as the children fondly called it, and they often begged him for a ride.

The Wachs offered us the use of their larger brick house on top of a hill, but we preferred the little stone cottage, known as the *kowandeh chip*, or middle house, for its location between the ladies' house and the Wachs' house. The small cottage would be less costly to heat in the cold winters, and we did not yet have a need for a big house for just the two of us. A beautiful large yellow rosebush stood in full bloom at the end of the front porch. From there, one could easily see the new Boys' School and the Mission Hospital adjacent to it. The buildings were within easy walking distance from the cottage. We were then invited to tour the medical facilities.

First, Dr. Kim and Miss Lund took us through the small hospital which in times of emergency could be stretched beyond its thirty-bed capacity. The hospital was housed in a two-story brick building with all space economically utilized, thanks to Dr. A. H. Norton's careful planning. The outpatient waiting room doubled as a chapel for the staff and was used by them the first thing in the morning before the patients arrived. When they did come, a layman evangelist or the

Bible woman took over the evangelistic work until the patients could be seen by the doctor. This seemed to be a good arrangement all around and allowed time for the team of evangelists to get personally acquainted with the patients and determine whether they would welcome home visitation or not. It was the policy of the Mission to invite the people to learn about the Gospel message, but not to force religion on anyone.

Miss Lund, I could see, believed that "cleanliness was next to godliness," and had seen to it that the hospital was kept spotless and neat. I could not even detect the so-called hospital odors, although later at meal time, when the patients were served their food, the penetrating odor of *kimchie* offended or pleased the olfactory nerves, depending on the individual.

The hospital laboratory was pitifully lacking in essentials. I knew that something would have to be done for I had no patience with the saying that "just a pill and a tract were sufficient" for our patients. The drug room was surprisingly well stocked, however, with the cheaper Japanese medicines. A lady pharmacist was in charge which especially pleased Marian. The outpatient clinic was in need of more instruments and equipment, some of which we had been able to bring with us. This news greatly cheered Dr. Kim.

Marian was especially interested in seeing the operating room. The mantle for surgery naturally fell on her, and she was game to accept it.

She observed that the operating room had its rather serious limitations. Perhaps the most outstanding was inadequate light. Though "King Sol" smiled cheerfully through the large window on most days, occasionally his beaming face was hidden by clouds. Even at best, he could not light up the mysterious inner recesses of the human anatomy. Thus, first on the list of needs was a good light for the operating room. Next would be a more adequate supply of instruments.

We were told that the Government Hospital recently had lost its Chief Surgeon because he had been run out of town for losing too many cases. This could be explained, in part, by the fact that he had never worn rubber gloves when operating, and bare hands are rather difficult to properly sterilize. In time, we were able to cooperate with the Government Hospital to our mutual advantage.

The city of Haiju with its picturesque tiled and thatched roofs was nestled in a valley at the foot of a fairly high mountain. Behind the cottage where we were to live was a steep hill covered with crooked pines, and on its summit was the so-called "devil house," the competitor to the Mission Hospital. Over this hill one could obtain a grand view of the harbor of Haiju, speckled with colorful junks replete with orange sails. Haiju, as capital of Whanghai Do, was a very important center. It was to become increasingly so when the branch line of the railroad connecting Haiju with Songdo was eventually built in the early 1930's.

Our introduction to the mission station seemed tantalizingly brief, but we realized we would be able to be of greater service to the Koreans with a better knowledge of the language to aid us. The return trip to Seoul with Pearl Lund would give us an opportunity to ply her with endless questions about the hospital, its staff and its equipment, and about the mission station in general.

Although Pearl had made arrangements to reserve an entire seat on the jitney for the three of us, we found this bench had to allow for a Korean mother and her brood of three squirming youngsters, with a live rooster thrown in for good measure. Marian generously offered to take one of the cute little children on her lap, but declined the same hospitality to the rooster because the latter was not provided with diapers.

Pearl interjected, "The babies don't have diapers either!"

However, Pearl had anticipated the situation from previous experiences and had come equipped with rubber sheeting which she had brought from the hospital.

The train reached Seoul on Monday, April 19, in the early afternoon and we hastened over to Morris Hall to register for Language School. Marian somehow found sufficient energy to read and discuss a paper on "Radium" at the Monday evening session of the Nurses' Association meeting which opened that day also. It was well received which made a gratifying conclusion to a very full day.

Emotions vied for attention inside of me during these first days of my return to the land of my childhood. And yet, I knew that I must resist the temptation to become absorbed in my own feelings and that I must try to be sensitive to what this early adjustment period would be stirring up in Marian. What was needed was objectivity and maturity.

I recalled Dr. Stone's astute counsel to me when Marian and I were visiting in his lovely home in New Rochelle, New York. He had told me in effect, "In Marian you have discovered a precious and rare jewel. She is talented, sensitive, vivacious, poetic, artistic and musical as well as beautiful. You must show her the same tender consideration and understanding care that a musician would give to his Stradivarius violin, if you hope to keep her that way."

I had treasured Dr. Stone's words in my heart. Here was certainly the time to apply them. At the same time, I was keenly aware of my own inadequacy and inexperience in such matters. I instinctively turned to another of my father's friends, Mr. W. A. Noble. He had known my parents before they were married and had been like a father to me since the passing of my own father. He had an innate sense of discretion and mature judgement. Because I thought that he might be more responsive to Marian's unstated inner uncertainties and homesickness than I could, I coveted for Marian the opportunity to talk with him now.

Marian readily agreed to my suggestion that we call on the Nobles, for she had often heard me speak of them and looked forward to getting to know them. Mr. and Mrs. Noble welcomed us cordially. As I had hoped, they filled us with reassurance.

"I can guess how you must be feeling, Marian," Mr. Noble observed, "for I recall when we first came to the mission field. This

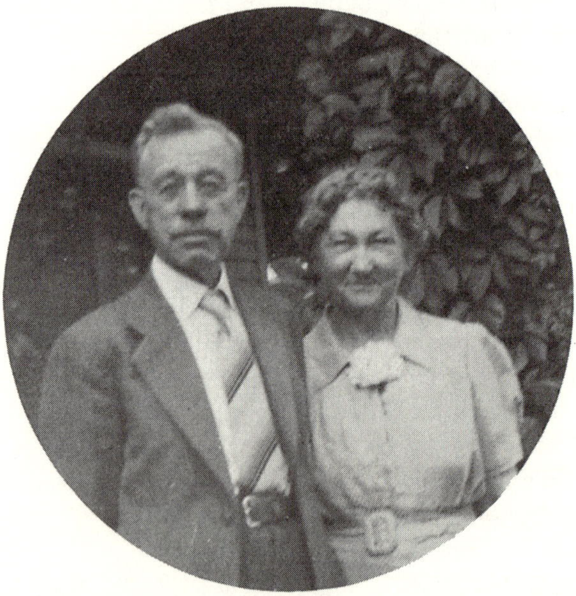

The Rev. and Mrs. W. Arthur Noble

Sherwood would not completely understand, for he was born and brought up here, and there was no abrupt change for him on his return. But for you, Marian, it is a sudden change and must come, at least to your subconscious mind, as a real shock. You are venturing into a strange and unchartered ocean. This is not just a brief and casual excursion from which you could opt out if you found the environment not congenial, but this is for life.

"All around you are strange people of another race, with different language, habits of thought, and behavior patterns. You have not been here long enough to know how friendly and congenial they can be. Even the white folks here are strangers to you, whose names it will take time to learn. But you are about to join a very different and unique society, unlike any other in the world.

"The Seoul community is indeed fortunate in that we so-called 'foreigners' are a very close knit group. There are no sharp lines here, as are sometimes seen in the Orient, between the non-missionary and the missionary community. For example, Morris Hall is named after J. H. Morris, a much loved and respected businessman here. You will soon meet him, his wife, Pearl, and his daughter, Marion.

"This unique hall houses the Language School you are now attending, as you know. It also houses the school for our children as well as the Community Church. Union services are conducted here, and you will want to hear Dr. Underwood preach on Sunday, for he is such a dynamic speaker. An ecumenical spirit is everywhere in evidence, and in actual practice here in our various union mission institutions.

"In due course, our children may inter-marry within this community as some have already done, including my own daughter, Ruth. She is married to Henry D. Appenzeller, the son of the first Methodist missionary to Korea, Henry G. Appenzeller. Sherwood's mother delivered Ruth and also delivered my son Alden.

"You will find that very soon your natural homesickness and feeling of being an outsider will disappear. This new kind of society that I speak of is also exceptionally open and cordial. I am certain with your own warm outgoing personality it will not be long before you feel that you, too, have lived here most of your life. And what a need we do have for you! I am personally so glad that you have joined our unique fellowship."

Just then Alden Noble and his wife stopped in and were introduced. It was apparent that they were looking forward to a happy event of their own soon.

Sure enough, not many days later, on April 24 at 8:20 P.M., Marian delivered Alden's wife of a daughter at the Lillian Harris Memorial Hospital! We had been invited that evening to dinner at Ruth and Henry Appenzeller's but that had to be postponed.

Already Marian was making her contribution to the fellowship of this "new kind of society" in a more immediate way than either Mr. Noble or I could have foreseen. It was only the beginning.

CHAPTER 13

Orientation

Newcomers to the mission field traditionally relied on older missionaries and printed self-study courses to learn the Korean language. However, in 1919 the Federal Council of Protestant Evangelical Missions instituted formal courses for Korean language study. Spring and fall sessions of two months each became the format of the curriculum. The intervening time was then available for home study and practice on the classroom material. This program took a total of three years to complete. New missionaries were expected to enroll in the first term of Language School before beginning their mission assignments.

Language School was to hold some surprises for me. My smugness about already knowing Korean would be short lived. I had thought the language would be a cinch with my previous background, and I was feeling rather sorry for poor Marian who would have to struggle through even the simplest "A B C" of Korean. How mistaken I proved to be.

As a boy, I would jabber away easily in Korean, but I used the "child talk" which was what we children heard spoken to us. We must have horrified many a dignified Korean who came calling on my mother by suggesting "*On-ja-ra!*" (Sit down) instead of the high form one is supposed to use with elders, "*On-ja-sip-si-o!*" (Your honor, please sit down). It would not have been quite so shocking even if we had used the middle form, "*On-ja-si-o!*" (Please sit down). But they must have excused us, for, after all, how could children of the Western barbarians be expected to show proper respect for the *yangbans* (gentry) the way their own children did? However, once when a gentleman ventured to reprove me for not using the respectful form to him, I fear I did not improve matters by suggesting to him that if he used the high form to me, I might better learn how to use it.

Now I found that I had to unlearn my boyhood type of Korean, which process I found harder and more painful than learning a new language. Marian, on the other hand, was skipping merrily past me and teaching *me* the equivalent of, "*Nai ga cham nab-e-o!*" in the more dignified adult idiom!

We had as one of our excellent teachers, Henry D. Appenzeller, who took his teaching and us seriously. Then there was Horace Underwood, also a whiz at speaking the language, who would fire questions at us in Korean faster than a super machine gun, the purport of which usually didn't dawn on us until after he had left the classroom.

Charlie Sauer was on loan to teach at the Language School from his northern Methodist mission station in Yeng Byen, Province North Pyeng An. He was truly a gentleman and a scholar. He cautioned us not to laugh at any quaint translation errors a Korean teacher might make because of his limited knowledge of English, for such loss of face would be extremely painful to him. We, therefore, geared ourselves to restraint while attending this class. Charlie Sauer had written one of the textbooks in Korean. He used to show endless patience in drilling us in conversation on familiar Biblical themes, such as the "Woman at the Well," and have us practice how many different ways we could tell it in Korean. Once, in my "best" Korean, I ventured, "the woman *in* the well," which drew forth hearty, and unrestrained laughter from the class, with total disregard for *my* loss of face, I might add.

The Director of the Language School, Dr. E. W. Koons, was also one of our teachers. A Northern Presbyterian missionary, he was the principal of the Kyung Sin Academy in Seoul. Dr. Koons proved to be a very popular and colorful teacher. He had the knack of helping to make things stick by his graphic and vivid presentations. I remembered that he had extra large ears which he could "flap" at will, especially when we made a translation error.

We were attending Language School, as it turned out, at an exciting and historic time. The 27th and last king of Korea's famous Yi dynasty, ex-Emperor Sunjon, had died in Seoul on April 25, 1926. Following Korean custom, the official state funeral was not scheduled until June 10. It promised to be a very majestic affair.

The Japanese feared that Korean patriots might try to use the occasion to stage a comeback to power as they had during the Independence Movement demonstration of March 1, 1919. This movement had surfaced just prior to the last royal funeral which had been for the late Emperor's father, Emperor Kojong, on March 4.

Emperor Kojong, the father of Sunjon, found the Japanese presence in Korea oppressive and had secretly dispatched three emissaries to the Second International Peace Conference which was meeting at the Hague during the summer of 1907. The appeal for removal of the Japanese was rejected, whereupon one of the emissaries (Yi Jun) is said to have disemboweled himself before the world delegates. Infuriated by news of this attempted appeal, the Japanese forced Emperor Kojong to abdicate in favor of the Crown Prince on July 19, 1907.

The official reign of the Yi dynasty came to an end on August 22, 1910 when Korea was formally annexed to Japan. Following World War I, however, Korean patriots became inspired by U.S. President Woodrow Wilson's advocacy of the principle of self-determination for all nations. They concluded that if the fact of Japanese oppression were brought to the attention of the world, which had just concluded the Great War, sufficient international pressure might be brought upon Japan to persuade her to relinquish her hold on Korea.

Thirty-three Korean leaders drew up and signed a declaration of independence which was secretly printed and circulated throughout Korea. Taking advantage of the fact that many people were sure to come from the provinces to throng the streets of Seoul on the occasion of the Royal Funeral, a non-violent demonstration was planned for March 1, 1919. On that day the 33 leaders, which included 15 adherents of Chondogyo, 16 Christians and 2 Buddhists, assembled in Seoul and publicly read the declaration of independence they had signed. It proclaimed to the world that Korea was of right a free and independent nation which had been unjustly annexed by Japan against her will. Copies were sent to the governments of the leading powers and it was also read in all provincial centers in Korea by local leaders.

Korean flags, forbidden by the Japanese, were waved by the crowds, shouting, "*Mansei!*" for Korea (long live Korea). The leaders then notified the startled Japanese authorities to come and arrest them. Brutal retaliation followed, despite the disciplined peaceful nature of the demonstrations, and many were arrested, jailed and killed. For the first time Koreans identified Christians as also being Korean patriots for they were jailed or killed in large numbers.

Although the Independence Movement did not bring the desired freedom, it moved the Japanese to change the military government that had been in power, for a civil one. Baron Makoto Saito was appointed to the position of Governor-General and the policies he followed were more conciliatory than his predecessors. His major interest was education. By the time we had reached Korea, the number of educational institutions had increased almost five times from the 250 schools in the country at the time of his appointment. By 1925, when he was raised to the rank of viscount, he had become widely respected for his open and genial manner of conducting the duties of his office.

Nevertheless, fearing another similar demonstration at the 1926 funeral of ex-Emperor Sunjon, elaborate police precautions were taken. We were advised to keep off the streets at the time of the funeral procession. However, such caution was not necessary for us, for we were staying with my mother at the East Gate Hospital compound which afforded a grand view of the proposed route. This was to be through the ancient city wall at the Great East Gate to the historic Royal Tombs at Kumgok, fifteen miles northeast of Seoul.

We later heard that some student groups had indeed planned a demonstration similar to the one in 1919 and had gone so far as to print anti-Japanese leaflets. Although the forbidden Korean national flag appeared on nearly every street corner in Seoul, the police had been alerted to the plan this time and successfully suppressed the demonstration.

My mother had been invited to the special farewell ceremony which was not far from East Gate and she had wisely decided to walk there. Crowds were already gathering on the hospital grounds and, we later discovered, the 2,000 or so people did considerable property damage. We had selected an excellent vantage point where Marian would be able to take snapshots of the colorful funeral procession. After the police had duly inspected Marian's camera to assure themselves it was not a bomb, we had a long wait. Marian took this opportunity to ask me to give her some of the historical background to the occasion.

As I tried to gather my hazy thoughts, there flashed before me the recollection of the time when, as a lad in Korea, I used to go over to play with the Hulbert children in Seoul. Their father was the famous Dr. Homer B. Hulbert, a recognized authority on Korean history who had initially gone to Korea at the request of the Korean King to help organize and teach in a government school established in 1886. Dr. Hulbert had resigned that position in 1893 and joined the Methodist Mission. However, he had remained a friend to the

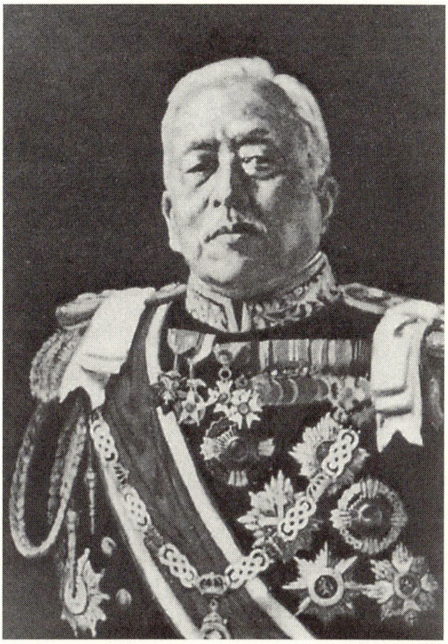

Viscount Makoto Saito, Governor-General of Korea

King and was one of three missionaries who stayed beside the King to protect him when he was afraid for his life in the days that followed the murder of Queen Min in 1895.

One of Dr. Hulbert's children, Madeline, was especially fond of recounting some of her father's stories about Korea to her playmates. She liked to play school and the rest of us were appointed the role of students, while she reserved the role of school mistress to herself. When she became stuck on remembering some date or historical event, she would call in her expert father to help out, and since he always concluded with a story, we children were more than delighted. This play-acting was thus a painless method of learning history.

Our play would go something like this:

"When did Columbus discover America?" Madeline would ask.

Someone would shout, "Fourteen ninety-two!"

"That is correct. Just remember the Yi dynasty was founded one hundred years before that. Can anyone give me the date?"

Perhaps I would volunteer (on the strength of the clue she had given us), "Thirteen ninety-two!"

Madeline would then say that I could move to the head of the class.

Upon that reflection, I proceeded to impress Marian with my knowledge that the Yi Dynasty was founded in 1392 and that King

Sunjon, the 27th king, had married the daughter of Marquis Yun, who, by the way, was related to our friends, Baron Yun, Tchi Ho and his daughter, Helen. Sunjon's queen was a year younger than I, and she was married at the tender age of thirteen.

Suddenly we heard the shout, "*Own da!*" (Here it comes), and we looked in the direction from which the funeral procession was due. We watched the distant white line grow closer and closer, and now could make out the sing-song wails of the hired mourners, "*Ay go. Ay go.*" Then, just as suddenly, everything stopped. We were wondering what had happened when someone suggested that they must be resting.

"Well," Marian remarked to me, "No need for you to rest. More historical data, please."

Although I had left Korea in 1910 and was not there to witness the events of the 1919 Independence Movement, I recounted to Marian what Dr. Hulbert had told me of them. I had visited the Hulberts in their home in New England during my college years, and he followed very closely what was happening in Korea. He had worked actively in behalf of the Emperor Kojong for Korean independence from Japan. His efforts included a personal, although unsuccessful, appeal to President Theodore Roosevelt to intercede on Korea's behalf before the Treaty of Portsmouth was signed on September 5, 1905, at the conclusion of the Russo-Japanese War. As a consequence, the Japanese had banished the Hulberts from Korea with orders never to return. Dr. Hulbert still continued to work hard for the independence of Korea by means of lectures, writings, and interviews with key persons in prominent places. He was to have the eventual satisfaction of witnessing Korean independence and of returning to that country before his death in Seoul in 1949.

Again we heard the shouts, "*Tassee own da!*" (They are coming again). The ancient gates in the city wall had always been focal points or places for meeting and gathering and none more so than the picturesque Great East Gate. For centuries it had served as the final exit gate of Korea's monarchs, as they were taken to the Royal Tombs where they would be enshrined. This time it was not just the passing of an emperor, but the end of a grand era in Korea's history.

First came a squadron of mounted police. Then, like a swarm of hornets, their stings in the form of sheathed swords, followed police on foot, dressed in black uniforms. Rattling their swords, these police interspersed themselves in the dense crowd, black spots against the white clothed spectators who had gathered along both sides of the street and at the open space before the Great East Gate. (White, not black, is the Korean color of mourning.)

Again, we were carefully scrutinized, but evidently judged to be harmless. As it turned out, there was no serious disturbance at that location, only a scuffle here and there when someone stepped out too far from the viewing line. The people really seemed to be too sad for protest, and we could see tears trickling down the faces of some of the old-timers standing near us. Evidently they recalled Korea's proud history and sorrowed at the passing of this royal dynasty.

Now we heard the "*Ay go! Ay go!*" lament of the hired mourners more clearly. Soon we saw more military police on horseback. The procession had evidently resumed its course.

Banners and scrolls carried aloft on bamboo poles bore eulogies to the deceased. To frighten away the evil spirits, there were several masked men, each pulled in a cart. The three-feet wide masks bore grotesque features with bulging eyes and a toothy leer guaranteed to scare off the most intrepid demon.

To further outwit the evil spirits and to facilitate transporting the coffin through narrow gates or down steep inclines, a second bier, about half the size of the main catafalque, was included in the procession. The evil spirits were supposed to be kept guessing as to which one carried the body of the deceased.

Our gaze was soon fixed on a magnificent spectacle, the giant red colored bier containing the casket of the late ex-Emperor Sunjon. The chief hired mourner in front was dressed in light straw-colored grass-cloth with high peaked headgear of the same material. Dressed similarly were crowds of hired mourners who walked alongside the bier.

The royal catafalque rested upon an elaborate network of wooden poles interlaced with flat cloth ropes. These were woven of hemp and were padded, to enable the one hundred and ninety pall-bearers to support the heavy superstructure. The ropes were passed under two parallel beams and seventeen cross poles. The bier itself was roughly ten feet long, five feet wide and six feet high and was painted red, the color for royalty.

Long ropes extended fore and aft of the bier, manned by additional men. For practical purposes these were to help control the heavy load whenever inclines had to be negotiated. However, while those in front pulled forward, those in the rear pulled back constantly in symbolic regret. Two men stood on planks on either end of the bier, facing outward in opposite directions. Each one had a bell with which he rang out the rhythm of the funeral march so that the pallbearers could keep in step.

There followed the palanquins containing ex-Empress Yun and female relatives of the royal family. They were, of course, veiled and not in public view. Just behind the palanquins came rickshaws carrying men of the royal family and state officials.

What most attracted our attention were the six floats of paper horses wheeled on individual carts. They stood about fourteen feet off the ground and were constructed by pasting a strong type of homemade Korean paper, prepared from mulberry tree bark, onto bamboo horse-shaped frames. These models were supposed to be the riding horses for the late king in the next world. Four were saddled and presumably ready to ride, while the two unsaddled ones were kept ready in reserve. These would all be burned at the tomb site. They helped to make the more than a mile long funeral procession very photogenic.

Marian and I felt privileged to be witnessing Korean history enacted before our very eyes. We were keenly aware that a significant chapter had just been concluded and that this spectacle of a royal funeral was the last of an ancient tradition.

Two days later, Mother, Marian, and I attended the Seoul Women's Club annual entertainment on the lawn of the U.S. Consulate. With summer just around the corner, many of the conversations centered upon vacation plans. The group appeared equally divided in their recommendations to us to vacation at one of two beaches: Sorai Beach on the west coast and Wonsan Beach on the east coast.

The senior Avisons and one of their sons, Dr. Douglas Avison (a schoolmate of mine at Toronto University Medical School) said we simply must go to Sorai on the Yellow Sea. The Underwoods were also great Sorai enthusiasts. Horace Underwood insisted that we must have a sail with him just as soon as the "Black Duck," the sailboat which he had designed and was having built, was completed. Since Haiju, our assigned station, was on the way to Sorai, we invited the Underwoods to stop off and see us en route.

Gordon Avison, Jack Boots, and others were just as insistent that Wonsan Beach on the Sea of Japan was *the* beach, and furthermore, if one went there, one could easily go on a camping trip to the fabulous Diamond Mountains nearby. Henry Appenzeller also

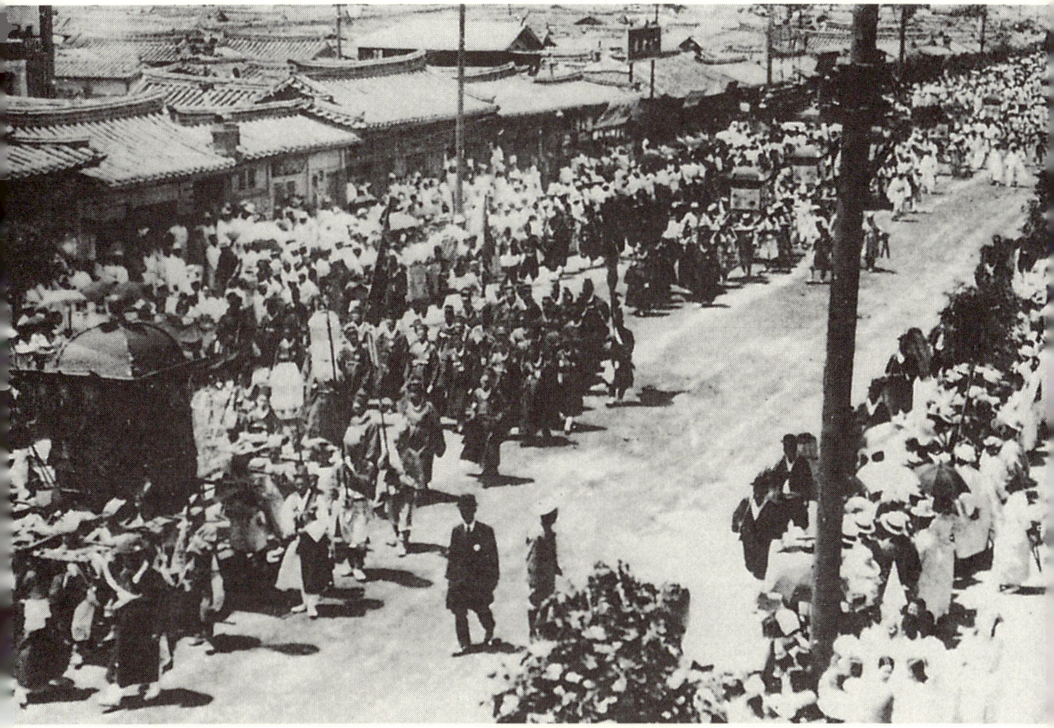

Funeral procession of ex-Emperor Sunjon, June 10, 1926

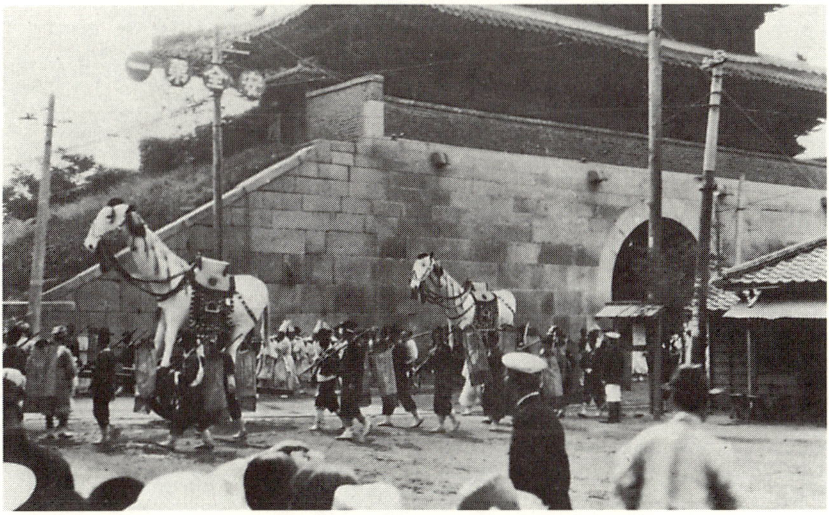

Floats of paper horses saddled in readiness for late King to ride in next world

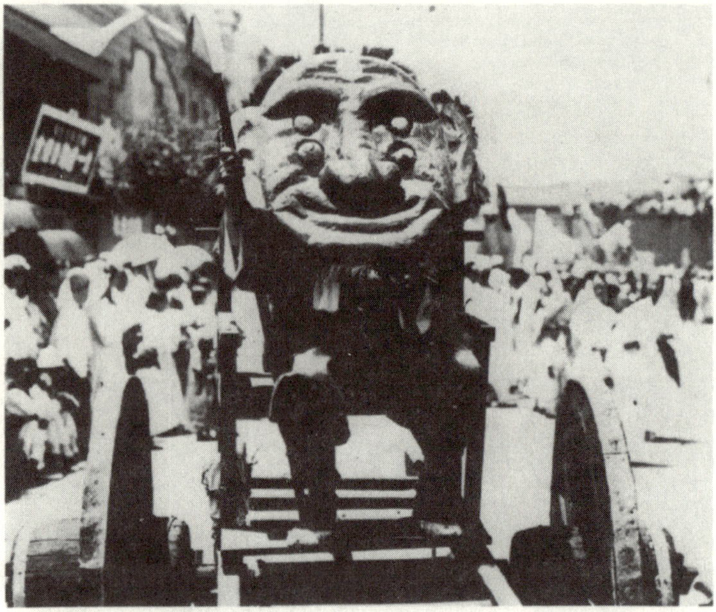

Masked man pulled in cart to frighten away evil spirits

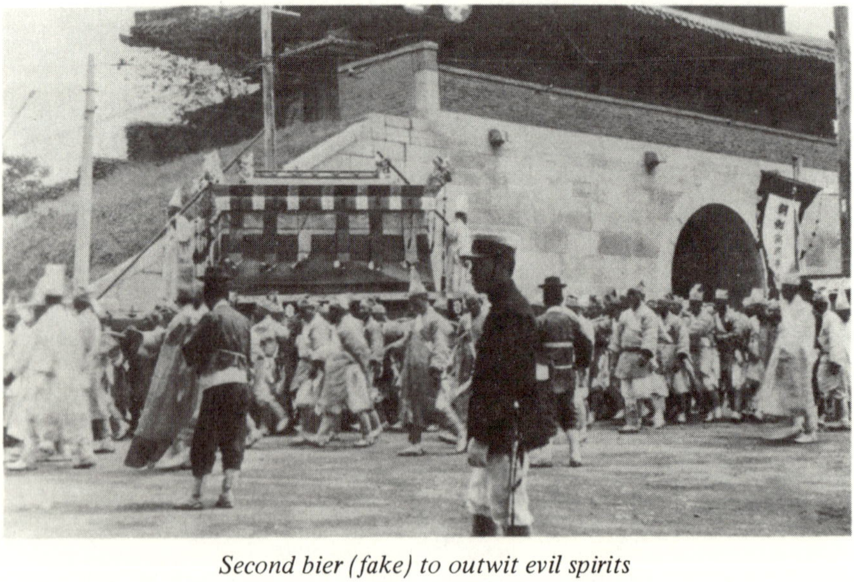

Second bier (fake) to outwit evil spirits

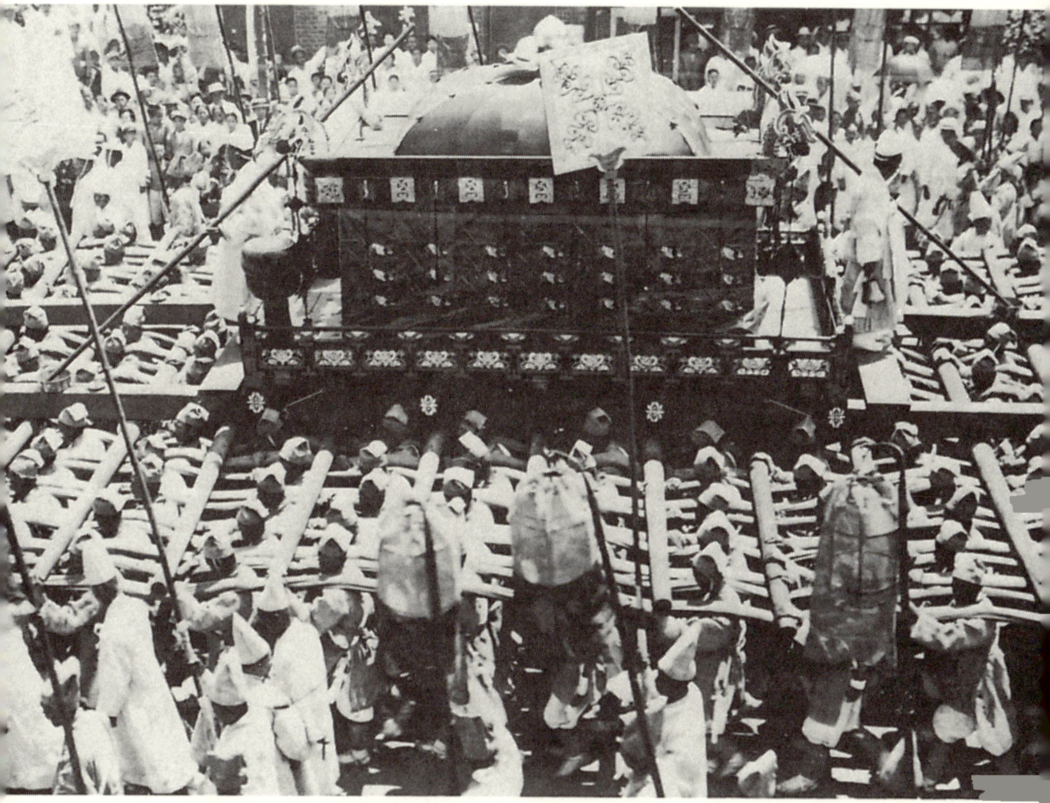

Masked man pulled in cart to frighten away evil spirits

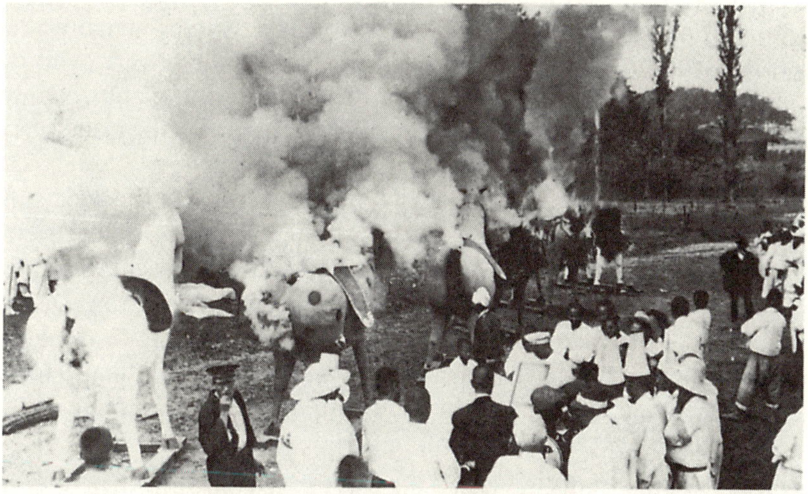

Second bier (fake) to outwit evil spirits

offered to take us for a sail if we went to Wonsan Beach. He noted that the famous harbor at Wonsan was one of the largest in the world and could shelter an entire fleet of ships.

Another "Wonsanite," seeing that we seemed interested, spoke up. "I have just learned that one of the cottages at Wonsan Beach, complete with a small boat and the only outboard motor on the Beach, is up for sale. The present owner actually believes that the world is coming to an end imminently, and has already taken his children out of school. He has started to pack for home."

Immediately I became all ears, excited at the prospect of possibly purchasing a cottage very cheaply. I could easily persuade such a person that if the world was soon coming to an end, he would have very little need of money.

Marian, then, in true wifely fashion, applied the brakes by simply asking me, "How do you propose to finance it? By the interest on our college debts?" She added in a more conciliatory tone, "Anyway, don't you think we should see both beaches before coming to a decision?"

I realized, of course, that Marian was right and agreed. "Yes, Sorai Beach is only fifty miles from Haiju," I replied. "We could easily take a run up there some weekend and visit Wonsan later at the first opportunity. In the meantime, there is much work to be done which naturally must have first priority, for we have yet to dust and air our stethoscopes."

During the party at the Consulate, Dr. Ludlow, Chief Surgeon of Severence Union Medical School, said that he wanted to visit us at Haiju and learn the Roger's treatment for liver abscess which we had been taught in London. He later did so. Dr. Mary Stewart, who was Surgeon for Women at the Korean Royal Palace in Seoul, wanted Marian's advice and assistance on a difficult operation for one of the palace ladies, which later, Marian was able to give.

Everyone pronounced the party a huge success. We received some very cordial invitations to stay at the homes of newly made friends when we returned to Seoul, which in time we were able to accept.

The first term of Language School ended on June 18. Despite hard study, those days were really happy school days which launched many lasting friendships. We were a little reluctant to see the session come to a close, but we would be back in October for the second term.

The Annual Conference of the Methodist Mission in Korea was held at the end of the month and on June 24 the new appointments were announced and the new missionaries were formally introduced. Along with us, a vivacious young lady, Miss Maud Keister, was presented to the Conference. Maud had arrived in Seoul on June 10, the same day as the funeral for the ex-Emperor of Korea, and we complemented her on her sense of historic timing. She proved to be a friend who became very dear to us during the ensuing years, along with the man she married two years later, the Reverend Kris Jensen. Maud served as assistant treasurer for the Mission and later as treasurer. Kris was an evangelistic worker, assigned to cover the central provinces, when he and Maud came to Korea as man and wife on their first wedding anniversary, July 13, 1929. We were to enjoy many happy visits together in our future years in Korea.

There was still one important thing that I had not done, Marian gently reminded me, and that was to show her the home where I was born. Mother advised that I had better not wait until the next time we came up to Seoul, for by then it might be torn down. She had heard that a more modern structure was soon to be erected in its place. Marian was as keenly interested in seeing my old homestead as I had been in seeing hers. So she insisted that I take her to it forthwith.

The home was not large or pretentious, but it had a touch of Oriental beauty all its own. The roof was of tile and gracefully curved upward at the corners. On the very top was a small gable effect. The ceilings were not flat, but the counterpart of the sloping roof with the large central beam and rustic rafters all exposed. It resembled ribs coming off a central vertebral column. The outside walls back of the veranda had evidently been repeatedly plastered with clay, and imprints had been made there before the walls had dried. There were interesting Oriental designs, such as crooked pine trees, the stork and the tortoise, all symbols of long life.

We saw the room where I was born and where my father had died. The partition was partly broken, so one could see the broom-stalk lath that had been used so effectively. It was a comfortable Oriental dwelling, a counterpart to the log cabin where my father had been born. My parents had shared it with the Nobles during those early years, and it was here my mother had delivered Ruth Noble. That was the evening on which my parents and I had returned to Seoul from Pyong Yang at the outbreak of the Sino-Japanese War.

Our conversation turned naturally to the Nobles and I commented to Marian that I held Mrs. Noble in very high regard. "Two of her children, Cyril and May, died in infancy," I told Marian, "and despite grief and heartaches in her life, she remains an optimist. It was always a tonic for me to talk with her as I was growing up, for she believed, along with Rabbi Ben Esra of the poem, that 'the best is yet to be.'"

Marian suggested impulsively, "Let's call on the Nobles right now. I'd like to see them before we leave for Haiju."

Mrs. Noble was out when we stopped at the house, but Mr. Noble invited us in cordially. We thanked him for his helpful words and understanding the other evening. Marian urged him to speak more about "the new kind of society" he had alluded to then.

Mr. Noble seemed pleased that Marian had asked him about one of his pet subjects. I recalled that what he told us that day was a particularly helpful introduction to missionary life.

"Money may have seemed a very important factor in one's personal life, before coming to the mission field. But from now on, it will appear less and less so to you, except as it relates to your work. In the first place, missionaries in the same mission are all on the same basic salary. Notwithstanding the fact that you are both doctors, you will not be getting any more than had you both been merely high school graduates. The educational requirements established by the Mission Board are now higher, it is true. You will find that most missionaries today are college graduates and are working towards doctoral degrees when they go on furlough. There is some extra financial allowance; however, it is not based on education or training, but on the number of children you need to support and on seniority. It does not amount to much extra, even so.

"Since you both have your college and medical diplomas and are so well qualified, you no doubt could really 'go places' at home in the United States. You will see many of your classmates eventually sporting fancy cars and costly private yachts and living in sumptuous homes. Indeed, some of your classmates and friends may even offer you their discarded clothes. Accept such gladly, for by doing so, you will be both materially benefitted and giving them an opportunity for vicarious service through you.

"While on furlough, you will be going among your friends with what the Buddhist monks here call the 'begging bowl,' but it will not be for self, as in the case of the monks. It will be, rather, to seek help for supporting the work you are trying to build up, in the name of God, for stricken humanity, making the coming of His Kingdom on earth that much sooner.

"Here you will not be labeled by your income, as in the States, where a person might be labeled as a 'ten thousand dollar man' or a 'twenty thousand dollar man,' and the wife is ever urging her husband to get a better position. Even in the so-called classless society of Russia, there are different gradations and privileges for those on top. However, here on the mission field, all such competitive tensions are eliminated since we are all on the same income level. It is true that one missionary may decide to put his small savings, if any, in books and skimp on clothes, or vice versa. However, we missionaries are truly a classless society, not only in name, but in fact. The rat race of trying to keep up with the Jones is virtually non-existent. In Haiju, even the Jones won't be there. Such a system spares the nerves to that extent.

"There may still be a race for power or prestige. However, for the most part, even that does not occur, since the rewards are not any increase in money, but only an increase in headaches. Thus, there will be few missionaries attempting to bypass his fellow missionaries. The sincere and honest missionary, nevertheless, will always strive to do his best, since he is entirely working for God and service to man, and not for personal ambition or gain.

"Herein lies the real satisfaction of life on the mission field. It makes it immensely worthwhile and marks its genuine uniqueness. Those of lesser motivation, religious cranks, or fanatics, will soon tire and automatically drop out. If you do drop out, you can be sure that there will not be a long line of those who want to take your place, as would occur at home. There is little likelihood that there will be anyone covetous of your job, and so God's work in that particular sector will suffer. You can see that you have, indeed, a great responsibility both to God and to suffering humanity, and you will need to call upon Him constantly for strength and guidance in the task He has given you. I have every confidence that you have what it takes and will serve Him faithfully and loyally."

On that statement of faith, we were ready to roll up our sleeves, supported by this "unique society" in which we were eager novitiates.

CHAPTER 14

The First and the Sixty-First Year

With Annual Conference over, our future was awaiting us in Haiju. We needed to arrange for our heavy baggage, hospital supplies and equipment to be shipped by a small coastal vessel to the port of Haiju on the Yellow Sea. Since we had already tried the journey ourselves overland, we decided it might be well to make plans to accompany our baggage and go by way of the scenic coastal route.

This could sometimes be hazardous as well as scenic for sudden storms caused many a wreck on that rocky coastline. It was such a storm which caused the death of missionary pioneer, the Reverend H. G. Appenzeller, when he tried to save the life of a Korean child and was himself drowned. That had happened in 1902 and we were on furlough when my mother received the news.

Before we left Seoul for Haiju, I needed to obtain an Imperial Japanese Medical License so that I could legally practice medicine in Haiju, or for that matter, in any part of the Japanese Empire. This I was readily able to obtain, for under a reciprocal agreement between Japan and the United Kingdom, my Canadian medical license was officially recognized. We learned that Marian would be able to obtain a Provincial License, which would adequately serve our purpose.

We left Seoul for Chemulpo the evening of June 29 in order to catch the steamer which sailed at 6:00 A.M. the next day. We were blessed by good weather and thoroughly enjoyed our trip. The boat followed the rugged Korean coastline and weaved in and out among the numerous islands which clustered near it.

As soon as we arrived in Haiju, Dr. Kim suggested that we call on the important officials of the city which was the provincial capital. When we were in Seoul, we had had calling cards printed for us as was the custom, so we were prepared. It was really a pleasanter task than we had expected. Somehow it had been noised abroad that we were friends of the Governor-General, Viscount Saito, so we were especially well received everywhere we called.

Then, on top of this warm welcome, I made the discovery that the Governor of the Province, Governor Luther Pak, had known me as a boy. My mother and I had once been guests in his home at 'Nampo where his father was Magistrate. This was the town where we had stayed at the time of the incident when I took up a collection in my cap for the first church there. Governor Pak seemed really delighted to see us.

Another person who was especially cordial during the course of our calling, was Mr. C. Sasaki, the Japanese Chief of Police. He told us that his family was rather isolated socially. There were very few in Haiju with whom it was considered proper to fraternize, and his wife was finding it rather lonely. Glad to be of any service, we invited this lovely family to our home and were often guests in theirs. We grew increasingly fond of them and with the passing years our friendship became stronger.

We were off to a good start and, in time, both our work and ourselves were to benefit. Some day, although we could not have known it then, we were to be in personal danger and in dire need of these friendships.

Marian was still unpacking when an emergency call came from the hospital for her services. She unsheathed her stethoscope and then was led posthaste to the maternity ward where a poor woman had been in labor for some time but was making no progress. On examination it was found that the babe was a breach presentation. Marian's stethoscope told her that the child was still viable, and after some deft manipulation of the fetus, the mother was safely delivered. In this case the baby proved to be a boy, and although Marian claimed no credit, she received it anyway. The news of Marian's "achievement" spread quickly, especially that she was expert in delivering boy babies. I knew then that Marian was in for sleepless nights, since most babies seem to prefer the nocturnal hours for their début.

In the meantime, I had had quite a different sort of emergency call that was not yet cause for unsheathing my stethoscope. The head teacher at the Boys' School, Mr. Kim, came over from the school and said that I must please come at once to fire one of the teachers. He

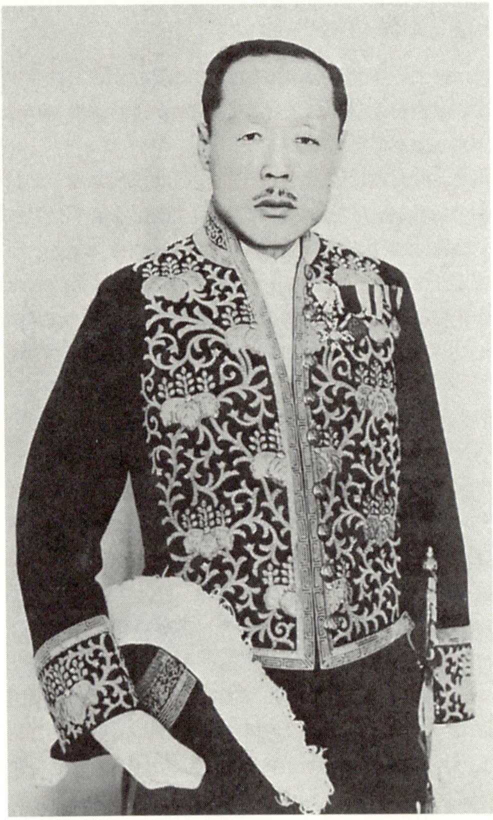

Governor Luther Pak of Whanghai Province

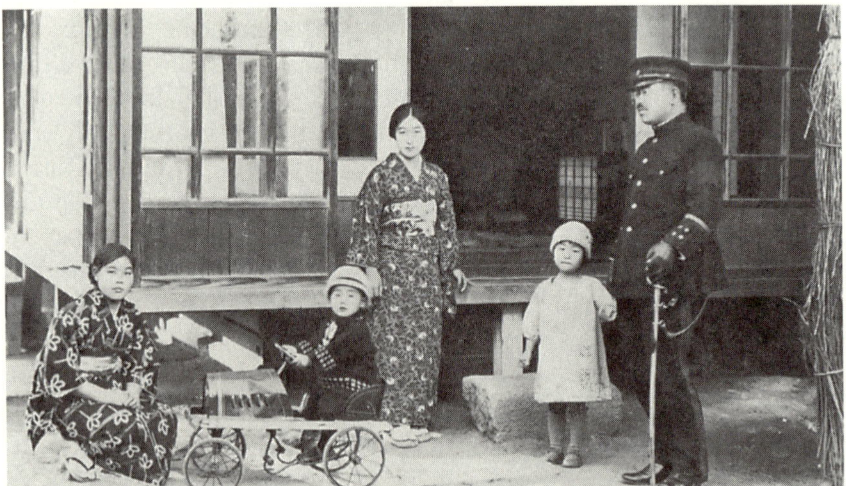

Mr. C. Sasaki, Japanese Chief of Police in Haiju, with his wife and children

had been repeatedly absent from his classes; therefore, as principal, I should do the firing. I was not very keen to start off my new career by firing someone, so I am afraid I was not as quick to run to the school as Marian had been to run to the hospital. On the way I tried to figure out how best to handle my new assignment, for I knew that my reputation as principal was also at stake.

Upon entering the school office I could feel that the room was charged with emotion. Anger was written on the face of Mr. Kim, and bitter resentment on the countenance of the one to be fired. Under these circumstances I could see that it would not be easy for me to be objective and just, and to demonstrate loving understanding to both individuals. I prayed a silent prayer for guidance, for this was not in the realm of medicine and I knew I was on unfamiliar ground.

I could see that Mr. Kim expected me to make short work of the confrontation; that since the facts were self-evident, I should fire the teacher at once. I was, of course, expected to uphold the head teacher's position and not cause him to lose face with the other teachers and students. In this way I would help to uphold school discipline. My task, from Mr. Kim's view, seemed clearcut and relatively simple. He was certain that the entire matter would be disposed of in no time.

To the surprise of them both, however, I said with a smile, "This is a strange welcome to your new principal. Let us all relax and have a cup of tea together and get acquainted. I presume you have facilities for serving tea here?"

Mr. Kim nodded, as he clapped his hands, which is the Oriental way of calling the serving boy. So with puzzled looks they sat down to tea.

After exchanging a few brief pleasantries, I inquired about the family of Mr. Kim and learned that he had a wife and four children, for which I congratulated him. Then, I asked about the family of the one to be fired. He hesitated at first, and looked to Mr. Kim for permission to speak and received a rather reluctant nod. He spoke slowly and his eyes filled with tears. I could see that he was struggling to express himself and I encouraged him to go on.

He then revealed, "My wife died recently of *pay pyung* (tuberculosis). Now my only son is also stricken and there is no one to care for him. This is what explains my absence from my classes."

I interposed, "Why on earth did you not tell this to Mr. Kim before, for I feel sure he would have understood and excused you?"

This time Mr. Kim nodded vigorously. I could see that the heat was off and we all became more relaxed.

Then the one to be fired explained, "*Quochang* (Principal), you know we Koreans in the North are ashamed of having tuberculosis, just the way the Koreans in the South (where the incidence of leprosy is high) are ashamed of leprosy. We are thus reluctant to admit to anyone that there is tuberculosis in the home."

I asked Mr. Kim to please have the serving boy at once take a note, which I had scribbled, to Dr. Kim. (The surnames, Kim and Yi, or Lee, are the most prevalent family names in Korea, as similarly, Smith or Jones are in the United States.) The doctor came right over and I explained our problem to him and asked if it might be possible to admit the sick boy into the hospital.

Dr. Kim hesitated, for he noted, "It is against the policy of our hospital to take TB patients, for we would then be swamped with them and have no room for other types of patients."

Upon seeing my disappointment and the acute distress of the poor father, he quickly added, "I suppose, as a special case, we could put him in our outside isolation ward, since it happens to be empty just now."

We all breathed sighs of happy relief, for everyone's face had been saved, and I had successfully passed my first school hurdle. That very evening I sat down by a pumped-up Coleman lantern and wrote an appeal letter to some of our special friends for funds with which to build a small TB ward for such cases as our teacher's son. I realized that my dream of establishing a TB sanatorium for Korea would take time for fulfillment. It would require a great deal of spade work because the Mission itself was not in a financial position to help. I also realized now that my new vocation of principal, which added responsibility I had at first been reluctant to assume, would dovetail into my medical duties to the benefit of both the school and the hospital.

The next day, Marian and I were invited to go on doctor's rounds at the Mission Hospital and to start seeing those so-called "difficult cases" which had been lined up for us. Although it has been facetiously said that "a doctor buries his mistakes," we did not care to have to do so, especially on our first day and with the limelight on us. Here, too, I breathed a prayer for guidance. As I took my stethoscope from its case, I came to the realization that the battle had begun.

Overnight, the importance of my stethoscope had increased, for there were no x-ray and other diagnostic aids to fall back on. It would be my constant companion and mentor as I acquired greater and greater experience in detecting, and above all, in correctly interpreting the various sounds it would amplify to my ears. There would be the clear, resounding "rub-a-dub" of the healthy heart, and the various types of muffled sounds coming from a damaged heart, growing fainter and fainter, until no sound at all might be detected, and we would have to pronounce the patient dead. Over the abdomen, the stethoscope would aid in the differential diagnosis between fluid, flatus and fetus, the latter producing the delicate sounds of the fetal heart.

From the lungs could be elicited the coarse rasping or fine gurgling or other types of "rales," so essential in the diagnosis of lung diseases. These rales have to be heard to be fully appreciated. Some sound like rubbing hair between the forefinger and thumb close to the ear. Others sound like tires going over a wet pavement. Also important is the exact location from which one hears the rales: whether they come from the base of the lung, or from its apex. These factors, and more, had to be kept in mind almost simultaneously as the patient was ausculated by stethoscope, or percussed, or palpated. At the same time one had to keep a careful eye on the patient's facial expressions, ever on the alert to detect the slightest change from normal, which observation often could make the hair-splitting difference between a wrong or a right diagnosis.

Although I knew that our training in the best recognized schools had been thorough and sound, I could not help but wonder how we would meet the challenge when we actually had to face it entirely on our own. Here we would not be able to ask the advice of our chief, or refer the patient to a specialist, or even to a medical conference. Everything had seemed so simple before, but now we alone often held the life or death of the patient in our hands. Right or wrong, we were the final authority. There was always, too, behind our backs the menacing, gleeful threat of a witch doctor who would hasten to broadcast any serious errors in diagnosis.

Suddenly I felt professionally very alone and, for a moment, well nigh overwhelmed. Then an inner voice seemed to quiet me with, "You are not alone, for the Lord your God is your helper and stay." From that moment, I felt reassured and went forth in confidence.

Dr. Kim reminded us that the patients he had lined up for us to see had come. Marian took the women and children, and I, the men. Out came our stethoscopes, and for the next few hours they were put to constant use.

A patient who had been badly mauled by a tiger was brought in. He had been cutting wood on a mountainside when he was attacked. Usually a tiger will leave a man alone if not provoked. However, if the tiger has been previously maimed, and so forced to seek easier prey, it is likely to become a "man-eater." Fortunately the other woodcutters nearby had heard the stricken man's yells and rushed to his rescue, but not until he had had an eye gouged out and had been badly clawed. I realized that the immediate danger was infection and treated him accordingly.

There were several cases of snake bite. In one instance, the farmer had been transplanting young rice plants in the paddy fields and had inadvertently stepped on a snake hidden among the seedlings. Actually it was not so much the snake bite that had to be treated, as the resultant gangrene that had set in because the tourniquet had been kept on too long. A number of the gangrene cases were so severe that they would require amputation.

Then there were the enlarged abdomens, not due to adipose tissue, as is so often seen in the West, but to intestinal tuberculosis, enlarged spleen (usually indicative of chronic malaria), or enlarged liver (often due to liver abscess). These abscess cases I was able to aspirate, as taught us at the London School, with very happy results.

I had barely started my examinations when Marian called me over to see one of her cases. She wanted to know if I could hear the two heartbeats she thought she had detected. I applied my stethoscope to the patient's abdomen, and, sure enough, there were the hardly audible sounds of two distinct fetal heartbeats. We concluded that the patient was carrying twins, but I cautioned Marian to watch out for triplets, recalling my previous experience at the Stetson Hospital. She laughed and promised to keep a sharp lookout.

Marian also found other types of swollen abdomens: enlarged uterine fibroids, tumors, and a surprising number of huge ovarian cysts which would have to have surgery. Fortunately, however, she found few cases of carcinoma. We discovered that cancer was less prevalent here than in the West.

As the day went on, my stethoscope told me that nearly every other patient had tuberculosis, many of them advanced cases, and that meant there was little hope for them without hospitalization.

All this underscored more than ever the urgent need for a TB sanatorium. I prescribed palliative treatment for such patients. Of more importance, however, was the advice I gave that the patient be kept in a separated room and be permitted as little contact as possible with other members of the family, especially the children. Although I did not tell the patient, I felt it best to inform his adult family of the sad prognosis for their loved one. This news proved very hard on them for they had set their hopes in my ability to restore the stricken one to health. This part of the clinic work I found very depressing, and I felt sick at heart that I could do so little for these TB sufferers.

However, there were a few bright spots in all this gloom. Despite alarming hemorrhages and the chorus of sounds relayed through my stethoscope, some of the patients did not look as ill as their symptoms implied they were. They often brought up bright frothy blood, which would indicate that it was coming from the lungs. If it had come from the gastro-intestinal tract, the appearance of the blood would not have been frothy and its shade would have been dark, due to the discoloration caused by hydrochloric acid of the stomach. Dr. Kim had been puzzled over these cases, for the medical textbooks had mentioned that such cases were apt to be TB. I asked Dr. Kim if he had examined the sputum for lung fluke and he replied that he had not.

Fortunately, we discovered that some of these patients were suffering from distoma and not from TB and that the lung fluke could successfully be overcome by emetine treatment. What a joy it was to be able to tell these patients that there was a specific cure for them, and they were not victims of *pay pyung*, for which they had such feelings of shame.

At the close of the long clinic session, we had found that these so-called "difficult cases" had not been as difficult to diagnose as we had anticipated. Of course, the ultimate cure of some was quite a different story.

"The first operation must be a real success." So announced Marian. "Though the lighting may be inadequate, the instruments insufficient, my assistants not yet used to working together as a single surgical team, and your surgeon still rather inexperienced, yet we must not fail." These were braver words than Marian realized when she had uttered them, as she entered the operating room on that fateful morning.

The day previous, Miss Lund and her nurses had been as busy as bees, dusting the ceiling, scrubbing the floor and other objects with disinfectants, and making everything spotlessly clean. The gowns, drapes for the patient, rubber gloves, and instruments had been twice sterilized to be doubly sure that no lurking germ might spoil everything. Even the orderly had been posted outside the surgery, armed with a fly swatter to prevent any offending insect or unwanted intruder from entering.

Marian had selected with meticulous care the first patient for her series of operations at Haiju. She had asked me to examine the heart and lungs of her patient and had ordered the necessary laboratory tests. Except for the patient's ovarian cyst, she was found to be in the pink of health. Even the relatives had signed the necessary document for the operation, which, if anything went wrong, might prove to be only a worthless scrap of paper.

The patient's family had previously pleaded with Marian to please remove the huge bulge in their daughter's abdomen. It made her look even larger than a full-term pregnancy and was so unsightly and uncomfortable that it prevented her marriage. In fact, some had even taunted her, claiming that she had lost her good reputation and was, in fact, pregnant. Yes, much was at stake for the patient, the hospital, and us. Even the chaplain was not permitted into the operating room. He offered his prayer for the patient in the hallway, just before she was wheeled into the surgery.

All procedures went like clockwork at first. The patient had been sedated and appropriately draped. Doctors and surgical nurses had scrubbed, been gloved, gowned and masked. The anaesthetist had gently placed the mask for the ether over the patient's face and his little ether bottle was poised, awaiting the nod from the chief surgeon. Then, like a bombshell, a disturbance seemed to explode outside the hospital. It was the roar and shouting of a crowd which was gathering outside the operating room, and the noise grew louder and louder.

Someone burst into the surgery unceremoniously, yelling, "*Sunsul comontoo, comontoo!* (Stop, stop the operation!) The family demands that a photograph of the patient must first be taken for they find that they have no portrait of her, and if she should die without a portrait, evil spirits will plague the family. If there is no portrait taken of her, then there will be no operation."

Yes, it was just as simple as that. Marian and Miss Lund looked at each other in consternation. "This is all nonsense and should not be tolerated," declared Marian. What of all the previous careful sterile preparations? What would Marian's former surgical chief, Dr. McGuire, think about her now, allowing outsiders into the sacred precincts of the operating room at the time of an impending operation?

Dr. Kim and we three had a quick huddle. He knew how the angry crowd outside might vent its wrath. Miss Lund, seeing Dr. Kim's worried face, hastily mentioned that if we postponed the surgery that had been scheduled for tomorrow, enough sterile materials would be available to re-drape the patient, and start all over again. It was decided that I, as Medical Superintendent, should make the final decision.

I well knew the temper of a Korean mob, so I gave a reluctant "yes" to the messenger at the door, knowing it was a calculated risk. However, I insisted that only the photographer and a member of the immediate family would be allowed in, and both had to be out in less than ten minutes before the effects of the sedation on the patient wore off. This decision seemed to satisfy all, including the crowd waiting outside, and they gradually melted away.

The dopey patient was quickly propped up on the operating table, and steadied by a relative, while the photographer clicked his camera. The resultant photo must have presented a ghoulish appearance, well calculated to drive away any evil spirit.

The contaminated items were soon replaced by sterile ones, and after a disinfectant had been duly sprayed, the operation proceeded without further interruption. Some of the new Korean surgical nurses performed remarkably well and were quick to anticipate Marian's needs, but two of the nurses became confused and handed Marian the wrong instruments. Here, Marian was not as outspoken as Dr. McGuire would have been. Miss Lund, however, quickly had these nurses exchange places with those holding the surgical retractors.

The operation was successful, and in this case, the patient neither died nor became infected. Later, in contrast to her original girth, she was able to walk out of the hospital a slim young thing, admired by all and as happy as could be. In the future, however, we practiced the precaution of inquiring of all surgical cases whether or not they had had a photograph taken recently.

Days were kept more than busy with patients and various hospital and school problems. The evenings were used in writing to friends and sending out "appeal letters" by the glaring light of the Coleman lantern, which needed frequent pumping.

At first the nights were rather hard on Marian, for besides her obstetrical cases, she found the night noises of Korea especially trying. It was like someone used to a quiet country atmosphere moving to a noisy city. Only the noises here were not ordinary "big city sounds."

There was the monotonous "rat-a-tat-tat" of the ironing sticks on the rollers, as industrious Korean women folk made sure their husband's white garments were kept beautifully ironed for use the next day. There was the sad howling of dogs mourning the loss of their mates, which creatures might have been served up in soup the day before. It might be their turn next.

The sound hardest to bear, however, emanated from the tom-tom drums and the clanging, ear-splitting cymbals of the *mudongs* (witch doctors). The sound screeched to an ever increasing, frenzied crescendo, at which point it would suddenly stop altogether, only for the entire process to repeat itself again and again throughout the long, eerie night.

Processions of people on their way to the "devil house" would pass up the steep hill behind our home. These patients, who had previously been "needled" to let out the evil spirits, or burned by red hot irons in specified locations, were carried on men's backs or on donkeys. The use of unsterilized needles in this acupuncture treatment often resulted in infection and painful inflammation. The poor wretched victims were clinging to the forlorn hope that the *mudongs* would be successful in driving out the evil spirits responsible for their illness. Marian could not help being perturbed by the thought that when these patients failed to get relief, some of them would come to us at the hospital as a last resort and when it would be too late to save them. The question she kept turning over in her mind was how to get these people to come to the hospital, first.

On the other hand, my sleep was plagued by disturbing dreams. I seemed to be ever hearing the ominous sticky rales through my stethoscope, like tires running on a wet pavement, until the sounds became louder and louder, waking me up with a start and in a cold sweat. Or in my nightmares I would see some wretched TB victim going from hospital to hospital but being refused admission; then, appealing to friend after friend for help and being denied on the

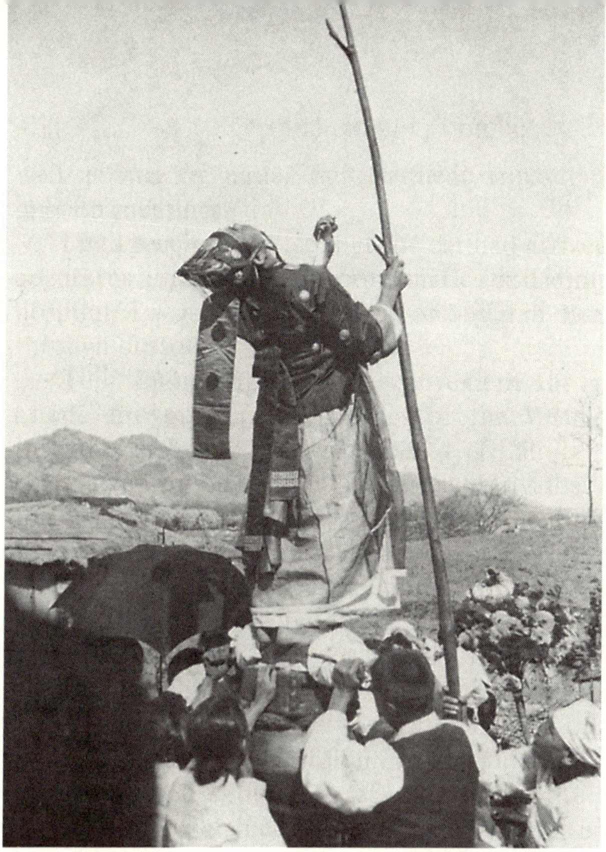

Mudong (witch doctor)

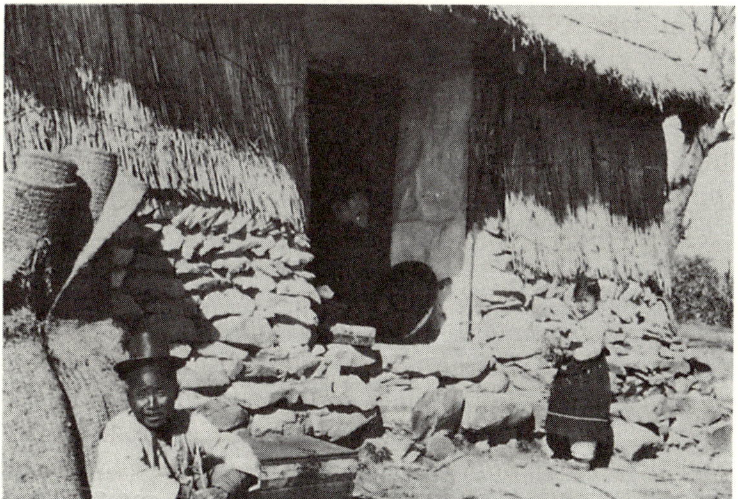

Devil house on hill behind Hall's residence

grounds that he had a "shameful disease." To spare his family from his offensive sputum, he would swallow it and develop agonizing intestinal tuberculosis.

Such were the impressions which haunted me. Marian, then, by gently placing her hand on my shoulder would waken me and ask, "What is troubling you so?"

One morning Pearl observed, "You do not seem to be your usual cheerful selves. You both look so worried. Have you been trying to carry the burden of this responsibility in your own strength? Remember, we all have a loving heavenly Father. He really cares. We should go to Him, for His yoke is easy and He can lighten our load."

We realized that Pearl was right and expressed our gratitude for her timely reminder. After our evening prayers, we both experienced a good sleep that night. It seemed we were back on the right path.

At long last we received word that the remainder of our freight had arrived. Not everything had been shipped together and so immediately following Clinic, I went down to the Port to arrange for this delayed shipment to be brought to our house, a distance of about four miles. The cheapest and best way was by slow moving ox cart. Marian eagerly greeted the arrival of our things and began to unpack. Carefully she checked each item against her packing lists and found everything there. Thanks to her careful packing, only a few items were found to be broken.

We had been having our meals with the ladies until the arrival of our things, so now the question of servants arose. An experienced cook, Sinsie, and an outside man, Songsabang, who had previously worked for the Wachs, were available. We had incurred some rather heavy expenses, and Marian, who always kept a careful watch on the pennies to our mutual advantage, at first felt that we should dispense with the idea of having servants. It was at this point that Miss Barlow adamantly declared a flat, "No."

She explained, "That would be a tragic waste of the time of two physicians. Servants in the Orient are not a luxury but a necessity. In the West you also had servants, in the form of running water, electricity, gas, and such fixtures as washers, sweepers, and flush toilets. These did the work for you. In Korea there are not such conveniences to save both labor and precious time. Yes, here, in order to accomplish anything worthwhile, one has to have servants. It is a clear 'must.' Besides," she added, as if to clinch her argument, "servants are comparatively cheap, and to do without them you would really be depriving these poor people of the income they so desperately need."

So Marian rather reluctantly consented. In this decision I concurred more readily, knowing what was to be in store for her and which secret we thought the time was not yet opportune to divulge, especially to Miss Barlow. Then we might be in for a dissertation on a different subject which would not find us in agreement with her.

Some time after this, Miss Barlow had returned from an interesting itinerating trip and wanted to tell us about some of her experiences. Pearl suggested, "Why don't we all go on a picnic?"

This seemed like a fine idea to us and the others heartily agreed. Miss Barlow took charge of the drinks, which, in this case, simply meant tea. She had the brewing of tea down to a fine art and would have detested tea bags. Pearl and Belle agreed to provide the sandwiches, and Marian offered to make a salad and bake a cake.

Miss Barlow had rested sufficiently from her trip to be in a happy frame of mind. At such times, she was really a good sport, and I was pleased to see that she and Marian were getting along famously. They were the life of the party. Miss Barlow amused us with an anecdote from her recent trip.

"The Korean word '*mal*' can mean one of three things: a bushel-like measure, a speech or a horse. I had intended to congratulate a young Korean lad on his fine speech but he mistakenly thought I had been referring to his horse, of which he was very proud. He promptly ran to fetch his steed and insisted that I take a ride on it!"

Belle was the quiet one, but on drawing her out about school work, I could discern that she had much wisdom. I knew she had a rich background of experience from which I could well profit.

Many wild flowers grew on the mountainside where we were picnicking. In the spring, Belle told us, it was covered with purple azaleas. We noticed an abundance of *halmanie gawt*, or "grandmother" flowers, which I have seen only in Korea. The flower is so named from its white hair-like exterior, but it has a rich velvety purple interior. In great profusion, also, were the wild violets, both white and colored.

After we tired of gathering flowers, the ladies brought out their game of "Anagrams," in which we all participated, but at which I did not distinguish myself, for I have always been poor at spelling. However, Marian saved our reputation by winning easily. I had a private theory that one had to have a musical ear to be a good speller, which nicely let me out.

Through this most enjoyable and relaxing outing we came to know one another better. We concluded that Miss Barlow was not such a bad sort, after all, and not as difficult as she had at first appeared. We had not yet put her to the crucial test, but for now, she approved of us, and all was well.

"Three Underwood dogs arriving," announced the telegram delivered by the telegraph messenger boy one day, not long after the picnic. This had us puzzled. Although we had invited the Underwoods to stop off and see us when they were sailing the "Black Duck" to Sorai Beach, there had been no mention made of any dogs. Moreover, we had had no experience with dogs and were at a loss to know how we were expected to entertain them and how much meat we should provide for them.

Fortunately, before we had the opportunity to purchase the meat, Dr. Underwood and his two sons arrived, solving the mystery. It seemed that the local telegraph office somehow had garbled the message, and they had substituted the word "dogs" for the word "boys." (Dr. Underwood had included himself as one of the boys.)

The weather was hot, so Marian proffered our guests some grape juice which she had been making from the delicious wild grapes we had gathered the day of our picnic. She was certain that this drink would serve to greatly refresh them. Dr. Underwood took the first sip, and since he was standing where I could see his wry face, I began to suspect that something must be wrong. Before I could say anything, he gallantly asked Marian to have a toast with him, and filled one of the empty glasses. After touching glasses, they raised the dark drink to their lips, but this time only Marian took a sip. She was off like a flash to the kitchen sink, while they all began to laugh.

Our cook had filled one of the grape juice bottles with soy sauce. Since the bottles of both the grape juice and the soy sauce looked similar, by mistake, Marian had proffered a salty drink of soy sauce to her guests, which would be anything but refreshing. Dr. Underwood had been quick to turn the tables, and had given Marian a drink of her own medicine. On later occasions he enjoyed teasing Marian by reminding her of her unusual formula for quenching thirst.

The Underwoods wanted us to go with them to Sorai, some 50 miles distant, in their new boat. Since we were not free to accept their invitation then, we promised to join them later during the weekend.

We found Sorai Beach to be delightful. It had the most beautiful sand we had ever seen, and from which the Koreans made crystal clear glass. Although we were very favorably impressed with Sorai, there was no cottage up for sale at that time. Besides, we had promised my mother we would visit Wonsan Beach before making up our minds about a regular vacation area.

The second term of Language School was due to begin on October 5. October 1 had been declared a national holiday in Korea by the Japanese to commemorate the annexation of Korea by Japan. Mother suggested, therefore, that before we began school, we should take advantage of the holiday to visit Wonsan Beach for a few days. My mother shared a cottage there with two Canadian missionaries, the McCully sisters. We had been urged to visit the beach by other Wonsan enthusiasts also, and this did appear to be an opportune time to do so.

We stopped overnight in Seoul with my mother and then traveled by train a distance of some 140 miles northeast. At that time it took about seven hours to reach our destination from Seoul. Elizabeth and Louise McCully, sisters, whose missionary work was in the town of Wonsan, met us at the station and took us to their pleasant home on the hill, overlooking the harbor. They arranged for us to go to the beach in the afternoon.

As soon as we saw the beach, we were biased in its favor. Impulsively, we decided to pay a visit to the Reid cottage which the McCullys told us was still up for sale, and now at a lower price than originally.

The modest wooden frame house favorably impressed us. We were especially taken with its location: the sea and distant isles in front, and the outlet of a small river on one side. This made a haven for the small outboard motorboat (which came with the cottage) as well as a safe channel for it when there was a storm at sea. The cottage was so constructed that the sides, in convenient sections, were hinged from above. In good weather, these could easily be opened to let in the refreshing sea breezes and to allow an excellent view. In the event of a storm, they could be tightly closed, and glass windows provided in each section still permitted light to enter.

Dr. W. T. Reid was a physician and son of C. F. Reid, founder of the Southern Methodist Mission in Korea. Dr. Reid had taken special precautions to have the cottage well screened against possible malarial mosquitos by night and flies by day. Also supplied was a pump and a good fresh water artesian well.

We noted that the cottage was conveniently situated to the auditorium. This building housed the church on Sundays and became a lecture, game, and entertainment center on weekdays. In addition, it was the meeting ground for various summer conferences. Most of the other cottages were fairly near, yet no cottage at the resort had been built too close to another. We could not help but conclude, "This is it!"

Upon later contacting Dr. Reid, we found him to be very reasonable and the delayed payment terms he offered us were so generous that we felt we would be foolish not to accept them. This simple cottage was to become a vacation center for us and for our children to enjoy in the years ahead. My mother felt that we had made a sound investment and viewed it as a form of health insurance which would offer us a place to go for respite when we needed rest from our work. We returned to Language School with a feeling of elation over our "find."

Although my mother's sixty-first birthday fell on September 19, a conflicting meeting of the Federal Council of Protestant Evangelical Missions had prevented any special celebration of it on that day. Korean friends, however, would not be letting such an important day slip by unnoticed, for in Korea, the 61st birthday holds a very special significance. It is called the *hankap*. A celebration had been planned for the first available date, October 22, 1926. The *Liberty Gazette*, the newspaper in my mother's home town, printed the following account of the event which Marian had written for them:

"Dr. Rosetta Hall Honored in Korean '*Hankap* Party'"
"By Dr. Marian B. Hall

"It was my privilege to be one of the honored guests at mother-in-law's '*hankap*.' It is a Korean custom to celebrate the sixty-first birthday of one's parents by a big feast to which many friends are invited and at which eulogistic speeches are made telling of the notable things done and important events in the life of one so honored. Many beautiful gifts are sent by friends and all kinds of good wishes made. Supposedly this marks the termination of active labor and the sixty-one-year-old settles down thenceforth to enjoy his remaining years in peace.

"The selection of the sixty-first year has its own significance. It marks the completion of a cycle in the Korean calendar, a cycle being sixty years and the *hankap*[1] the beginning of the second cycle. It works out as follows.

"The Korean calendar has ten years named respectively, *Kap, Ul, Pyung, Chong, Moo, Kee, Kyung, Sin, Im,* and *Kay*. These correspond in length of time to our years. In addition they have what they call twelve hours named after animals or reptiles. These are *Cha* or rat, *Chuk* or cow, *In* or tiger, *Myo* or rabbit, *Chin* or dragon, *Sa* or snake, *O* or horse, *Mau* or sheep, *Sin* or monkey, *Yu* or rooster, *Sul* or dog and *Hay* meaning pig. Each year is given one of these names. For instance the first year would be *KapCha*, the second *UlChuk* and so on. But since there are more hours than years the second decade would start a new combination and instead of *KapCha* we get *KapSul*, then *UlHay*, and the *Cha* or rat appears this time with the *Pyung* year. A little simple mathematics shows that it is sixty years before the same hour and year coincide again and when this happens a new cycle is begun. And since a Korean baby is one year old the minute it is born instead of a year later as with us, the *hankap* marks the sixty-first year, which corresponds to our sixtieth year.

"With the missionaries, the Koreans play the part of sons and daughters and few of them pass the sixtieth milestone without a feast being made in their honor.

"Dr. Hall's *hankap* was really due last year but she was loathe to celebrate it until the arrival of her son and his wife and persuaded her Korean friends to wait until this year when they could be present. However we had nothing to do with the arrangements, as all plans were made and carried out by a committee of thirty-three of the most prominent Koreans, among whom was Baron T. H. Yun.

---

[1] [The word *hankap* means "returning to the new cycle." The Chinese lunar calendar adopted by Korea in 1433 forms the basis for the calendrical system traditionally used in determining dates for rituals and holidays. Chinese ideographs for the celestial and terrestrial signs are given Korean phonetic pronunciation.]

"At 6 P.M., an automobile came to take us to the restaurant where the feast was to be held. We were taken to a room where the other guests were already assembled and seated on the smoothly polished floor against the gaily decorated walls. Leaving our sandals, for which we had previously exchanged our shoes, at the door we stepped on the spotless floor and were led to the end where thick padded mats and cushions were arranged. Dr. Hall's place was marked by a large blue gaily embroidered cushion for backrest and other cushions on either side on which to rest her arms. Sherwood and I were placed beside her and were introduced to the guests as they came up to mother Hall to pay their respects.

"These formalities being over we were taken to the dining-room where a delicious Korean feast was laid out on low tables. There was a special table for Dr. Hall and her children and across the front of this forming a gay barricade, were plates of brightly colored Korean candies, cakes, and fruit piled high in tall cylinder formation. These were not eaten at the feast but sent to the house later for Dr. Hall to distribute amongst her friends who could not be present. Much of this went to Pyong Yang to be enjoyed by the girls in the blind school which she had started there.

"The rest of the food was the same at each table. First there were the bowls of "*kuksoo*" a meat soup with spaghetti-like strings of buckwheat flour put in it. On being eaten it sounds like the s-o said on inspiration instead of expiration for unless one inhales it no end of trouble arises in getting the strings to separate themselves politely at the esthetic juncture. But it tastes mighty good and is the one Korean dish I can truthfully say I enjoy. To go along with this were innumerable side-dishes of various combinations of preparations of fish, meat, rice, honey, nuts, vegetables and fruits. It would take a Korean epicurean to do justice to the description so I won't attempt it.

"During and after the feast many speeches were made by prominent Koreans and others referring to Dr. Hall's work during her thirty-six years in Korea. The two things which called forth their greatest praise and appreciation were her work for the blind, in establishing a school and adapting the

New York Point system into Korean print, and her training Koreans as medical doctors.

"Both of these groups were represented in the speech makers and their words of gratitude were such as only an Oriental can express. One of the most spontaneous talks was made by a girl of over twenty who said that the only reason she and her grey haired mother were alive today was because Dr. Hall had saved both their lives at the time of her birth. Other speakers referred to the time when she had taken her own skin to graft onto a burned child and to the woman who was so grateful for what had been done for her that she cut a large piece of flesh from her own body and gave it, with a letter written in blood, to Dr. Hall begging her to be sure to return from America after her last furlough.

"The following is the translation of a song which was composed by the husband of one of the doctors at the hospital and sung by the staff at the feast:

'Deep in the mountains lie hidden
    silver and gold.
Pearls rest on the deep ocean floor,
But through the grace of God,
Dr. Hall has been placed by Him here.
The toil and tears of sixty years
Are given without stint,
And this her life so freely given is
    indeed her true memorial.'

"At the close of the speeches one of her women doctors walked up the aisle between the tables bearing a box from which trailed bright pink ribbons. This she presented to Dr. Hall as a gift from the Koreans. It was a beautiful silver vase entirely of Korean workmanship and art, having cost, as was announced to the audience, Yen 150 ($75). In Unman was written the occasion of the presentation while the pattern on the vase was made by a design of ancient Chinese characters inlaid in the silver in a contrasting metal.

"Dr. Hall made a suitable speech in reply and following this the guests gathered around to see all the gifts which had been piled on the table in the dining room and consisted of silver and brass articles, silk Korean clothes, framed embroideries, and useful embroidered linen articles. The silk Korean dress she wore for the occasion was given Dr. Hall by one of her blind women who had earned the money herself through work she learned to do at the school.

"Over a hundred guests were present at the feast and amongst them were prominent Japanese and Koreans as well as representatives from amongst the various denominations of missionaries. One of the Koreans told us that it was the first time that such a group of prominent people, both Christian and non-Christian, and representing so many groups and organizations, had so united to plan and arrange such a function as this.

"The automobile was again waiting to take us home at the close of the meeting and we were more than happy in the joy that all this demonstration of love and appreciation of her efforts, had brought to our mother who has accomplished so much in the face of opposition which would have discouraged and broken one with less courage or fainter vision of the needs of Korea, the country she loves and where her loved ones are buried.

"A fitting memorial of her work would be the establishment of a Korean Women's Medical College where Korean girls could be trained in their own country and under Christian influences, for lives of service to their sister women who so greatly need their care. The Koreans feel the great need for such an institution and are already making plans which, if they receive the support and help of the missionaries and friends in the homeland, give every promise of making this dream come true. Then, indeed, would Dr. Hall feel her cup of joy running over for in this work is all her heart."

Only two years later, this dream was to become a reality. The Woman's Medical Institute, founded by my mother, opened in Seoul on September 4, 1928, as the first medical school for women in Korea.

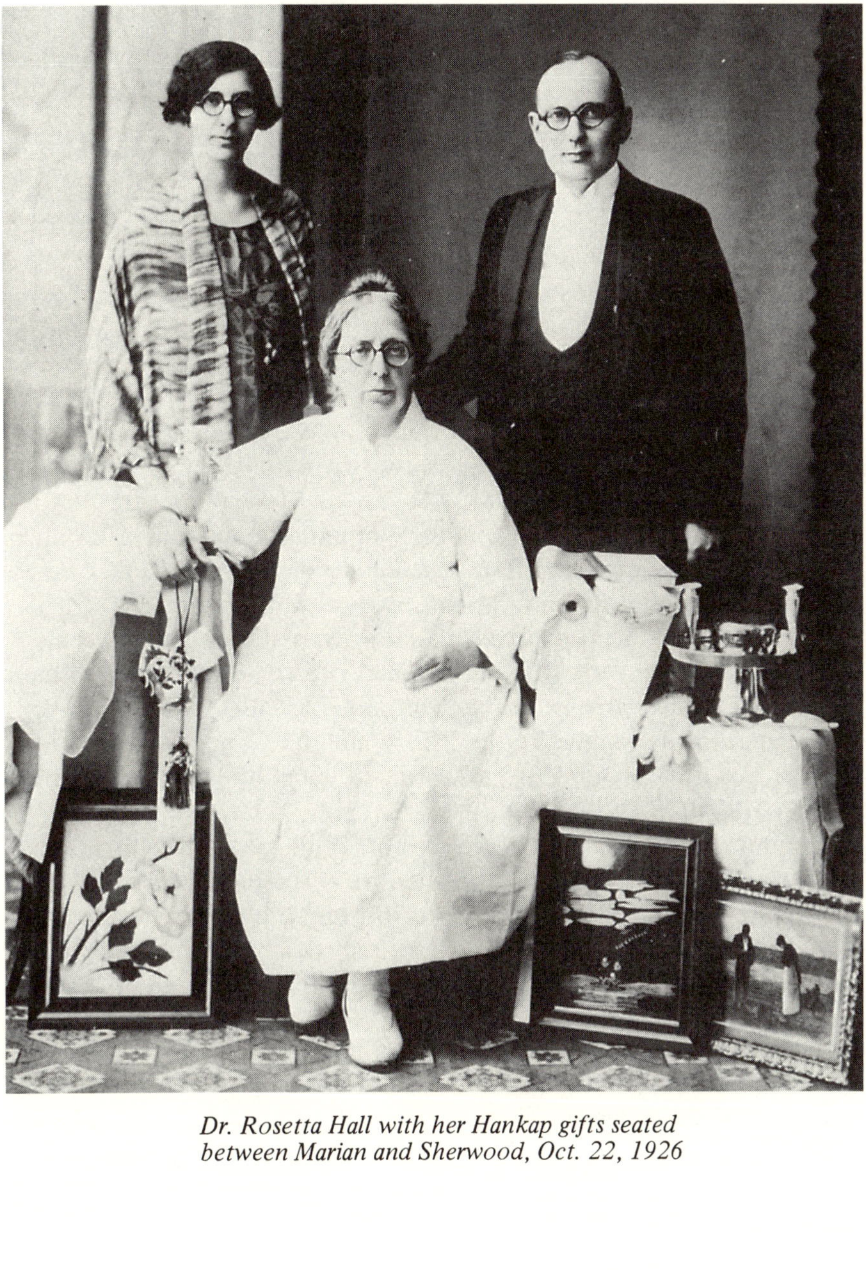

Dr. Rosetta Hall with her Hankap gifts seated between Marian and Sherwood, Oct. 22, 1926

CHAPTER 15

First-born

On our return from the second term of Language School, Miss Barlow greeted Marian with the exclamation, "Well, I never! You must be expecting!" She went on, "I am sure it must have been accidental. Now your usefulness on the mission field will be severely curtailed."

Stunned, Marian was at first going to give Miss Barlow a spirited reply. She chose instead to turn away sorrowfully, saying under her breath, "What is the use?"

The other ladies gave Marian a sympathetic and understanding look, and warm embraces. Later, Belle started to knit a lovely baby blanket right under the disapproving eyes of Miss Barlow.

If there had been a mixed reaction from the missionary ladies, there were only cheers from our Korean friends who were more than delighted at the prospect of a white baby. Miss Helen Yun had returned from her studies in the U.S.A. and had come to Haiju to try to start a private school for girls. She explained the Korean point of view to Marian.

"Your Korean lady friends were really disturbed that after several years of marriage you still had no offspring. They knew that inevitably your husband would take to himself a concubine and you would be displaced. I tried to assure them that your husband would never do that, but they simply shrugged their shoulders and said they knew better. Because they really like you, they did not want this to happen. Now they are greatly relieved.

"Many hold you in high esteem and, out of their respect for you as a professional woman, have set you on a pedestal. However, there has existed a chasm between you and them which no gestures of friendship on your part could bridge. Almost overnight, all this has changed. Motherhood will now be a strong common bond between you which will draw you ever closer to them, especially with the birth of your son.

"'Of course, she will have a son,' everyone says, 'for does she not almost always deliver sons? She will most certainly see to it that her own child is a son!'

"No longer will you be just 'the nameless one,' but elevated to the exalted position of 'the mother of "so-and-so."' Moreover, being assured of a son, you will have an heir to worship at your grave and bring you joy and peace in the next world. Henceforth, your service to the women of Korea will automatically be greatly augmented."

Marian grasped the point. She exclaimed, "So Miss Barlow is wrong! Having children will not impede my usefulness here but will increase it. I wish, Miss Yun, that you would kindly explain all this to Miss Barlow, for it might change her attitude."

Miss Yun nodded. "Yes, we unmarried women in Korea are still looked upon with suspicion and lifted eyebrows, for traditionally from ancient times the only unmarried women were dancing girls. It is one of my aims to change this view and to help in the emancipation of Korean women. The single missionary ladies are rendering noble service in elevating the status of the single woman. They are brave souls, and I know that God will bless their efforts."

Although we had no way of knowing, for sure, whether Miss Yun had talked to Miss Barlow, the latter called on Marian soon after that and told her how sorry she was for her hasty remarks. She had just returned from a hard country trip. Besides being unsuccessful in making any new converts, there had been several "back-sliders," all of which led to her feeling very depressed and out of sorts. Marian accepted her apology graciously. Miss Barlow remarked, in parting, "I have ordered a complete layette for your baby. I only hope that it will arrive in time for the event."

Miss Barlow's change of attitude made us both feel much better. In a small mission station it meant much for one's peace of mind to be in harmony with one's co-workers. We admired Miss Barlow for she had come to the mission field well past middle age and had mastered a foreign language. Coming from a background of luxury, she could have remained at home in comfort, but instead, she had chosen and adjusted to a rough, new life.

Christmas was suddenly at hand. My mother had hoped to be with us for Christmas, but her furlough instructions from the Mission Board decreed otherwise. She was to leave for the U.S. from Kobe, Japan on December 12. I knew that this first Christmas in a foreign land, far away from loved ones and old friends and associates, would be a difficult one for Marian.

Overseas mail was very irregular. For long intervals there would be no "home mail," and then when it did finally come, there would be a huge pile. It was a case of either feast or famine. How I wished for a feast of mail this particular Christmas to cheer Marian. I was having some staff troubles at the hospital, from which I tried to shield her, and so felt the need of cheering myself.

Moreover, we were having heating difficulties. In the basement of our house was an old coal burner furnace which provided heat to the living room through means of a single hot-air vent. The other rooms could be warmed to a lesser degree if we kept all room doors open. The furnace had an annoying habit of periodically belching forth smoke and soot, in addition to hot air, when sufficient gases had been built up within it. This caused our eyes to burn and blackened the walls and curtains. However, at the moment, our regular delivery of coal was late. We did not have to contend with the smoke for there was nothing with which to fuel the furnace. Instead, we huddled around a small kitchen wood fire to keep our teeth from chattering.

Marian spied some loaded ox carts coming up our driveway and called to me in happy relief, "At last our coal is coming." But when they arrived, it turned out to be, not coal, but more cold! This was in the form of cakes of ice to be stored for summer use, for of course, we had no refrigerator.

It certainly appeared that Marian's first Christmas at Haiju would be rather dreary. From time to time I could see her glance furtively down the driveway when she thought that I was not looking, for she did not want to add to my worries. After much searching, I was at least able to find some fairly straight Christmas trees for the hospital, the school, the ladies and ourselves. Marian busied herself in decorating some of them with homemade decorations and with her artistic ability, she was able to make them look very attractive. I only wished that there were more packages to place under the trees.

The day before Christmas the creaking of wheels and the sound of crunching snow in front of our cottage, accompanied by shouts of exhortation from drivers to oxen, heralded the arrival at long last of our coal! Soon thereafter, we heard grunts and exclamations of, "*Mao magupso!*" (Very heavy!) on our front porch. The postmen appeared bearing parcels!

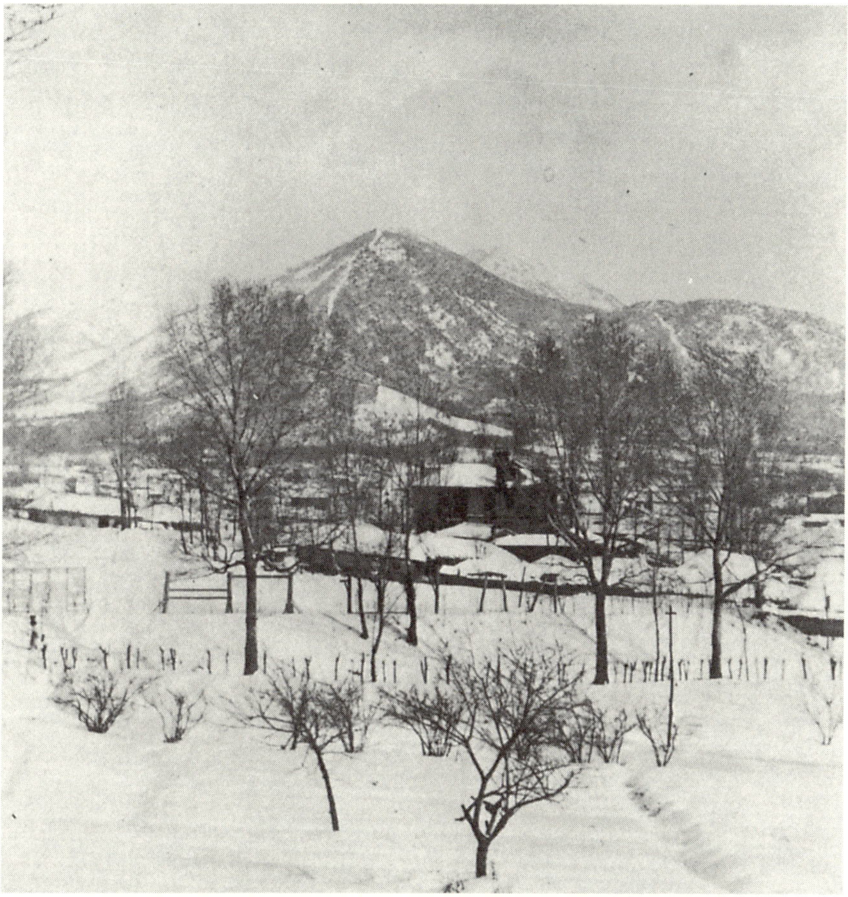

View of Norton Hospital from stone house, Haiju

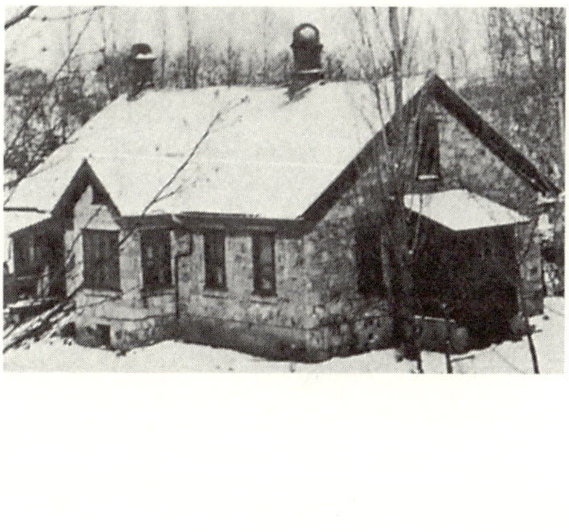

How they timed it to meet our Christmas wishes and provide us with such joy we have never been able to explain. We now had gifts to put under the Christmas tree and an exciting pile of Christmas mail to read. There were cards from friends and patrons to decorate the mantel of our imaginary fireplace.

To accompany the warm glow in our hearts, hot air from the furnace soon began to warm our bodies. The loving remembrances and thoughts of generous friends erased the miles between us as if by magic. There was even an occasional gift for our unborn infant, and his mother insisted that she could feel him kicking up his heels for sheer delight over his gifts. Like children, we eagerly unwrapped the lovely packages, finding real happiness in this first Christmas at Haiju after all.

As time went on, I had to restrict Marian's activities at the hospital more and more. She was over-ambitious and eager to do too much. However, all the staff members were considerate. When Marian's condition was explained to the women patients who usually clamored for her services, they too were understanding and allowed me to see them instead. Marian, however, was not one to put her physical comfort above the needs of others. Shortly before our baby was due, an emergency call came which she did not wish to refuse. Later, she wrote of the incident to our supporters back in America, and I shall let her own words describe that memorable night:

> "It had been an unusually tiring day and I had promised myself that just as soon as I finished a certain little task, I would go right to bed and lose my weariness in sleep. But it was not to be. Providence had chosen this night to give us one of the real thrills of medical missionary life. Just as I was turning down the bed covers the telephone between our house and the hospital rang. It was a call from the country thirty miles out where a man was lying with a strangulated hernia and had been suffering since early morning. Would we come out and operate on him?
>
> "For the medical missionary there is only one answer to such a plea. Someone was in distress and if we did not go to his assistance, it meant that he would die, for no other help was available for such an emergency. Dr. Sherwood Hall went over to the single ladies' home and roused Miss Lund, our

nurse, who was just as eager as we to answer the call. He then went to the hospital to start preparations for the trip and by the time I got dressed and over there, the Korean head nurse had the instruments all ready for me to O.K. before she put them in to sterilize. Miss Lund arrived in a few minutes and, before arrangements could be made to get a Ford jitney to take us, we were all ready and waiting . . .

"It was a beautiful moonlit night but a bitter cold wind was blowing and before we reached our destination it was snowing. The road, thanks to Japanese road-building, was very good most of the way and we rattled through village after village at a good speed. It was a novel sensation to go speeding through a Korean village. In the daytime it is a problem to get through the streets at all. The street is the children's playground and the adult Korean considers it beneath his dignity to hurry out of the path of a noisy Ford. Then the bullock cart assumes the right of way and whether it will turn out on the right or left is not for you to presume to prognosticate. A missionary who itinerates with a motorcycle answered my query as to which side of the road you take in Korea, by saying, 'You take the left, whether what's left be right or left,' and it is certainly true. Someone else told me that the reason the Korean lets a car shave past him is because he believes he is followed by an evil spirit, and if he lets the car just miss him, it will catch the evil spirit and carry it away from him. I can't vouchsafe for the truth of this but it certainly would seem to explain some of the needlessly narrow escapes which keep your heart in your mouth all the time.

"But no such problem prevailed at this midnight hour. The Korean villages lay quietly and picturesquely sleeping in the moonlight. Only occasionally did some white clad Korean, returning late from an evening with convivial friends, pass by us or was overtaken . . .

"Finally, just as we were beginning to feel pretty much frozen, we entered a village where a ghostly figure blocked our path, holding up a signalling hand. As we drew up before a Korean house, the door slid back, revealing a roomful of men warming themselves about a charcoal fire. We said with relief, 'We are here,' but we were far from right. Four of these white clad men attached themselves to the sides of the car and on we started again, looking I imagine, like a Ku Klux Klan expedition. They ventured the cheerful news that when the car had gone as far as it could, we should have to walk 3 *li* (1 mile) through the rice fields . . . we found the actual distance to be 5 *li*.

"The walk helped to warm us, however, and we were relieved of all bundles by the men. After almost two miles of stumbling along the donkey-paths between the rice fields, looking then like terraced skating rinks, we came to a miserable mud dwelling set back in the hills by itself. After being hauled up one of the highest steps I ever attempted, we found ourselves in the *sarang*, or men's quarters, a tiny low-roofed room with bare mud walls and grass mats on the floor. The only heat seemed to be a charcoal burner feebly glowing, and the only light a tiny oil lamp on the wall with a flame about the size of a green pea. I said to Miss Lund, 'How thankful I am that Dr. Kim thought of the lanterns and that I put my flashlight in my pocket just as I was leaving.' A herniotomy with only that tiny flickering flame would have been a miracle beyond my performance.

"Having divested ourselves of our wraps, we left them on the *sarang* floor with the hope that not too many vermin would find a resting place therein, and went into the next room where the sick man lay surrounded by a host of relatives and friends, at least it seemed a host in such a small room.

"The *wesang* (native doctor who is a licensed undergraduate) got his training under Dr. Norton when he was here, and learned enough to get his license and set up practice in this country place. He was amongst the group and he it was who advised them to send for us. His diagnosis of strangulated hernia was correct. The man had been suffering since early in the morning and was now groaning with pain. It was out of the question to reduce the mass by taxis and we immediately made preparations to operate, the first step being to clear all but two men out of the room. I glanced around the room at the mud walls, the dusty beams, and the patient lying on a mat in the dirtiest clothes I had ever seen, and under the dirtiest covers, and wondered how, kneeling on that dirty floor beside him to operate, it would be at all possible to observe sterile technique.

"I started scrubbing up and after a few moments glanced up, to discover that what had before seemed a solid wall had disappeared and there, gazing at me intently, were three sadfaced Korean women seated on the floor of an adjoining room. They probably thought the foreign lady in the queer white head-dress must be very dirty to have to wash herself so long. Dr. Kim scrubbed up to assist me and Dr. Sherwood gave the anaesthetic, while Miss Lund did multitudinous things. One of them was to hold the flashlight so that I could see what I was doing, for the light from the oil lanterns, held by two Koreans at a safe distance, was quite insufficient. You should have heard the exclamations of these same two Koreans when I released about five inches of greatly discolored intestine and restored it to its normal habitat. The cocks were crowing before our job was done, but finally the last suture was put in and we could stretch our cramped and aching legs and backs, and had the satisfying knowledge that we had given the man a chance of life.

"We returned to the *sarang*, which by now was blue with smoke, and found that not one in the group was a Christian. Miss Lund took the opportunity to teach them something about Christ . . . and the new life that comes from serving Him. Dr. Sherwood, too, was giving the message in the other room and here he learned that in all the village there were no believers. So another door has been opened, for those men told him that if only this man recovers, the whole village would believe . . .

The patient made a good recovery and as a result, two villages petitioned for churches and for us to hold a regular country clinic there."

After our night emergency call, I ventured to suggest to Marian that since jitney rides seemed to agree with her, even when pregnant, that we go up to Seoul for the delivery, for usually it is the first baby that is the hardest.

Marian was quick in her reply, "Do you want me to have our baby in a public jitney? You know I have every confidence in you. I have not even felt the need of checking the instruments and supplies you and Pearl have prepared for the event. I am not the least bit worried."

I confess that I was not quite so confident. To deliver a patient to whom one is unrelated is all the difference in the world to the responsibility of delivering one's own wife! Pearl and I had been going over all our meticulous preparations for the "nth" time, for I did not want to leave anything to chance. Finally, in near exasperation, Pearl exclaimed that I was as fussy as an old maid.

I noted that for a young maid, she had herself been very careful to select the very best supplies available.

"You know, none of the Koreans consider me young because of my blonde hair," responded Pearl. "To them it is white and they associate it with old age. Some even call me "*halmanie*" (grandmother) and give me the respect and veneration they give to the aged. I used to try to correct them, but after all, it is safer here that way. The Koreans are always asking me why I never married. They wonder why I did not allow my parents to select a bridegroom for me. When I tell them that I consider other objectives in life just as important as matrimony, they simply laugh in disbelief."

"I respect your point of view, but I am certainly glad I chose matrimony," I declared.

We had decided on a joint plan of action for the baby's delivery which was to take place in our home. My focus would be to care for the mother and the actual delivery, and Pearl was to look after the baby as soon as it was born. But if the baby was slow to cry, I was to administer his or her (Pearl was one who was not convinced that the baby would necessarily be a boy) first spanking, and other appropriate measures to insure that we had a "cry baby" with fully expanded lungs. I knew from past experience that Pearl was a competent nurse and capable of quick and correct action in any emergency. Both Marian and I had every confidence in her.

Miss Barlow had gone on one of her long country trips and we all knew the stage was now set for the happy event. We knew that Miss Barlow preferred to be away. It was shortly after she had left, as if by prearranged signal, that Marian's labor contractions began and we were off to a good start.

"Natural childbirth," so-called, had not yet come into vogue in the delivery room, although it did often occur in the rice fields. However, painless dentistry was growing in popularity, as was painless childbirth, despite some religious cranks who felt that women were ordained to suffer pain. The method for painless childbirth then in use was known as "twilight sleep" for which the chief drug used was scopolamine. This was an alkaloid, extracted from salts of a plant called "scopolia." This drug was both hypnotic and sedative in its effect. It had the great advantage of stopping the sensation or memory of pain, while at the same time permitting normal muscle action and the cooperation of the patient.

Everything went beautifully and according to plan. As predicted by the Koreans, the baby was a boy. I could not resist the temptation of giving Pearl a gleeful wink as soon as the baby's sex had been determined. Through my stethoscope I heard Marian's heart beating correctly and with strength, although she drowsily asked, "When do you suppose the baby will arrive?"

I motioned to Pearl to bring over our boy, and as I placed him tenderly in Marian's arms, I replied, "Here is the answer to your question."

"I can hardly believe it. I felt nothing." Marian placed a hand on her now flat abdomen. Her next question was, "Is it a boy?"

"Yes, we have a son," I replied with a broad smile. Pearl came forward to give him the attention he needed as the little fellow began to cry lustily.

It had rained that early memorable morning in Haiju, February 18, 1927, and then everything had frozen over solid, a slippery, glassy sheet of ice. It was then that I sallied forth to the telegraph office to announce to our world the glad tidings that we had a son; that his name would be "William James," after his grandfather Hall; and that both his mother and he were doing well.

At first, I was so overjoyed that I felt I was walking on air, but I soon discovered that I was actually walking on very slippery ice. The proverb, "*Pride goeth . . . before a fall,*" became more than mere words as I skidded and fell flat on my back.

After struggling to maneuver over the icy road on which I kept slipping, I finally reached the telegraph office bruised and dishevelled and suffering considerable injury to my dignity. I was, nonetheless, still able to beam with pride to the telegraph officer, announcing that we had a boy, and to please be doubly careful in spelling the word "boy" correctly over the wires. I recalled the telegram sent us by the Underwoods in which the word "dog" had been inadvertently substituted for the word "boy" and I didn't care to risk that error on this occasion.

He assured me that he would never be guilty of such a mistake, for had not my wife taught him perfect spelling?

Under my breath I remarked, "I hope you have proved to be a better pupil than I, for despite her strict tutelage over a much longer period of time, I still can't spell!"

Things soon settled down to routine in our home, with plenty of baby noise to remind us that our baby's voice box and lungs were developing well and that he must not be neglected. Much later, when Miss Barlow called to admire our son, he protested so loudly that she hastily excused herself, saying she would call again when he was napping so that we could all talk in peace and quiet.

Even before our baby came, we had resolved that our son would be brought up properly. We would not pick him up every time he cried, for this was only his way of expressing himself and developing his lungs. This discipline seemed to work well for a short while, but once he cried so persistently that his cries got on our nerves. Although we were still determined not to pick him up and spoil all our previous good training, we finally could stand it no longer.

When at last we went to him, we found that his head was wedged in between the slats of the crib. In fact, because of the swelling so caused, we had great difficulty in extricating him from his dilemma. After that episode, William joined all the other plebian "picked-up babies" of the world, to the great delight of his *amah*, who had previously been highly distressed at what she felt was our extremely cruel treatment. The one exception was that, crying or no crying, he was always fed on schedule.

At the same time that I was discovering that parenthood was not always smooth sailing, I was learning that neither was directing the course of a mission hospital. It seemed there existed in Haiju a rather active anti-foreign and anti-Christian organization, reminiscent of the Tonghaks. They lost no opportunity to attempt to discredit our Mission efforts both at the hospital and at the school.

It was often said that with the advent of the Japanese control of Korea, the latter had changed from a "Hermit Kingdom" to a "Permit Kingdom," for permits were needed for almost everything, from building, clearing land, owning or driving a car, to publishing anything or even holding a public meeting. Various lower echelon officials were given control over granting such permits in their particular area, and it was here that we began to feel the effects of the anti-Christian group. In our efforts at public health education, for example, we found that we were blocked by endless red tape whenever we wanted to give a public health lecture out in the villages. By means of a combination moving picture and magic lantern machine, that we had received as a gift for the work, and the public health charts we had developed, we felt we could do much in the way of preventive medicine through education. However, we were always mysteriously blocked, or if granted the permit, then the meetings were subjected to harrassment. This was particularly true if we attempted meetings that were strictly evangelistic in character.

Permits were also needed for inoculations against certain diseases. While we were finally granted permission to inoculate against typhoid in our Mission schools, we were flatly refused permission to do so elsewhere. We had over 200 students in our schools and none of them developed typhoid. During the same period, however, several cases developed in another school of similar size where we had been prevented from inoculating the students.

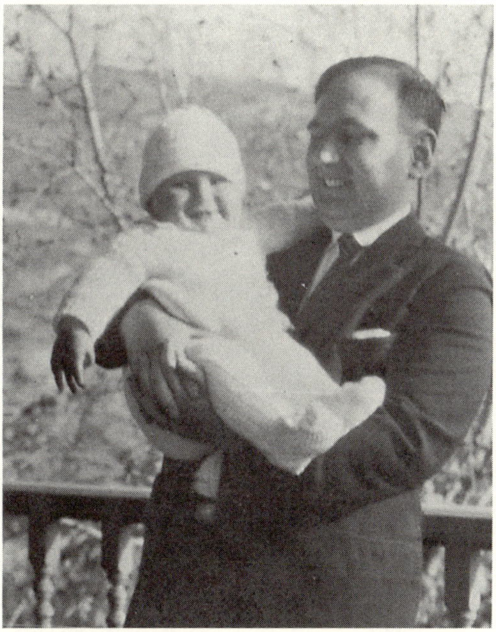

Sherwood holds first-born son, William James Hall

It was all very frustrating and did not bode well for the big plans I had in mind for the future. Even before leaving the United States, I had already developed some strong convictions about the vital need for establishing a tuberculosis sanatorium in Korea. I would talk of it often to my co-workers at the Suffolk County Tuberculosis Sanatorium at Holtsville, Long Island. I suppose in the naiveté of youth, I was so fired with zeal for the idea that I convinced others that I would bring this dream to fruition, despite the unlikely financial realities of the day. One of the first gifts I received for the as yet non-existent institution was the combination moving picture and magic lantern machine. It was given to me by Mrs. Jessie T. Skidmore, whom I had met at the Suffolk Sanatorium. She was so sure

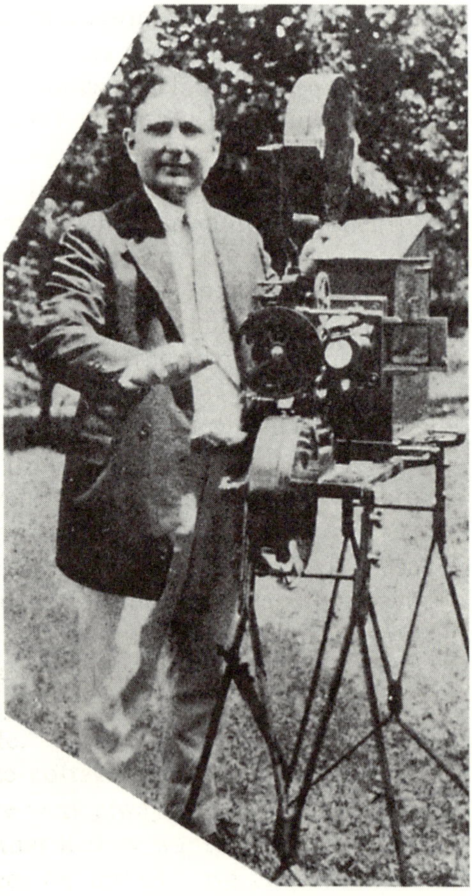

Sherwood with combination movie and magic lantern projector

my dream would be realized, she told me, that she wanted her share to be ready to do its part in public health teaching by means of pictures. The staff and patients at Suffolk encouraged me still further by taking up a collection of forty dollars to go towards the purchase of a quartz light and x-ray apparatus.

Bishop Welch had listened to me tell of my plans to attack TB in Korea, even before there had been any assurance that Marian and I would be able to raise sufficient salary to support ourselves on the mission field. He did not scoff at what must surely have seemed the foolish outpourings of youthful idealism. His eleven years as president of Ohio Wesleyan University before he became a bishop may have given him his special tolerance for visionary schemes. All he had said then was that the Mission Board had been notified of a bequest left by Mary Verburg for a new hospital in Korea. It was being held until a plan should be proposed which satisifed the executor as fulfilling the terms of the will, which stipulated a public health education emphasis. With an encouraging smile, Bishop Welch had commented, "Your project just might appeal to a hard headed business man."

However, the anti-Christian opposition I had encountered in this very area of public health education was most discouraging. I was therefore surprised one day to see among my clinic patients one of the officials who had given us so much difficulty whenever we had needed a permit for our public meetings.

"What brings you here this morning?" I asked him.

"I have this very painful cough which does not permit me any sleep," he answered. "I have tried the treatments ordered by the *mudongs*, but it keeps getting worse."

I listened to his chest with my stethoscope. It did not take me long to explain his wracking cough.

"Regretfully I must inform you that you have *pay pyung*," I told him. "We do not have facilities at the Norton Hospital for treating this disease, for we would need to isolate you from the other patients until your sputum is negative. That might take a long time."

The official's face registered both shock and fear.

"If the chest disease demon is in me, then I will surely die," he moaned.

Suddenly he looked up with new alarm.

"Oh, Doctor, I now have a great concern about my only son. He has been coughing all night long. I hear him when I am kept awake by my own coughing. Is it possible the chest disease demon is in him also?"

"It is very possible that he has TB," I said, "*Pay pyung* is very easily transmitted from one member of the family to another, especially when you are all living so close to each other every day." I added, "This was why I was so eager to get permits for holding meetings in the villages so that we could help the people understand how such diseases are spread and what they might do to help prevent this."

He ignored my pointed reference. In obvious distress he begged, "May I bring my son to you for examiantion to learn if he also has TB?"

"Yes, I shall be glad to examine him. In the meantime, you would be well advised to try to avoid too close contact with your family members, for their sake."

He returned to the next clinic session with a thin sickly looking boy in tow. My stethoscope confirmed my worst suspicions.

"Your son too has *pay pyung*," I told the worried father. "It seems that not only does he have TB in his lungs, but it has also infected the glands in his neck. In one so young the prognosis is not very good, for he has developed very little resistance to fight the disease."

"He is my only son and very precious to me," the distraught father sobbed. "Won't you please use that magic skill from your Christian God that I have heard some of the people in Haiju say you use here. They call this place 'Salvation Hospital.' Please will you save my son?" he implored.

How readily I could understand the man's distress, especially now that I had a son of my own. I excused myself momentarily and motioned to Dr. Kim that I wished to consult with him privately.

We discussed what we might do. Dr. Kim proposed that since we had used the isolation ward for the school teacher's son, perhaps it might be feasible to temporarily turn it into a TB ward until we could begin to build a sanatorium. He suggested that now that this official was experiencing the problem first hand, he might even bring his influence to bear on the other city officials to respond more favorably to our public health education efforts.

"But what if either he or his son die while they are in our care?" I asked.

"We must simply turn the matter over to the Great Physician," Dr. Kim smiled. "Is that not what our own fathers did when they faced difficulties?"

I called the official to my office and informed him that after consulting with my colleague, Dr. Kim, I had decided to admit both him and his son in the fervent hope we could help them.

Tears of gratitude flowed down the man's cheeks.

I felt in this instance there was more at stake than just the life of a boy and his father, important as that was. Upon their cure hinged the climate of acceptance that was needed if I were ever to be effective in waging my war on TB in Korea. I turned to our Christian prayer groups to seek their help in prayer, for those Korean Christians had the type of faith that moved mountains.

The prayer groups were so arranged that they were praying day and night, around the clock, in cottage prayer meetings. Korean Christians loved to pray out loud and at the same time, each one choosing his own words. So it was a babel of voices that struck the human ear, although I am sure that God heard each individual person, as he or she poured out their heart in fervent supplication.

Having seen and experienced many answers to prayer, I am a firm believer in its power. I also believe that God gave us intelligence with which to respond as intellectual men and women, putting to wise use our specialized training.

Of my two new patients, the young son seemed to be more severely ill than his father. Medically speaking, I knew that successful treatment would not be easy in one so young, frail and reduced to almost skin and bones. Remember that in those days we did not have the advantage of the modern "miracle drugs" against TB.

Nothing was left to chance, or to relatives. The latter might try to sneak in their special remedy against TB, such as snake soup, which might still contain unremoved portions of the poison glands of the reptile. This meant that our nurses had to be on duty around the clock, for everyone realized that this boy was a very special medical patient. Meals for him would need to be prepared with a higher content of protein, minerals and vitamins than was provided in his usual diet of highly polished rice, the food of the rich.

The wracking cough, which prevented his rest and sleep, had to be controlled with a special cough mixture containing a touch of codeine. Sunshine must be administered internally in the form of vitamin D, as found in cod liver oil. This also provided him with another much needed vitamin, A, often found to be deficient in those with TB. To make the cod liver oil more palatable, I mixed it with *yut*, a malt candy which I used to enjoy so much as a boy. When our patient grew stronger and afebrile, we gave him carefully graduated doses of real sunshine, which rapidly melted the TB infected glands of his neck, to the amazement of all.

The young boy soon began to put on weight, so now we had difficulty counting his ribs which before had been so noticeable. His father too was making good progress. Different members of the prayer group were now allowed to visit them, and they came away much encouraged and determined to continue to pray unceasingly.

Meanwhile, I did not rest on my oars but persisted in my treatment. Both patients received calcium gluconate injections, since they refused to drink milk because of the natural aversion of the Korean to its source. However, they did not seem to object to the frequent injections for they were accustomed to needles used in acupuncture, a time-honored native treatment method.

The young lad became the hospital pet, and as he grew stronger, he became more and more mischievous and difficult to keep in bed. His cough gradually disappeared and my stethoscope could discern no more tell-tale rales.

One day Dr. Kim suddenly burst into my office, excitement replacing his usual composure. He announced that a former magistrate of Pyong Yang was in town; and more significantly, it was the one who had been largely responsible for the persecution of our parents in those pioneer days.

The Reverend Kim, Chang Sik had retired in 1924 and was living with his son in Haiju. By chance, Mr. Kim had seen his former persecutor at the marketplace, but did not think he had been recognized in turn. It was uncertain whether the ex-magistrate's presence indicated good or evil intentions towards us.

We did not have long to wait for an answer. At our very next clinic, the former magistrate appeared. He asked if he could visit his son and grandson who, he understood, were patients in our hospital. To our great surprise, it turned out that this former magistrate was none other than the father and grandfather of our two special TB patients!

After he had visited with them, he asked to speak to me privately in my office.

"You probably do not know me, but I know of you," he began. "You are the son of the man I tried to have killed, and whose helper,

Kim, Chang Sik, I almost succeeded in having beheaded. I had him in the prison death cell in Pyong Yang. In fact, he is about the only one who ever came out of that death cell alive.

"We who persecuted you Christians have since grown weaker, while you Christians have grown stronger. Governor Min banished me from Pyong Yang after that incident. Under my code, it was now the Christians' turn to wreak vengeance on their former persecutors. But you Christians have shown only love and kindness, as your care of my son and grandson have demonstrated.

"I have grown to respect the Christians, when before I hated them. In Pyong Yang I tried to force them to deny their Christian God and say that Christianity was a bad religion. I have come to see that I was wrong."

The happy sequel to these events was that both the official and his son were eventually discharged as arrested cases. The former

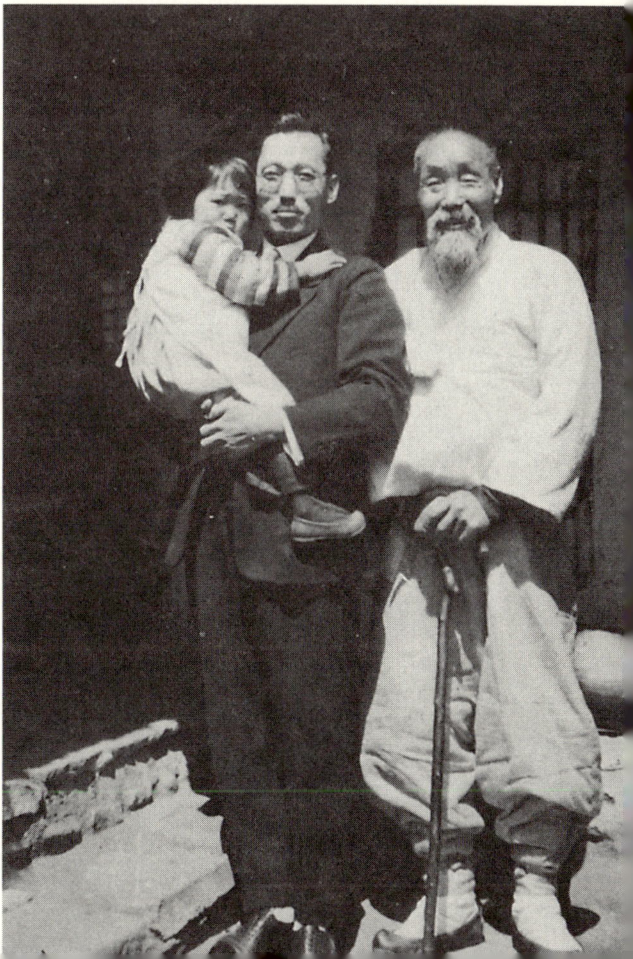

The Rev. Kim, Chang Sik (right) with his son, Dr. Kim, and grandchild

Pyong Yang persecutor and his son could not do enough for us and our work and even offered to protect us and our church property. The young lad was sent regularly to our Sunday School. On an occasion when there was to be a representative gathering of people from all over the province and we wanted to put on a lantern lecture on the Life of Christ, the Haiju official enabled us to get a permit from the government on short notice and was himself present at the meeting.

I took this series of miracles to be a clear mandate from Heaven to make immediate plans to bring to fruition my long cherished dream, the founding of a TB sanatorium in Korea. The Mission Hospital at Haiju was on a firm basis and the Boys' School was going well. The climate of acceptance for our Mission efforts had undergone a miraculous change. Although money was needed, I viewed that as less of a hurdle than the one I must overcome at the next meeting of the Annual Conference. Before I could make any application for the Verburg bequest, I would need to gain permission from the Mission on the "field" and from the Board at "home" for me to branch out on such an undertaking.

The Annual Conference of our Mission had been scheduled to begin June 19, 1927 in Seoul. We decided that this would be an appropriate time to have young William James baptized by Bishop Welch. The baptism was to take place at the Conference session in the First Methodist Korean Church following the ordination service. William and a number of Korean babies were to be baptized.

Bishop Welch conducted the ceremony with impressive dignity. The service seemed to be proceeding routinely when suddenly a Korean man in his snow white attire jumped up amid shouts of, "*On-ja-si-o! On-ja-si-o!*" (Please sit down!) from those seated near him.

Ignoring their shouts, he declared, "I must speak! How many in this congregation know that the white baby who is being baptized here this morning is no ordinary baby, but is the grandson of '*Harak*' and bears his name? It was '*Harak*' who picked me up out of the gutter, for I'd been a beggar and a petty thief, and he put me on the shining path of salvation."

The shouting gave way to solemn silence broken only by an occasional exclamation, "God be praised!"

The ceremony now took on added meaning for us, and we happily greeted those who gathered around afterwards. William was the center of attention, as many who had known my father came up to speak to us. I felt my father's benediction fortifying me for the pioneer endeavor I was about to launch.

CHAPTER 16

Wonsan Summer

The Executive Meeting of Annual Conference was ably presided over by Bishop Welch. When the matter of building a TB sanatorium was proposed, a lively debate ensued.

Some asked, "How can we possibly support a new work when we are having such difficulty in simply continuing the maintenance of our well established endeavors? Medical work begun by Methodists at Yeng Byen, Kongju, and Wonju all had to be discontinued because of either a lack of funds or personnel. In fact, the only rural hospital of the Methodist church now operational is the one where Dr. Hall now works at Haiju."

I pointed out that such statistics only underscored the great need for rural medical work since eighty percent of the Korean population was rural.

Another said, "While we all recognize the urgent need for such a service and are in hearty sympathy with Dr. Hall, this is hardly the appropriate time to branch out on a new venture."

I could see my fond hopes vanishing before me. Had Bishop Welch not been sympathetic, he could have easily allowed the matter to stop then and there and moved on to the next item on the agenda. However, he permitted the discussion to continue.

My old friend, Mr. W. A. Noble, then proposed convincingly, "Why not let Dr. Hall continue as Medical Superintendent of the Mission Hospital at Haiju but permit him, during his spare time, to work on the sanatorium project? Of course, this would be with the proviso that he not seek a capital grant from the Mission or Board, nor ask for annual appropriations."

With this suggestion that neither the Mission nor the Board would be held financially responsible, most of the previous objections were withdrawn. Fortunately, it was ruled that I should be allowed to approach individual donors in both Korea and the United States and that funds so derived could be channeled through the Board.

With this first hurdle cleared, I was elated and felt confident that I could interest friends and patrons in this venture of faith. Although

I did overhear one member of the conference remark, "It will, of course, die a natural death, but there is no harm in letting him try," my spirits were undampened.

Later, when I was walking by one of the meeting rooms, I heard my name mentioned. "Dr. Hall is just a wild visionary and an idealist. He has had only two years' experience as a missionary and only one of those on the field. How on earth does he expect to move the Orient, with all its red tape, so soon after arriving here? The officials will never listen to one so young. Perhaps if we give him sufficient rope, it will come to a sudden end. It would have been kinder to him to have referred it to a committee which could have disposed of such a matter in the least painful way. Isn't Dr. Hall aware that we are on the verge of a depression?

The brief reply came back, "Perhaps Dr. Hall feels that with God, there is no depression."

I was glad that I had overheard this discussion for it increased my awareness of my human limitations and heightened my realization that "*with God all things are possible*."

Although many expected that I would be discouraged, I was walking on "Cloud 9" and a conversation with Bishop Welch helped to keep me there. He assured me that the way was now clear for me to make my application for the bequest of $3,850.00 left by Mary Scott Verburg for a special form of public health type of mission work. Although practically all the Mission hospitals had applied for it, the trustees seemed hard to satisfy. Bishop Welch suggested that I submit to them details of my plans, giving facts and approximate figures of the incidence of TB in Korea, and just how I proposed to combat that scourge.

That very night, working into the small hours of the morning, I drafted my appeal to Mary Verburg's nephew, Mr. Bennett, who was the executor of his aunt's will. I carefully stated the facts and figures, hoping that the wording would prove persuasive. A friend typed out my figures and the accompanying letter, and it was in the mail to the United States forthwith. It would take my letter almost three weeks to reach its destination so all I could do was wait in a spirit of prayerful optimism.

Back in Haiju, we found a cable waiting for us. It contained the sad news that Marian's mother, Mary Bottomley, had died on June 25, 1927. It was a great grief to Marian.

It was also a great grief for me. I had enjoyed a special closeness with my mother-in-law, especially during the year I spent at the

Suffolk Sanatorium. My position there as assistant physician included quarters designed for a family. Since Marian was interning at Pittsburgh that year, she was unable to be with me in Holtsville. Consequently, I had invited Mother Bottomley to come stay in the extra room assigned to me. She was a deeply Christian woman and a most enjoyable companion, and her presence had helped to make my separation from Marian more endurable.

Several weeks later another cable was delivered to our door. I was a little leary about opening it for fear it would bear more bad tidings. Marian watched my face anxiously as I opened the pink envelope. She could see by my expression that this time it was good news. The message read simply, "Your project approved. Money now available." I hugged Marian and she let out a cry of joy. The glad tidings spread quickly among our friends. Bishop Welch seemed especially gratified.

I lost no time contacting certain Korean friends who would be knowledgeable about land purchases. They directed me to various locations where they thought land might be available and Marian and I took long walks to examine the properties. Sometimes we made a picnic of it and brought William along.

At last we discovered an ideal location just on the other side of the hill from our house. It was a clearing in front of a pine grove on the southern slope of the mountain, protected from high winds by elevations on either side. It commanded a magnificent view of the

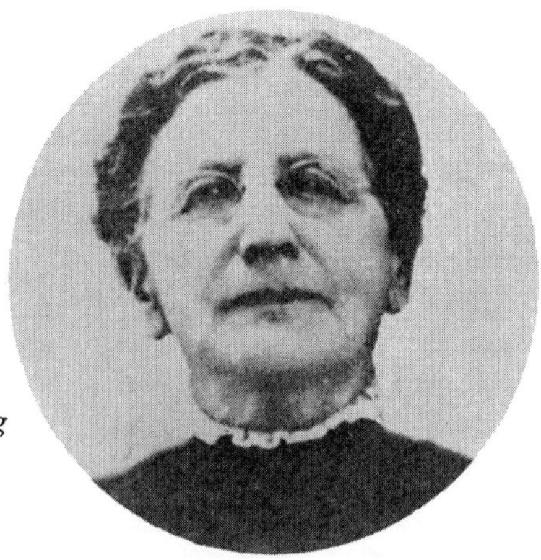

Mary Scott Verburg

bay and the port of Ryongtang and the many beautiful islands studding this arm of the Yellow Sea.

Sufficient funds had been received from our appeal letters that we felt it would be safe to proceed with negotiations to purchase the land. We were advised that it would be less expensive if the buyers were our Korean friends, for as soon as it became known that the foreigners were in the market for land, the price was sure to go up. It was decided that the opportune time for our friends to make the purchase arrangements would be while we were away on vacation later that summer.

Knowing how long it usually took to obtain equipment from the United States, to say nothing of the delays of getting it through customs, I also took care of another priority matter before leaving on our holiday. Although my stethoscope served faithfully as my ears, I felt the need of fluoroscope and x-ray machines to serve as my eyes. I therefore decided to place an order for the x-ray apparatus at this time. Some were highly amused that I would take this action before there was even a sanatorium building in which to house such equipment. They were also somewhat skeptical that in these financially hard times I would be able to raise enough money to pay for the x-ray machine when the bill came due. However, I felt that God had so richly answered our prayers up to now, that it would be showing a lack of faith not to assume the funds would be there when we needed them.

The skeptics came very near to being right, however, for I had no way of anticipating all that I would be up against before the sanatorium ever became a reality. Had I known, perhaps I would not have been so bold.

At the hospital we observed a marked falling off in the numbers of patients. We knew then the summer rainy season was upon us. Many of our patients came from the rural areas where the temporary wooden bridges had been taken down over the smaller streams, now swollen to roaring rivers, and side roads were impassable due to knee-deep mud. Besides, these were rush times for the farmers who worked in the rice fields, for they were needed to clear and build the irrigation ditches. Everyone seemed too busy to be sick. What was more likely, no one could take time out to bring their sick to the hospital.

We found the sticky, humid, wet days and the consequent heat very trying. Dr. Kim and Pearl Lund finally suggested that this would be the best time for us to take our vacation, and we were eager to be off. With the school on vacation and the work at the hospital slackened, we could visit Wonsan Beach with a clear conscience.

Until we could furnish and fix up our own cottage, we stayed at the McCullys. We painted our boat and named it the "*Chamie*," which is the Korean word for "fun," and, indeed, it gave us and our friends much pleasure. Many of the folk we had met at Seoul had come to the Beach. They expressed delight that we had chosen Wonsan and made us feel right at home. Our group became known as the "Younger Set," and that name clung to us, even when we became older.

The Jack Boots, who were now our near neighbors, seemed particularly glad to welcome us. They arranged a breakfast picnic for us on one of the islands. The sea was usually calm early in the morning which made this an ideal time for such an outing.

We were to provide our little motorboat, the "*Chamie*," and the drinks (which Marian, being of English background, assumed to mean tea), and they would provide the rest. A jovial spirit abounded until Marian poured the tea. We observed Jack's revealing face, and it was then that we realized we had committed a major blunder. We had not brought along any coffee for breakfast! Neither of us drank coffee so it simply had not occurred to us to supply it. Thereafter, Jack enjoyed kidding us on making such a serious error of judgment. It was one lesson we were not allowed to forget.

There was a medical clinic set up in the basement of the Auditorium and the doctors who were vacationing at the Beach took turns officiating. When my turn came, what was my surprise to find that the leather case of my stethoscope was all moldy. I realized that it was high time I put it to use again. Although my white patients were relatively free from tuberculosis, I found considerable TB among the Koreans even here. I had to advise several of my compatriots to make other provision for some of their TB infected servants, lest in time, members of their own families also become infected.

One morning, we awoke to find that our fine sandy beach was cluttered with debris. Wreckage from houses, and even the dead bodies of people and animals littered the sands. There had been a disastrous flood inland. The evidences of the damage had been swept into the river north of us and then carried to the sea.

Almost before we were able to fully comprehend the scene, beachcombers descended in force and staked out claims to the loot on the beach. As word spread of what was happening, the authorities came and, after removing the bodies, taxed each beachcomber what was considered a fair price for what he had claimed. Although the funds so collected were to be sent to help the devastated villages, the action was greatly resented by some of the beachcombers and fist fights ensued. Eventually order and a clean beach were restored.

This proved a busy time for those of us who were doctors. We feared that the epidemics of dysentery, cholera, and typhoid that were raging in the city might come here. For the sake of prevention, we gave inoculations, warned everyone against eating any uncooked fruit or vegetables, and cautioned that all drinking water should be boiled.

On the brighter side, the summer afforded a number of good impromptu entertainments. On one occasion, we husbands put on dresses taken in secret from our spouses, and were so disguised as to become almost indistinguishable from the wife we were supposed to represent. (This was possible then, for we were slimmer than we are now.) I had donned a very gay dress of Marian's and proved myself to be such an excellent mimic of her mannerisms, and her position in staunch support of the feminist movement, that I was awarded one of the prizes, amidst the joyous merriment of the audience. The children and our respective wives seemed to enjoy the spectacle.

Henry D. Appenzeller had not forgotten the invitation he had extended when we first arrived in Seoul to take me out sailing with him at Wonsan. So one fine day when the wind was just right, he asked me to go for a sail with him in his boat, the "*Sea Gull.*" Marian was invited to bring William over to their cottage and to have tea with Ruth and watch our exploits with binoculars from the beach.

Henry seemed to have the sails and boat under excellent fingertip control and the craft obediently went just where he directed. It was a real thrill to skim so fast past the various islands on the bounding deep. I could see that Henry was thoroughly enjoying it. I, too, was beginning to have a sense of real pleasure from the experience and wished that Marian could enjoy it with me.

I called to Henry that he should name *his* boat "*Chamie-go-mal-go*," (a lot of fun). The sailboat must have made a pretty sight as viewed through the field glasses by our women folk. I began to wonder if perhaps I had been mistaken to invest in a motorboat, with its occasional starting trouble, its vibration and motor noise which made conversation difficult. Here I could converse softly and still be heard. Here there was quiet and peace. The only sound was the musical note of the gentle breeze on the billowing sails, and the swish-swash of the waves against the boat as the tiny craft cut like a knife through the water.

Then all became too quiet and still. We were becalmed. The sails flapped listlessly at first then, not at all, and the turning of the rudder had no affect in changing our course. Here we were, far out at sea, almost motionless and helpless. Henry looked at me with a sheepish smile, and I began to wish that we might be having a cup of refreshing tea at Ruth's.

All of a sudden there was a slight gust of wind which began to billow out the sails. Henry now had a pleased, triumphant expression on his face as he exclaimed, "This is it! We shall be back for that cup of tea after all."

He had hardly finished uttering these cheering words when the gust of wind turned into a terrific gale, and no matter what Henry did, we were being driven out to the open sea at express-like velocity. The roaring wind at our stern pushed us farther and farther from the fast receding shore, until it soon appeared as only a thin line on the horizon and then disappeared completely. Henry had immediately taken down the sails, leaving only enough up to enable him to keep out of the trough of the waves, which by now were assuming mountainous proportions, towering over our pigmy craft.

At such times of personal peril, it is amazing how many and how rapid are the thoughts which race through the mind. Some of these thoughts, I recall, were at first rather amusing. I could see in my mind's eye, the big headlines in the papers: "Medical Missionary Dies While Battling Waves on a Pleasure Cruise," while I was sure the Mission Board would have preferred: "Medical Missionary Dies in Harness While Battling Disease and Superstition."

Then my thoughts began to take a more sober turn. I recalled things not done and sentiments not expressed. These recollections filled me with remorse.

Henry was too preoccupied with trying to keep the wildly tossing craft afloat to torment himself with such thoughts. Fortunately, after a time the wind died down as suddenly as it had come. Then, "believe it or not," as Richard Haliburton would say, the wind actually changed direction, right about face. It began to blow us back toward shore with equal force and speed.

Before we knew it, the rocky coasts of the islands, smothered in white foam spray, sprang into view. The islands quickly lost their charm for us as we realized the hazard they had become across our path. Henry knew better than I that we must not be tempted by these outreaching white arms of land that seemed to lure us to them like tempting damsels. Somehow, we had to by-pass the hidden sharp rocks that lay just below the surface of the water if we were to reach the safety of the sandy mainland shore and the loving arms of our waiting wives.

Henry negotiated a sudden sharp turn which barely avoided the rocks that protruded ever so slightly and could have caused our frail craft to be dashed to pieces. As we streaked past the rocks, the crest of a huge wave broke over us and nearly swamped the boat. We had to do some frantic bailing to stay afloat.

The wind continued to blow us toward the shore, and with considerable relief, we found ourselves once again on the sandy beach. The eager and anxiously waiting Wonsanites pulled the boat and us from the angry breakers, which seemed loath to give up their prey.

Marian and Ruth embraced us warmly and all was well. They told us how they had seen our sails disappear below the far horizon and how worried they had been, until the sudden change in the direction of the wind brought us back into view. They believed this was an answer to their fervent prayers. Indeed, some of the other Wonsanites had prayed too, for all of them were deeply concerned for our safety. Ruth, at first, had been more sanguine than Marian, for she had inherited some of the optimism of her mother, and was more habituated to Henry's sailing exploits. However, toward the last, even she was not able to maintain an unruffled calm.

The season closed with a fine inspirational conference. Thus fortified for the work ahead, it was now time to return to Haiju and make it possible for the other members of our staff to go on their vacations. On our way back, since Mother was on furlough, we accepted the kind invitation of Dr. and Mrs. J. Earnest Fisher to stop off with them at Seoul.

Dr. Fisher was a brilliant professor at the Chosen Christian College, and his good wife, Bessie, was the daughter of the Hardies. In fact, Dr. Hardie was my spiritual mentor, whom I held in deep affection. It was thus a double joy and privilege to get to know the Fishers and to enjoy their gracious hospitality. Their home was beautifully situated in a pine woods near the college.

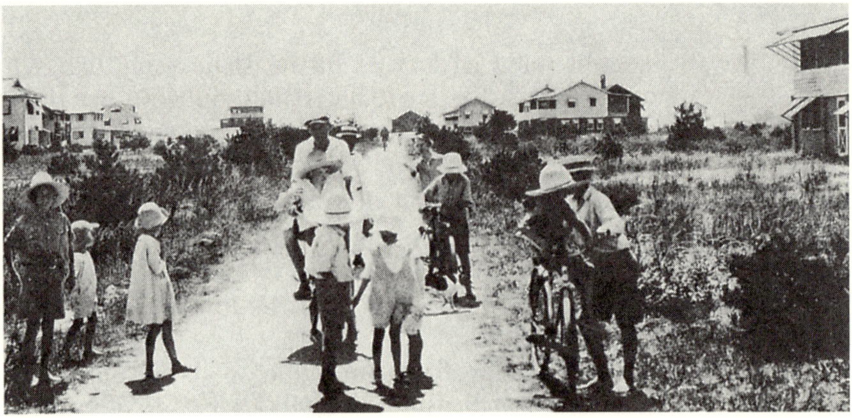

Houses and main road at Wonsan Beach

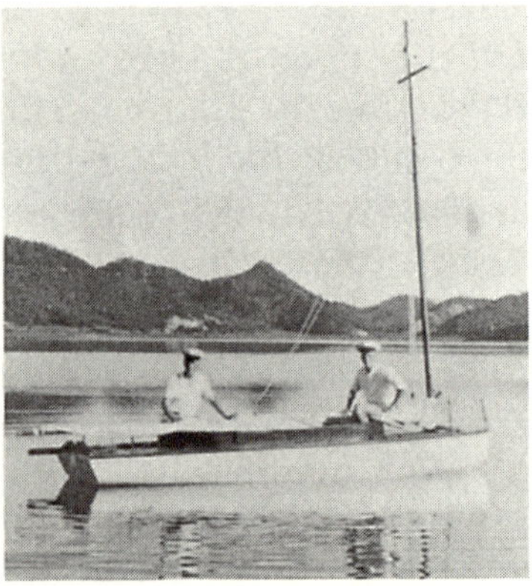

Henry D. Appenzeller's sailboat, the "Sea Gull"

Important among the other tasks needing attention while we were in Seoul was the procuring of food and supplies for both ourselves and the hospital, to last for a period of at least three months. Essential supplies were simply not available in Haiju. Shopping was time consuming and tedious, for there were no supermarkets nor department stores. One had to progress from one small store to another, accompanied by a *jiggie kun* (coolie with a carrying rack) or a woman with a big round basket on her head, until the desired article could be found. For the overflow there were always small boys eager to carry what they could. By the time one had finished a morning of shopping, one's entourage included a parade of all types of coolies and carriers trailing behind, a sight that would have made an amusing movie.

Dr. Kim was able to leave for his vacation, along with several other staff members when we returned from our holiday. There were still a lot of so-called "summer complaints" among the hospital patients, mostly children who had become ill due to eating such things as cucumbers, unripe melons and other unripe fruit. The increased number of flies in the summer also brought an increase in infection. This all kept Marian especially busy in addition to her obstetrical and surgical work, and other regular duties which now included the care of our son. She had organized a flourishing "Mother's and Children's Welfare Club" and now being a mother herself, her instruction was more respected.

Serious epidemics of typhoid and dysentery had developed in our absence, and I, too, had my hands full. Our hospital soon earned a good reputation for treating dysentery, for our Korean patients responded quickly to the treatments we had learned at the London School. In fact, many Japanese patients who had been attending the Government hospital transferred to us when they heard of our good record.

Then I became puzzled, for these Japanese patients proved to be bad risks, and at best made very slow recovery when given exactly the same treatment we were giving our Korean patients. Adequate facilities to conduct proper research were not available, and the only explanation I could come up with was empirical. Our Korean patients had been accustomed to consuming hot, red peppers in their relish of *kimchie*, so hot, in fact, that it would bring tears to their eyes. I therefore assumed that their gastro-intestinal tract must have reacted in a similar way, and had mechanically washed away the amoeba before they could get well imbedded in the intestine. The Japanese, on the other hand, abhored peppery foods, and strictly abstained from them. Although it was, of course, too late for my Japanese patients to start on peppery foods when the disease was already in progress, many of them found later that my advice to include *kimchie* with their diet proved very helpful. Less came down with dysentery or, if they did, seemed to make a faster recovery.

The lot of the patients with a terminal disease was pitiful in the extreme, both with regard to their own suffering and the anguish of their relatives. At first we had had to be very selective with our inpatients, taking only those who had a reasonable chance of recovery. However, as the hospital gradually built up its reputation, we could afford to take patients who involved greater risk. Eventually we reached the point of taking some of these terminal cases on the grounds of Christian compassion alone. We did not hold out any false hope to them or to their relatives. Indeed, some later surprised us by making remarkable recoveries. With the others, we were able to ease their pain and protect them from the primitive witch doctor treatments, which included unsanitary acupuncture and burning the flesh with red hot irons.

Frequently, these patients were suffering with ascites (fluid in the abdomen), pleural effusion (fluid in the chest) or edema (fluid in the tissues). One could often make these patients comfortable by means of simple paracentesis (removal of the fluid) or the administration of diuretics which caused faster elimination of the fluids. These treatments might have to be repeated often and could be likened to removing water from a well, only to have more water accumulate. However, in the meantime, relief was afforded the patient and there was much subjective improvement, which was beneficial despite the fact that little could be done from the objective point of view. Where necessary, analgesia was given to these patients to relieve their suffering. There was no point in refusing such patients sedatives, for one did not need to be concerned with a problem of addiction in terminal cases.

Although the Oriental patient is perhaps not as afraid of death as are many Occidental patients, they are human and certainly suffer mental anguish, particularly if there is the prospect of being turned out on a refuse heap to die. I would remind our staff of our Christian guidelines that we must ever comfort our patients, since we had the firm Biblical assurance that God "*. . . comforteth us in all our tribulation, that we may be able to comfort them which are in any trouble, by the comfort wherewith we ourselves are comforted of God.*" (II Corinthians 1:4) Our hospital evangelist would pray for and with our patients. Often we found them receptive and invariably, grateful. They seemed to then be able to meet death with a sense of peace, and many would pass on with smiles on their faces.

Staff in the terminal wards had to be rotated, for I found it just as necessary to understand their needs as those of the patients and relatives. Even at best, these terminal patients were very hard on the emotions and attitudes of the staff. They often felt their efforts had been in vain. At times they became frustrated and depressed over the failure of their patients to recover. To maintain their balance and cheerfulness, they needed to care for other types of patients.

For the good image of our hospital as a place in which to get well, and not a place in which to die, I had to keep to a minimum the number of terminal cases admitted. It was hard to turn these cases away, for I knew the fate that awaited them without nursing and medical care to ease their painful and often terrifying end. The picture ever haunted me.

CHAPTER 17

Groundwork

"You can't build a sanatorium here. I don't want my city crowded with tuberculosis patients," said the Mayor of Haiju. "To have an institution that harbors such a shameful disease so close to the city would be intolerable. Since it would be the only hospital of its kind in all Korea, victims of this fatal sickness would just flock to Haiju and die and spoil the good name of our fair city."

I had come to the Mayor's office to obtain a permit to purchase the site we had chosen for the sanatorium. Our Korean friends had negotiated a reasonable price for the land with the owner while we were at Wonsan. I was not prepared for this outburst of opposition. The Mayor was not finished.

"You have chosen a place right beside the Government pine grove which we plan to make into a park. It simply would not do to have your TB patients go strolling there."

I tried to point out to the Mayor and the city Elders that it would be much better for the patients and the city if the former were segregated in an institution like the one we proposed where they could be taught how to care for themselves.

Knowing the Korean veneration for schools, I told them that I had decided not to call it a TB hospital or sanatorium, but a "School of Hygiene for the Tuberculous." There TB patients would not only be treated, but also would be taught. They would learn how best to burn their sputum, and use paper handkerchiefs over their mouths when coughing, in order to prevent droplet infection. I added that I was already engaged in preparing booklets in the Korean language on the special hygiene of such patients and the steps that could be taken to prevent the spreading of tuberculosis.

"Haiju has more than its share of tuberculosis victims right now," I added, "and they are far more dangerous scattering their germs promiscuously in the streets, shops and public places than if they were in a sanatorium."

The Elders laughed rudely in my face. "This talk of germs is just a figment of your imagination," they scoffed. "Who ever saw these germs anyway?"

I offered to show to any representative they might appoint, the little red eosin stained TB assailants, readily visible under our microscope. They coldly turned down my offer, dismissing this germ theory as "ridiculous." Their answer remained a firm, "No"!

I saw that I was up against a solid wall of ignorance and superstition, and would have to find another approach at a more propitious time. I was very frustrated. I could not seem to quiet the conviction that this country desperately needed a sanatorium where tubercular Koreans could go for treatment.

Tuberculosis was sweeping unchecked through the country at that time. One out of five people fell victim to the disease as opposed to one in twenty elsewhere. Where Korea was beginning to feel the change from the old order of civilization to the new, tuberculosis was taking its toll. It stalked the new lines of travel and communication, scattering its microbes from isolated country villages to big cities and back again.

The factory workers in the cities, where the conditions of a new sort of labor had not been met with a proper regard for health, were easy prey. Once these microbes reached into the Korean house there was little hope for the occupants. The foul, dungeon-like dwellings, on the whole, permitted no sunlight. So widespread was the disease that it attacked indiscriminately the farmer, the city worker, the educated, the old, and the young.

Added to the normal deaths from the disease were countless suicides. Viewing *pay pyung* as invariably fatal, the average Korean preferred death to the period of isolated misery to which fear and superstition would ostracize him. Truly then, the task of a sanatorium lay not only in curing tuberculosis, but in the area of education.

The School of Hygiene for the Tuberculous that I envisioned would teach its patients a common sense knowledge of the disease, its treatment and the preventive measures that could be taken. This would be done in the hope that when they recovered, our patients would return to their homes and teach others how to either avoid or treat TB, thereby helping to control the spread of this illness.

To be thwarted in my desire to begin such an urgently needed institution left me with a feeling of deep discouragement. I saw my boyhood dream vanishing into thin air just at the threshold of realization. I felt depressed enough that I could begin to understand why some people hoped for the end of the world.

However, I was soon shamed into action. Our faithful Korean Christians began organizing prayer groups, which served to bring me to my senses and made me realize that once again, I had been trying to achieve things through my own puny strength.

During this anxious period we began to wonder indeed if "the old-time religion" was going to work. No glimmer of a solution seemed in sight, and even some of our staunchest supporters seemed to be losing their optimism. Just at the point of apparent success, after a green light from the Mission Board, and cash in hand to start the sanatorium, were all my fond dreams now to be dashed to pieces?

It was on a day during this period of diminishing hope that I felt a strong inner prompting to pay a visit to Mr. C. Sasaki, the head of the provincial police, whom we had met when we first arrived in Haiju. Up to this point I had scrupulously avoided working through my Japanese friends. I had wanted the Koreans themselves to first give their consent and then, with their endorsement, I could approach the Japanese officials to help expedite matters. However, the thought that kept crowding out all others was that I should call on Mr. Sasaki.

I finally arranged for an appointment. Mr. Sasaki greeted me cordially and graciously inquired as to what matter he owed the honor of this visit.

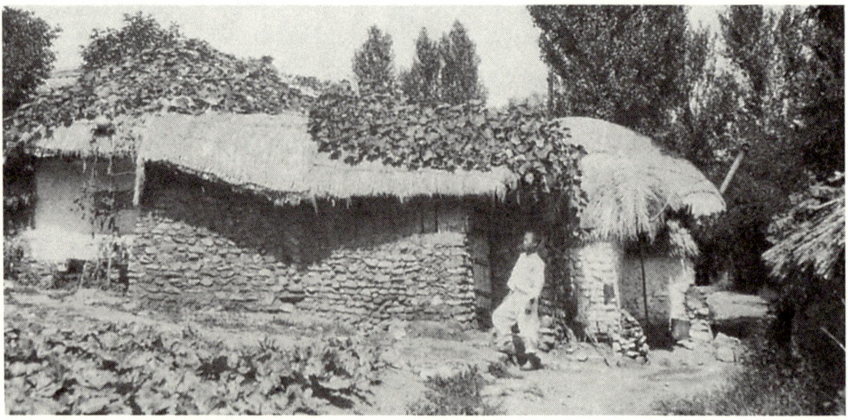

Korean country dwelling with dark, airless interior

At first I hesitated. Then I decided to present my dilemma to him frankly. I told him about my boyhood dream of establishing a TB sanatorium and how I had been refused permission to purchase land for this purpose by the Mayor and his city Elders.

He appeared genuinely interested and much concerned, so I went on to say that it was my fervent hope to have the needed facilities soon. I told him that we had received the essential financial backing to begin work on the first building but that we were encountering much resistance to our attempts to purchase the necessary land.

Mr. Sasaki had been listening to me intently. "I would advise you to look for another site," he suggested. "I do not believe that you will then have any trouble obtaining permission to build your sanatorium."

Although Mr. Sasaki had made me no promises, I sensed that he had chosen his words with studied care. I did not feel the need to push him to elaborate further and left his office, feeling light-hearted for the first time in weeks.

It did not take us long to locate a new site. It was several hundred yards further on from our first choice with the same southern exposure. Just above was a fine mountain spring where we could be assured of a good supply of running water. The land sloped down gently, by rice terraces, to a plain below, which would be an excellent location for a sanatorium site. It was near enough to the city to enjoy its facilities, yet far enough away to avoid its dust and smoke. The owner seemed happy to sell us the property.

When the Mayor and Elders permitted us to purchase the new site, I was sure that Mr. Sasaki had intervened. Everything seemed to be falling into place. I felt an inner assurance that the sanatorium dream would now become a reality. With deep humility I offered my gratitude to God.

During this time, the Norton Memorial Hospital was growing in reputation and often attracted outside visitors, including several from America. One of the first guests was my own cousin, Miss Emily Haskins, who had come from visiting the Dr. Mary Stone Mission in Shanghai. She conducted a series of Gospel messages at the hospital when she was with us that proved an inspiration to staff and patients alike. She expressed genuine interest in our work and promised to return some day and bring her Binghamton, New York family with her.

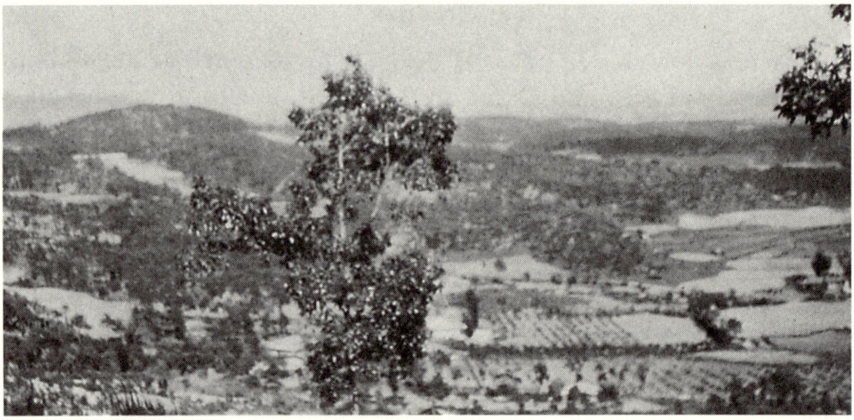

The new sanatorium site

Also, because of the need for drugs in the hospital, we would often entertain representatives from various American drug firms, including Eli Lilly and the Parke-Davis Company. One of these representatives from the latter firm was Mr. H. V. Stokely. He became more than just a drug salesman to us and we enjoyed his personal friendship and generous support of our work down through the years.

One day we received a letter from Bishop Welch announcing that the Mission Board Secretary, Dr. Ralph E. Diffendorfer, was visiting Korea and wanted to see a rural mission station in action. Bishop Welch wondered if it would be convenient for us to have them visit our work at Haiju at this time. Of course our answer was yes. We felt honored that Haiju should be the mission station selected, and it might mean much for the future development of the work. A welcoming committee was formed to arrange for the appropriate display of our evangelistic, educational and medical activities. Miss Barlow and the pastors headed the evangelistic section, and Pearl and Dr. Kim were on the medical team. They chose me to be the coordinator, while Marian had charge of the entertaining and arrangements for transportation.

Marian was of the opinion that if our honored guests should arrive at Haiju, stiff and bruised from being bounced around in the public jitney during the trip over the pot-hole scarred road from Shariin, they would not be in the best frame of mind to assess the Haiju mission. Some maintained that they should "rough it" like the rest of us.

However, Marian's idea prevailed. In her most persuasive language and beautiful penmanship, she drafted a letter to Mr. Sasaki, the only man in the province who owned a comfortable, large American car, an Essex. As the Chief of Police, he was the most powerful man in the province.

In her letter, Marian gently and diplomatically led up to her request. She wondered if he would kindly let us rent his lovely car so that our honored guests might be met at the railway station northwest of Songdo at Shariin (the Koreans called it Sariwon), and be brought all the way to Haiju.

This was a distance of some 40 miles by road and the request was, in fact, a bold one. Only Marian would have had the nerve to make it. We all waited a little anxiously for the reply, which was delivered almost immediately by special courier.

It was written in large script by Mr. Sasaki's own hand on specially scented notepaper. The first page simply read, "Very sorry, I am unable to rent you my car."

Someone remarked, "Did I not tell you so?"

Marian, chagrined at the thought of being rebuffed, turned the page and continued to read: "I shall, however, be very happy to give you free use of my car for meeting your guests." Marian paused, then gleefully went on, "Also, my car will be put at your disposal during their visit here. In addition, I should like to take you and your guests all on a fishing trip on the bay in my police motorboat. Please let me know the date and time that will best suit you for this picnic party." It was signed, "Yours sincerely, C. Sasaki." A postscript was added, "You need not worry about baiting the hooks. My men will do that for you."

The limousine with its official pennants flying drove up to our home. Having been alerted from the hospital that the guests were on their way to our residence, Marian awaited them on the verandah. As Bishop Welch came up the steps with his hand outstretched in greeting, Dr. Diffendorfer called out, "Remember what you said, Bishop, that you were going to kiss her."

Marian seemed flustered as Bishop Welch asked her, "How did you do it, Marian?" He had remembered previous rides by jitney.

Marian replied, "I told Mr. Sasaki that you were getting on in years and that Dr. Diffendorfer was distinguished!"

Bishop Welch looked momentarily stunned and Dr. Diffendorfer looked elated. As Marian blushed, Dr. Diffendorfer kept urging on the Bishop, saying, "Remember, you said you were going to kiss her for getting the car. Don't go back on it now just because she called you an old man!"

Bishop Welch thereupon gave Marian a fatherly kiss and as the guests were led into the house, he turned to Dr. Diffendorfer and said, "Come along, young man!"

Thus, beautifully, the ice had been broken. Formalities were thrown to the wind, and we all had a jovial and thoroughly enjoyable time together during our guests' visit.

Before they left, we reminded Dr. Diffendorfer that Mrs. Woolverton's three-year pledge for our support would soon be up. Dr. Diffendorfer told us the Board was still not in a financial position to assume payment of our salary as originally envisaged. He promised to see Mrs. Woolverton on his return to the United States and inquire if she would extend the original arrangement for another three years.

CHAPTER 18

Emergency Assignment

The promise evidently slipped Dr. Diffendorfer's mind. We waited (rather impatiently, I fear) for some word from him about our future, but no letter came. Although we had tried to go through the proper channels, finally in desperation we wrote directly to Mrs. Woolverton. If we were unable to remain in Korea and had to return to the United States, we needed to know in advance. Ship reservations took a long time to secure in those days and we had the added responsibility of a son.

About that same time, we received a proposal from the Oriental Consolidated Mining Company at Unsan which we were considering as a possible alternate plan. The mines at Unsan were the same American gold mines that I had visited as a boy. It seemed that Dr. E. L. Power, the physician at the mines, felt that he should go home to the United States with his family for health reasons. He had submitted his resignation. Thus the manager of the gold mines had written to us requesting our services.

They offered a most attractive financial arrangement. Since they were aware of our deep concern for medical missionary work, they said we would be able to devote our free time to it, and they would provide us with free medicines and supplies for such a charity clinic.

Such a liberal offer at this crucial time was indeed very tempting. It would mean that we could stay in Korea, and still do some medical missionary work. But I also realized that we would not then have either time or opportunity to realize my dream of establishing a tuberculosis sanatorium. Besides, I knew that I could not serve well two masters, and that either the mine's work or the Mission's work would suffer.

While we were in this difficult dilemma, a letter arrived from Mrs. Woolverton of New York. She wrote that she was glad that we had communicated with her, for she had had us on her mind. She then declared that she would be glad to continue our support for the remainder of the five-year term, including our passage money back to the United States, but could make no further commitments after that. This wonderful news was indeed a godsend to us. We conveyed Mrs. Woolverton's promise to Bishop Welch and Dr. Diffendorfer, and gave the American gold mines our answer that we would remain at Haiju. We felt certain that this happy turn of events had been God's leading.

The good news about our personal financial support ended one aspect of this impatient period of uncertainty. However, we still had the frustration, common to the "Permit Kingdom" these days, of waiting for the necessary building permits which would enable us to begin construction of the sanatorium on the site we had purchased. A communication from the Bishop's office in Seoul was to distract our attention from these irritating delays. It read in effect:

"Would you two consider helping out in the emergency at the American gold mines in a temporary capacity? Dr. Power, their physician, has been advised to take a sick leave of at least two months. You would remain under our Mission and on missionary pay. They will see that the Norton Hospital does not suffer financially. Please reply immediately. Bishop Welch."

I sensed that this request from our Bishop was in the nature of a polite command, but wondered how wise it would be for Marian and our baby to take the trip north to a fairly remote area known to become extremely cold. However, Marian felt that we could trust ourselves to God's care. Since the American gold mines had come so close to helping us out in our own dilemma, it did seem only fitting that we should help them out in theirs. It would, after all, be only for a couple of months to allow Dr. Power to regain his health.

That settled it as far as we were personally concerned. Therefore, I hastily summoned our Norton Hospital Board. They were not too keen about letting us go, but since the request had come through Bishop Welch, they reluctantly agreed. As far as the Sanatorium plans went, we would not be able to proceed in any event until the permits were processed. So our reply telegram was, "Yes!"

Previously we had taken a rather dim view of some of the commercial enterprises in the Orient. Several appeared to be based on a theory of "dog eat dog" and only committed to pleasing their stockholders by giving them high dividends at the expense of the workers. Although we realized that our own good Bishop would not likely be sending us to such a mining company, we did have some private reservations. However, these were completely dispelled the moment we reached Unsan.

Our journey took us considerably north of Haiju into the winter cold and snow of the wild mountain country. The introduction to our emergency assignment is perhaps best described in a letter Marian wrote to her sister Emma on January 30, 1928 soon after we arrived at Unsan:

"My dear sister,

"I'm seated before a big blazing fire in a cabin in a gold-mining camp way up in the north of Korea, just sixty miles from the Manchurian border. Last night the thermometer registered 9 below zero and for four days we have been without mail due to a snowstorm which blocked the roads. We got here, fortunately, just two days before the snowstorm or we should have been held up at Mochuri [Maengjoongri], the station where we got off the train to come here. We are here for two months, loaned by our mission, to substitute for the mine doctor who is ill.

"While we feel much more isolated than in Haiju both the work and the place are interesting, and as there are over forty white people here, there is considerably more social life than in Haiju. Our cabin is more suited for a summer camp than a winter residence but wood seems to be plentiful and two stoves and a fireplace going full blast serve to keep out the cold pretty well.

"We left home last Monday morning, arriving at Mochuri that evening where we stayed all night at a house the company keeps there for such purpose. The company's car was there to meet us and we started on the sixty mile drive to the mines early next morning. It was a beautiful trip through snow covered valleys or high up in the mountains. We went through the pass where in 1916 a young American was killed in a holdup in which a gang of Koreans made an unsuccessful attempt to steal the money being brought back to the mines after a trip to take the gold bullion out. The spot is marked by a stone erected by the company. Along one windswept valley the trees bordering the road and the grasses in the fields hung heavy with ice which, sparkling in the early morning sunshine, made a dazzling fairyland picture of diamonds everywhere.

"Great curiosity was evidenced in one village where we stopped to give William his bottle. The hot water in the thermos bottle seemed a mystery at which I am not surprised, for though thermos bottles are not scarce here, they are Japanese made and no earthly good, as we have since had reason to experience. (Someone let our precious thermos bought in England, drop. The water kept just as hot in it for sonny's 6 A.M. feeding as when put in the night before, but the bottle we have now would make a good ice-chest by morning.) I offered one little shaver who stuck his head through the side curtains, a sandwich, but he was afraid of foreign food and wouldn't take it.

"We reached here in time for one o'clock dinner and found a warm welcome awaiting us. The folks here are most cordial and we've been invited out almost every evening. There is a lovely clubhouse where they have all kinds of good times. Indeed the clubhouse is so much better built than the houses. However we are in a makeshift, unoccupied for a long time. If we had accepted this job permanently we should have had Dr. Power's house which is very comfortable. Since the company spends $15,000 a year on the hospital and all the work done is charity, they have many more patients than we do in Haiju and so a much greater opportunity for missionary work.

"Everything considered, it was not easy to turn down such an attractive offer for we could find many places for the extra cash available in a salary twice our present one, but this offer coming just a few days before Mrs. Woolverton's renewal of her gift and the fact that the sanatorium proposition had gone so far that we expect to start building as soon as we return, made it seem that our duty was to stick by the Mission now, though on Mrs. Woolverton's death (and she is 76) we shall be left high and dry. Perhaps we've been foolish to turn this down but we believed we were doing what God wanted, so if we did, we need not worry about the future.

"Someday we are going all through the mines but we must first recover from our first visit to the mill just the third evening after our arrival. We get our meals with Mr. Woodford in the house just below us. After dinner on Thursday evening he suggested that we take a little walk to the village. We were game and after seeing the G.P.O., the general store (a stuffy little Chinese shop where they sell foreign canned goods etc.) and making a date with the little Japanese barber to come up and trim what little our Haiju barber had left on my dome, we went back by the mill.

"Mr. Woodford was anxious to show us around and not being able to get in the regular entrance, he tried taking us through the engine room. He was gallantly hanging onto my arm, for the road was slippery in places with mud and ice, while Sherwood was picking his steps gingerly in the rear, mindful of a nasty fall he had in Haiju. The light in the engine room was dim and we were making for a door at the other end of a stretch of cement floor when suddenly we found ourselves sprawling and I was conscious of a sickening pain on my left shin. The cement that was, was not, and in the dim light we had not seen the big hole in the floor.

"I just thought, 'Well, Sherwood will see our plight and won't get in the hole anyway,' when on he came at a run to pick me up and landed bang into the hole himself sustaining a badly sprained ankle. He was as much surprised as we, for he turned the corner just in time to see Mr. Woodford trying to lift me up, saw a couple of long pipes near me and thought I had tripped on them.

"Two huge lumps came on my leg with surprising swiftness but I know Sherwood was most hurt and we finally got him home up the hill. I strapped his ankle. Mr. Woodford only got a scratch. His feelings were most hurt because he got us both hurt. We had a regular clinic though before we got all fixed up. Sherwood stayed in bed all next day and has been going round on crutches since (except when his pride only permits a cane). He says after this I'd better depend on his arm as the consequences of depending on another man's arm are too painful. I agree.

"Since they have heard a woman doctor is here the women come every morning to see me and I have a growing clinic. However, as there is no nurse to help me it's rather difficult to take care of them. So far there is no place for me to see them but the operating room and it certainly isn't good policy to see gyn. cases there. At best I can only help them a little for I haven't time to give the part of their treatment usually relegated to a nurse, and it is sort of slipshod work which leaves me feeling dissatisfied. I've sent to Seoul for special instruments I need which are lacking here and expect to do a few operations later. Dr. Power has an interesting case he wants me to help him with when he comes back from taking his rest and I'll be glad to assist an experienced surgeon again and getting some experience without all the responsibility. When I see where the patients have to go, though, I wonder how an operative case ever pulls through. They lie on mats on heated floors, like their own houses, and with only relatives to take care of them (no nurse to provide even a semblance of care) and the rooms look and smell like pigsties. We are not starting out to revolutionize things as our stay is so short."

Marian had been delighted with the beautifully equipped hospital and was openly envious of the efficient surgical lamp. The business manager assured her that she should have one for the Norton Hospital surgery and that the company would provide her one to take back. We were shown row upon row of all types of surgical instruments protected in a lovely glass case, and noted their large assortment of hypodermic needles. When we were told that once used, they were not resharpened (as we had to do in our hospital at Haiju) but were discarded, I asked if we might have the discarded ones. I was assured that the Norton Hospital would be welcome to them.

We viewed with interest the many shelves of costly American drugs and supplies, including some new ones I had not seen before. In Haiju we were forced by our budget to rely on the much cheaper Japanese manufactured drugs. This hospital was indeed a sight for sore eyes, and a virtual paradise to medical missionary doctors. Although we would use discretion, we could see that we were going to have the time of our lives in using the very best, without always having to count the cost. The business manager seemed pleased with our excitement.

Dr. E. L. Power was evidently a modern version of the old-time country doctor. We soon became aware of how attached to him the mining community felt. He treated both American and Korean patients with kind and equal consideration. However, now that their beloved physician was seriously ill and they were without an American trained doctor, our welcome to the community was especially warm. We were made to feel right at home.

When I had visited this mine as a child with my mother, the families did not accompany the workers. However, over the years that had changed. The mining company had wished to attract top engineers and other high grade personnel to that remote mountain location. In order to do so they supplied these medical facilities for the mining families. The younger children were provided an American teacher, and the older ones could attend the excellent Pyong Yang Foreign School, which now had boarding facilities and a high school.

We had not been at Unsan long when Marian had her first experience of witnessing a Korean custom which, until then, she had only heard about, but which to a Westerner is quite a shock. We were being driven to tea at the Thomas W. Van Ess home when a Korean crossed the road dragging a live dog with a rope around its neck, slip noose fashion, the dog bleeding and suffering. The Koreans ate dog meat and this method of slaughter, where the dog was put to a slow agonizing death, was believed to make the meat more tender.

When we arrived at the Van Ess cottage, Marian was too upset for tea and the conversation turned on what we had just seen. I recalled as a boy seeing men killed in the same way who had been found resisting the policies of the old Korean government.

Mr. Van Ess then shared his experiences with us, observing that he had risked considerable unpopularity with the Koreans because whenever he had come across a dog being dragged in this manner, he had shot the dog to put it out of its misery. He added wryly that his response of mercy had recently given him more than he had bargained for.

"The other day when I was riding on horseback through this town," he told us, "I saw a man dragging an almost nude young woman by the hair over the sharp stones which tore into her bleeding flesh. I dismounted, indignant that one human being would treat another (and a woman at that) so cruelly. Whereupon I ordered him to desist from his torturing and let the woman go. He refused and kept saying that she had been unfaithful to him and deserved to die. This infuriated me so, I horsewhipped him until he finally released the terrified woman.

"The next day, this very man, if he can be called that, had the nerve to show up at my place with this wounded woman.

"He yelled, 'Here she is! You must have wanted her for yourself.'

"I realized that it would be useless to argue with such a brute, and if I did not take her, he would kill her. We had adopted a couple of young children and so always have a lot of extra laundry. Therefore, we decided to employ her as our washer woman. She is so grateful that it almost hurts."

A big difference between "heaven on earth" from "heaven above" seems to be that on earth it does not last as long. However, we rejoiced over Dr. Power's recovery and returned to our hospital at Haiju in March, enriched by our experiences and with a deeper appreciation for commercial enterprises.

Our baby seemed to have thrived on the love lavished on him at Unsan, but both he and his parents had been terribly spoiled. Marian was especially pleased with her fine new lamp for the operating room, and I with my huge supply of used, sharpened hypodermic needles which I knew would be welcomed by Pearl.

Dr. Kim greeted us with the usual announcement that he had accumulated some more difficult cases for us. We smilingly retorted that we were now better equipped to handle them.

CHAPTER 19

Launching a Dream

Soon after our return from the gold mines in March, 1928, the permission to build the sanatorium and the approval for the plans were granted. The documents were signed by Governor Luther Pak, friend from my boyhood days in Pyong Yang.

On Easter Sunday, April 8, 1928, soon after this favorable turn of affairs, a party of my cousins from Binghamton, New York, came to visit Korea. Cousin Emily Haskins had returned as promised, bringing her mother with her, Mrs. Fred H. Haskins (Grace). Emily's sister, Polly Williams, had come too, along with her husband, the Reverend Robert Williams. They could not have come at a more propitious time, for with many of the hurdles now overcome, a glorious and happy day dawned for us.

It was April 13 and the occasion of the ground breaking ceremony for The School of Hygiene for the Tuberculous, only two years after we had arrived at Haiju. Mrs. Haskins, as honored guest, turned over the first shovel of sod, and the Reverend Williams gave the address.

Shortly thereafter, on May 28, 1928, my mother, Dr. Rosetta Hall, laid the cornerstone which commemorated the founding of the first tuberculosis sanatorium in Korea. Retired District Superintendent Kim, Chang Sik delivered an inspiring message. Mother had returned to Korea from her furlough in January and it pleased me that she was able to officiate at this historic ceremony.

Later we were all invited to dinner at the home of Governor Luther Pak, who was happy to see my mother again. It was at this dinner that Marian was first persuaded to try some *kimchie*. Marian had been content until now to limit her acquaintance of this Korean dish to merely sniffing it. However, when the Governor placed a carefully selected morsel of *kimchie* on her plate, Marian realized she could not refuse without offending her host. Figuratively clamping down her nostrils, she was startled to find herself actually enjoying

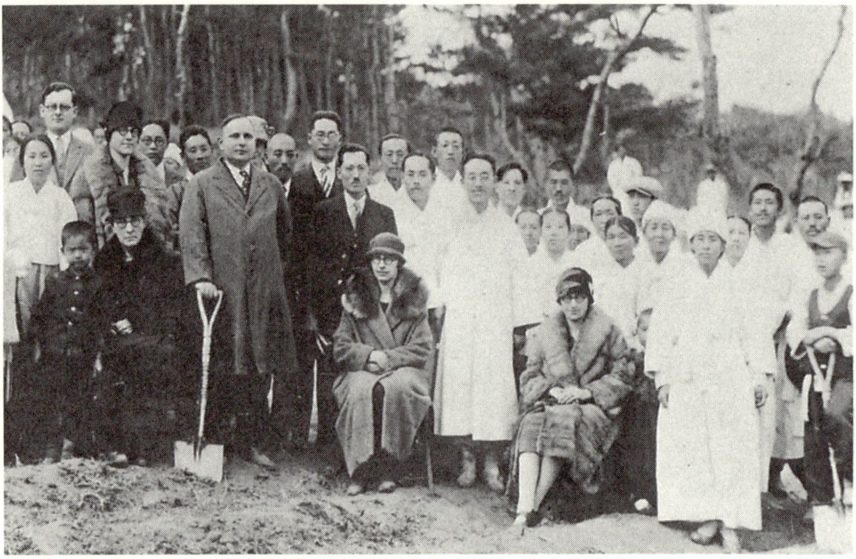

Ground-breaking ceremony for sanatorium

l. to r.—The Rev. Robert Williams, Mrs. Polly Haskins Williams, Mrs. Fred Haskins (Grace) (seated), Dr. Sherwood Hall, Dr. Kim, Dr. Marian Hall (seated), Miss Emily Haskins (seated)

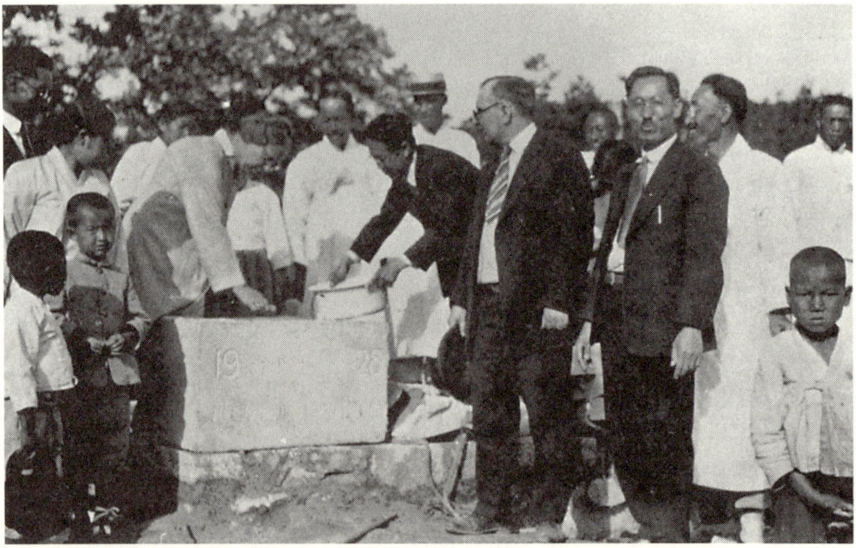

Dr. Rosetta Hall lays the cornerstone:
"1928—Commemorating the First Tuberculosis Sanatorium in Korea"

the taste of this particular concoction. Governor Pak was delighted with her surprised admission that she found it so delicious.

My mother returned to Seoul to continue her efforts to establish a medical college for women, and I turned my attention to building a sanatorium. I found that the path ahead still had its obstacles. Anxious periods and unexpected difficulties continued to test my mettle. Often they provided more excitement than I might have wished.

It was not easy to find a contractor who could or would put up the desired building for the sum available. Finally, however, a Chinese Christian contractor offered to erect the building at cost in memory of his wife who had died of tuberculosis. The first sentence of his contract stipulated that there should be no work done on the Sabbath day, and this was kept.

The Chinese contractor let out to the local Koreans as much work as he could and was beseiged with men wanting to furnish him stone for the foundation. A selection was made and all was going well, the stone being broken into large or small pieces according to requirement. Some were already in the foundation and the rest lay in piles ready for placement. Naturally I was pleased at the good progress being made and began to wonder if I were truly in the Orient where everything usually took so long.

My mind was soon disabused of this fancy, for I was hastily called from my hospital clinic to meet an irate crowd. I could see by their wild gestures, shouts, and the rocks in their fists, that they were ready to hurl more than mere invectives at me.

At first, I could not imagine what all the fuss was about. Then, one yelled louder than the rest, saying something about this foreign devil desecrating the graves of their ancestors, and as he did so, pointed to the pile of foundation stones. I knew that he could not be referring to the actual site of the proposed sanatorium, which was on a former paddy field. It finally dawned on me that these stones must have been taken from the graves scattered on the mountainside, not far from the sanatorium site.

These Korean graves were mounded hillocks and before each, whether ancient or more recent, lay a polished stone table on which food was offered from time to time to the departed spirits, in keeping with the Korean practice of ancestor worship. This was, therefore, a serious matter indeed.

Sure enough, upon investigation, we found that some of the rocks in the pile bore carving characteristic of the decoration sometimes found on the sides of the stone tables. The rascal who had sold them to our contractor had apparently fled long since.

One table was in too many pieces to be restored to the owner of the gravesite from which it had been robbed, but some of the others had not yet been broken. I apologized profusely and assured the irate gathering that all the gravestones would be restored, and if any had been broken, compensation would be given. This seemed to appease them and the angry outbursts subsided. How relieved I was that these stones had been discovered before, and not after, the building had been built.

Everyone concerned was working at fever pitch. I had to personally attend to many of the finishing details, such as showing the masons how to make the unique Manchurian style beds for the wards. These I had encountered on my trip across Manchuria in 1910. They consisted simply of a raised platform of slate slabs and cement which was covered with heavy Korean oil paper. Under the raised platform passed flues for smoke from the fireplace in a sunken kitchenette. Thus the heat and smoke passed directly under each concrete bed to the chimney at the opposite end of the room.

There was a damper in each flue which could be turned off in warm weather so that the smoke then traveled directly to the chim-

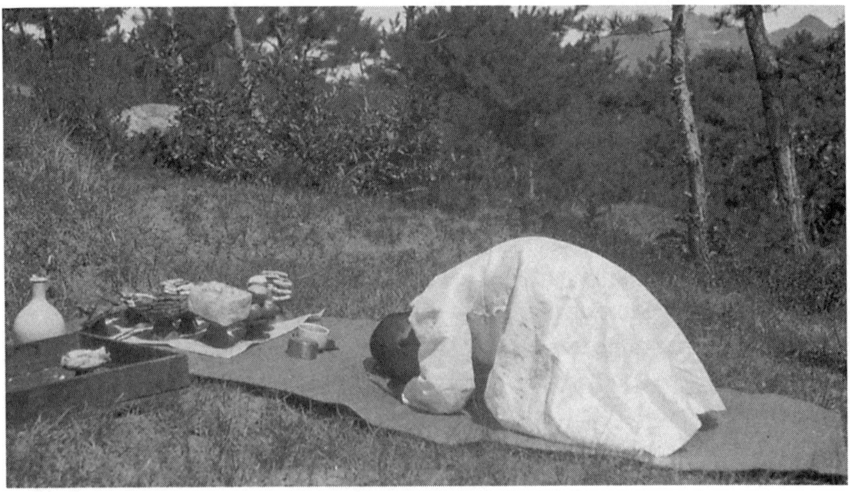

Ancestor worship

ney, instead of via the bed. The effect was as warm as lying on a large flat hot water bottle. The same fire that cooked the patients' food would also heat their beds in winter, while the stone slabs retained the heat till the fire for the next meal was made. This method was not only an economical one for keeping the patient warm, but allowed good ventilation at the same time.

The Koreans had similar arrangements for the floors in their homes, and what I did was to combine the systems: the heated Korean floor and the heated raised platform beds. The latter made nursing and the examination of the patients much easier, and proved less back-breaking for the medical staff. The smooth polished oil paper covering for these beds made them easy to clean and disinfect, and above all, free of bedbugs, for there were no crannies for such insect pests to hide.

This was the first time that this type of bed had been introduced to Korea, or, for that matter, to any sanatorium in the world. In addition to being cheap, permanent, and easy to maintain, the bed was well suited to the Oriental patient, who preferred a bed without springs, and was content with a thin mattress on a solid surface.

To permit the admission of ultraviolet rays a special material called cellu-glass was used. While another material called vitaglass admitted a higher percentage of ultraviolet, the cellu-glass had the advantage of not deteriorating as rapidly and of being cheap enough to be within the means of the average Korean patient. In this way the patient, when he returned home, could put into practice what he learned at the sanatorium without feeling that he must have a foreign style house to be able to progress in health. The idea was not to make Koreans into foreigners, but to show them how to take from Western knowledge what would benefit them and apply it to their own style of living. In other words, they could incorporate the best from the West with the best from the East.

Although we would not be able to complete the entire layout of our proposed design until further funds became available, we had ultimately planned for two eight-bed wards. Wings would extend from each side which would house a solarium for each ward. A central wing was designed wider than the two side wings. It would divide the two ward units and would accommodate x-ray and dark rooms, laboratory, drug and treatment rooms, reception room and doctor's office. The total plant would be formed in the shape of an "E" facing the bay.

Our current funds only permitted the construction of one ward unit and sun room wing plus the central main wing. This initial building was to be constructed of bricks which were made from local clay and were therefore relatively cheap. The Chinese were better masons, and so were assigned the brick laying, but I preferred to use Korean carpenters for the woodwork. I found throughout this venture that my boyhood experience of being the supervising foreman for the building of my mother's hospital was an invaluable asset.

Nursing, as a profession, was a relatively new concept for Koreans. In fact, when Miss Margaret Edmunds began the first Nurses' Training School in 1903 under the sponsorship of the Woman's Foreign Missionary Society in Pyong Yang, there was not even a word in the Korean vocabulary for such a person. A scholarly old Korean gentleman had helped the missionaries to decide on a Korean name for a nurse, *kan-ho-wun*, one who cares for and protects the sick. Miss Edmunds assisted Miss E. L. Shields in organizing The Nurses' Training School in Seoul in 1906 in connection with the Severance Hospital there, but even with these two training schools, nurses were in short supply. Koreans of that day did not believe in the education of women, let alone educating her to take care of sick people who would be both men and women.

The custom common to many medical institutions in the Orient, therefore, was that when a patient came to the hospital, relatives came along also and provided food and care for the sick one, under the instruction and supervision of the medical staff. Even after institutions had nurses for patient care, the families of the patients still provided the meals. Thus, the wards for our TB sanatorium were designed with individual kitchens for each two-bed room.

Temporary huts were built nearby to house the relatives who accompanied the patient. These huts were rather crude, but we wished to discourage the entire family from moving in on a permanent basis. Their purpose was to serve as a convenience for the person who prepared the patient's meals. The other option open to the family was to find quarters at a local inn in the city.

Friends and relatives from my mother's home town in Liberty, New York had followed her missionary career with interest that had always been backed by concrete generosity. They extended both to our work in Haiju also, and we were thrilled to be told that they had raised money so that we would be able to have a car. What a blessing this would be to the rural clinic work I was trying to establish, as well as making easier our frequent trips to Seoul for medical or mission meetings.

I had received notice that the car had arrived along with the x-ray apparatus I had ordered from America and some special drugs for the hospital. I would need to go up to Seoul in order to clear these items through customs.

The timing proved most convenient for me, for I was able to attend the opening ceremonies of the Woman's Medical Training Institute in Seoul on September 4, 1928. It was a day my mother had longed to see and she had struggled against many odds to achieve this initial step towards a full-fledged medical college for women, which it later became. Her teaching staff were all volunteering their services without financial compensation. As the school grew to the point of receiving accreditation, it had achieved its financial backing and endowment almost exclusively from Korean support. It was a triumphant day for my mother and I was glad I could share it with her. Even the downpour of rain could not dampen the elation surrounding this happy occasion.

I next set about my task of getting the hospital supplies and equipment through customs. It would save us considerable expense if I could persuade the customs officials to pass these things duty free. I knew it would not be easy but our finances were tight. We had not even had sufficient money to build the west wing of the sanatorium. Two sets of officials would need to be involved, for the Japanese handled hospital equipment and supplies, while the Koreans handled drug imports. The approach I would need to use for each group would be different.

I decided to tackle the more costly equipment first. Presenting my official calling card, which was printed in Japanese and gave my designation, hospital and address, I was ushered into the offices of the Chief Inspector. There I was formally received with much bowing and sucking in of the breath, and offered green tea from a cup without handles.

After some preliminary pleasantries, and some incidental "name dropping" on my part, referring to some of my Japanese friends in government circles who had helped our hospital in various ways, I thought the time was ripe to make my request. However, the official evidently did not think so, for he began a long tirade of how ungrateful the Koreans were for what the Japanese had done for them. He talked about how backward, stubborn, and generally unprogressive the Koreans were, and he very much doubted whether I could prevail on them to use this costly equipment anyway.

I attempted to change the subject and only did so with difficulty, for he seemed to have a lot on his chest. I gently reminded him that in our different ways we were both here to help Korea. I was fully aware that the Japanese had done much for the country in improved communications, reforestation, *et cetera*, and especially in public health. I noted that smallpox, which used to be so prevalent here when I was a boy, had now, thanks to the Japanese, been practically eradicated.

The Inspector's manner gradually changed and his face beamed with pleasure. This was the time, I decided, to ask him to pass our equipment duty free for the sake of the common good. Due to my limited knowledge of Japanese, I could catch only a few phrases, as he conferred with his assistants, such as: "*Ikaradiska?*" (How much the cost?), and, "*Sodiska?*" (Is that so?). Finally, after much apparent reluctance and sucking in of breath, he stamped his official seal, "Passed free of duty," on my papers in the appropriate place.

After this long drawn out "touch and go" negotiation over the equipment, I decided to freshen up a bit and gather my thoughts before I approached the Korean customs official. I was well aware that there was no love lost between the Koreans and the Japanese and that it would make the Koreans see red if I even mentioned that the Japanese had passed the equipment duty free.

My approach to the Korean official, though dignified, was less formal. Absent was the manner of sucking in the breath and there was less bowing. In contrast, I was made to feel more at ease, as we sat comfortably on cushions around a small low table. My calling card was also different, for it was printed in Chinese characters with some Korean script thrown in. Neither was I offered any Japanese tea, but instead, a sweet drink of boiled rice water, and a Korean malt confection. I had removed my shoes at the entrance, and noted that the oil papered floor was scrupulously clean.

Hardly had I begun to exchange a few pleasantries, before the official started to decry the barbarian Japanese overlords, who were no better than savages. He commented that although they were so contemptuous of Koreans, it should really have been the other way about, for had not the Koreans been the ones to introduce fine porcelain, ancient culture, and the Buddhist religion to the Japanese? He seemed to relent a bit as he noted with a smile that at best, the

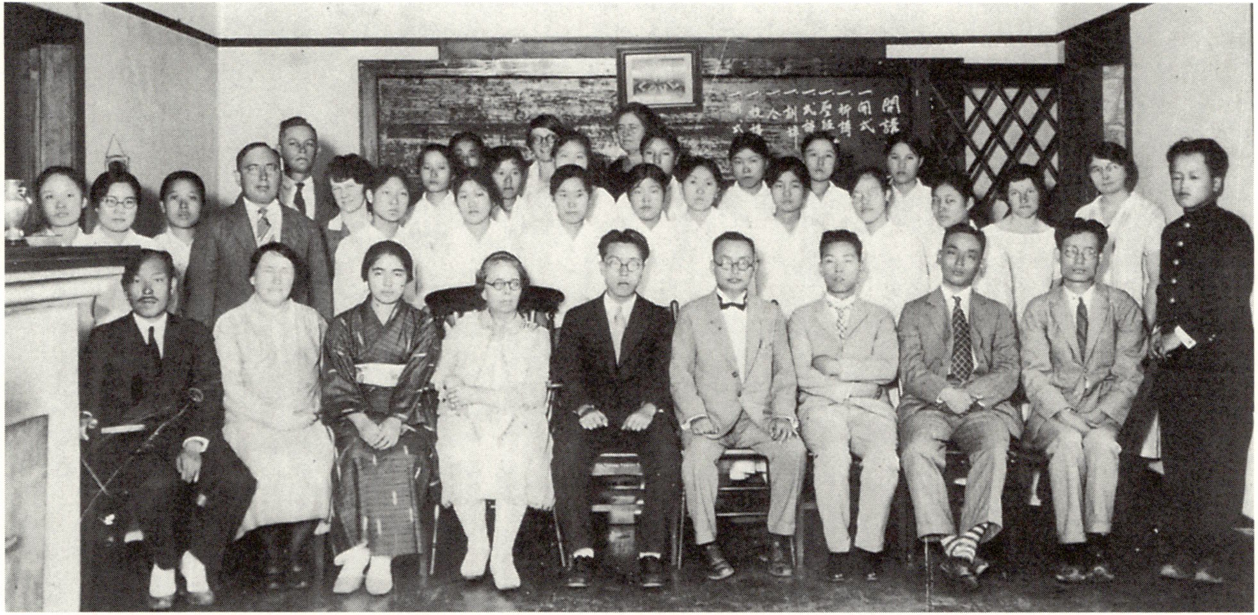

Official photograph on the opening of the Woman's Medical Training Institute, Seoul, Sept. 1928
(Dr. Rosetta Hall, founder, 4th from left, seated. Standing left: Dr. Sherwood Hall, the Rev. Henry D. Appenzeller and Mrs. Ruth Noble Appenzeller)

Ilbon nome (Japanese rascals) were really just imitators, appropriating from Korea, China and now from the West. I could hardly get a word in edgewise, but perhaps it was just as well, for I saw that he needed to blow off steam and he realized I would do him no harm.

He then startled me with the direct question, "Why are you importing all these costly Western drugs when we have far superior Korean medicines that have come down from the ancients and have stood the test of time? Where could you obtain a more powerful medicine than powdered tiger claws or a better bitter tonic than from the gall bladder of a leopard, or the snake extract which can cure all manner of diseases?"

I feared he would go on and on, so I interjected, "Yes, I am aware of many of these Korean remedies, for I was born in Seoul. I know some have special virtue such as resarpine for lowering blood pressure."

He looked startled. "So you know, and I am not telling you anything new!"

"Yes. I have found the Korean governor of Whanghai Province very understanding and helpful in our medical work and I hope that you will also be generous and pass free of duty these few Western drugs, which are quite different in content and effectiveness than the ones you mentioned."

With a smile he reached for his *tojang* (seal).

The Sanatorium building was essentially completed by the end of September. I looked upon it with great satisfaction as it nestled there among the crooked pine trees. It was located in an ideal spot with plenty of room for future expansion. The patients and staff would be able to derive inspiration from the peaceful view of the Yellow Sea below, dotted with the bright orange sails of the fishing craft. The environment was restful, away from the hub-bub of the city, its dust, and morning and evening smoke. I felt that God had answered our prayers beyond our fondest expectations.

The program committee had been giving much time and thought to the official opening of The Haiju School for the Tuberculous. This was scheduled for October 27, 1928, right after Annual Conference. Key speakers were to be invited and arrangements made for their accommodation. The program was planned in detail. Invitations would need to be sent throughout Korea to those most likely to have a special interest in this occasion. The actual dedication ceremony was to be conducted by Bishop James C. Baker, who by then had

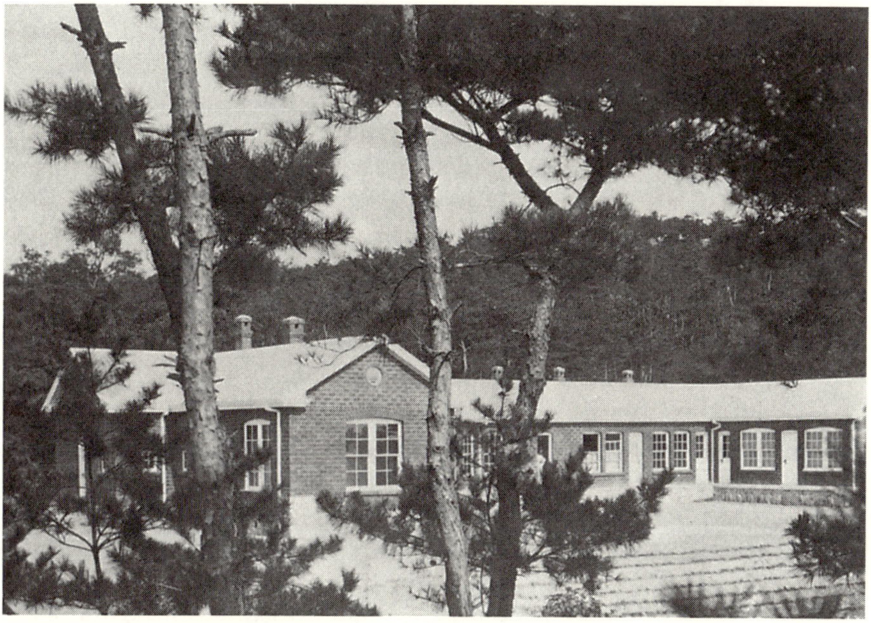

The initial Sanatorium building, side and rear view

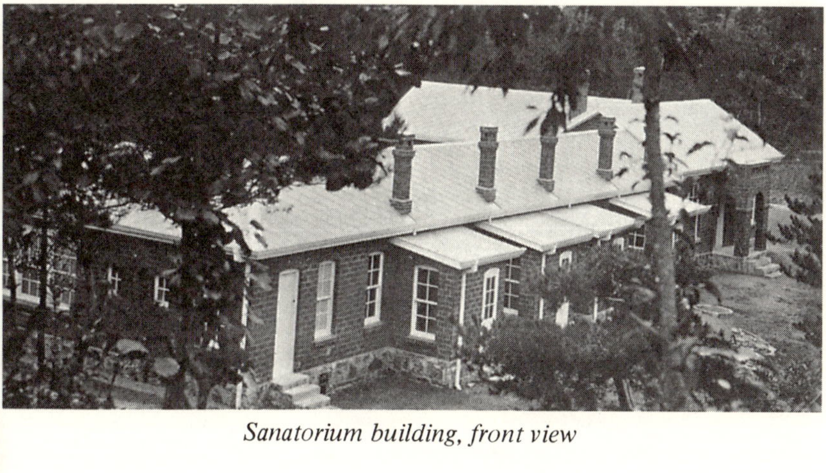

Sanatorium building, front view

replaced Bishop Welch as Methodist Bishop of Korea. He was to be assisted by Mr. W. A. Noble and Dr. B. W. Billings. Our own staff member, Dr. Y. J. Kim, who knew me so intimately from my boyhood days and knew the background of the recent trials and tribulations was to give the historical sketch.

The committee insisted that Dr. Marian be the one to cut the ribbon at the ceremonial opening, although she felt that this honor should go to one of the VIP's. However, the committee's wish prevailed, and I was glad.

As Marian approached that ribbon, I saw the launching of a dream that could usher in a dramatic new era for tuberculosis sufferers in Korea. No longer would the Esther Kim Paks of Korea need to be doomed to a tragic death. Marian cut the ribbon, and "The School of Hygiene for the Tuberculous" was declared open for business.

Governor Luther Pak was there, resplendent in gold braided uniform. Representing Japanese officialdom was our good friend, Mr. C. Sasaki, this day bedecked with medals and ceremonial sword. Both of them gave congratulatory speeches.

Dean K. S. Oh, of Severance Medical College in Seoul, spoke of the great need for the work that would be done here. Bishop Baker in his dedication address compared the work beginning in Korea on the slopes of South Mountain in Haiju to the work of Dr. Edward Livingston Trudeau. With little more than faith and enthusiasm to sustain him, in 1885 Dr. Trudeau had founded the first sanatorium for tuberculosis in America at Saranac Lake in the Adirondack Mountains. The ceremony concluded with a choir of Korean girls in their colorful garb singing a song composed in honor of the new sanatorium.

The guests were then shown through the building. The x-ray machine was at that time still in packing cases in the x-ray room awaiting the arrival of the expert to install it. A quartz lamp was ready for use in the treatment room. Some basic supplies were stocked on the shelves of the room that would serve as the sanatorium store where patients could purchase incidentals.

The Mayor took special note of this and commented, "I see that this will keep your patients from the temptation to come into the city and infect my citizens."

I nodded politely, inwardly delighting in the observation as a sign of progress in his understanding.

Plans for the construction of the west wing to match the present east wing, as well as plans for various cottages to dot the mountainside near the main building had already been drawn up by Mr. Edwin L. Campbell. Mr. Campbell was a civil engineer and a Northern Presbyterian missionary teaching at a boys' academy in Syen Chun near the Manchurian border. He had designed the original building for the Sanatorium. His blueprints for future construction were on display in the hope that some visitor might become interested in contributing funds for a cottage or two. A cottage could be built for about $800. Such units would provide accommodation for private patients whose fees would help defray the expenses of the charity cases. Additional cottages would serve as separate residences for the staff.

After the guests had all departed, I slipped away quietly to my favorite rock above the Sanatorium for a few moments of reflection. I was overcome with gratitude to God and to our friends for what had been wrought for us in only a little over two years on the mission field.

I viewed below me the new buildings where only a short time ago were pine trees and rice terraces. What a physical transformation had occurred in such a short space of time. Soon, cozy cottages would be joining the other buildings, dotting the mountainside. Streams of hope and health would issue from them, and the pain and despair of their occupants would be replaced with joy and a forward look to a bright future.

I permitted my imagination to run wild for a moment as I gazed upon the pine clad slopes of South Mountain. I envisioned the entrance to the Haiju Sanatorium as though it were a gateway on which there appeared to be emblazoned in large sunlit gold letters a message which spoke clearly to the aching hearts of Korea's TB victims: "Cast out your fear! Put on the garment of hope, all ye who enter here."

Tuberculosis sufferers of all types would flock through these open gates. At first we might anticipate that only a few would hear or heed this call, and only a trickle of hopefuls would climb up the sunbathed mountain to this haven of health. But, in time, that trickle would swell to a stream of such large proportions, that many such havens would have to be built to succor these victims.

Here would come young maidens, who had been trying in vain to rid themselves of blemishes due to skin TB, by the use of "beauty creams." Wracking coughs and stabbing pleuritic pains, so severe the victim hardly dared to breathe, would mark another host of sufferers. Or one might see, slowly crawling up to the sanatorium, the unsightly ones afflicted with intestinal TB, who claimed that snakes had sneaked into them and must be instantly removed. Striking to any onlooker of this scene, would be the hunch-backs, although such patients would have a good prospect that their bent backs might be straightened. For this, such appliances as the "Bradford frame" could be used in combination with ultraviolet light treatment, and in the more severe cases, a spinal fusion technique. Most dramatic of all would be the hemorrhage cases which would require prompt pneumothorax treatment and other emergency measures.

I rose to leave and to return to the world where those challenges I had envisoned awaited me in reality. I felt the presence of a greater Power infusing me with strength and a courage not my own.

CHAPTER 20

The First Sanatorium

In the first three weeks following the official opening of the Haiju School for the Tuberculous, there were only three patients and these were women. Soon, however, applications began to pour in from all over Korea and by the end of the month the building was full. In order to accommodate more than the eight-bed capacity of our single ward, we began to use the sun room, the treatment room and the doctor's office as patients' rooms.

The original intention was to take only one sex, but as it did not seem right to discriminate on that basis, the available space was divided so that men were at one end of the building and women at the other. We felt sorely pressed for the greatly needed west wing which would not only double the accommodation for patients, but provide for a more satisfactory separation of the sexes.

It was not long before we had a lengthy waiting list of patients clamoring for admission. Because the accommodation was so limited, we could not take advanced or hopeless cases. It was a heart-rending task to turn people away, especially since there was nowhere else where they could be referred for treatment in Korea. One young man had traveled a six-days journey all the way from northern Manchuria at an expense of sixty-five yen (about $22.00), but we simply had no place to put him and therefore were forced to refuse him admission.

With so many applicants and so little space, it seemed wiser to concentrate our efforts on those whose TB had a good chance of being arrested. This was especially the case with students, who by virtue of their education, might be the logical leaders of the future. It was reasoned that they could most intelligently apply the hygiene principles taught them at the Sanatorium and disseminate the public health facts about tuberculosis.

As November days began to show the signs of cooler weather approaching, a practical difficulty forced itself upon my attention.

Although the patients' ward rooms were warm, the treatment room, dispensary, drug room, x-ray room, laboratory and doctor's office had no heating system other than the registers for a furnace. This we had no immediate prospect of getting because there were no funds. I had advanced out of my personal income all the money I could possibly manage and simply did not have the means to advance anything for a furnace.

A renewed sense of urgency drove me to seek additional help from friends and supporters in the United States and my appeal letters laid bare our most immediate need for a furnace, and our almost equally urgent need for property and building funds. In the meantime, we tried to keep the patients warm in our "overflow" rooms by means of small stoves.

There was great rejoicing when a cable came in response to our heating dilemma announcing a gift of the necessary amount. By good fortune, or the hand of Providence, depending on one's point of view, we found that a furnace ordered from America for an institution in Pyong Yang was immediately available. The Pyong Yang Mission had a unit which was unsuited to their needs but an answer to our prayers. The furnace was installed in December and the heating problem was solved.

On January 9, 1929 at 6:30 P.M., my father's faithful Korean colleague was called to glory. The Reverend Kim, Chang Sik had died at the age of 72. The funeral service was held on January 15. His had been a life of remarkable service. I recalled his saying that in working for God for over thirty years, in appointments at some 125 centers, he had never once been sick or missed a Sunday service. His eldest daughter had married a minister, the Reverend Kui Soon Pang. His only son, Dr. Y.J. Kim, was a physician at our Norton Hospital. HIs youngest daughter, Dr. Rhoda Kim Pak, was a physician at the Lillian Harris Memorial Hospital in Seoul.

Even though the Sanatorium had been operating only a short time, we already had a "graduation class" of four arrested cases from our School of Hygiene for the Tuberculous. Their places were immediately filled. The location seemed to be proving highly conducive to good progress towards health. Every patient seemed to gain weight rapidly from the time of admission and to show improvement in symptoms.

In January 1929, I received an unexpected honor. On one occasion the previous fall, Mr. Sasaki had asked me many questions about the Sanatorium and wrote down the answers in Chinese characters on an official looking document. Apparently this document bore fruit in the form of a letter from the Governor-General of Korea, accompanied by a check for 300 yen ($100) for the Sanatorium.

I had been thrilled to receive this recognition from the Governor-General for the work we were trying to do. A still greater honor awaited me only a month later when, at a special ceremony in the Haiju Government Building, I received at the hands of Governor Luther Pak a Certificate of Merit from His Imperial Majesty, the Emperor of Japan, and a gift of 100 yen ($35) for the Haiju School for the Tuberculous.

My mother wrote in her diary on February 22, 1929, after receiving my letter:

> "Sherwood's letter . . . had word of a great honor done him. The Emperor sent him a Certificate of Merit by the hand of our old friend Governor Pak who handed it to him with great ceremony before representative citizens, like Governor Matsunaga did mine 15 years ago. But I had to work 25 years in Korea to get mine while Sherwood gets his before 5 years! And so the second edition surpasses the first, as it should."

It was consulting hour at our new Sanatorium, and I had before me a most unlikely visitor. "What can I do for you, sir?" I asked.

The Mayor of Haiju looked at me with obvious uncertainty. One could almost read aloud the thoughts going through his mind. Here was the doctor whom he had opposed—of whom he had made an enemy—and now he must ask him a favor.

"Dr. Hall, it is about my son," the Mayor began haltingly.

"Your son?" I gently prompted the apparently tongue-tied man.

"Yes, my son. I am afraid he has tuberculosis. Will you look him over and if it is as I think, could you take him here for treatment?" The request came out awkwardly. There was genuine fear in the Mayor's eyes.

"Bring him up," I told the Mayor. "We're crowded, but we'll find room for the boy somehow if he needs us."

The boy was indeed infected, but fortunately he was in the very early stages of the disease. He therefore responded well to treatment and improved so rapidly that I felt he could safely complete his rest cure at home. I visited him there frequently until there was no doubt that the boy's case was arrested.

"What can I do for you, my friend, in return for your great forgiveness and kindness?" the Mayor asked me on my final visit.

The Mayor's opportunity came later. When the responses to my appeal for building funds began to trickle in, I had decided it was time to buy the strip of land which adjoined our present building site. I had found that in order to build the west wing the same size as the east wing, all the presently owned land would be utilized, leaving no space for a driveway to the front.

Furthermore, we needed a hard surfaced road built to the Sanatorium, and the most direct route was through the very Government pine grove which the Mayor had planned to turn into a park. Permits would have to be obtained to remove any trees on government property. The Japanese were very particular on this score, for they had

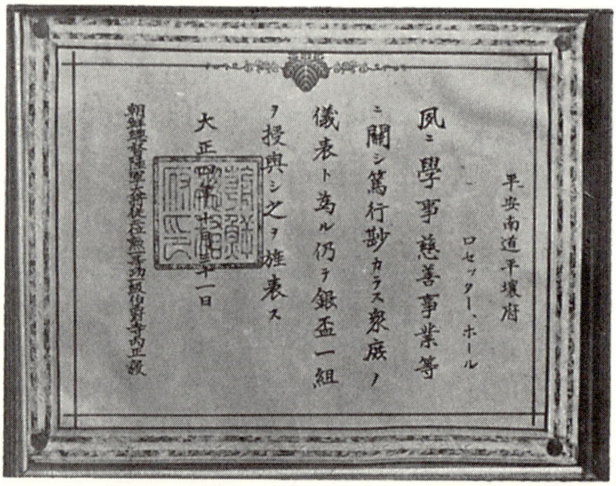

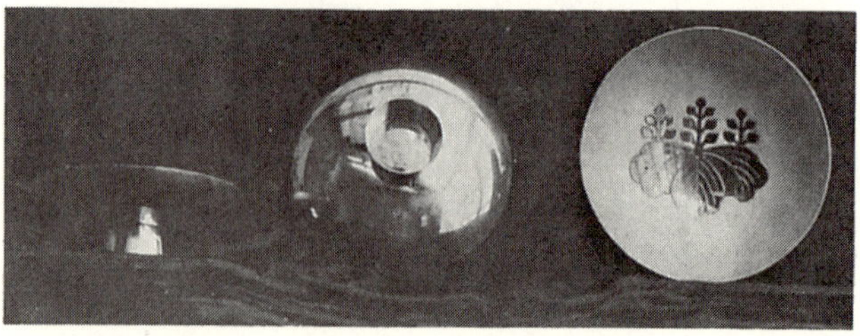

Certificate of Merit and silver cups given to Dr. Rosetta Hall by Emperor of Japan, 1914

concentrated on a program of reforestation for Korea and did not look favorably upon the cutting down of any trees, even on one's own property, let alone on government land.

I knew the Mayor would not object to the property purchase this time. I even thought that he might be able to offer us valuable assistance in the matter of obtaining a permit for the road.

Some time later, the Sanatorium doctors received a rather mysterious invitation from the city Mayor and his Council of Elders to attend a picnic in the vicinity of a remote Buddhist temple. Some of my good Korean friends strongly advised against our accepting an invitation from a group that had been formerly so hostile to us.

If the invitation indicated a change of attitude that might favor our road permit, the last thing that I wanted to do was to offend them by not accepting such a friendly gesture. So we went. We were greeted cordially and were served a ceremonial feast of friendship. This included a special dish prepared before us and presented with much formality, to signify special honor and confidence.

The Mayor gave me a welcoming speech. He said, in effect, that they were sorry for the obstacles which had been put in the way of a project which had become a great blessing to many of their people. What they could do to help in the future they would do.

The Mayor was as good as his word when he accepted the responsibility for getting us the needed permission. Not only was he successful on that score, but unbidden, he later contributed 400 yen ($135) toward the cost of the road construction, which was a large share indeed.

I had anticipated that the road permit would be our biggest hurdle and that the property purchase would be no problem at all. I found soon enough that just the reverse was the case. The owner was approached but refused to sell. He declared that in the center of the land was a grave of an ancestor, and to sell a strip of it, even though it did not include the gravesite, would be selling his family's blessing. Could a man sell his blessing? Impossible! As the landowner was wealthy and not apparently tempted by money, it seemed that an impasse had been reached.

The months passed. Then the landowner's daughter became ill and I was called to see her. Every day I walked back over the hills to her home to see my patient. As she began to improve, the father began to think over his attitude in regard to the land. Finally he decided that rather than hinder the good work being done by the Sanatorium, he would sell the strip of blessing.

His change of heart did not go deep enough to either donate the land or even offer it for a fair sum. He drove a hard bargain and asked the top price for the property.

This was more than the available funds would cover. One of the patients heard of the dilemma. Out of her own money she paid the difference, while at the same time soundly berating her fellow countryman for trying to make money out of the need of an institution built for the care of its own people.

We were thankful to be able to get the land at all and felt that God had opened a way which had seemed tightly closed. Perhaps He had had another purpose in mind, for this patient's gift was one of the very first gifts to the Sanatorium from a Korean. Chinese, Japanese, Americans and British had given, but it was especially encouraging to see this demonstration of genuine interest in the work by a member of the country for whom it was being developed.

Although we had obtained the desired property and construction had begun on the road, we still did not have sufficient funds to warrant proceeding with the building of the west wing. We would just have to wait.

In the beginning period of the Sanatorium, I found that it was extremely difficult to convince our admitted patients that a sanatorium was not a hospital, and that they could not be discharged as soon as most other hospital patients were, because their illness required an extended period of treatment. Both patients and staff had to learn the fine art of patience and perseverance. Indeed, we tried time and again to get across to them that "patient" was a term with a double significance at a sanatorium, for they must not only be patient in name, but also in fact.

The local press featured the tragic story of one of our more disappointing cases, a student by the name of Hyung. He had initially done so well that he thought he did not need to follow the rules of rest and graduated exercise laid down so strictly at the Sanatorium.

Hyung had been referred to me by our mutual friend, Henry Appenzeller, Principal of Paichai High School (founded by Henry's father). Hyung had been a student at the Paichai School. He came to us a very sick lad, with high fever, wracking cough, and was averaging a cupful of sputum per day. My stethoscope revealed that his right lung was affected, while the left lung appeared normal. This was confirmed by x-ray.

Pneumothorax treatment (air into the pleural cavity) on the right side was initiated at once, as well as other palliative measures. He showed a very favorable and rapid response. Because he had such a thin chest wall, his lungs showed up especially well on screening with the fluoroscope. Active lung movement on the left side could be seen and very little movement on the right side, due to the air pressure of the pneumothorax treatment. Our young staff members were excited to see this contrast demonstrated so vividly in front of them.

All of Hyung's symptoms eventually abated: his fever and cough disappeared, followed by a marked decrease in his sputum output until it was practically nil. His appetite increased and he began to gain rapidly in weight and strength. He claimed that he felt like a new boy and his appearance bore this out. I was able to considerably increase the intervals between his pneumothorax treatments.

Hyung was a very friendly and likeable lad and was spoiled by the Sanatorium staff. He enjoyed basking in this sunshine of love and affection. However, Hyung soon grew restless and wanted to try out his own strength, although I warned him against too hasty a return to normal activity. He became very homesick and began to talk of leaving us. We pointed out that his treatment was incomplete and it was still too early for him to be safely discharged. He kept shaking his head at this and insisting that he never felt better in his life.

One morning, when I was making my rounds, I found that Hyung had packed his few possessions in a *pojake* (a large square of cloth, tied at the four corners). He had decided to return home. I strongly protested and told him he might thus undo all the good we had been able to render him. He refused to listen to reason and insisted we call a jitney at once to take him to the station. Our staff members then tried their best to dissuade him, but to no avail, although in the past he had always been cooperative.

The Sanatorium was not a jail, and so, under the circumstances, we had no choice but to reluctantly let him go. He heartily thanked us and as he waved us a wistful good-by, I saw tears begin to trickle down his cheeks. My staff were all greatly moved.

"Good-by, Hyung. We shall miss you. You've been a good patient."

"Thank you again, Doctor. I've tried to tell you how much I appreciate everything. I can't."

"You have, Hyung. We know. But remember that the best sort of thanks you can give us is to take care of yourself. You know what to do. Do it, and as soon as you are well and strong, teach others. Let us hear from you. Good-by."

Hyung leaped into the jitney and it headed for Sariwon, 40 miles by road, where he would catch the train to Seoul. Five hours later his train pulled up to a familiar station platform. He was home.

"Better walk up to the house," he thought to himself. "Those streetcars are filthy, and this is just the hour the factory workers and other workers will be coming home. Many of them are tubercular."

Hyung walked the long distance to his home slowly. He rested often, but he was tired when he arrived. The family assembled to greet him, but there was no warm welcome. They stood around him in a distant circle, eyeing him suspiciously.

"Did they give you snake soup or the blood from a live deer?" demanded Hyung's grandmother.

"No. I had special treatments of air into my chest to give it rest while it got better. I had rest and sunshine and even learned to drink the milk of a cow."

"I knew it!" His grandmother turned triumphantly to his father, "You had better call the *mudong* at once to give him needle punctures to let out the evil spirits he must now have inside him from being in that place run by foreign devils."

Hyung cringed from his grandmother's words, for now he knew them to be all nonsense. Suddenly, he felt very tired and discouraged. He went into the dark house.

Later, he heard his father and a neighbor talking.

"I see Hyung has come home."

"Yes," his father answered gruffly.

"Is he all right?"

"He says he is."

"Well, see that he doesn't come over here. He may be all right, but I'm not taking any chances with my family."

His father entered the house hastily and slammed the door shut. "You sleep out there in the shed," he addressed Hyung bitterly.

It was damp and cold in the shed. There was no fresh air. Hyung remembered the doctor's parting words. He could not sleep there. But argument with his family was useless. They had been taught that drinking snake soup and deer blood were the only cures for tuberculosis. They simply could not accept that anything else would do it.

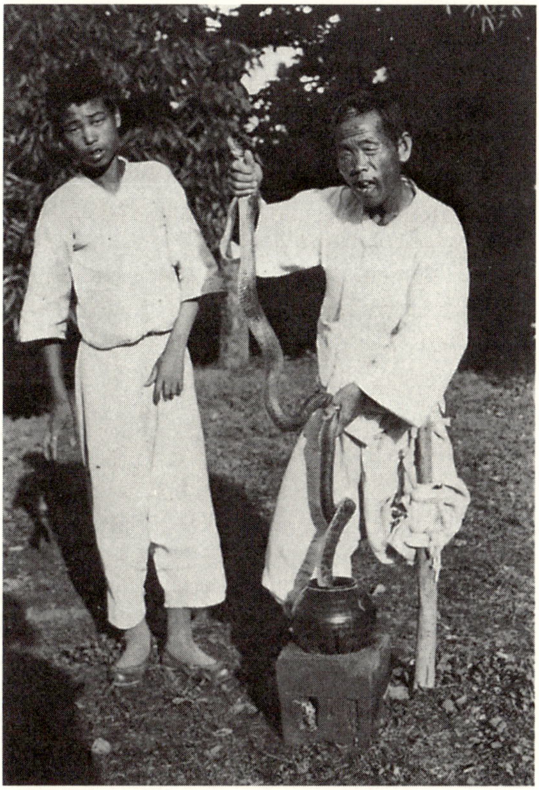

Making snake soup, thought to be a cure for TB

The following weeks were unhappy ones. Hyung's family could not overcome their awful fear of the disease. His old friends shunned him. Everywhere he went he felt unwelcome. His food was wrong. The house was foul, and he was avoided if he went outside. His discouragement was so complete that when his father told him to go to work, Hyung seized the opportunity. Anything would be better than that atmosphere of suspicion.

Several months later, Hyung wrote to the Sanatorium saying that he was again very ill and that he wanted to come back. But there was absolutely no room at the time and we had to write to tell him that he was on the waiting list. Alas, only a short time later, we heard that Hyung had joined his ancestors.

Hyung's case was typical. There was also the young farmer who had made good progress at the Sanatorium. He became an ardent Christian while there, and was so anxious to give up his place to other more serious cases that there was trouble holding him until we were sure he was strong enough to leave. The farmer finally returned to his village to face a lot of accumulated work on his farm. He felt well, and was eager to make up for lost time. There was no doctor in the village to check up on him. He did too much. He too died an untimely death.

Cases like these made it abundantly clear that something must be done. There must be some place within reach of the Sanatorium and its doctors where the critical transistion days from "all-rest" to the "work-all-days" of the active world could be bridged under care.

Since over eighty percent of Korea's population at that time was rural, I had long felt that a model farm should be connected with the Sanatorium. During the necessarily long period of convalescence for our patients, they could be learning modern methods of farming of a less strenuous variety. These patients, and especially the farmers among them, would then be enabled to teach others when they returned to their remote rural areas in different parts of Korea.

For the sake of better health, a program of re-education was needed. Due to the Korean's aversion to milk, milk cows and goats were still not popular. The udder of the Korean cow, compared to Western standards, was an extremely modest affair, and the milk yield, insignificant.

Now, when it came to the Korean chicken, the contrast was even greater. It truly had to "scratch for a living," so that the toughness of the bird for eating purposes rendered that a task for only those with good teeth. The eggs were extremely small. Vegetables fared little better. The Korean diet was nutritionally unbalanced, for it consisted primarily of grain foods, mostly rice.

Thus, if we were to have real tuberculosis control, and did not wish our patients to bounce back to us, we must not just tell them what they should eat, but show them how to obtain it. The sanatorium farm seemed to be a very practical means of doing this at a level suited to the peculiar needs of the Koreans.

My dream extended beyond the farm to a model village that would be sanitary and wholesome, where convalescents could be taught how to live in health. Here would be sunshine-flooded houses, instead of the usual windowless, smoke-filled hovels. Families of the convalescents could come and participate in the program with them.

In the center of such a village I envisioned the spire of a church. There could be a schoolhouse and a clubhouse. The latter could be the public health education center. Movies, lectures, mothers' and babies' club, housewives' club, boys' basketball games and girls' sewing circle, all could be centered in such a building. The village would have its own store, post office and playground. The houses would be built of material of which the average Korean house was built. They would be built so simply that the model villager could later build houses like them in his own village. They would have air, sunlight and septic tanks.

I knew that my dream of a farm and model village would have to be a long-range project, but I made up my mind to begin the effort at once. Not long afterward, we had the opportunity to obtain twenty-five acres of land adjacent to the Sanatorium. It would be ideal land for growing crops for the patients. The soil was fertile and already supported persimmon, chestnut and cherry trees.

This orchard had been the hobby of a young Korean man who had died suddenly. Because his father, in his grief, wanted to quickly dispose of the property which so reminded him of his sorrow, he offered to sell it to us very cheaply. A gift, given in memory of Harold Willis Moore, made it possible to purchase the orchard. The farm project was started.

The Sanatorium attracted frequent visitors. On one occasion we were privileged to entertain romantic guests. Willard Price, a free-lance writer, and his bride were on an extended honeymoon. They came to Haiju on the recommendation of Bishop Welch, who had told Willard, "That's where the action is."

Willard Price was well known for the articles he contributed to various magazines. He had served as a managing editor for *World Outlook*, a magazine published by the Methodist Board of Foreign Missions. Willard was ever on the lookout for new material. Thus, he was especially keen on going with me on outcalls, or to visit officials, or to watch Marian perform some interesting operation. His illustrated writing on these subjects gave our work some fine publicity. This kind of helpful exposure for our program won it many new friends.

The resulting increase in financial aid helped to expand the Norton Hospital and the Sanatorium facilities. Mrs. Bennett, the niece of Mrs. Mary Verburg, sent us a beautiful Zeiss microscope for use in the Sanatorium laboratory. It was another evidence of the active interest taken by the Bennetts, their relatives, and friends, ever since the granting of the Verburg bequest made the Sanatorium financially possible.

The tests performed in the laboratory were a significant help in diagnosis. The sedimentation test helped us in prognosis. This procedure involved observing the patient's blood in a test tube. The rate by which the red blood cells agglutinated (clumped together) seemed to reliably forecast a positive or negative prognosis quite early in the examination.

The tuberculin skin test proved to be a more useful diagnostic tool with children than with adults, for in the Orient practically all the adults had a positive reaction to the tuberculin. This was injected just under the skin.

Of the diagnostic procedures we had learned in medical school, the guinea pig test proved the least practical in its application to an Oriental setting. In this test the guinea pig was injected with the patient's sputum. After six weeks, the animal was killed and its organs (such as the liver, spleen, etc.) were examined for pockets of tuberculosis. However, we found that by the time the results were available, the average Korean would have long since vanished.

Our individual quartz (ultraviolet) lamps were eventually replaced by a beautiful large revolving Swiss solarium. Here about twelve bed patients could be treated simultaneously on a revolving table under a single large overhanging ultraviolet lamp while the technician was protected behind a glass screen. She could see that each patient received the correct dosage prescribed. A very strict record had to be kept of each patient with regard to duration of exposure, and whether the patient experienced an elevation in temperature following treatments. This prevented an overdose of ultraviolet, which could prove fatal.

The treatment generally started with a three minute exposure, gradually increasing the time by three to five minutes, depending on the patient's reaction, until about two hours could be tolerated. If a poor reaction was observed, the treatments would be discontinued for a day or so and then reinstituted gradually. The solarium provided better controls than when patients were left to administer the ultraviolet treatment themselves by sunshine. Patients with TB of the lungs did not respond well to this type of therapy so it was only given to patients suffering from TB of the bone, abdomen, or lymph glands.

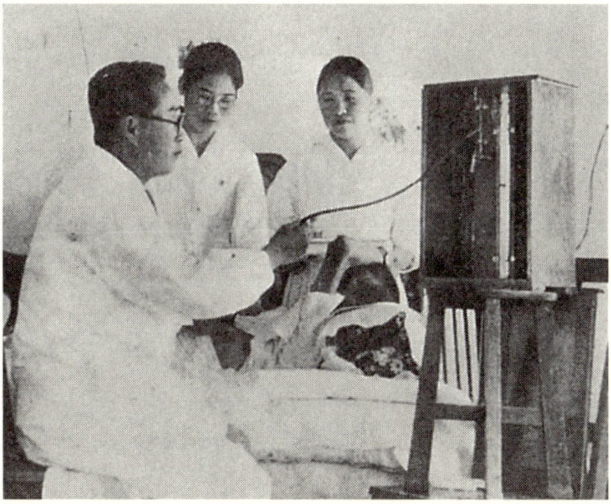

Pneumothorax treatment on a TB patient

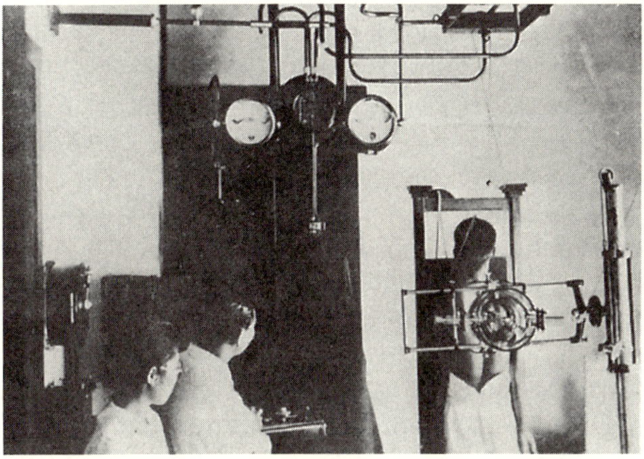

Patient x-ray

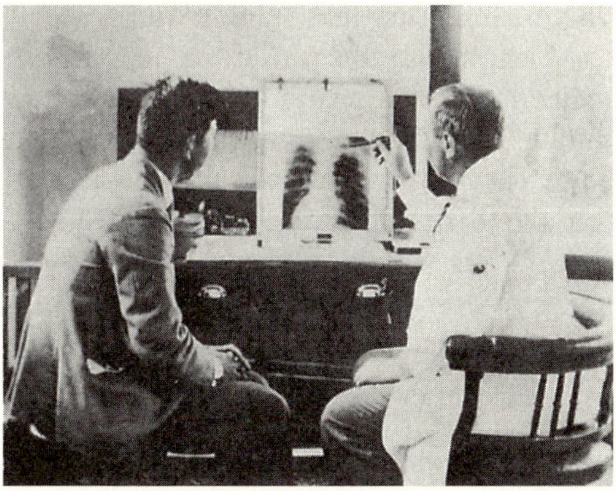

X-ray plate examination

We were especially proud of our new pneumothorax apparatus. This was used for introducing air into the intra-pleural cavity in graduated quantities to collapse the affected lung. This air served the same purpose as a splint by immobilizing the diseased lung. The enforced rest enabled the affected portion to recuperate by the restorative forces of nature. This mode of treatment, except as a supplementary aid in postoperative cases, has now been largely replaced. But we did get some excellent results and had very few complications. One possible complication, however, was pleural shock which could prove fatal to the patient and a devastating experience for any physician. For the bilateral cases, where both lungs were involved and therefore considered almost hopeless, we had excellent experience with pneumoperitoneum (air into the peritoneal cavity). Of course, all this pre-dated the day of the so-called "miracle drugs." Nonetheless, these earlier methods proved remarkably successful in many cases.

Our reports to our patrons in America continued to yield fruit. In November of 1929 we finally received word that sufficient donations were on the way to enable us at last to build the west wing on the property we had acquired with so much difficulty. Since spring, we had had money in hand to build a cottage for women to be known as the Edith Margaret Memorial. This was a gift from my mother and her friends.

However, it was not economical to build just one cottage at a time, for the contractor lived in Seoul and preferred to come only when there was enough work to justify his travel expenses. By the time we sent for him, we had funds guaranteed for two cottages besides the additional wing. We could also provide for some of the landscaping that had been in our original plans.

Adding to the variety of artisans employed, we had been fortunate in locating a good Japanese landscape gardener to design and build a miniature park. It contained goldfish ponds, arched bridges, and tea houses for our patients. A suitable lawn for croquet was also prepared for the use of those who had reached a convalescent stage. Later, Mr. Sasaki gave a gift to the Sanatorium of 100 Japanese cherry blossom trees which each spring were to add their unique touch of beauty to the Sanatorium grounds.

I was very proud of my fledgling sanatorium which I sometimes referred to affectionately as "my baby." Despite periodic growing

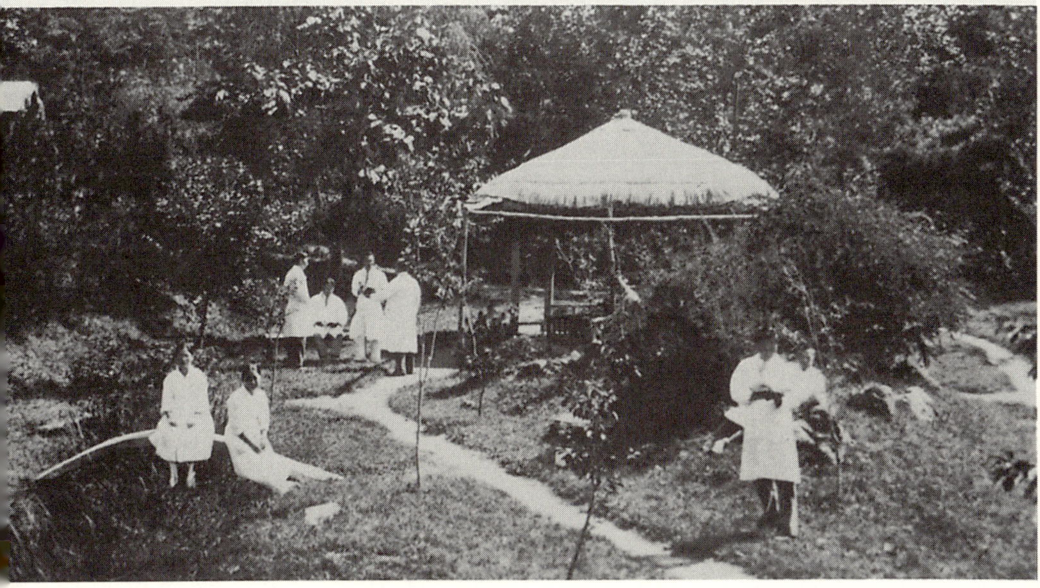

Sanatorium park

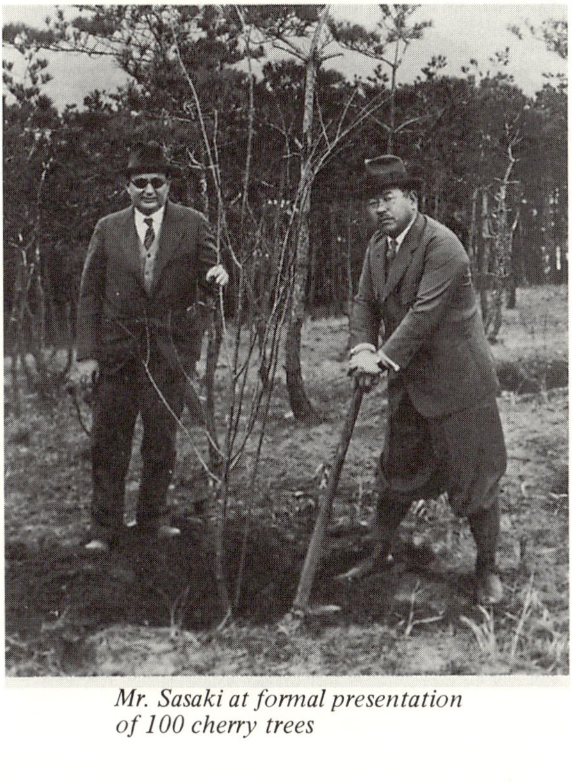

Mr. Sasaki at formal presentation of 100 cherry trees

pains, it was doing well. Although it appeared at first that my promise not to call on either the Mission or the Home Board for help would prove a serious handicap, as things worked out, it actually proved a blessing in disguise. It had, in fact, given me the freedom to build up what might be termed an almost "instant sanatorium."

Rarely in the history of missions had a first-term missionary been given so much latitude. I was allowed practically a free hand, and this by-passed much red tape and saved much precious time. Since I did not receive Mission grants for the Sanatorium, I did not need the Mission's permission to construct new buildings.

Had I been required to follow customary procedures, it would have been necessary to submit estimates and plans to the Finance Committee before embarking on a building program. If these plans were approved, they were referred to a Building Committee. This could mean deferment to allow for questions to be raised and points clarified. The Mission Field Committees would then submit it all to the Mission Board in the United States which, in turn, would repeat the whole process of committee review. In the meantime, construction costs could go up while waiting for the slow delivery of sea mail.

Furthermore, it was the rule that before anything could be built, one had to have all the cash in hand, which accounted frequently for still more postponement. In my case, since the Mission was not supplying the building funds, I could, with one stroke, cut out all these frustrating delays. This meant that I was able to build when the timing was best, although I always had the advice and help of our local Sanatorium Board.

For example, if we needed to build a cottage, all that I needed to do was to give out the plans to various contractors, and accept the bid. It would not necessarily even be the lowest, but rather, from the one I had found to be the most reliable. The builder could then proceed at once, and before the cottage was completed, I usually would have the money on hand. But if not, there was still no worry, for he trusted me, and would gladly wait, knowing that this would give him a better chance of getting the next contract. We were a going concern, and in this way cottages and wards sprang up like mushrooms on the mountainside.

Many of the gifts for these cottage units were obtained locally from the richer Koreans. As we were always short of beds, I would suggest to our rich applicants that if they wanted to get in without delay, they could build cottages on the sites we chose, under our plans and specifications, and agree to bequeath them to the Sanatorium when they left. Thus, from the rent of these cottages, we were ultimately able to help support our charity patients. Of course, for the larger buildings, such as the big wards, we had to continue to solicit help from our patrons at home who often responded generously.

Naturally there were times when I had my anxious moments. To have an excellent staff, one had to always pay them well and promptly. I never failed to meet the deadline of payday for the ever increasing staff, although it was sometimes nip and tuck. Still, personnel matters were my greatest headache. Harder to solve than the fiscal problems facing the institution was the considerable prejudice which still existed against working in a TB sanatorium.

There had not yet been time to develop our ex-patients in the roles of doctors and nurses. Even though a staff member had become convinced that with precautionary measures, such as the use of masks, there was relatively little risk, the friends or relatives would prevail upon him to quit. The public also needed to be educated, but this could not be done overnight. Yes, the staff problem was our weakest link.

Often I was advised to build up a good financial reserve for a rainy day, but I preferred to plow back any extra into the institution for the purchase of good equipment and medicines. This proved an incentive to keep us on our toes, as well as to increase our efficiency and the future potential of the Sanatorium. More importantly, I believed that it should not degenerate into a money making institution bent on profit alone, for then it would lose its original purpose.

A different sort of problem would soon be requiring our attention. Mrs. Woolverton's support was due to terminate as our term was drawing to a close, and the Mission Board was still not in a financial position to undertake it. We needed to return to the home base to try to make other arrangements for our continued financial support on the mission field. Besides, it was time for our furlough.

First-term missionaries were required to go on furlough on the completion of a five-year term on the field, not only on health grounds, but for taking some refresher courses and doing deputation work among the churches. So we had no choice but to go, and it was also to our personal liking and advantage.

What about the Sanatorium during our absence? The Norton Memorial Hospital and the Haiju Boys' School had older and deeper roots, but the Sanatorium was still in a developing, almost experimental stage, with a very young and inexperienced staff. Some of the nurses were threatening to leave. It was said no one would marry a nurse who had worked in a TB institution for fear of contracting tuberculosis.

I had promised our Mission that I would not call on them for help. They were very short of medical workers anyway and other missions were no better off. Even if a short-term doctor could be brought out, there would be the language and adjustment difficulties, and in those days there were just no such doctors available. There were a few Job's comforters, but most shared our deep concern. The whole problem weighed heavily on me. While there was never a thought of letting the Sanatorium down, humanly speaking there did not seem to be even one ray of light, although I had probed various possibilities. Always I seemed to come up against a stone wall.

Before dawn one morning, in sheer desperation, I slipped out of bed and climbed up the slopes of South Mountain, until I stood on the huge rock overlooking the Sanatorium. There I sat down to struggle with the problem. At first I felt utterly alone and more frustrated than ever. Then, as I looked toward the East, I saw unfolding before me a glorious sunrise. I said to myself, "The sun's rays are directing me to God's power and to hope. The sun never ceases to shine, even when hidden behind the clouds. My clouds will soon melt away."

My "mountaintop experience" was nothing unusual; even the sunrise was not special. There was no burning bush, no ten commandments, not even one commandment. Yet, as I gradually relaxed and let go, I could feel my anxiety and tensions being lifted. Although there was still no solution in sight, I did experience a strange peace of mind and a definite feeling of assurance that all would be well. I still did not have the faintest idea how. Nevertheless, now I found myself able to contemplate the serene scene before me with considerable pleasure, when only a few moments before I was totally preoccupied. I felt as if a big load had been taken from my shoulders.

Sure enough, in a few days, I received word that Dr. and Mrs. Ernest M. Ewers were about to leave their work at the American gold mines at Unsan to return to the States and might be available to help us out while we were on furlough. This good news came as no surprise to me and I lost no time in contacting them.

After being driven out of China, Dr. Ewers had accepted a call to help out as physician for the Oriental Consolidated Mining Company when Dr. Power had found it necessary to return to the United States for his health. It was the Ewers who had been able to fill the emergency need that we had been asked to fill, prior to learning of Mrs. Woolverton's renewal of our support. The Ewers were therefore not unused to responding to an S O S like ours, and to our unspeakable joy, we found they would be glad to serve.

Our Bishop and the Executive Committee readily agreed to the Ewers' coming, although, I heard later, a few had questioned how I could possibly raise the salary for them in these difficult days in addition to raising our own salary. The Committee feared that they would have the financial problem dumped in their lap. Here Mr. Noble spoke out strongly and said that I had never called on them for a penny for the Sanatorium and he was sure that they could count on me to keep my pledge.

So it was that we welcomed the Ewers with deep gratitude, and I felt convinced that they had been truly sent by Heaven to save the Sanatorium. They fitted in nicely and were well received by our patients and staff.

Getting ready to leave on furlough proved to be something of a juggling act. We were due to leave Haiju on June 13, 1930. We had a most gratifying send-off, however, in the form of visitors from Pittsburgh, Pennsylvania, the Reverend and Mrs. Paul. I drove up to Seoul to meet them on May 30 and on June 2 returned with them to Haiju.

On the following day, the Reverend Paul dedicated the Woman's Pavilion which he had given in honor of his wife, the new West Wing, and the Edith Margaret Memorial Cottage. We entertained the Pauls

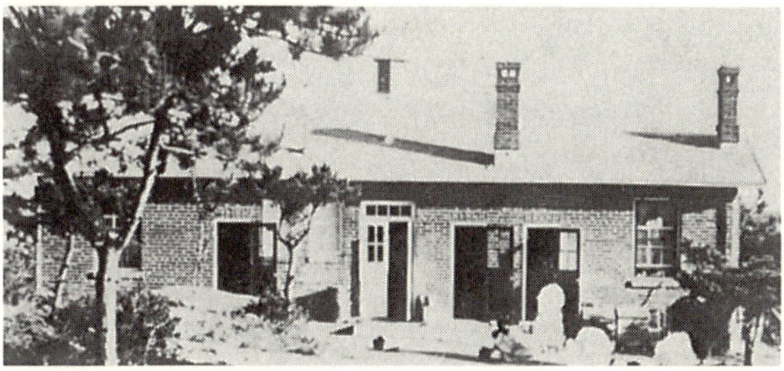

Cottage for TB patients

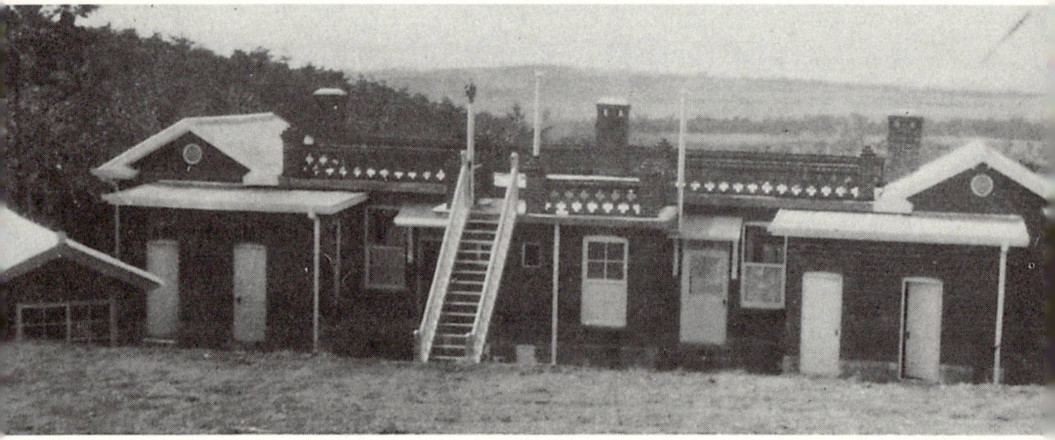

Woman's Pavilion

with sight-seeing and a fishing trip and then saw them off for Pyong Yang on June 6. My mother had been incapacitated by a bad fall and had been recuperating with us. We made arrangements with the W.F.M.S. ladies to have her spend the rest of the summer in their home and then bade everyone *adieu*.

Our first term in Korea had proved a challenging and rewarding one. We looked forward eagerly to our furlough as our ship, the *Totsuta Maru*, pulled away from the Japanese coastline on June 27, 1930.

CHAPTER 21

Furlough

Our trans-Pacific Ocean voyage to the United States proved to be extremely pleasant, and the ocean true to its name. To our delighted surprise we found that the "honeymoon couple" who had visited us in Haiju, the Willard Prices, were fellow passengers. Upon reaching San Francisco, we boarded a train for the trans-continental rail journey to New York. William especially enjoyed this trip.

We were saddened, however, upon reaching our destination, to learn of the passing of our good friend and benefactor, Mrs. Woolverton. This meant that we were again on our own, and must lose no time in trying to find a future source of income.

It was natural that we should first turn to our Cousin Grace Haskins at Binghamton with our predicament. She did not disappoint us. Although she could not provide our full salary, she had assured that her portion of it would continue to come to us by making arrangements with the Binghamton Tabernacle Methodist Church to assume her share in the event of her death.

Eager to get the matter of our full support settled, as well as the support for the Ewers while we were on furlough, I consulted the Mission Board in New York for any suggestion they might have for securing the balance. At that time, the head of our Mission Board was none other than the internationally famous hymn writer, Frank Mason North. His hymns were favorites of mine, particularly the hymn, "Where Cross the Crowded Ways of Life." I felt impelled to call on Dr. North, even though I had made no previous appointment and knew him to be a very busy executive. The man whose hymns had given me so much help during some trying times might also have some helpful advice for solving the problem which now confronted us.

As it turned out, I did not have to wait long in the anteroom of his office located at the Methodist Mission Board Headquarters at 150 Fifth Avenue. Soon after I called, his secretary showed me into Dr. North's presence. He greeted me warmly.

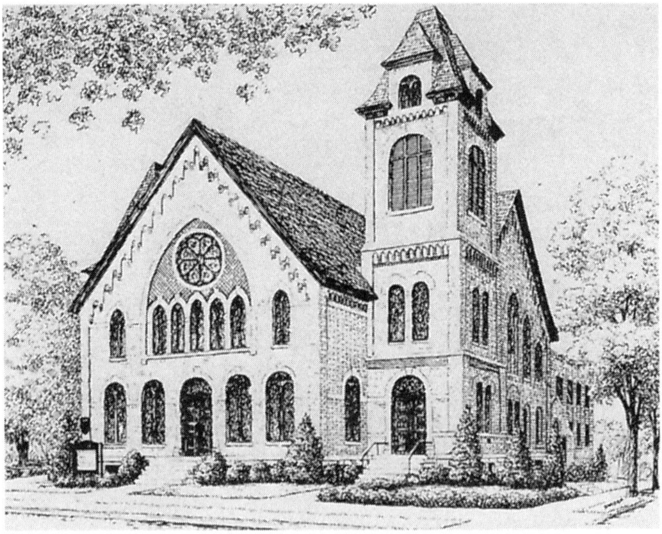

Tabernacle Methodist Church, Binghamton, New York

"I almost feel as if I already knew you," Dr. North commented. "Every time I hear your name mentioned by Bishop Welch and others, there is a stirring of my recollections of the personality and work of your father, Dr. William James Hall, to say nothing of your remarkable mother and her influence in Korea, as well as here in the homeland.

"When I came to New York as the Directing Secretary of the City Mission in 1892, your father had been serving on the New York East Side. Your father's name and lasting influence were among the familiar facts with which I dealt immediately upon coming into the work. I was confronted with the almost impossible task of finding someone who could take his place.

"Of course, his subsequent unparalleled activity on the field, until he was taken into the larger ministry above, is now a matter for the record. His magnificent medical missionary work now belongs to mission history and to you, who are giving yourself to such noble work in Korea. It is indeed a precious legacy."

Such a welcoming speech nearly took me off my feet. In my surprise and embarrassment I almost neglected to tell Dr. North of the help that I had derived from his hymns.

With regard to our further support Dr. North proved most encouraging. He said that the Board had long felt that there should be closer and more personal contact between the supporting church and the missionaries on the field, and so had proposed a plan known as "the Parish Abroad." He had just received a request from The Church of the Saviour in Cleveland, Ohio, and he was sure that they would be glad to have us as their representatives on the field, particularly since we had both graduated from Mount Union College, not far from Cleveland.

This arrangement was no sooner proposed than accomplished. In due course, another fine church, the Appold Church of Baltimore, Maryland, also became one of our supporting churches. This plan gave us a firmer financial base, for there was some security in numbers.

The Pennsylvania Medical Missionary Society which had helped us with scholarships during our medical student days, now offered us free use of one of their comfortable "furlough cottages" for missionaries, at Ventnor, New Jersey. So we made our headquarters there and took turns making deputation visits among the churches, as well as commuting from this point to our postgraduate studies in New York and Philadelphia.

Fortunately there was a small private school nearby under the capable direction of kindly Miss Josephine Zimmerman where we could enroll William in kindergarten. Thus, we settled down for a profitable and restorative furlough after those sometimes rather hectic and strenuous days in Korea.

I enrolled in the Graduate School of the University of Pennsylvania to take an excellent course in TB at the Henry Phipps Institute. I commuted to Philadelphia daily for the classes. On the completion of these studies, I took my turn looking after William. This freed Marian to take special work in surgery at the New York Post Graduate School.

One Sunday I was doing deputation work in one of the Philadelphia churches. At the close of the service, as was customary, a number of people came up to shake my hand. A gentleman, who appeared to be more knowledgeable about TB than most, introduced himself as Mr. Philip P. Jacobs, an officer of the National TB Association headquartered in New York. He told me about a special course which the Association would be giving later, entitled, "How Best to Inform the Public on TB," and he wondered if this might be a course with special interest for me. It was.

"In the meantime," Mr. Jacobs added, "there are two very good friends of mine I want you to meet. They would be most interested in the story you told this morning about your TB patient, Hyung, and how better public health knowledge might have spared his life.

I shall be glad to give you letters of introduction to them. One is Leigh Mitchell Hodges, editor of one of America's leading newspapers, the *North American*. He lives right here in Philadelphia. The other is Miss Emily P. Bissell of Wilmington, Delaware. These two have been instrumental in introducing the Christmas Seal idea to the U.S.A."

Mr. Jacobs went on to say, "It is now the chief source of income of our Association, yielding over five million dollars annually, and what may be significant to you, the Seal Campaigns have not been seriously affected by the financial depression, so should prove especially suitable for the low income countries of Asia. Between 1907, when the seal idea was introduced in the U.S.A., and 1930, over sixty-one million dollars have been raised. Vastly more important is the fact that it has been the greatest single factor in the record reduction of TB in the U.S.A."

These facts and figures I felt to be truly significant. I thrilled to the prospect of meeting those who had helped initiate the great Christmas Seal Movement in the U.S. The letter of introduction proved to be an "Open Sesame," for I was ushered right in to Mr. Hodges' elegant office. Although he was now getting on in years, I could see by the huge pile of work on his desk that he still must be very active.

Mr. Hodges greeted me cordially, and after the exchange of a few pleasantries, he came right to the point.

"I see you want to get my side of the story, but the real credit goes to that remarkable lady, Miss Bissell, who gave me the Christmas Seal idea. Each year our paper selects and promotes some worthwhile cause, for I believe we should be more than just a news medium.

"I well remember, as if it were yesterday, back in 1907 when Miss Bissell came to my office. I was extremely busy that morning and had a sign on my door marked, 'Do Not Disturb,' which was respected by my senior staff. Perhaps my office boy had failed to see the sign. Anyway, he knocked on my door and announced that there was a young lady waiting outside who insisted on seeing me personally. I looked at the stack of papers still awaiting my perusal. Perhaps I wanted a breather. I paused for a moment to ask, 'Is she pretty? If she is, show her in.'

"Evidently, the boy thought she would pass, for he ushered her right in. For a moment the young girl was speechless with embarrassment, so I gave her an encouraging smile and helped her tell her story. I shall let her tell you the details herself. In short, she wondered if our paper could help the small sanatorium in Wilmington, in which she was interested, by sponsoring the sale of health stamps or seals, since many of the TB patients there came from our area.

"I could not help but admire the plucky young girl before me. She had already won my sympathy for her cause. As a newspaperman I could see that with proper publicity, the Christmas Seal idea, though new here, had possibilities. So I promised the persistent young lady to see what I could do.

"The success of the first Christmas Seal here is now a matter of history. The little Brandywine Sanatorium in Wilmington was not only kept from closing its doors, but was enlarged and enabled to render increased and better service as a result. The idea grew by leaps and bounds, and it was not long before the National Tuberculosis Association was glad to take it over. That about wraps up my part of the story."

I heartily thanked Mr. Hodges and withdrew, wondering indeed how best I could apply this type of plan to Korea. I could hardly wait until I could see Miss Bissell and get the full picture. The opportunity came sooner than I had expected, for I had a speaking engagement in Wilmington.

Miss Bissell received me most graciously. Like Fanny Crosby, she gave the impression of frailty, so that I marveled at how such a petite and unassuming girl had been able to get her ideas across to the mighty Mr. Hodges. Even now, after her noteworthy achievements, she seemed rather reticent and shy. At first I had to coax her to reveal her wonderful story, but once she began, she showed plenty of animation. Her eyes sparkled with excitement as she recalled the past.

"Near my home was a small struggling sanatorium which had been suffering sorely for lack of funds and was daily obliged to turn away patients. This institution had not been able to attract the interest and help of patrons, and we who were friends of the sanatorium were growing discouraged.

"Just about this time, I happened to read a magazine article by Jacob Riis telling about a humble postal clerk in Denmark, Einar Holboell, who had observed how both rich and poor alike bought postage stamps, and though the value of each stamp was not much, the total income from the sale of these postage stamps was considerable. There was a small TB sanatorium in Denmark, near the home of the clerk, which was having difficulty in keeping its doors open. He wondered why a special stamp could not be issued that everyone, regardless of their means, might be able to purchase and so help this deserving institution. These stamps, or seals, would cost so little, that men, women and even children might all become working partners in the fight against TB.

"After considerable effort, permission was finally granted for these seals to be issued for the holidays. With the spirit of Christmas in people's hearts, the seals were widely sold and the struggling sanatorium was put on its financial feet. The idea worked so well that it was gradually enlarged so that all TB sufferers in Denmark benefitted through the sale of these Christmas Seals. What was still more important, the death rate from TB dropped in Denmark to one of the lowest in the world.

"Jacob Riis, who had lost six of his brothers to TB, pleaded in his article for someone to use the Christmas Seal idea in America. Since reading his plea, I could hardly sleep nights. I repeatedly tried to interest friends in the idea, but they were skeptical, and did not think it would work in the U.S.A. 'Anyway,' they said, 'it would have to be done by some large organization or group.'

"I approached the National TB Association, but they did not think the idea suitable for raising large sums of money, so they did not care to sponsor it. The Red Cross was somewhat more encouraging in that it would allow its name to be used, but it seemed impossible to get any group to initiate it, and in the meantime, my beloved Brandywine Sanatorium was suffering. There was no apparent relief in sight.

"Someone had told me that the *North American* had often sponsored worthy causes. So I grasped at this straw, and rather timidly approached its fine editor, Mr. Hodges, and you know the result."

Miss Bissell had told her story simply, but this marvelous woman had left a deep impression on me. I went out from her presence with a new vision and the resolve to see if something similar might be done for Korea.

The course offered by the National TB Association followed soon after this, and I was doubly glad that I had already been able to meet Mr. Hodges and Miss Bissell, pioneers in the Seal Movement in the U.S.A. The National TB Association course, led by Mr. Jacobs, included helpful pointers in public health education and on how best to gain a more sympathetic and understanding approach to TB victims and ex-TB patients from a reluctant public.

This was just what I needed to know. I was particularly interested in learning about Christmas Seals in more detail: design methods, printing and distribution. I had always been a stamp collector, so I now found it natural to add seal collecting to that hobby. My collection soon included seals from all the nations which produced them. I found this both fascinating and educational and it gave me an additional rich resource of ideas for future application.

Our furlough was fast drawing to a close. While there had been little rest, we had found it very stimulating. I had some big plans for the future and was eager to get back to Korea to begin work on them. I wanted to launch a campaign of health education and TB prevention on a large scale. This, I knew, would not be as popular as treatment, important as it was. I recalled a poem I had learned as a boy in school in which it was noted that the appeal for an ambulance down in the valley was more attractive to the public than for a preventive fence on the precipice above.

Before we sailed, we had been invited to attend a special commissioning service for us by The Church of the Saviour in Cleveland. This beautiful church, cathedral-like in appearance, had been hard hit by the depression. However, under the able leadership of Dr. J. McCombe, and its loyal members, it was fast coming back. Later, under the guidance of Dr. Howard Brown, its good work in all fields continued to flourish. We found the members exceptionally warm-hearted, and they have been our fast friends down through the years. Their beautiful send-off did something for our morale that was hard to express. Their prayers and encouraging letters were to strengthen us during some of the trying times that lay ahead. Some of these days were coming sooner than we knew.

Shortly before we returned to Korea, we received a very gracious letter from Dr. North:

> "I have thought much concerning you and your work since we last met. I have a very profound interest in you both. Your ministry to the Koreans is so sane and genuine. It has been prompted after so unique a medical preparation by you both, and is carrying into effect such definite scientific and spiritual ideals that I am stirred to enthusiasm by it.

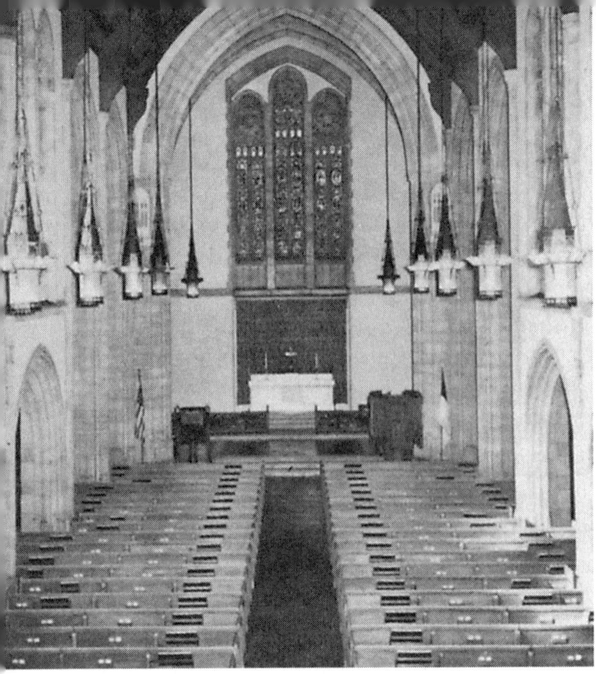

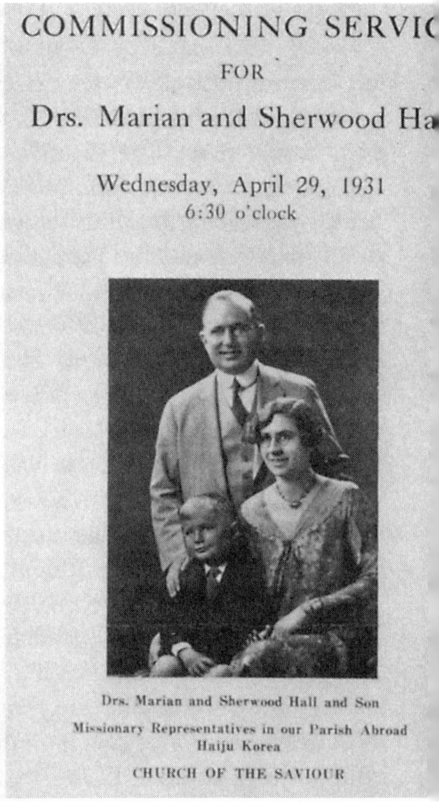

COMMISSIONING SERVIC

FOR

Drs. Marian and Sherwood Ha

Wednesday, April 29, 1931
6:30 o'clock

Drs. Marian and Sherwood Hall and Son

Missionary Representatives in our Parish Abroad
Haiju Korea

CHURCH OF THE SAVIOUR

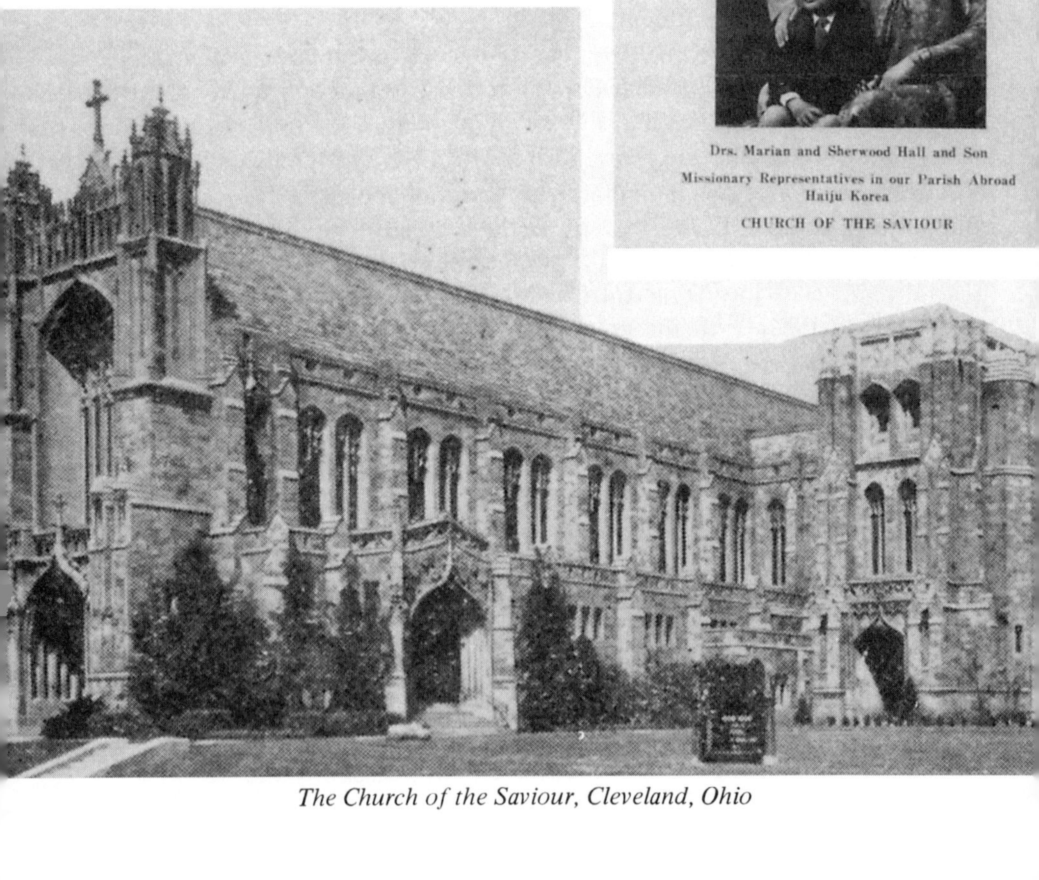

The Church of the Saviour, Cleveland, Ohio

"I earnestly hope for each of you, the large success of your fine sacrificial, far reaching enterprise."

One of the fastest routes back to Korea from the east coast of America at that time was not by water, but by land, via Trans-Siberia. We decided to take this so-called shortcut. I had traveled it as a boy, and I thought it might be easier now. That proved to be an erroneous assumption.

We had been advised by the travel agency at New York to get through tickets to our destination and to take as little cash with us as possible. Although I had some misgivings at the time, we took their advice feeling they must surely know best.

We reached Berlin in the early fall of 1931. The Hitler menace had not yet reached Berlin, although it was fast approaching. The shops were well stocked and prices were moderate. We knew that in Russia and Siberia there would be a short supply of what we considered essential items, so we stocked up. Especially important on our list was powdered milk for William and other light food supplies that we could carry easily and that would keep. I saw an attractive hat for Marian, which took my eye and suited her. We purchased this luxury item at a fantastically low price.

Soon we were on our way from a green land, then "*flowing with milk and honey*," to the drab, brown land of the Soviets. In Russia the ladies wore "mini skirts." They were very short for the times—well above the knees. However, the extreme shortness of the hemline was not due to either fashion or fad, but to dire necessity. There was hardly sufficient cloth available for decent covering, and everything was severely rationed. There were even long lines to be seen waiting for a small loaf of bread.

The train en route had been crowded at first with laughing well padded Germans, although, as we approached the Soviet border, most of these had been replaced by a few sad faced, rather scantily dressed Soviets. There still remained one well dressed gentleman, who was pacing restlessly up and down the train aisle with a rather worried expression. When he passed us his face always lit up with a friendly smile, which seemed to be directed chiefly toward William. As we started to eat our lunch, we noted the envious look in our fellow traveler's eyes.

We invited him to be seated next to William and offered to share our food. He gratefully accepted. He then told us that he had not brought anything to eat because he had assumed that on an international train such as this there would be a dining car.

As we talked, we learned that our new friend was a New Yorker who had previously left the Soviet regime as a young man and had since made good in the United States. His name was Mr. Samuel Fine. He was returning for the first time to visit his relatives and former friends, and to share with them some of the good things he had brought from his adopted country, the land of plenty. He confided that he was not sure how the Soviet authorities would receive him, but he knew he would get a warm welcome from his kindred. He had brought them parcels of items no longer available in the land of the Soviets. By the time we had reached Leningrad, we had begun a friendship with Mr. Fine which was to last down through the years and would later include his wonderful family.

When we reached Leningrad, the large station was bleak and almost deserted, as were the streets. There was not a single taxi nor a drosky in sight. We had been assured by our travel agency in Berlin that there would be someone to meet us from the hotel where we had been booked. Mr. Fine kindly helped us pile up our luggage on the station platform and strongly warned us to keep our eyes glued on it. Under no circumstances were we to wander off, leaving it unguarded, he cautioned, or it would vanish. In the meantime, he had gone off to telephone our hotel. After some time, he returned

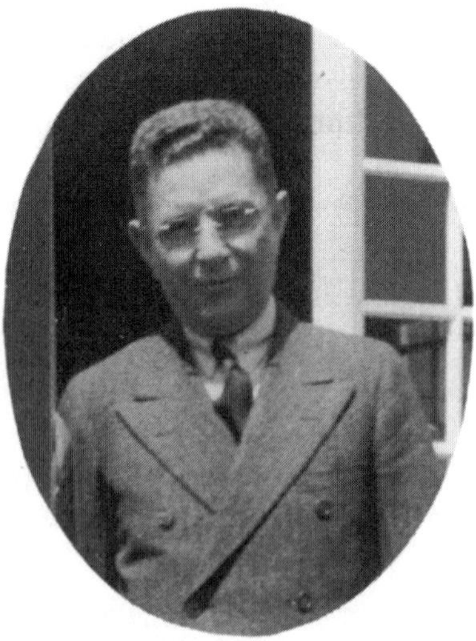

Samuel Fine

with the report that he had finally made connection with them and they would be sending a drosky for us soon.

We counted ourselves very fortunate to have met up with such a friend as Mr. Fine, who spoke Russian fluently and knew all the potential pitfalls for a foreign traveler. In fact, he became our guardian angel while we were in Leningrad, and we wished later that we could have had him with us all the way to our journey's end.

Usually, getting a bath in any large hotel is not noteworthy. Here, it was different. There was no bath in our suite, nor was one a few steps down the hallway. The communal bathroom was located several flights down the stairs, which we had to descend by foot. Since there were no towels provided in our room, we assumed there must be towels in the bathroom. But not so. We then had to go all the way down to the main desk, only to be referred to the hall porter on still another floor. Triumphantly returning to the bathroom, now armed with towels, we learned that we had to provide our own soap. Furthermore, a hotel guest emerging from his shower warned us that there was only about a bucketful of warm water left before it ran cold. After all that had transpired, we decided to resort to sponge baths.

Mr. Fine met us later to show us the sights. He thought we might be interested in seeing the Court House, where in one room, instant civil marriage was performed, and in the adjacent room, instant divorce was granted. The clerk assured us, however, that they were not necessarily the same couple.

The next place that Mr. Fine took us to see was a rehabilitation center for former prostitutes. Here they were being taught the art of weaving. The center seemed to be doing a very commendable job.

We also visited a factory restaurant where Mr. Fine thought we might be interested in seeing just how this classless society performed at meal times. On the first two floors we saw how the common worker fared. He was ladled out just a bowl of *borscht* (Russian beet soup) and black bread. The "top brass," the bosses, dined on the top floor. They were dining on choice Russian dishes which they washed down with vodka.

In the evening, Mr. Fine took us to see a popular Soviet movie. This was a propaganda film to show how the Soviet worker could now take his vacation at the famous Black Sea resort where previously only the rich could go. The jolting train ride was depicted very realistically and gave us a foretaste of what we soon would be experiencing on our trans-Siberian trip.

Next on Mr. Fine's selective list was one of the famous large collective farms in the country. As foreigners were normally not allowed to visit these farms, we felt privileged to have the opportunity. I found it most interesting, and observed with amusement that their pigs had special paved sidewalks which denied them the enjoyment of wallowing in the mud. William announced that he felt sorry for the pigs.

Modern machinery was pointed out to us with pride by the manager of the collective farm. Later we were told privately by one of the farmers that they were not happy with this collective system, and would prefer to return to their own farms and their crude implements, which were not always breaking down. We were struck by the fact that since our arrival in the land of the Soviets, we had not heard a spontaneous laugh nor seen a happy face.

We bade our new found friend, Mr. Fine, good-by as we boarded the train for Moscow. We had not gone far before we had a rather unpleasant encounter with a Soviet soldier who had evidently imbibed too much vodka. He insisted on trying to come into the small compartment where Marian and William were sleeping. To this I strenuously objected. I finally was able to contact a train official who claimed that this was a common practice, and with great reluctance ordered the intruder out. The remainder of the trip to Moscow was without untoward incident.

Moscow station, by contrast to Leningrad, was a bustle of activity. Around Red Square and the Kremlin there were large crowds. An especially long line of Soviet visitors waited to view Lenin's tomb. Later, we were assigned an Intourist guide, a Latvian girl, to show us the usual sights selected for tourists. We missed Mr. Fine's help and his more discerning tour. However, our guide did the best she could.

She solemnly pointed out to us how Lenin's beard had grown after his death (facial skin retracts in death, thus giving the appearance of elongation of the hairs). She said all the "correct" things when there was anyone within earshot, but on the quiet, she admitted to being very unhappy at what had happened in her beloved Latvia and wondered if we could suggest how she might escape to America. We sensed at once we were on uncertain ground, and although we felt sorry for her, we ceased further sightseeing.

We headed for the Intourist Travel Agency and en route, saw in a main store, a marvelous display of fine linens, silver and dinner sets, which had been confiscated from the rich, and were now being sold at a low price to attract U.S. dollars.

We hurried on to the travel office. Our through tickets would need to be endorsed by them. However, we were shocked to learn that due to the recent trouble at the Siberian-Manchurian border, this could not be done. We were told we would need to purchase tickets for the final leg of our journey at the Manchurian border. Of course we demanded a refund and were rather reluctantly paid the balance due us in Russian rubles, which then were almost valueless outside of Russia.

We strongly protested that since we had paid at New York in good U.S. dollars, we should be refunded accordingly. But all our protests fell on deaf ears. We then insisted that they should give us an official statement, to the effect that, since our tickets had been originally purchased in dollars, the refund granted us was in lieu of our dollar purchase.

After much talking and their initial refusal, we were finally given the precious statement. Later, we learned how very lucky we were to have obtained this scrap of paper and how priceless it was.

We were traveling on two separate passports: the photo of Marian and William together on one, and mine on the other. We were now assured at Intourist headquarters that our passports had been duly endorsed with Russian exit visas and our tickets were all in order as far as the Siberian border. We were wished a pleasant journey across their vast domain. They suggested that we return after a few years to note the great progress being made under the Soviet regime which would soon be outdistancing the capitalistic world. We did not linger to express our reservations. We had had enough of red tape.

The mighty trans-Siberian express train engine was puffing at the Moscow station as if anxious to be off. We were traveling "Russian hard," and the benches now seemed even harder than I had remembered them as a boy. In the beginning the train was very crowded, and from the bites we were receiving, not all the passengers were people. We had unfortunately neglected to bring any flea powder with us, so like some of the chickens we saw at the station, we scratched for a living. Crawling things were not the only diversion. Again, a Soviet soldier, filled to the brim with vodka, could not understand why Marian objected to "his endearing young charms." However, fortunately for us, an Intourist guide sized up the situation and came to the rescue.

This guide was en route to Vladivostok and so it meant that he would be with us to the border, for which we later had reason to be more than grateful. He spoke rather broken English and was very eager to learn how to converse more fluently. Marian's teacher instinct asserted itself, and she had a self-appointed task the rest of our Siberian journey. The progress he made in those few days was amazing.

As we crossed the Siberian steppe, the number of passengers on the train steadily decreased. At some of the longer stops we would get out to stretch our legs and to draw some of the boiling water from the engine for our tea. In the first-class coach were a couple of young Englishmen, rather "stand-off-ish" at first, but William soon engaged them in conversation, in which later we all joined.

They were fuming because, although they had been allowed to take pictures, the Soviet authorities had demanded that all film must be developed in Moscow. In good faith and ample time, they had turned over their film, but the authorities failed to return it. They had no pictures to show for all the trouble they had taken to get some good shots.

So it was that they tried to retrieve a measure of their loss by taking a few pictures from the train window. Somehow, the ever alert Cheka (N.K.V.D.) informers had spotted them doing so, and at the next station their baggage had been thoroughly searched. Fortunately the Cheka could find no film nor camera equipment, for our English friends, by some sixth sense, had managed to conceal such in the ladies' room. The Cheka must have concluded that someone had simply turned in a false report and they gave the Englishmen no further trouble. The taller Englishman dearly loved his liquor and had some bad words to say about the Soviet variety.

Our powdered milk supply for William was beginning to run low, so our new friends offered to share some of theirs. They, too, were worried about the border trouble and had been told it was worsening. We then recounted our difficulties of not being able to get through tickets and wondered if the Manchouli (Lupin) station would accept our rubles. They tried to assure us that most border towns accepted money from just the other side of the border, although, no doubt, we might lose heavily in exchange rates. Thus, we decided to husband our meager resources and purchase no more provisions at the stations.

As we later exchanged views on our experiences, I noted that the trans-Siberian railroad was now double-tracked, an advance from when I traveled it as a boy. However, we concluded that the Soviets, despite the fine new schools which were springing up everywhere, still had a long way to go before they caught up with the West.

Our Intourist friend, in due course, announced sorrowfully that the train was nearing the border station of Manchouli where we would have to part company. He thanked Marian heartily for her great help in improving his conversational English. We were genuinely sorry to have to bid him farewell.

Fairly soon after that, the train jerked to a halt. Then some heavily bearded Soviet officials swooped down on us. As nearly as we could make out, they demanded that we should surrender our precious rubles, which we had been hoarding so carefully. They claimed that it was forbidden to take such currency out of the Soviet. I became alarmed and hunted up our Intourist friend. I explained through him that these were special rubles, refunded to us on our through ticket, to enable us to purchase our tickets for the rest of the journey. I showed them the slip of paper which confirmed it.

That only brought forth a coarse laugh, and they immediately separated me from my travel funds. I then tried to insist that they at least give me a receipt for what they had forcibly taken from us; otherwise, it was no better than a train robbery. After considerable bickering, they begrudgingly gave me another scrap of paper on which the spokesman had scribbled something. Our friend assured us that it was in the nature of a receipt and that we were lucky to have been able to obtain even that much.

While we were still smarting over the loss and wondering how we could raise funds to buy our tickets for the rest of the trip, another group of Soviet officials demanded to see our passports. One started to shake his head at Marian's and then gave Marian and William a rude shove toward the exit. William, although too young to realize the full significance, was aware that something was drastically wrong and began to fight back with his puny fists. His mother restrained him with difficulty. Of course, I started to follow, but the official roughly pushed me down onto the seat.

By this time I had become thoroughly alarmed and, in desperation, again sought out our Intourist friend. It seemed that by some oversight, the Moscow authorities had failed to stamp the exit visa on

Marian's passport, although they had stamped mine. Thus, according to our inquisitors, Marian and William had to stay behind. On the other hand, I was given no choice but to go, and leave my family to their fate at this wild Soviet outpost in the middle of nowhere. They insisted that I should proceed the best I could across the border into Manchuria without the funds which they had taken from me.

All this seemed to us an impossible situation. We beseeched our friend to convey to the guards that under no circumstances could our family be separated. Anyway, I felt that surely this must be just a clerical oversight, for since my wife and child had had an entrance visa, they certainly would be entitled to an exit visa.

At first they seemed adamant and refused to listen to reason, and I could see were even berating the Intourist guide for befriending us. They evidently had not realized his position, for when he threatened to inform on them, they finally relented. After these agonizing several minutes, we were one family again and allowed to leave Siberia and enter Manchuria. It was with a great sense of relief that we were rid of that vile atmosphere of oppression and breathed the comparatively free air across the border.

In the meantime our English friends had become very anxious about us. They had attempted to get back to investigate, but had been roughly turned back by the Soviet guards. It was about time for the departure of the Manchurian Express. Had we missed it, we would have been stranded indefinitely in the inhospitable border town of Manchouli.

When our English friends saw us coming, they shouted, "Hurry, hurry! You have very little time left to get your tickets."

We shouted back, "We have still less money with which to buy them."

After a hurried explanation of what had happened to us, the tall Englishman, who dearly loved his liquor, began to count his money rapidly. He found that he would be able to loan us just enough to buy our third-class tickets. We knew that this meant real self-sacrifice on his part, for now he would not have enough to purchase his drinks. We were very grateful to him.

We barely caught the train and were more fortunate than we realized at the time. This proved to be the last train on that line for a long time to come, due to the so-called "Manchurian Incident."

We later learned that the train which had just preceded ours had been held up, and the engineer had been shot and killed. The train guards were expecting more shooting that night. At the time, we were blissfully ignorant of all this and were relaxing in our fancied security. Our English friends, however, were in the know and came to invite us to their first-class coach ostensibly for a cup of tea. Their real motive was to avoid alarming William and Marian, although they conveyed to me a little later the possibility of more shooting occurring. They wanted us in their coach where the windows were curtained, a luxury not supplied in the third class.

However, Marian, with her womanly intuition, sensed that something must be very wrong, especially when William was not allowed to look out of the window. The shorter Englishman seemed so upset and agitated that he made what would have been a strange request under normal circumstances. He gave Marian his sister's name and address and said that if for any reason he did not reach his destination, would Marian please write to her. Then an embarrassing silence fell upon them. Marian tried to continue conversation, but for the most part it was one-sided. To cover up her concern lest William get upset, she actually talked herself into a laryngitis.

We finally reached Mukden, the hub city of Manchuria, to find that the streets there were being heavily patrolled by Japanese soldiers. We were later told that a popular Japanese army officer by the name of Major Nakamura had been killed that June by Chinese soldiers. This had inflamed Japanese public opinion so that the situation was already tense. When word reached Japanese military officials that a bridge on the Japanese Manchurian Railroad line had been blown up, just north of Mukden, Japanese troops took over the city, accusing the Chinese of planting the bomb. Our train must have passed over that very bridge just moments before the explosion, which occurred the night of September 18, 1931. All rail service behind us had been disrupted.

Under all these circumstances, we met with considerable difficulty in sending a telegram to our Methodist District Superintendent, the Reverend William Shaw, in Pyong Yang. We wired him to please meet our train with the necessary money to repay our generous English friend. Evidently our telegram got through all right, for Mr. Shaw was at the Pyong Yang railway station with the appropriate funds when our train pulled in. Marian was still "speechless," and I had to do the talking for both of us.

Mr. Shaw was the one who told us that our train had been the last to get through, due to the "Manchurian Incident," and confirmed that a bridge had indeed been blown up and the rails removed. This incident proved to be the seed of another China-Japan war, which began with the Japanese military takeover of Manchuria (renaming it Manchukuo in 1932). Fighting between Chinese and Japanese forces continued sporadically during the mid-1930's and finally culminated in Japan's invasion of China in 1937.

We were congratulated on getting through by such a hairsbreadth. How fortunate we had been. We had our English traveling companions to thank for our present safety, and it was very good to be back.

CHAPTER 22

Christmas Seals and Poultices

We received a tremendous welcome from Christians and non-Christians alike when we arrived back in Haiju. Our institutions had flourished during our absence, and with Dr. Ewer's help, there had even been a couple of new cottages added to the Sanatorium.

I laughingly told our welcoming friends that perhaps we should go away again, for much had been accomplished during our brief absence. However, they did not seem to see it that way. We were sincerely glad that they had been able to achieve so much on their own. It would now free me to work on the new dream that had begun to preoccupy my thoughts during our furlough.

As soon as I could I began putting out feelers about the possibility of having a Christmas Seal campaign for Korea. Most of the reaction was indifferent. Some were flatly negative and said that such an idea might be all right in the West but would never work in a "have-not" nation like Korea. They claimed that the idea would be too foreign to Koreans even if they could afford the expense.

I countered by pointing out that stamps had once been foreign to Korea but were now very popular, even in remote villages. The use of greeting cards in Korea was also comparatively new, but the Post Office had reported that the postage revenue on these cards the year before was 247,700 yen ($82,567) and was steadily increasing at a rate of 49,000 yen ($16,667) per year.

We were scheduled to attend a Mission meeting in Seoul which would provide an opportunity to pursue the seal project further. Also the trip would enable me to call on the British Consul General in Seoul, Mr. Oswald White, to see if he could look into the problem of retrieving our lost funds from our Siberian trip.

Mr. White expressed his pleasure that we were safely back, and hoped that we had had a good trip. I related to him how our money had been forcibly taken from us at the Soviet-Manchurian border and how we had been able to secure a receipt from the Soviet border guards, as well as a statement from the Moscow authorities of how much they had given us on our travel refund. While fearing they might be no more than scraps of paper, I had wondered if there would be any chance of getting our money returned.

Mr. White was all attention now and asked to see these "scraps," for he felt sure they would be just what was needed to send to the British ambassador in Moscow. The reason for all this excitement appeared to be that many trans-Siberian travelers like ourselves had suffered similar losses and had been unable to secure any receipts. Thus, when their loss was reported to Moscow, a refund had always been denied. The Soviet authorities claimed that such reports were without foundation, since there had been no documentary evidence. Therefore Mr. White was delighted to have our receipts, for here at last was the proof that was needed. He congratulated us on being able to obtain them. Of course, at the time, we had not realized that extracting a receipt from the Soviets was so unusual.

The sequel to all this, however, did not occur until over two years later, when mysteriously, our credit in the local bank one month rose an amount equivalent to what we had lost on that fateful trans-Siberian trip. Upon inquiring at the bank, all the information that they would divulge was that a man who wished his name withheld had given the *Dai Ichi Ginko* (The First National Bank) this sum and had asked them to have it credited to our account. We never could understand all this secrecy unless it served the purpose of saving face for the Russians. Nevertheless, we were grateful to be reunited with our treasure which we had long ago counted as lost.

While in Seoul, I decided to start the wheels in motion for obtaining a Government permit to issue Christmas Seals, as well as to try to get my first design approved. I was well aware that such matters, especially ones that have no precedent, would take much time in the Orient. I had a good friend in Japanese government circles, Mr. Yasuma Oda, who was English Secretary in the Foreign Affairs Department. I sought his advice and help.

He personally was most sympathetic to the Christmas Seal idea and promised to do all he could to secure the necessary permit to issue the seals. However, when I showed him my proposed design for the first seal, he gave me a flat, "No!"

I had wanted the first seal design to catch the enthusiasm and imagination of the Korean public. Ancient Korea had invented the world's first ironclad battleship and had won a resounding victory over the wooden and less protected ships of the enemy. As English children never tire of hearing about Admiral Lord Horatio Nelson's famous naval victory, so Korean children never tire of hearing their elders tell the story of Admiral Yi Sun Sin and his "tortoise boat," which the Japanese could neither board nor burn. With a fleet of these tortoise shaped armored vessels, Admiral Yi Sun Sin attacked a huge flotilla of Japanese ships in Chinhai Bay in 1592 and drove out the Japanese.

Thus, I had figured that a seal design featuring this armored ship would immediately insure popular support. The salvos from the guns of the armored battleship in this case, however, would be directed against the national enemy, TB. What I had left out of my reckoning were the present overlords of Korea.

As Mr. Oda feelingly pointed out, such a design would be rejected from the start. The enemy in this battle had been Japan's mighty wooden battle fleet. Despite all of Japan's recent victories, the Japanese people still smarted from this historic Korean conquest. It

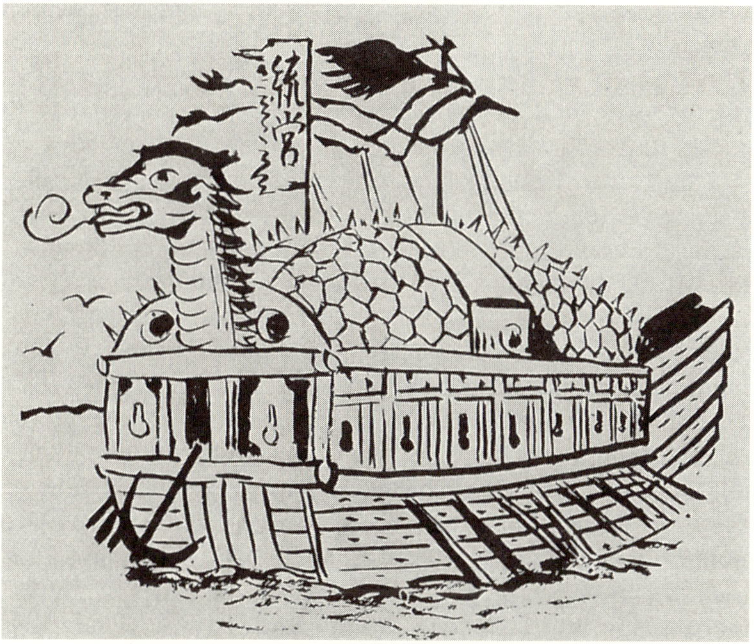

The "Tortoise Boat"–replica of ironclad battleships used by Korea against Japan in Chinhai Bay in 1592

would simply be unrealistic to expect the Japanese authorities to issue a permit for a design which symbolized their defeat at the hands of Korea. Mr. Oda diplomatically suggested that I submit a design that would be pleasing to both sides.

After much thought and consultation with my Korean and Japanese friends, I came up with a safer, though far less dramatic design—the historic Great South Gate of the City Wall of Seoul. This was a familiar landmark to all in Korea. Like the Rock of Gibralter, it represented to the Korean a citadel of strength. In this case, as a Christmas Seal design, it would represent a bulwark against TB.

In due course, thanks to the sincere efforts of Mr. Oda behind the scenes, we had Japanese approval for both the seal campaign and for the design of the first seal. By the fall of 1932, despite the misgivings of many, I felt that the necessary spadework had been done to enable me to launch the Christmas Seal idea for Korea. The introduction of Christmas Seals to this Land of the Morning Calm seemed to be a counterpoint to the introduction of TB seals in the USA. Governor Han was then governor of Whanghai Do. He took the role of a Mr. Hodges, while I, in a manner of speaking, took the role of a Miss Bissell in telling the Governor the Christmas Seal story, Korean style.

The account of the seal pioneers in America and their direct message of good will for the success of a similar experiment in Korea so impressed the Governor that he called a citizens' meeting, which met in the Town Hall of Haiju. In the meantime, I had called on some of the leading citizens to personally insure their attendance at the gathering, as well as to acquaint them with some of the important aspects of the Christmas Seal campaign. I did not want to leave anything to chance for the initial launching of the project. When the seal idea was presented to the representative citizens, I wanted a sufficient number present who were prepared to accept it.

There was good attendance at the meeting and a reasonably favorable response. A Christmas Seal Committee was appointed, with Governor Han as Honorary President and myself as Chairman. The first action of the Committee was to suggest to the Korea Medical Missionary Association that they handle the distribution of the proceeds to those institutions doing special work in TB, for by now several mission hospitals had a TB ward or unit. There was no National Tuberculosis Association at that time and one was not established until many years later.

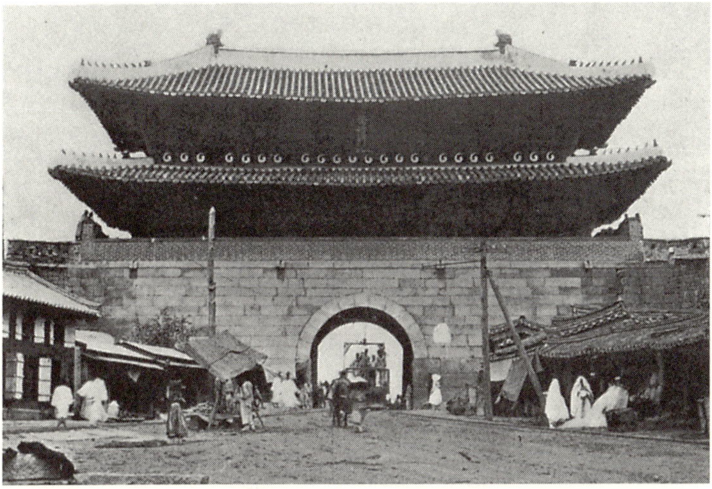

FROM HULBERT, "THE PASSING OF KOREA" (DOUBLEDAY, PAGE)

Great South Gate, Seoul

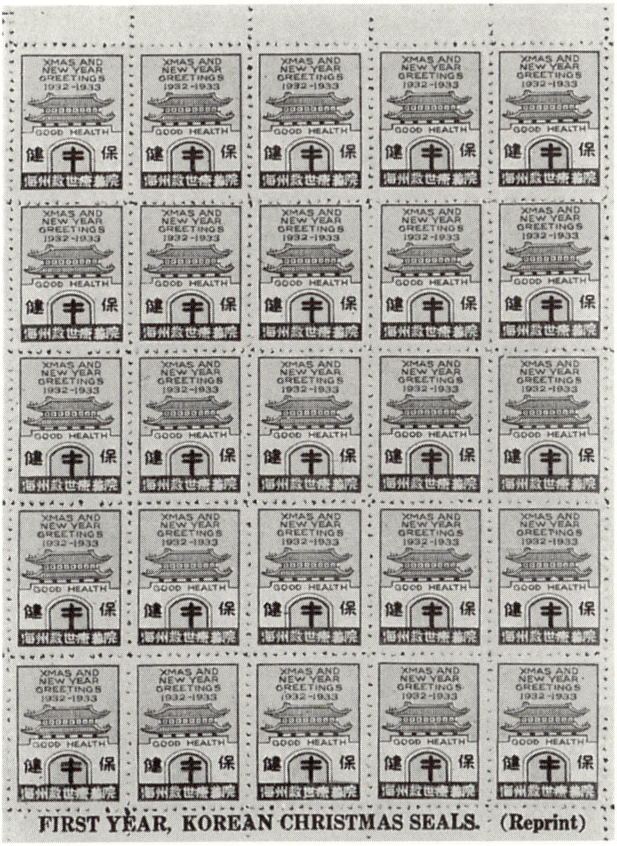

First Korean TB Christmas Seals

Korea's first Christmas Seal campaign, however, was not to be all smooth sailing. At the outset, some misunderstanding arose over our permit and we were ordered to suspend all activities until it could be straightened out. Frustrated and much concerned over the ruinous effect the delay would have on the campaign, I sought Governor Han's help.

After the Governor was finally able to see me and had heard my problem, he replied with an encouraging smile, "Probably it is just some technicality. Leave the matter to me. I will attend to it personally. You need have no fear of the outcome for such a worthy cause. I believe you advocate 'peace of mind' to your patients. Why not take some of your own medicine?"

The Governor proved to be as good as his word, and work on the campaign was resumed.

In the midst of all these pressures, which came in addition to my regular hospital, school, and Sanatorium tasks, I was jolted to awareness of a very important fact of life, namely, that time, tide and even babies do not wait for seal campaigns. Marian was "expecting" and we were to have another baby in our home.

Although Pearl Lund was away, we did have the privilege of being able to secure an expert English nurse, Miss Cooper, who happened to be visiting her brother, the Right Reverend Bishop A. Cecil Cooper. This time, to spare Miss Barlow's feelings, we had informed her earlier than would have been customary about the coming happy event. To our surprise, she seemed genuinely delighted and said that William needed a companion.

Marian had taken a photograph of William, blowing a toy trumpet, to joyfully announce the arrival of his sister or brother, whichever the case might be. This would be inserted later in the birth announcement. Now the stage was about set. I commented to Marian that I was glad that this time there had been no last minute night call to tempt her on a hazardous jitney ride.

Ironically, not long after I had made this remark, an urgent request did come for Marian. This call, she reassured me, was different for it only involved a short trip into the city. To this I could hardly protest.

On Marian's arrival at the home of an obviously well-to-do family, she was led through the courtyard to the women's quarters. After removing her shoes, she entered a poorly lighted and ill ventilated, odorous room, where she found the groaning patient lying on a *yo* (mattress) on the waxed, warm floor. Three months before, according to the patient's history, her seventh baby had "refused to come out," so had been removed bit by bit by crude instruments. The patient now had abdominal symptoms, which caused Marian to fear that peritonitis might have set in. The scaphoid abdomen was tender all over, but it did not show the expected rigidity. Her pulse was rapid and weak and she had fever.

Marian found that in order to make a proper examination, she would have to get down on her knees, since the patient was on the floor. Although this was not easy in Marian's pregnant condition, there was no choice. After Marian had made the necessary physical examination, she advised that the patient be admitted to our hospital for further observation and symptomatic treatment.

It was then that Marian discovered to her amazement that she was the fourth doctor active on this case. Each doctor, however, had been attending and prescribing separately and without the knowledge of the other. The family wanted Marian to join this anonymous group, assuring her that her visits would be timed when none of the other doctors would be present.

Marian, of course, gave an indignant and emphatic, "No thank you!" She further added that since "too many cooks spoil the broth," she was sure that too many doctors might spoil the patient by submitting her to the different types of concoctions each one would be administering.

Marian withdrew rather disgustedly, telling them in no uncertain terms that she would have nothing further to do for the patient unless they agreed to admit her to our hospital and give Marian sole control. This they would not do.

Not long afterwards, Marian received another hurried call to go to the home. They pleaded with Marian, claiming that the patient's abdomen had now grown so distended that her mother had to sit on it to keep it from bursting. This sounded like nonsense. Since Marian did not seem to be impressed, they added that the patient was also severely bleeding from below. Marian realized that this might be an emergency, but again insisted that the patient be admitted at once to the hospital. This they now meekly did.

Surprisingly enough, the patient's bleeding turned out to be her menstrual flow, which stopped the next day. They gave Marian the credit anyway. Since the tympanites (distension of the abdomen due to gas or air in the intestine or peritoneal cavity) soon yielded to treatment, Marian received high praise for being a wonderful doctor. Marian was not so sure the patient was cured for the mysterious abdominal pain persisted. The patient kept begging for an operation which Marian did not think was indicated.

The next morning the nurse came in with the results of an enema given the patient. Lo and behold, the specimen showed a dozen wiggling, separate tapeworm segments, although previous stool examinations had been negative. Marian excitedly called me from my clinic in the adjoining room. In the past, we had of course seen many specimens of the intact tapeworm, but this was the first time we had witnessed these very lively and active segments. These would, at times, elongate and thrust up what seemed to be ventral suckers, as if trying to attach to something.

We began to wonder if perhaps they might be flukes, about which we had studied in London. We decided to give the patient the therapeutic test with "Felix Mase." We soon had our answer, for this treatment resulted in yards and yards of *tania saginata* (tapeworm). On careful examination, we fortunately found its head, for if the head had not come out, it would have continued to grow more segments.

Although the patient seemed impressed when we showed her this lengthy parasite, she still pleaded for an operation, although we tried to assure her that she soon would be well. The family also still seemed skeptical, so Marian thought up an illustration that the Koreans could readily understand.

"When a Korean has managed to acquire wealth, as you have done, no doubt some of your poor relatives wished to take advantage of you, and take up residence with you. They, like the tapeworm," Marian explained, "were uninvited guests who took their food from the host."

We saw by their knowing smiles that the illustration was hitting home. Marian turned to the husband and continued, "While your wife was well, she could harbor this worm without serious symptoms, but when sickness came, she could only support this uninvited guest with difficulty."

The husband saw the point immediately.

Soon after this episode, Marian began to have abdominal pains of her own. Although I tried to reassure myself that I was now used to delivering my own offspring, I was not entirely nonchalant.

However, everything went beautifully. On October 8, 1932, at 5:45 P.M. Marian presented me with another fine baby boy, and

William had the companion of his choice. We named our second son Joseph Keightley, after his maternal grandparents. In due course, at another impressive ceremony, he was baptized by our good friend, Mr. W. A. Noble.

Our non-Christian friends, who looked upon sons as paid up insurance policies, congratulated us in the Oriental way as they exclaimed, "How fortunate you are! Now you will have two sons to worship at your graves, and offer your departed spirits food at the polished stone tables there. You will also have daughters-in-law to slave for you during your lifetime. May it be a long one!"

These Korean friends thought we now had the status symbol of choice—sons. It is true we had no daughter yet, but time was on our side. Among the Koreans, however, the prevalent idea was that daughters did not count. In fact, when asking a Korean how many children he had, he would proudly enumerate the number of his sons but fail to even mention his daughters. When asked about the adorable girls, clinging to his ballooned out trousers, he would invariably reply, "Those? They are only girls, to be betrothed at an early age and automatically removed from our household." As an afterthought, he might add, "I suppose they are really a financial loss, for I shall have to provide for their dowry, according to my wealth. You can be glad you have no such liability."

I could now turn my attention back to the Christmas Seal Campaign activities which had been so abruptly, but agreeably, interrupted. At this point, many of my Korean friends, and even some others, were strongly opposed to my branching out any further. They would often ask me, "Why do you want to assume any more responsibility and take on that crazy Christmas Seal project, which no one really wants? If you fail, who will reimburse you? You surely must have enough headaches with a school, a hospital, and a fledgling sanatorium still in the experimental stage and hardly on its financial feet. You are already spreading yourself out very thin. If you should crack up under the pressures, what will happen to your growing family?"

There were those who still insisted that Korea was not ready for such a seal campaign. The country was not at all happy over its domination by Japan and the Koreans could think or talk of little else. The chief preoccupation was not on health matters but on how they might achieve independence. All other causes were relegated to the background. Tuberculosis was an age old problem and the general feeling was that little could be done about it. Surely there were more pressing problems.

The average Korean still viewed TB as a shameful disease that fate had decreed for those who had offended the evil spirits. Rather than buying TB Christmas Seals, it would be better for the afflicted ones to placate the evil spirits by casting a few stones on a pile beneath a special "spirit tree" or by tying a bit of red cloth on its branches. If there was no result from this effort, it would clearly indicate that the sick were doomed. Why interfere with fate when those who did might receive a worse punishment?

Such talk made me fume with indignation. No, in the face of these attitudes I simply could not remain silent and passive. I had to try to help change the old entrenched ideas about TB, as well as the unsympathetic and cruel behavior, both toward the TB patient, and now, toward the ex-TB patient.

Treatment was always more appealing and dramatic than prevention, but it simply was not getting at the root cause of the trouble. If the TB education campaigns were directed especially to the younger

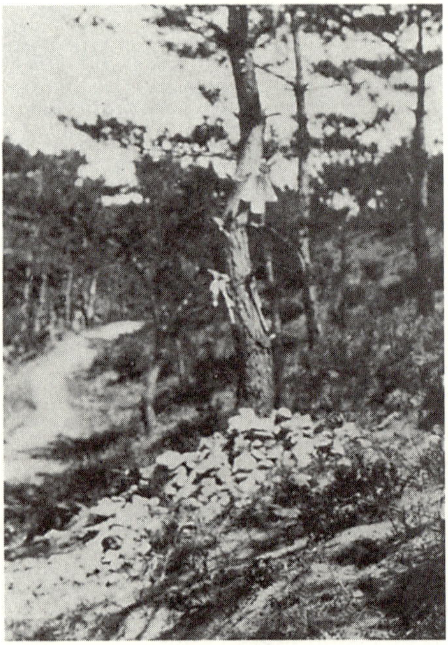

"Spirit tree" on the path to Sanatorium–red cloth tied to branch, or stone cast at base to placate evil spirits

generation, who would be more receptive to new ideas, perhaps the eradication of this disease was not an impossible goal.

The Christmas Seal Committee had appointed three doctors, two pastors, and two laymen, all voluntary workers, to carry the Christmas Seal message to all the provinces of Korea. I had been cautioned by Mr. Jacobs in New York that correct timing was vital in Christmas Seal promotion. The seals must not arrive at their destination either too early or too late. Already there had been delays due to the necessity of a change of design and the question over the permit. Now another postponement threatened.

My desire for a representative committee of the various missions in Korea to sponsor and distribute the Christmas Seals had not taken into account the time element required for each mission to give its respective approval to the endeavor. The deadline for the printing was fast approaching. I feared that we might have to repeat the history of both Denmark and the U.S.A. and have the first Korean seal issued only by our Haiju Sanatorium.

This turned out to be the case. I was especially eager to get our very first seal out on time, and considered it unwise to wait any longer. Reluctantly I issued orders for the printing to start, with the name of the Haiju Sanatorium imprinted on the bottom of the sheet of seals as the sponsor. The first edition of the Korean seals was issued on December 3, 1932, and our first purchaser was the Rev. Henry D. Appenzeller of Paichai Haktang (Paichai High School). Before many seals got off the press, I received the sanction of the individual missions. I was then able to have the Haiju Sanatorium name deleted from all subsequent printings.

The question arose of how best to dispose of those few remaining sheets of seals with the Haiju Sanatorium imprint. The Seal Committee decided that, under the circumstances, rather than waste such seals, it would be best for me to send them to the U.S.A. for the special benefit of the Haiju Sanatorium patrons. As time was of the essence for mailing seals to our patrons abroad, this was done at once. (Seals so marked are now rare and have been highly prized by collectors.)

The Christmas Seal Committee's initial team of workers began spreading the Christmas Seal message in early December and the last group did not return until late February after the Korean New Year. We found that the Koreans preferred to use the seals for Korean New Year which occurred in February and therefore, more were sold to Koreans after Christmas than before.

The teams traveled as far as Fusan in the South, and to Songjin in the North. They had distributed seals and told the Christmas Seal story to over 9,000 students and almost 3,000 adults. At every location, leaflets telling about TB and its prevention had been sold at cost. Our Committee felt that the public health education aspect of the campaign was even more important than raising money. Our own staff member, Dr. M. K. Moon, gave his full time to the students. He was a natural orator and knew how to effectively arouse the students to action.

The Committee gave me the task of contacting the editors of various leading newspapers and periodicals throughout the country to persuade them to print articles on the campaign. The assignment also included encouraging companies to donate advertising space to the cause. I was also expected to contact as many of the foreign residents as possible and gain their sympathetic cooperation.

From the first, it was fully realized that our small group of workers could not hope to reach the whole of Korea, except as we could stimulate interest and encourage other volunteers to carry the Christmas Seal message to remote regions and to other groups. In this we proved more successful than we could ever have anticipated at the time.

One very significant result of the campaign was the keen interest manifested by the patients of our Sanatorium and their earnest desire to help and to participate in every way possible. The patients repeatedly beseeched me for permission to go out and do personal work for the cause. Of course this could not be granted. However, each one of our patients who was able wrote letters to his friends in various parts of Korea. Our Christian patients organized prayer groups to pray for the success of the campaign.

The patients themselves succeeded in securing some sizeable gifts for TB work in addition to selling many Christmas Seals. Although a great many "seal letters" were sent out by our Committee to prominent Koreans, except for those which the patients personally had sent out, returns were negligible. We did receive some heartening mail such as this letter from a Korean:

> "I am writing you, hoping I can help the great cause. You may wonder why I am so interested. Well, the simple reason is that while in the United States, I came down with TB after graduating from Princeton and took the cure at a sanatorium

near there. So I am especially glad that, at last, Korea is also having this chance. Please send me many more seals to sell."

We also received a few letters in quite another vein, which showed us that we had hardly scratched the surface. One, especially, startled us:

> "I have bought the stamps you have advertised for helping TB sufferers. These stamps I have faithfully pasted on my chest as a poultice, night after night, but this plaster has not helped my terrible cough the least bit. I demand my money back."

Another letter written in Korean script read:

> "Please send some of that wonderful Christmas Seal medicine everybody is talking about. I shall pay you whatever the price is."

And still another read as follows:

> "Please send me some of those Christmas Seal tickets for free admission to your Sanatorium. I have a number of friends who want to go."

The trial balloon of our first Christmas Seal campaign could not be boasted about as an outstanding financial success. Nevertheless, after expenses had been met, we were able to turn in 350 yen ($117) for the Korean Medical Missionary Association to distribute. They had organized a Tuberculosis Committee to decide how this should be done and various mission bodies doing work in Korea on TB received the funds as follows:

Fifty yen each to tuberculosis units at Union Christian Hospital, Pyong Yang; Church of England Hospital at Yoju; and United Church of Canada Hospital at Hamheung; 75 yen to the Tuberculosis Ward of Severance Union Hospital, Seoul; and 75 yen to the Haiju School of Hygiene for the Tuberculous. Thirty yen was set aside for getting out TB literature and 20 yen towards research and laboratory work.

Most of the distributed funds were used to support charity patients who otherwise could not have received treatment.

In view of the fact that the campaign had been held up by the difficulties surrounding the permit, and that the idea was brand new to the Koreans, we felt that the results were most satisfactory. We had learned much that could be applied with benefit throughout the ensuing year and on the next campaign. We hoped to issue the next seals in October so that they would be out in plenty of time for Christmas mails abroad. We also hoped to do more in the way of TB literature printed in the Japanese vernacular for Japanese residents of Korea.

Korea's first Christmas Seal campaign had met with enough success that the Korea Medical Missionary Association agreed to take it over if I would continue to serve as Chairman of the Seal Committee. The Korean TB seals were the only tuberculosis seals in the world under missionary auspices. Much hard work lay ahead. There was the business of getting out more anti-TB literature, arranging press and radio interviews, lectures on TB, to say nothing of getting out the next seal design.

Since the inspiration for introducing the TB Christmas Seal idea to Korea had come from the United States, it seemed appropriate to me that a U.S. seal design should likewise inspire a Korean counterpart. The 1932 American seal depicted a boy and girl Christmas caroling in the snow. Since a carol is a song of praise or joy, caroling seemed to be a fitting symbol for our next Korean TB Christmas Seal—singing out good news of prospects for health to an afflicted nation. Mr. Philip Jacobs supported my suggestion and in behalf of the National Tuberculosis Association in America gave approval for the U.S. design to serve as a model. A staff artist at the Y.M.C.A. Press in Seoul was able to transform the American holiday snow scene to a Korean setting with Korean children singing the songs of celebration.

The 80,000 square miles of Korea were divided into thirteen provinces. There were mission schools in each province with important colleges in Pyong Yang and Seoul. Most of the white foreign residents in Korea were already familiar with the seal idea from their own respective countries. Many of the teachers had lost some of the best students in their schools to the ravages of TB. With the mandate from the Medical Association, an organization widely respected, I would try to enlist the support of these educators. If they became

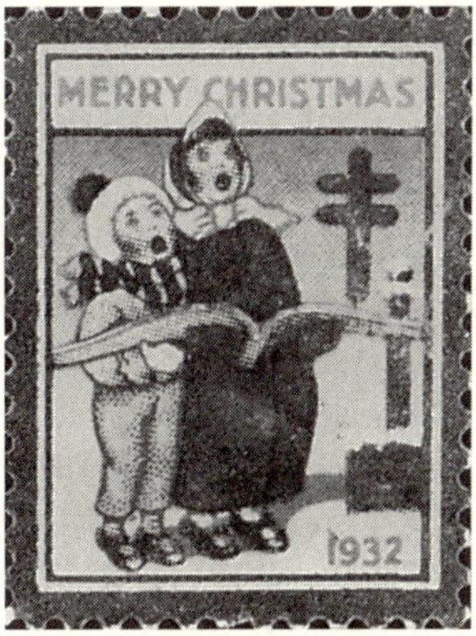

The 1932 U.S. TB Christmas Seal used as a model for the 1934-35 Korean Seal

enthusiastic, their zeal might fire their students with similar determination. This in turn might spark a flame in the more progressive elders. It had to become a chain reaction that would spread and grow into a worthwhile conflagration from city to village, from valley to mountain, in all of this beloved land.

Could the teachers be inspired? They already felt the pressure of too much work, caused by too few teachers and too many students. They might not take kindly to someone from outside telling them what to do. No doubt some would tell me, as a doctor, to mind my own business and they would mind theirs. Similar types of attitudes might be encountered in other groups, and even among the overworked doctors and nurses of the crowded mission hospitals. But the whole-hearted cooperation of all was a must if the project was even to get off first base. I saw it as a tremendous challenge.

There were only a few radios and, of course, no television at the time, so instant news communication was not available. Therefore, I had to depend on personal contact and the printed word, which latter ran the risk of being thrown into the waste paper basket. As in all new endeavors, inertia and skepticism were obstacles to overcome.

First, I engaged Korean artists to prepare an attractive and appealing series of anti-TB posters to be presented to the heads of the various leading schools and hospitals throughout Korea. I felt that even the most reluctant would not object to getting these posters for display in their respective institutions. The parcels would be clearly marked, "Gift, for free distribution." Then, before there had been time for them to lose interest, a brief follow-up circular letter would be sent. Where possible, personal letters would be mailed to key people to the effect that Christmas Seals were to be sent out soon, offering prizes to those institutions, according to category, securing the best sales. Mention would be made of the availability of simple anti-TB literature and progress report forms. It was felt by our Committee that a nominal price should be charged for the booklets to be sure they would be read. This would also help to defray expenses.

With our family expanding, we had decided to move to the larger brick house on the hill. Furthermore, I needed more office space to accommodate the increased paraphanalia connected with the seal campaigns. This office became a beehive of activity, and William would often join us to help with such tasks as stuffing envelopes or tying up parcels of seals.

The new Governor of Whanghai Do, Governor Won Chong Kyo, kindly agreed to officially open our next campaign. He called a public meeting and there was an especially good turnout to see and hear the new Governor. He began his address with what seemed to be anything but a cheerful note for Christmas. He said, "It is the Government policy to discourage extravagant funerals."

It seemed to be a semi-political address, and I wondered if I had failed to convey to him the spirit of the Christmas Seal idea which I had wanted him to give to the gathering. But as he warmed to his subject, I could see that my concern had been ill founded, for he went on to say:

> "Tens of thousands of yen are being spent in Chosen [Korea] for the funeral expenses of the tuberculous, but only a few yen are being spent for the prevention and cure of TB. The purchase of TB Christmas Seals should not be considered an act of charity, but rather a means of obtaining health insurance for the buyer, his family and his own community. Therefore, I consider it a great privilege to open this historic campaign which will help prevent needless funerals."

Copies of the Governor's pertinent address were sent to all on our mailing list, since it would strengthen their hand in enlisting other volunteers to help sell the seals. Soon progress reports and orders began to flood our office from all parts of Korea, and a few were received from Japan, China and Manchukuo. The seal idea was definitely catching on.

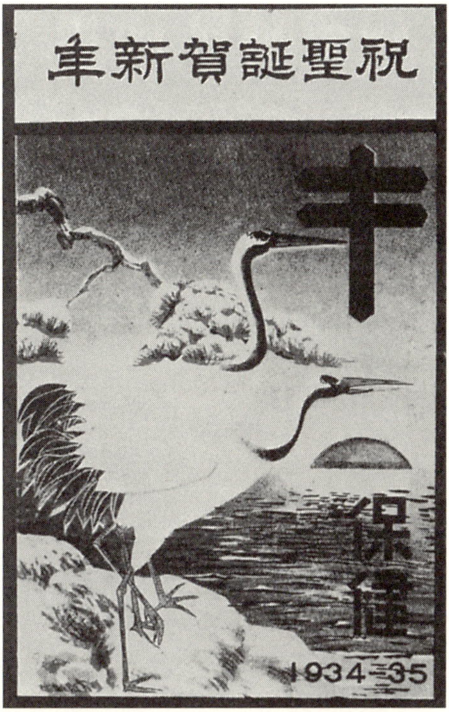

Anti-TB post-card–storks, Korean symbol of long life

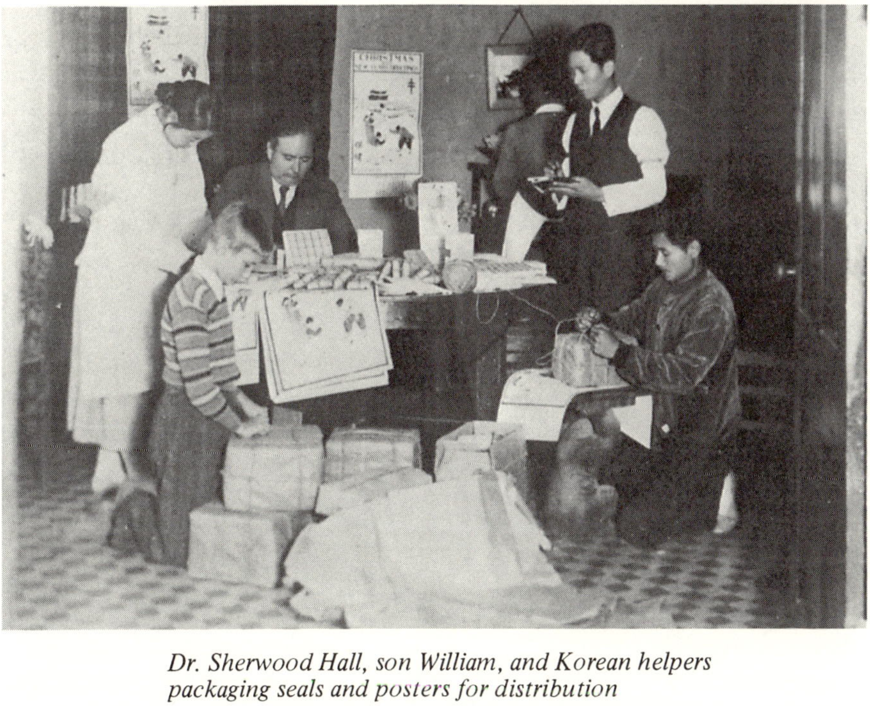

Dr. Sherwood Hall, son William, and Korean helpers packaging seals and posters for distribution

It was heartening to receive letters in our daily mail such as those below:

> "The design is most attractive. Mrs. Peters is an enthusiastic local leader and we have had a good rally. We are with you 100%."
>
> Marie Church

> "I enclose my check to help this pioneer TB seal work along. We are intensely interested in this splendid project. God bless and prosper it."
>
> (Bishop) Herbert Welch

> "I showed to a large group the international death rate graph, which you depict on the back of your health tract. There was a noticeable stir when they saw Korea's TB death rate was the highest. One of the girls in our school died of TB this week, and another is ill with it. It should make them think, and buy the seals."
>
> Allen Clark

> "Enclosed is a check for Yen 340 from the sale of seals. I am glad the Koreans are taking such a keen interest in it."
>
> Ada Sandell

> "The Pyong Yang Foreign School (which your mother helped found) is 100/120 strong helping sell the seals."
>
> Anna S. Dorriss

> "I am writing you unasked, but it is from deep interest in this thing you are doing for all Korea. I want to help you all I can. Wishing the cause every success."
>
> W. A. Wilbur

Not all the letters were so encouraging. Some said that they felt the poor Koreans should not be asked to contribute from their slender means and that everyone had enough burdens of their own without assuming any additional ones. However, such letters were surprisingly few, and year after year the campaigns gained popularity and momentum. In response to this reception, we developed for sale, in addition to the seals, matching Christmas cards, poster-size reproductions, calendars, post-cards, and even jigsaw puzzles.

Although the still-life scenes depicted on the first three seals were well received, I felt that our next seal design should have more animation and color. I conceived the idea of developing a series which would depict games and sports of Korean children, with a different one selected each year. Included in the series were designs to show kite-flying, playing shuttle-cock with the feet, spinning tops on ice, jumping on a see-saw Korean fashion, and swinging in the typically standing position.

Well known artists now came forward to offer their services. Among these was an English artist, Miss Elizabeth Keith. Miss Keith had spent ten years in the Orient from 1915 to 1925 studying Oriental design. She was particularly interested in learning how to make wood block prints from the Japanese who were considered experts in the technique. She often visited Korea and made several trips there in the 1930's, making my mother's home in Seoul her headquarters, as before. Miss Keith designed two of the seals and Mr. Watanabe, a famous Japanese creator of wood block prints, cut the blocks from her sketches for matching Christmas cards.

Two other seals were designed by a young Korean artist in his late 20's, Mr. Ki-Chang Kim, who had been deaf and dumb since the age of four. He had studied under such leading contemporary Korean artists as Mr. Y. M. Pack, and Mr. Eun-ho Kim, and his seal designs were made into wood block print Christmas cards by Mr. S. Sato. Mr. S. Y. Choi, a Korean artist from Pyong Yang, and the Reverend Esmond W. New, a missionary of the Australian Presbyterian Mission in Korea, contributed the designs for two more seals.

In dealing with the artists who were submitting their proposed designs, I sometimes found them a difficult group with whom to work. Their feelings were sensitive and easily hurt. I often discovered that I was lacking in proper diplomacy, for it seemed each artist needed a different approach, particularly if his design was not accepted. However, when these kinks were finally ironed out, I was pleased with the final results. Our patrons, too, seemed to respond favorably to the series and were generous in their compliments and financial contributions.

Each campaign represented a significant step toward the control of tuberculosis. I was glad I had not surrendered to the arguments of the skeptics but had gone ahead in pursuit of the goal of a Christmas Seal program in Korea.

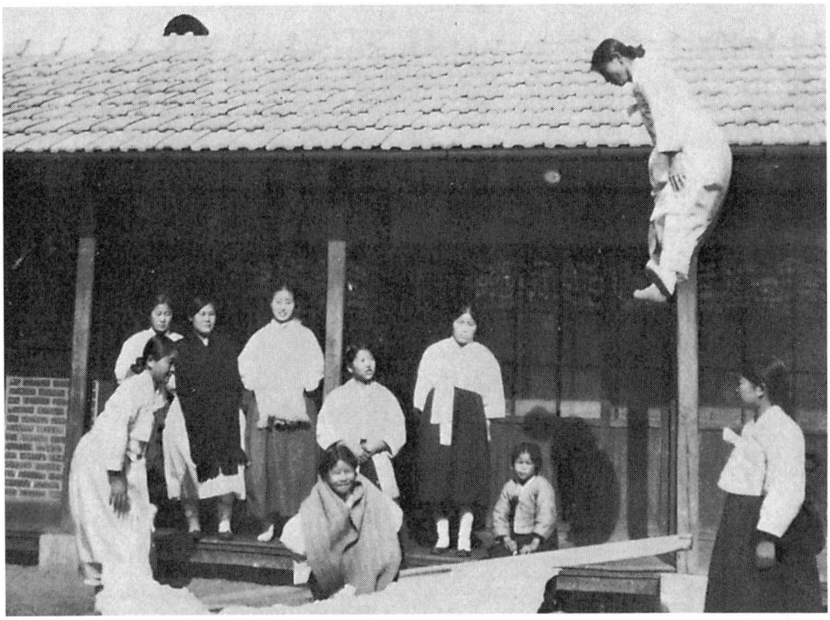

Korean girls playing see-saw

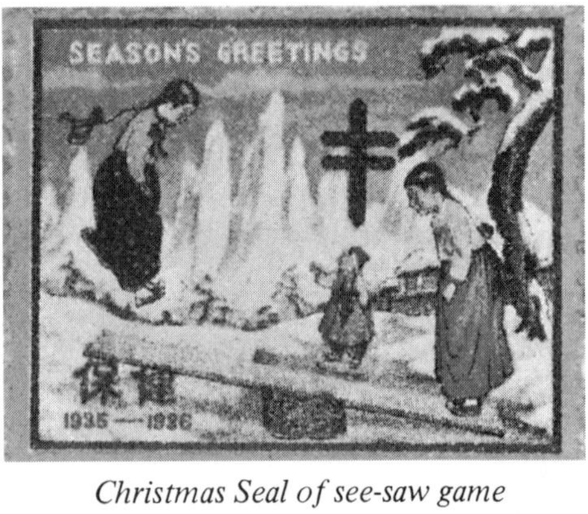

Christmas Seal of see-saw game

Tuberculosis Christmas Seals

of

Korea

Photographs Courtesy of Smithsonian Institution

Magnification 2x

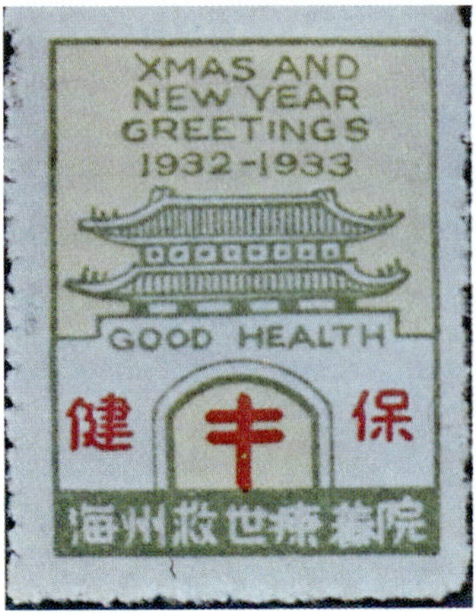

1932-33
Y.M.C.A. staff artist

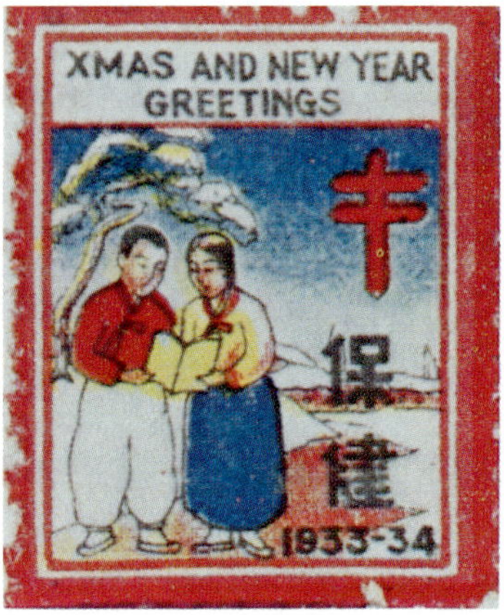

1933-34
Y.M.C.A. staff artist

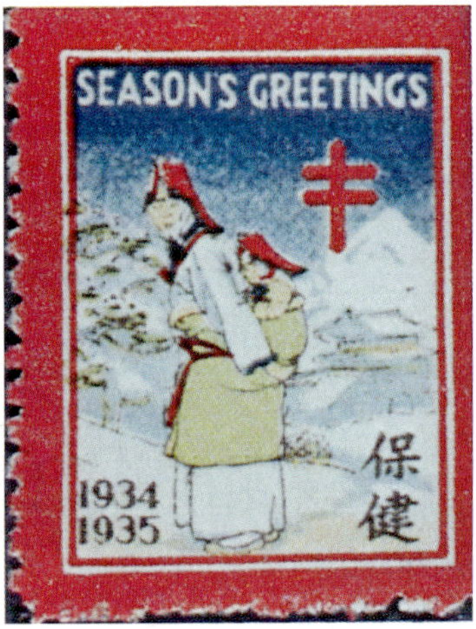

1934-35
Elizabeth Keith, artist

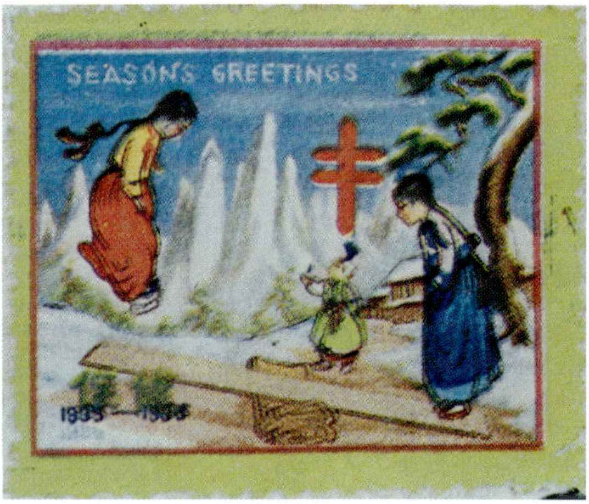

1935-36
S. Y. Choi, artist

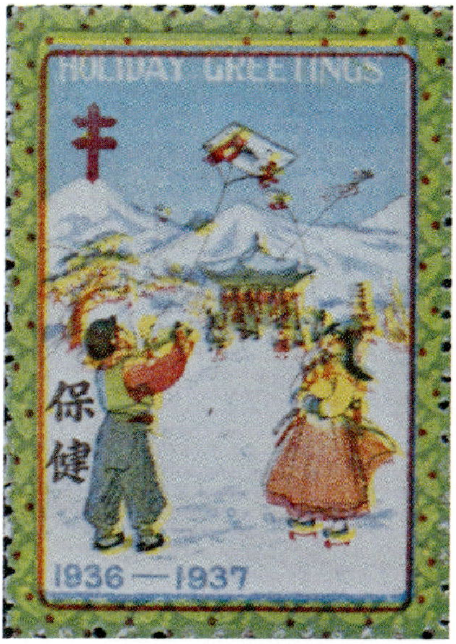

1936-37
Elizabeth Keith, artist

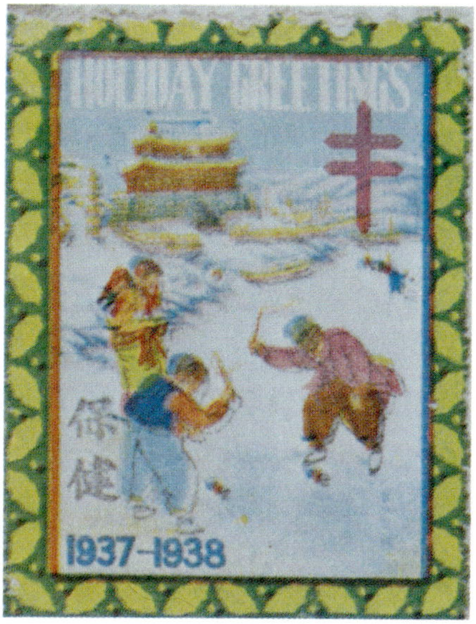

1937-38
Kim Ki-Chang, artist

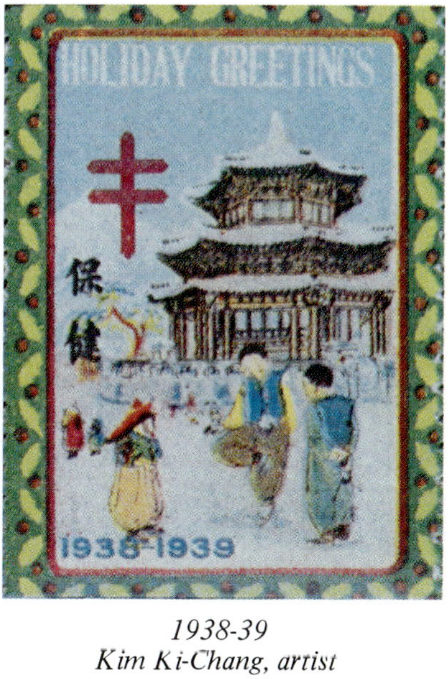

1938-39
Kim Ki-Chang, artist

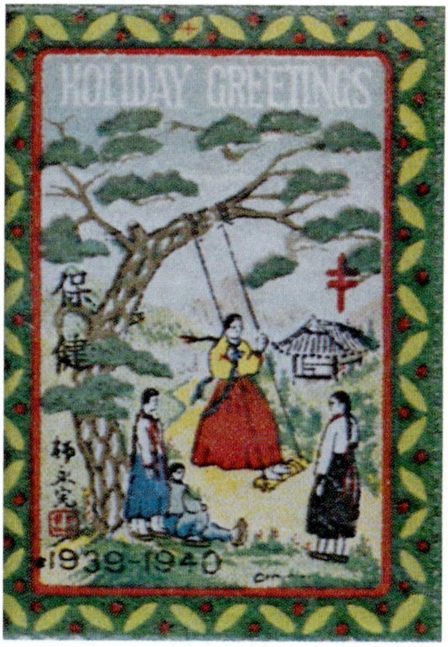

1939-40
The Rev. Esmond W. New, artist

CHAPTER 23

Landmarks

The Sanatorium continued to grow, strengthened by the seal campaigns. The initial eight-bed capacity had been expanded to accommodate over 60 patients, whose longer average length of stay at the institution was due in part to the public health education program that accompanied the distribution of the TB Christmas Seals. Most patients were by now convinced that their old snake soup cure was dangerous, the fresh deer blood useless, and that a long period of rest and treatment at a sanatorium was more effective.

Several attractive cottages had been added to the Sanatorium complex. As the Sanatorium grew, more and more young people were admitted. This caused a new kind of complication and concern.

Unlike the West, where mingling of the sexes was freer, in the Orient of that era such freedom was frowned upon. A girl became immediately suspect after any socializing. This could even prevent her future marriage, especially if there was any suspicion of physical involvement. A boy, however, could escape social censure with no serious consequences to his future. The decent Oriental girl of that day was very shy and reticent and instinctively very careful. It was the boys we found hard to control.

One of our male patients had been reported to the staff on several occasions for his advances toward a female patient. Even after repeated warnings, he showed no sign of mending his ways. Therefore, I had no choice but to discharge him. This would at least spare the girl. The youth in question happened to be very popular with the young male patients who sprang to his defense. I refused to yield.

Usually I finished my Sanatorium rounds by noon and then went home for lunch. As I concluded my rounds one morning, I left the main building by way of the male ward solarium as was my custom. Suddenly I heard the door slam shut behind me. I tried the exit door and found it was locked. I was astonished to find myself a prisoner in my own sanatorium.

In response to my call for help I heard angry voices outside the bolted door and soon learned that I had not been locked in the solarium by accident. Several of the male patients spoke to me through the closed door and voiced their grievance. They demanded that I reinstate the patient I had dismissed for his incorrigible behavior. They declared that they would not release me until I had agreed to rescind the discharge order.

I refused to do this, but I asked for the chance to explain to them more fully the reason for my decision. At first they would not listen and kept repeating, "Don't discharge him."

It was now after the patients' lunch hour and very few of the supervising staff would be on duty during the rest period which normally followed. Marian would just think that I must have been detained on a case, for I was often late for lunch. The patients certainly had chosen the best time for their purpose. My forced detention all seemed very silly and I felt the whole situation was quite absurd but they treated it as no laughing matter. How was it best to handle this totally unexpected dilemma?

I knew that at 4:00 P.M. the nurses would make their rounds to take temperatures. I even felt my own temperature rising. It looked as if I would have to wait it out until one of the nurses gave the alarm. After what seemed like ages to me, the leader unlocked the door and came in, although he stood defiantly in front of the exit. I could have perhaps forcibly shoved him aside but I knew it was never wise for a Westerner to manhandle an Oriental. So I decided to play it cool and try to talk my way out.

At first he did not seem to be listening, and I felt that I was just wasting my breath. Finally, one of my phrases registered with him when I said, "I was discharging the patient for your sake."

Somehow, that caught his attention and curiosity, for he blurted out, "What do you mean?"

This gave me the opening I needed. I then had the chance to explain how fatal it could be for a TB patient to indulge his emotions physically, especially as related to sex. If his friend got away with it for a time, others might be tempted to follow his bad example. This would result in quickly undoing the healing progress they had all worked so hard to attain.

I realized that my audience was hardly in the frame of mind to listen to a lecture on religion or moral values, but somehow my message got through. The spokesman apologized and stopped blocking the doorway. He also asked me to please tell no one what they had done. To this I readily agreed, for I realized my own dignity was also at stake. I was still feeling rather ridiculous and had no desire to lose any more face.

On a small scale, the Sanatorium Farm had become a reality. In developing this project, we were fortunate to have as our consultant a Northern Presbyterian agricultural missionary, Mr. Dexter N. Lutz. Mr. Lutz had come to Korea in 1920 and had initiated agricultural missionary service to rural Korea. He would come to our Sanatorium and give lectures which offered practical instruction on such topics as: soil analysis, the better use of land, especially on hills, growing fruits and vegetables, in addition to information on dairy farming and animal husbandry. Farmers from the surrounding rural area would be invited to attend these seminars.

The interest generated by these sessions and our own small effort begun in this area convinced me that a demonstration center was urgently needed. My dream of the farm and model village rehabilitation center for our convalescing patients persisted.

The men and women just regaining health could work in such a center for as many hours a day as strength permitted. They would be paid for their labor. Besides being housed comfortably, and under medical supervision, they would be receiving instruction in scientific farming, poultry raising, sericulture, carpentry, and handicrafts. No patient would leave the model village until he was thoroughly strong physically, self-confident mentally, and had mastered whatever line of work in which he had chosen to specialize. I estimated that the average length of occupation would be about two years.

As if in direct answer to prayer, we were blessed with an unexpected opportunity. Mr. J. C. Penney, founder of the Penney's Chain Stores in the United States, had a fine model farm in Florida under the expert management of Mr. F. O. Clark. Mr. Penney had agreed to loan Mr. Clark to the Korean Y.M.C.A. to introduce modern agricultural techniques to Korea. On learning of this, I wrote to Mr. Penney and to the "Y" about the possibility of establishing a similar model farm and village at the Haiju Sanatorium. I received an enthusiastic and favorable response from both.

It seemed that at the same time the farm and village project was developing in my mind, the Y.M.C.A. was considering the establishment of an agricultural demonstration center in some central location in Korea. At that time, prevailing methods of agriculture in Korea were primitive. Crude plows barely scratched the soil before the seed was put in, and scientific crop rotation was unknown. To their proposed demonstration center the Y.M.C.A. planned to bring interested farmers from all over Korea, teach them how to get the best results out of their land, and send them home to show their neighbors how things should be done.

When I wrote to Mr. Penney and the Y.M.C.A., my proposal happened to coincide very naturally with what had been their plan. The patients at the Sanatorium came from all over Korea and were just such a representative group as the "Y" itself might have chosen. Many were admitted to the Sanatorium because of their qualities of leadership. Their minds and attitudes were right to make the most of the vocational instruction and to teach others.

The Y.M.C.A., therefore, made its proposition to the Sanatorium: "If you can buy enough land, build your model village, and show us that you intend to make this project worthwhile, we will supply the stock, seed and fertilizer, and pay the salaries of the two men needed to supervise the farm and village."

This seemed too good to be true. The Sanatorium already had a twenty-five acre parcel of land which helped to supply food to the patients. I set about at once to raise the funds to purchase the one hundred adjoining acres that were available and that were varied enough to be ideal for experimentation. This especially appealed to the "Y". There were fields and orchards, mountain land (one whole mountain, in fact), and rice land. The great variety of crops that could be grown offered a practical advantage to the student-convalescent also, for he would be able to specialize in the sort of thing most useful to him when he returned to his home.

Mr. Clark came to us and helped in designing and constructing the farm buildings which were to be well stocked with high grade milk cows, Swiss goats, Belgian hares and white leghorn chickens. Not only would the farm provide occupation and education for the convalescents, but, in turn, would furnish fresh food at cheap prices to the patients in the Sanatorium.

What a chain of events the tragedy of Hyung's experience had set in motion! Hopefully it would deter like tragedies for his fellow Koreans in the future. Much still remained to be done, however, in the area of educating the Korean public to receiving ex-TB patients

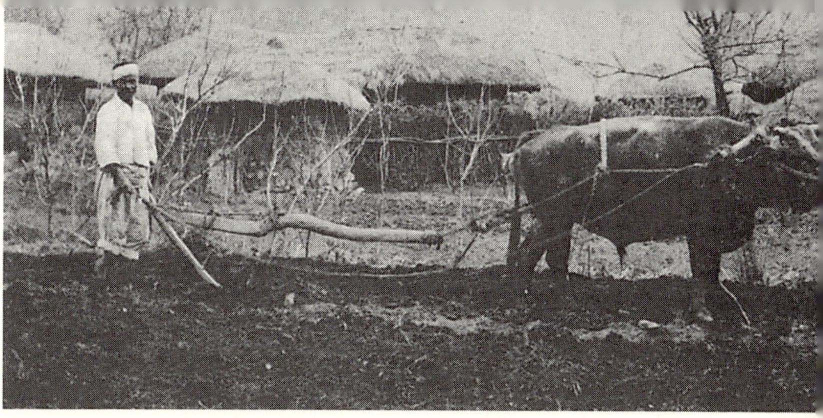

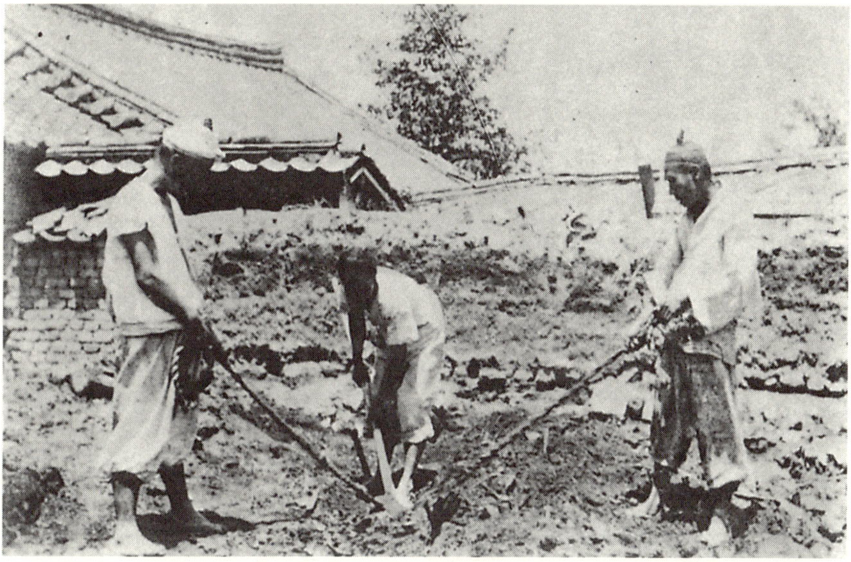

Korean ploughing (top); "three-man power shovel" (bot.)

back into the community and restoring them to happy useful citizens.

Mr. J. C. Penney had been following the progress of our Sanatorium Farm Project with increased interest, much to the delight of our "Y" friends, and especially Mr. Clark. Mr. Penney himself now saw this urgent need for extending the Farm Project to include a "Rehabilitation Center." To our great joy, he helped to make it financially possible.

While Mr. Clark directed the farm activities, Mr. Lutz, our missionary consultant, supervised the model village. His experience with model Indian villages in the United States proved particularly helpful. As a result of the work of these two experts, the Sanatorium Farm was extending its service both as a rehabilitation center and as a teaching center. Ex-patients and village farmers were showing con-

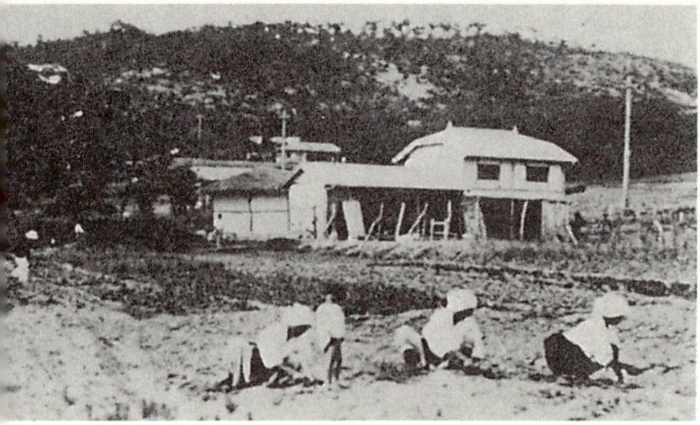

Sanatorium Farm

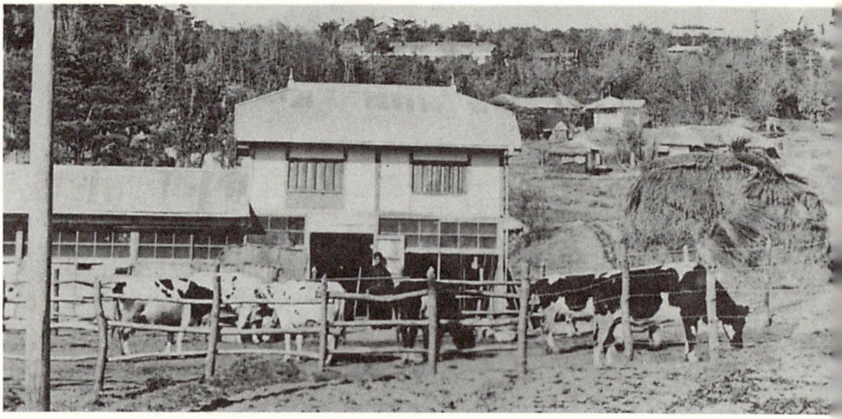

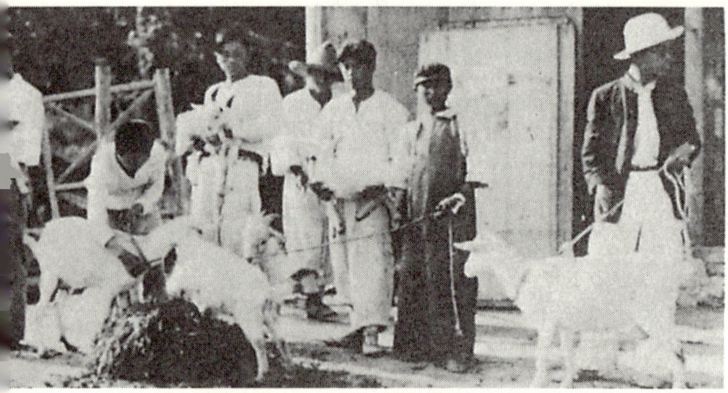

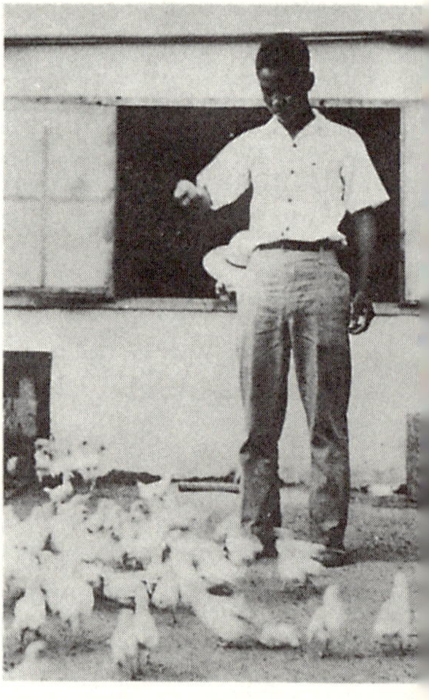

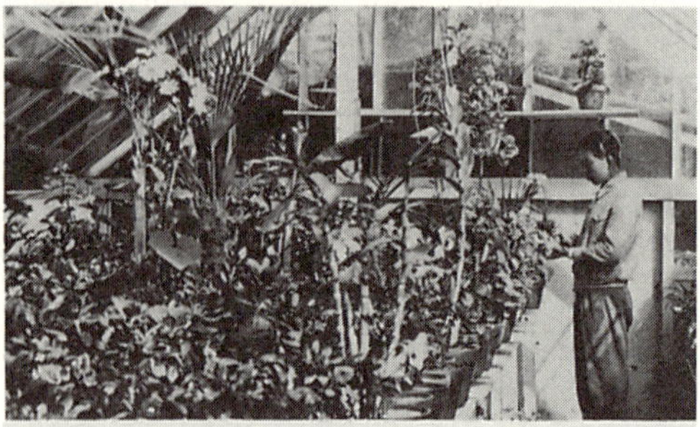

siderable aptitude in learning the modern methods of farming. A trucking service was initiated to carry garden supplies to a small store at Sorai Beach, only fifty miles distant, offering fresh provisions to the missionary summer vacationers there.

From the first, however, we knew the Sanatorium would never be complete without a chapel. This was very much in our hearts and prayers. It became still more pressing as our reception room became far too small to accommodate our increased load of patients and staff for the worship services usually held there.

Thus, I was led to appeal to another cousin, Mrs. Harold Moore (Mary Crary), the sister of Grace Crary Haskins. Cousin Mary was blessed with good works, which her wealth enabled her to better carry out. While we were on our furlough, Cousin Mary had invited us to stay with her at her lovely home in Denver, Colorado. Marian had taken movies of our work in Haiju and showed them to the members of Cousin Mary's church during our visit there. At that time I had voiced our need for funds for the construction of a chapel. My request fell on good soil.

Cousin Mary shared our dream of building a Sanatorium chapel and gave the largest single gift ($10,000) that we received for the work. Because she had long admired my mother, she requested that the chapel be named "The Rosetta Chapel."

Although I had had some experience in hospital planning and construction, building a chapel was beyond my depth. However, when I discussed my ideas with an architect who was visiting Korea at the time, he seemed to feel that what I envisioned was entirely feasible and would be in harmony with the landscape.

I had explored with him the possibility of utilizing the distinctively marked, rounded stones that could be found nearby along the seashore. He agreed that the stones would be more attractive than the usual brick, especially if set off by a red tile roof which would provide dramatic contrast to the evergreens on the mountainside.

Mr. Edwin L. Campbell, who had done the blueprints for our other buildings at the Sanatorium, drew up the design for the chapel accordingly. We contracted with a builder, Mr. C. Y. Mah, to construct it.

It turned out to be one of the loveliest chapels in Korea, and what is more, commanded a superb view of mountain and sea. We felt we had been true to the spirit of John Ruskin when he wrote:

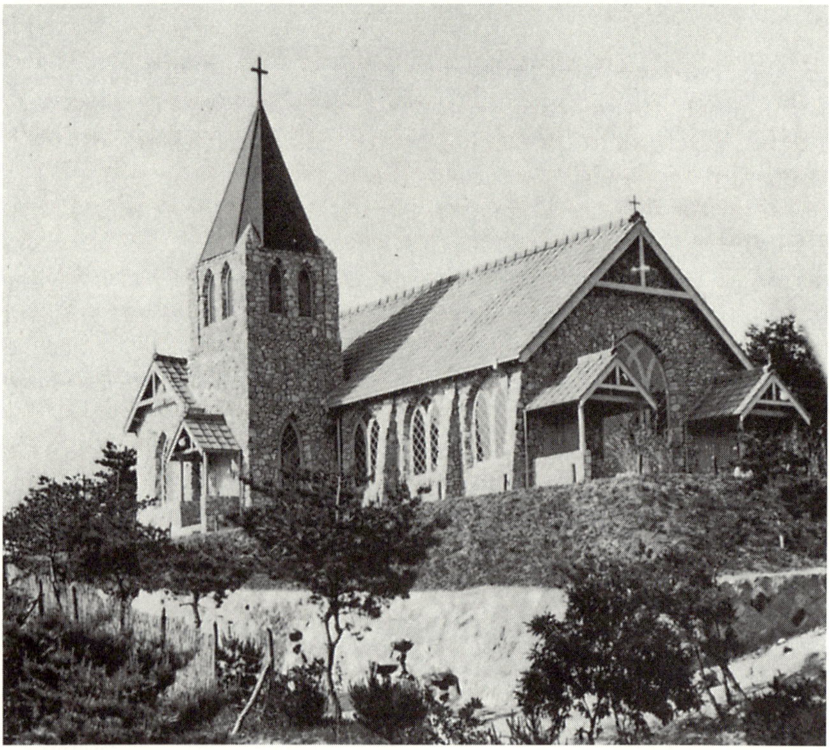

The Rosetta Chapel, Haiju

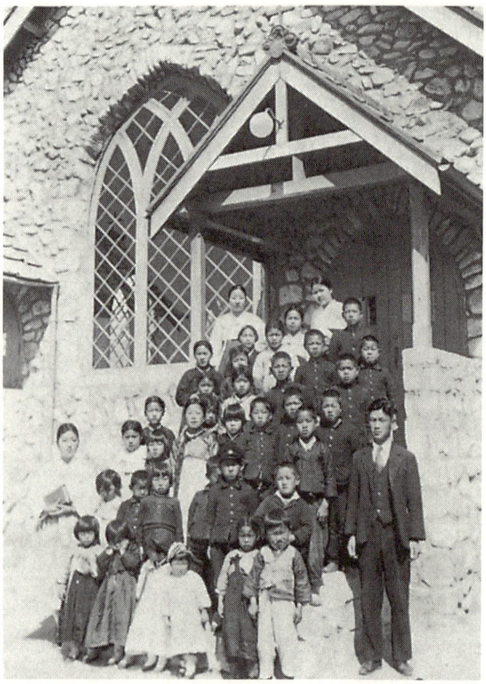

Sunday School students in front of chapel

> "When we build, let us build forever. Let it not be just for present delight, nor for present use alone. Let it be such work as our descendents will thank us for, and let us think as we lay stone on stone, that a time is to come when these stones will be held sacred."

Governor Won, Chong Kyo, who had been so very helpful in launching our 1933-34 TB Seal Campaign, was asked to participate in the dedication ceremonies of the Rosetta Chapel on September 23, 1933, just four days after my mother's sixty-eighth birthday. My mother was able to be present and was officially recognized for her forty-three years of service to Korea.

It seemed particularly fitting that, on the eve of my mother's early retirement from Korea, the Rosetta Chapel should be named in her honor. Although the Mission required compulsory retirement at age 70, she had felt compelled to return to America before then in order to take care of her ailing brother, my Uncle Frank Sherwood. He was a retired Methodist minister and a widower. Mother was scheduled to sail on October 2, 1933 for America.

At the time of the chapel dedication, I received a message from Mr. I. Yamagata, former editor of the *Seoul Press*, and it read as follows:

> "Korea, especially Korean *women*, will miss your mother very much. She has done a really splendid work for them, and deserves the highest possible honor.
>
> "However beautiful that chapel may be, it does not, I think, symbolize one-hundredth part of the great merit of her service."

One of the features of the dedication program which proved a delight to all was the special music rendered by the Salvation Army Band. Baron Yun Tchi Ho had very generously covered the expenses so that this group of Korean boys from the Salvation Army Boys' Industrial Home in Seoul could participate in various aspects of the weekend program. This also included a musical concert and drama, a health parade, and lectures and addresses commemorating the twenty-fifth anniversary of the Norton Memorial Hospital and the fifth anniversary of the Haiju Sanatorium. The Band played to a capacity audience of three hundred people in the chapel and the Korean fondness for music was reflected in their excellent performance.

The Korean church typically had no "comfortable pews" and in fact, the entire congregation sat on the floor, tailor fashion. In some Korean churches, there would be a screen running down the center of the church which separated the men from the women and children. Babies were offered "cafeteria service" by their mothers throughout the religious service. The luxury of diapers was not provided the children, so often the babies were merely held up just outside the windows to "do the needful." Small children were permitted to run up and down the aisle during the service, and when the screen was used, would venture around it to inspect the men's section and disrupt their concentration on the sermon. The sermon might also be interrupted by the loud wails of some baby who would then at once be comforted at the mother's breast. Even some of the older children were so indulged.

It seemed hard to see how the woman could get much out of the service in a Korean church, for she was kept so busy looking after her children. However, the ladies did not mind, for it was so much better than being confined to their women's quarters at home. They could compare their own children with other noisy youngsters, or could shyly observe other husbands as they were leaving the church and comment on how their own husband looked like a *yangban* (gentleman) in comparison to the others.

Although there was an active First Methodist Church in the city, our new chapel permitted wider participation in formal worship services for those not able to travel that far, and added much to the life of the Sanatorium. It was an inspiration to staff and patients alike. In fact, a former patient, the Rev. Y. S. Kim, served as the chaplain.

In years to come, it might be noted, this very chapel became the only one allowed to function freely and without interference when the Communists took over North Korea. They apparently conceded that the chapel services kept up the morale of the TB patients and thus helped in their cure. This was a remarkable admission on their part.

Early in October, soon after the dedication of the chapel, our chaplain, the Rev. Y. S. Kim, suggested that we visit the Diamond Mountains over the forthcoming holiday. This was the traditional occasion when Koreans took time out to visit the graves of their

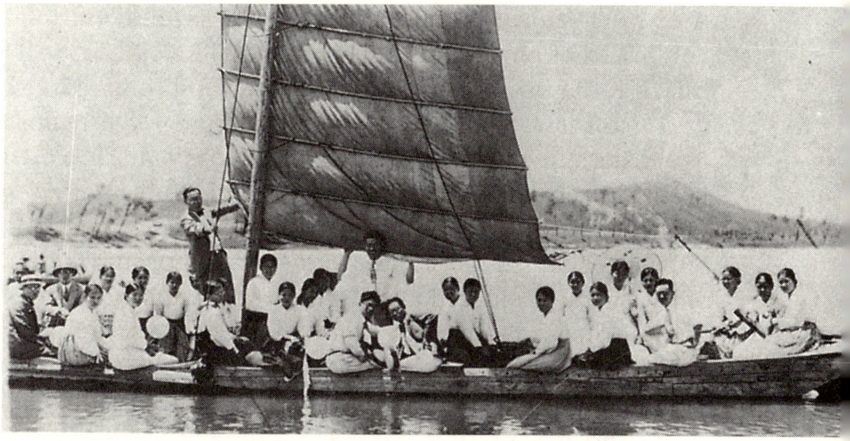

Faculty and students of Woman's Medical Institute on Han River outing

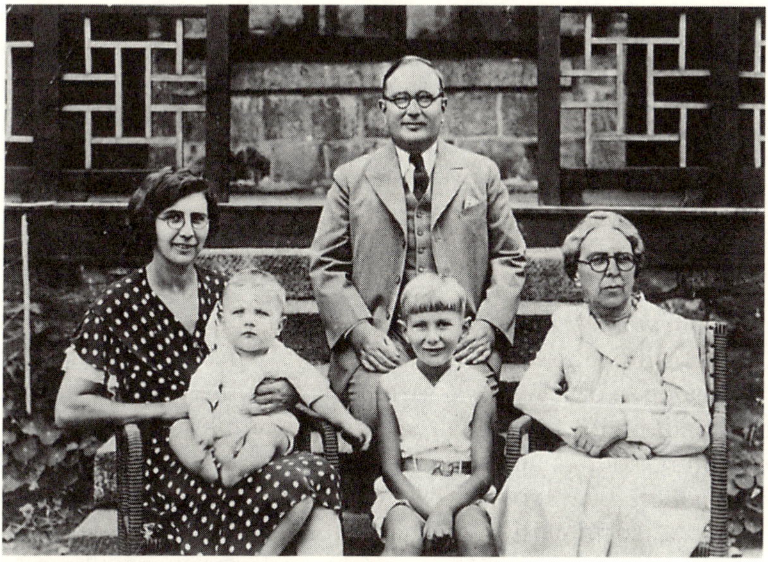

Dr. Rosetta Hall on her 68th birthday, Sept. 19, 1933 (l. to r.–Dr. Marian Hall, Joseph, Dr. Sherwood Hall, William, Dr. Rosetta Hall)

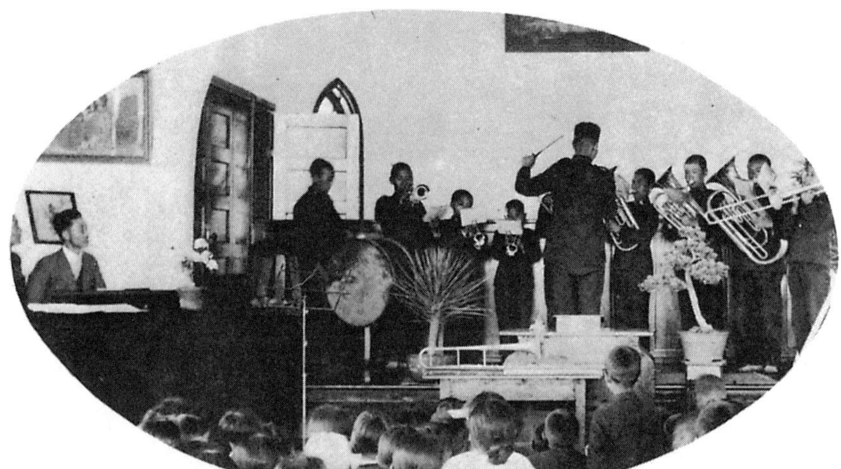

Salvation Army Band plays at Chapel Dedication Ceremony

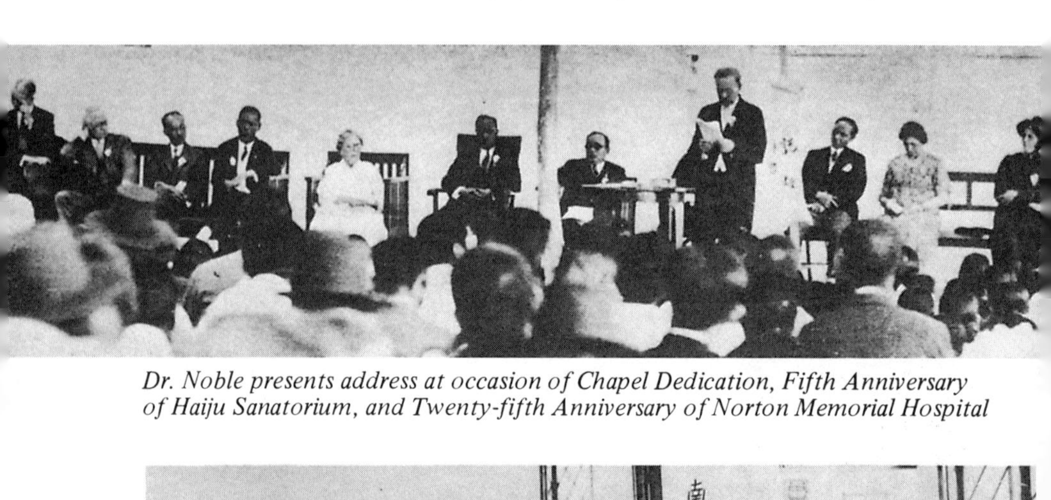

Dr. Noble presents address at occasion of Chapel Dedication, Fifth Anniversary of Haiju Sanatorium, and Twenty-fifth Anniversary of Norton Memorial Hospital

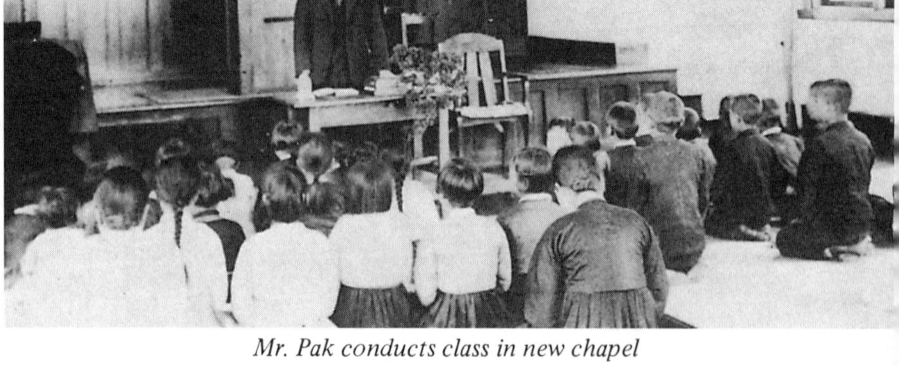

Mr. Pak conducts class in new chapel

departed relatives, and so it would give us an extended weekend. The timing would be good now also because the farmers were busy getting in their fall crops and this always meant a lull in the hospital work.

The Diamond Mountains were located on the east coast only a short distance south of Wonsan. Marian had taken a trip there with friends from Peking some years earlier and had reported that it had been well worth the effort. She encouraged me to go with Chaplain Kim for she did not like the idea of leaving the children with the *amah* and preferred to stay home with them.

Our Sanatorium laboratory technician, Mr. Kim, Pyung Si, and I had once made the drive by car between Wonsan and Haiju by way of the Diamond Mountains in July 1929. The hazardous road conditions we encountered that summer, however, were sufficient to discourage any plans to drive there directly on this occasion. The road skirted the Diamond Mountains and the only way to really explore them was on foot.

Chaplain Kim and I decided to take the train towards Wonsan via Seoul. From Ampen, three stations south of Wonsan, we would transfer to a jitney to travel to the starting point of our trek. There we would need to secure *jiggie kun* (coolies with carrying racks) to carry our gear.

Our Korean friends believed these particular mountains, in this land of mountains, to be the most scenic. They even claimed that the Diamond Mountains had been given by the Creator to Korea as a mark of His special approval. They were a place of pilgrimage and had been so from ancient times.

The head man of the village also proved to be the chief merchant and we approached him to hire our coolies and purchase our supplies. At first he grumbled at our request and feigned reluctance at having to make any arrangements for us. He finally agreed and we could see that he was really quite pleased to do so. His manner, however, conveyed contempt for the scenic grandeur above us.

"Why do you wish to bother with such a trek?" he asked us. "Those mountains are just piles of rock, of no use to anyone. It is almost impossible to grow anything there. The Buddhist priests and priestesses, with shaven heads, have to come down to our village during the winter months with their begging bowls. We are compelled to fill them lest, by not doing so, we incur bad luck. I never go up there. These mountains can never stop one's hunger pains, nor fill one's empty belly."

It was obvious that he liked a full one, for he patted his bulging abdomen with pride, saying as he did so, "*Pai pulla!*" (full stomach).

He now offered us some helpful suggestions. "It will be warm enough in the daytime in those mountains, but it gets very chilly at night. You may wish to take along quilts for each of you from our stock. They have silk padding made from our silkworm cocoons. Unlike cotton-padded quilts, these are as light as a feather, but will keep you as warm as if you were sleeping on *on-dol* (heated floor). You will find them far more comfortable than the kind you get in the city." (This proved to be the case.)

When I paid the merchant, I could not resist pointing out to him how these beautiful Diamond Mountains that he claimed to so despise were actually benefitting him and his village.

He laughed good naturedly. He then offered us some large juicy Korean pears which were not pear-shaped like those seen in the West. They were as round as apples but had a pear flavor. "These will refresh you and help to quench your thirst when you toil up those steep, rocky paths," he assured us.

We thanked him for his thoughtfulness and began our climb. We had not gone far on the trail before we realized we were entering a different Korea. Here the style of clothing was still that of old Korea. The peasants carried bundles which were tied together with human hair ropes, probably made from the hair shorn off the heads of the Buddhist priests and priestesses. One of the mountain ridges received its name, *Tanpa Ryong* or Crophair Ridge, because novitiates to the Buddhist priesthood had their heads shaved when they reached this point.

The wild animals in this area seemed almost tame and game appeared plentiful the further we walked. Deer of various species often bounded across our path or would stand motionless as we passed, as if to look us over. Then they were off like a flash, their white rumps bobbing up and down as they disappeared into the thicket. A big black bear padded alongside the trail, unconcerned that he made us feel a little nervous. However, the least dangerous creatures gave us the greatest start. These were the pheasants and quail. We were almost upon them when they would take off, right in our pathway, with a resounding flutter of wings, swishing past us so closely that we could feel the breeze that their wing movements created. This natural game preserve existed because of the high regard the Buddhists had for the life of all creatures.

The terrain was now rocky and became increasingly rugged the further we went. A greater variety of deciduous trees than is usually found in other parts of Korea could be seen here. Their autumnal reds, oranges, and yellows bathed the landscape in a kaleidoscope of vivid colors that brought forth our spontaneous expressions of delight.

The scenery grew still wilder as the ascent became steeper. By late afternoon, we were getting foot sore and weary and wondering where we might spend the night, when a group of Buddhist pilgrims overtook us. They were friendly and slowed their pace to match ours. They suggested that it might be well for us to spend our first night in these wild mountains at one of the most famous of the Buddhist monasteries, *Chongansa*, or the Temple of Eternal Rest. There the priests were accustomed to accommodating pilgrims and visitors like ourselves. They assured us that this was only a little distance further.

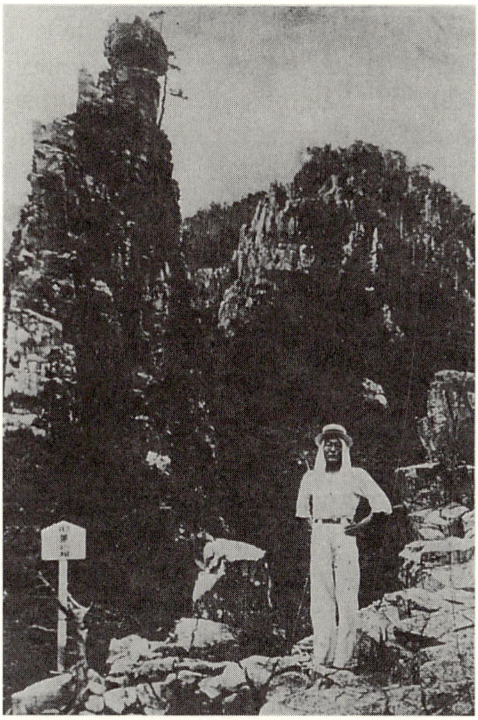

The Rev. Yung Syoon Kim in the Diamond Mountains

We received their suggestion gladly. Only, their "little" seemed to our tired and blistered feet like a lot.

The head priest at the temple was a merry, friendly sort and he welcomed us warmly. Our host at once ordered some water to be heated to bathe our aching feet. He sprinkled some powder from dried herbs into the water, which he claimed would heal the blisters and cuts. He had also ordered that an extra large helping of rice be added to the huge iron pot. He said that we would be welcome to all the rice and *kimchie* we could eat.

We soon found that the herb lotion had really given our sore feet much relief and the rice reminded us of our returned appetites. Noting that our leather shoes were inappropriate for the climb ahead, he offered to provide us in the morning with special straw sandals called *shin*. These were made by the monks and would be better for fording streams and climbing the stony paths. After spreading our bedding on the heated floor, with its oil-paper covering, we were soon asleep. Towards early morning the floor became extremely cold, so we reached for our silk cocoon quilts and were amazed at how warm they kept us.

The next day, we were treated to another meal of mountain rice and *kimchie*. As we ate, the priest asked us to look high up the mountain. As we followed the direction of his pointing finger, we could see a temple, built on an overhanging ledge, giving the appearance of a huge eagle's nest.

I asked in amazement, "How in the world did they get those huge timbers up there? If appears sufficiently difficult, if not impossible, that men should even be able to climb up those sheer cliffs!"

"It was not easy, I am sure," he answered. "If you will look carefully with your field glasses, you will note there are narrow slanting ledges on the perpendicular face of the mountain. If not inclined to dizziness, a man can work his way from ledge to ledge.

"Now, in regard to the big timbers which serve as the framework for the temple, they had to be planned with great care. Each log had to be sawed into small pieces. One priest would strap a piece to his back and carry it up. The pieces would then be reassembled and matched like a jigsaw puzzle up there. Actually, it took many years, and unfortunately, a few of the priests slipped and failed to make the next ledge, so fell to their deaths. However, there were always volunteers glad to take their places."

He then asked me with a twinkle in his eyes, "Would you like to go up there and meditate? I assure you there will be no one to disturb you. You might even find that our Buddhist Nirvana and your Christian Heaven are not so different after all."

His remark sparked my curiosity. Although we had often been told about the Buddhist religion, it had usually been from the perspective of a Christian. It was particularly interesting to me to have this opportunity to learn something of Buddhist philosophy from the vantage point of a Buddhist priest. Therefore, I asked him to tell me about his religion.

"Once we Buddhists were very powerful in Korea," he began, obviously pleased at my interest. "But unfortunately, we let temporal power go to our heads and we meddled in politics. This proved to be our undoing, and we were expelled from the cities and lost face in the country areas. We were expressly forbidden to enter any walled city in Korea. We found this region in the mountains was relatively uninhabited, due to the untillable land, so we sought refuge here. Gradually we have been regaining our lost spiritual strength, and are now in the slow process of building up a Buddhist center here."

He then went on to say in his whimsical way, "You Christians have an entirely different conception of heaven than do we Buddhists. We call our heaven, 'Nirvana.' This is the highest religious state of consciousness, where all desire and struggle are extinguished. Here the soul finally becomes absorbed in Deity. However, as I understand it, our 'Nirvana' would be 'Hell' to you Christians, for to you, the struggle is a major part of the joy of accomplishment. For the most part, you of the West already have food, clothing, and shelter, so you wish to go on to ever higher planes of individual achievement.

"But, you see, with us Korean Buddhists, our struggles for mere sustenance start almost at birth, and continue to an early grave. Our agonized efforts tend to make us heart sick and bone weary. We yearn for rest; the chance to cease from all struggle and to be absorbed in 'Nirvana.' We long for the time when we no longer have to go around from door to door with a begging bowl, often receiving nothing but insults.

"We of this temple are fortunate, since we are at the gateway to the Diamond Mountains and most travelers, like yourselves, stop here and leave something. But many of our other temples are not so conveniently situated.

"Your 'heavenly approach' is to go to ever higher goals with thought of others replacing thought of self. Our severe circumstances, on the other hand, force us to think chiefly of ourselves. Our philosophy of Nirvana is almost opposite to yours, for we love to sit in ever deeper contemplation."

Not only did I find the priest's remarks illuminating, but I was highly curious that he should be so apparently well acquainted with Christian beliefs. However, Chaplain Kim reminded me at this point that we had better get started on our journey.

Although we had expected to pay for our accommodation and service, the priest would not hear of it. He refused our cash but said, if we insisted, we could make a contribution to their temple fund. We were happy to do so.

As we continued our journey, the scenery became ever more breathtaking. We found that the path often led us to streams. These could only be crossed by means of stepping stones which sometimes lay under the water and proved quite slippery. We were more grateful than ever now for the straw sandals so thoughtfully given to us by the priest. Although they wore out after a certain distance, we would stop at one of the many little monasteries along the way to purchase new ones.

At the top of one hill we were rewarded with a view of the "Twelve Thousand Peaks" where we could see the saw-toothed range that may have suggested diamonds to whomever it was that named these mountains *Kumgang San* (Diamond Mountains). The Japanese called them *Kongo San*. Sunshine lit up the crystals in the rocks along our way and we wondered if it was their glitter that perhaps reminded someone of the sparkle of diamonds. Another theory which may have had some greater merit was that the Diamond Mountains received their name from the best known of the Buddhist scriptures, the Diamond Sutra. Whatever the source, we agreed that the name suited the splendor stretching to the sky before us.

Along the way we were reminded that this was a pilgrim route, for names had been painstakingly carved into the rocks. Besides the images of Buddha seen at the temples, we could see evidences of Korean Shamanism (demon worship) that mingled with the Buddhist effigies. Devil posts with their grotesque faces leered at us along the path.

At the southern approach to the Diamond Mountains, a Korean Christian, known to everyone as "Diamond Mountain Yun," operated a retreat house. Missionaries wishing to visit the famous Nine Dragon Falls from this approach often stayed at Mr. Yun's inn before proceeding on this trip. We did not stop there since our route was

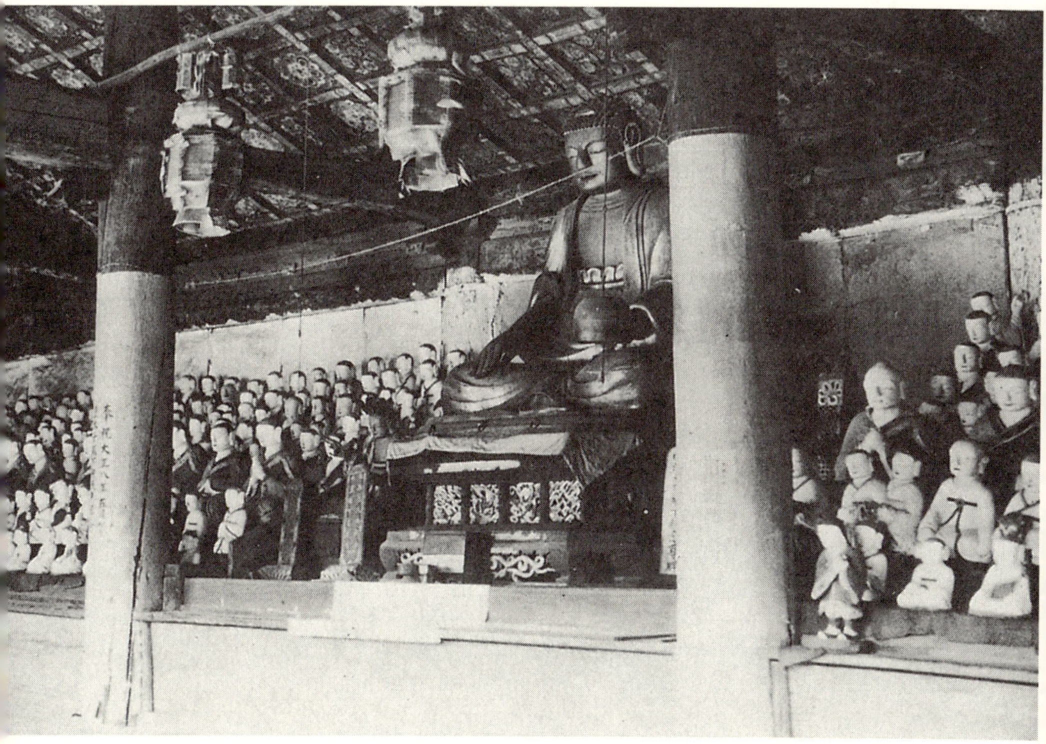

Buddhist temple with images of Amida Buddha and bodhisattvas

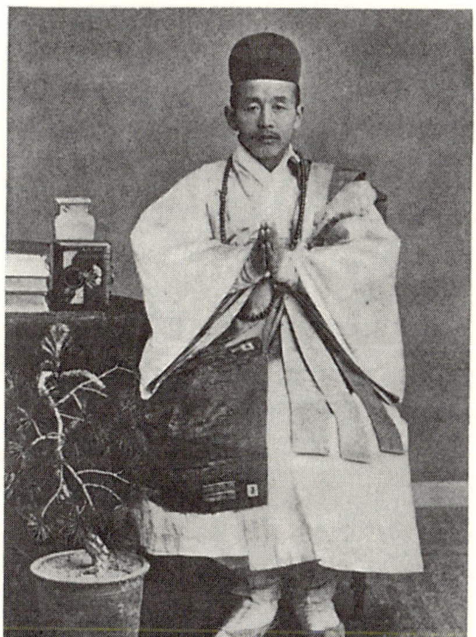

Buddhist abbot

FROM HULBERT, "THE PASSING OF KOREA" (DOUBLEDAY, PAGE)

from the North. As we neared the Falls, the scenery became ever more spectacular. A series of nine waterfalls descended in quick succession, dropping their foaming spray into deep pools below. In order to see them, we would need to ascend the rocky path which did not promise ease.

The "Dragons" nevertheless seemed to be beckoning us upward and onward, giving us a true *kananmom* (going mind), as the Koreans would say, to see them all. Each succeeding climb seemed harder to negotiate, and ever more rewarding. By the time we had reached the Ninth Falls, we were breathless both from the climb and more so from the wonder of it all.

We could now better appreciate the delicate Oriental brush paintings of thin transparent mist patches, enveloping the mountain like a Spanish bridal veil. With our own eyes we had seen one of the greatest sources of inspiration for Korean artists.

We, too, had been uplifted by witnessing this facet of God's heaven on earth. We returned to earth, at Haiju, glad of the opportunity to have seen this mountain treasure.

Another Christmas had come and gone and our Christmas Seal mailings had been winning us many new friends for the work. It was after the busy rush of the season had subsided somewhat that our Sanatorium chaplain approached me about one of our younger patients, a girl by the name of Haisunee. Chaplain Kim was concerned about her and asked me if I had any new suggestions to offer that might pull her out of her doldrums. Different ones had tried, but to no avail. Haisunee was convinced that her case was hopeless. She hardly bothered to eat.

It was then that I remembered we had received a box of very attractive used Christmas cards from the United States. These had been sent to us after the holiday season that year to be used by our patients in our occupational therapy work with them. I thought that the most recently received box of cards might have a special appeal to our discouraged patient. On that hunch, I gathered a handful of them from the carton which had come from the White House and went to see Haisunee.

"Look, Haisunee, these cards came all the way from America. They were first sent to the President of the United States, and he, in turn, has kindly passed them on to you patients. See, here is his name, Franklin D. Roosevelt."

There appeared, for the first time, a flicker of a smile as she asked, "May I please have one to keep?"

"Yes, you may select two or three of your choice. You may wish to give one each to your brother and sister, when you get well and can go home. You might be interested in knowing something about the President. He was once, like you, very sick but he made up his mind he would get well. The President did everything that the doctors told him to do, and, at last, after a long time he did get well."

"I did not know that people in America ever got sick!" she exclaimed. Then she added, "If I try very hard to get well, will you write and tell the President?"

"Yes, I shall be glad to do so, but I fear he will not be able to reply, Haisunee, because he is so extremely busy. But perhaps he will tell someone else to write us."

When the nurse brought her supper, Haisunee looked up with a happy smile as she said, "I must get well now." For the first time since her illness, she ate without coaxing.

It was not too long before we began to notice an improvement in her health. She could sit up several hours at a time after awhile. Then she began to walk a little. With satisfaction we observed that she was well started on the road to recovery.

Now I felt that I could write a letter to the President as I had promised Haisunee. I briefly told him her story. William was working at his stamp collection, while I composed the letter.

All of a sudden he blurted out the suggestion that he enclose some of his Korean stamps for the President. He had read in his home study lessons that President Roosevelt was an avid stamp collector.

I was on vacation at Wonsan Beach when I received a letter from the White House forwarded to me from Haiju. It bore a Washington postmark dated June 18, 1934 and had been readdressed to "Katsuma Beach, Gensan, Korea." (Gensan was the Japanese name for Wonsan.)

William shared my trembling excitement as I opened the envelope. How eager I was to get back to Haiju to tell Haisunee that her wish had been granted despite my skepticism.

When I returned, my first stop on sanatorium rounds was by Haisunee's bed.

"I have a surprise for you, Haisunee," I said. "I have a letter from America here in my hand."

"Is it from the President?" she asked in great excitement.

"Yes, it is, Haisunee, and it has even been signed by the President's own hand. See, here it says, 'Franklin D. Roosevelt.'"

Haisunee could hardly contain herself. "Read it to me, Doctor, please! I just knew he would write it himself."

Her tone was so compelling, that without further hesitation, I started to read, translating into Korean as I did so.

> "My dear Dr. Hall:
>
> "Thank you ever so much for your letter of May twenty-fourth. I was particularly interested in what you had to say regarding the little . . . girl. She has my very best wishes."

Then I paused to explain to Haisunee that our son, knowing the President to be a stamp collector, had enclosed some Korean stamps and a few of our TB Christmas seals in my letter to the President, so the concluding paragraph was in reference to that.

> "Please tell your young son, William, that I deeply appreciate his thought in sending me the . . . stamps. I am delighted to have them for my collection.
>
> "Very sincerely yours,
> "Franklin D. Roosevelt"

Haisunee clapped her hands in delight. "I knew the President would write to us and he did. He would be so happy to know he had helped me to get well!"

Some time later, Haisunee's brother came to fetch his little sister, now fully recovered. She danced along the mountain stream that irrigated their rice fields, as sparkling and radiant as its waters. She proudly showed her happy family the Christmas cards from the White House as she exclaimed, "The Americans have troubles and sickness, too, but they are always trying to help others." Her heart welled up in gratitude to the great President, who amidst all the affairs of state, had taken time out to remember a little girl in far off Korea.

As the story of Haisunee and President Roosevelt's letter circulated, it proved to be a real shot in the arm for the Christmas Seal Campaign. Increasingly too, we were receiving reports from doctors and nurses in medical centers all over Korea that they could detect a definite change in the attitude of the people. No longer were they ashamed to report tuberculosis, with the result that patients were coming in at a much earlier stage of the disease. Our Haiju Sanatorium also reflected this most encouraging new trend.

The Methodist Church was making plans to celebrate the Fiftieth Anniversary of Methodism in Korea. The selection of the date, June 24, 1934, was based on the arrival of the Reverend Dr. and Mrs. R. S. Maclay in Korea on that date fifty years before, with the specific assignment to secure property and permission to conduct a school and hospital in Seoul. In this they had proved successful and so opened up the possibility of future mission work in the Hermit Kingdom.

The Fiftieth Anniversary celebration would continue through 1934 and 1935. On April 5, 1935 a special program would be held in Seoul to commemorate the arrival of the first resident Methodist missionaries, the Reverend and Mrs. H. G. Appenzeller. A history of the Methodist Church was to be compiled and published along with other special publishing efforts in the way of articles and pamphlets and commemorative addresses.

The plans also included the printing of a special commemorative seal (not a Christmas seal) to mark this historic milestone. I was called upon to have such a seal designed and printed.

The design which I submitted depicted a map of Korea on which various locations of Methodist mission work in the nation were symbolized by pictorial sketches. The caption, "Korea for Christ, 1884-1934," summarized the spiritual emphasis which was being given to the commemorative year.

By now an autonomous Korean Methodist Church had been formed with its own Korean Creed delineating the essentials of Korean Christian faith. Bishop Herbert Welch had originally drafted such a creed based on his knowledge of the views of Korean Christians obtained during his twelve years of experience as Resident Bishop of Korea. This creed was approved in condensed form by the First Korean General Conference in Seoul in 1930. It is this same "Korean Creed" that appears as one of the four "Affirmations of Faith" published in the official American Methodist Hymnal and is repeated many a Sunday in Methodist churches across the U.S.A.

The Chong Dong Methodist Church in Seoul, usually simply referred to as "First Church," was the first foreign style church building in Seoul and had been completed in 1898. It was here that the Fiftieth Anniversary ceremonies were held. The first Korean

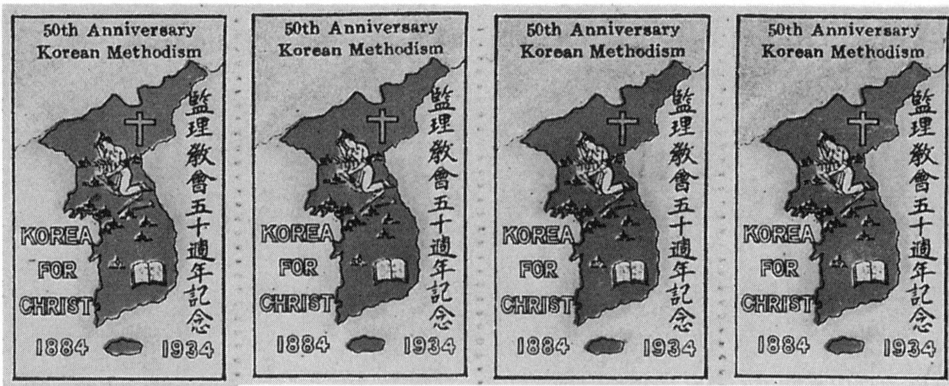

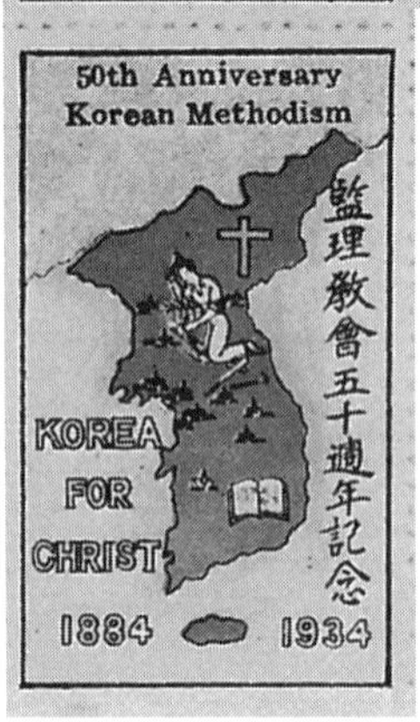

KOREAN JUBILEE SEALS

representing Fifty Years of Progress of the

METHODIST CHURCH IN KOREA

To be used by all who have helped to make this possible-churches, Sunday Schools, and individual in America, and by missionaries in Korea.

The artist has depicted churches, schools, and hospitals being built on the map of Korea. This work is shown to be still in progress and one in which all may share in winning Korea for Christ.

Seals commemorating 50th Anniversary of Korean Methodism and seal packet cover

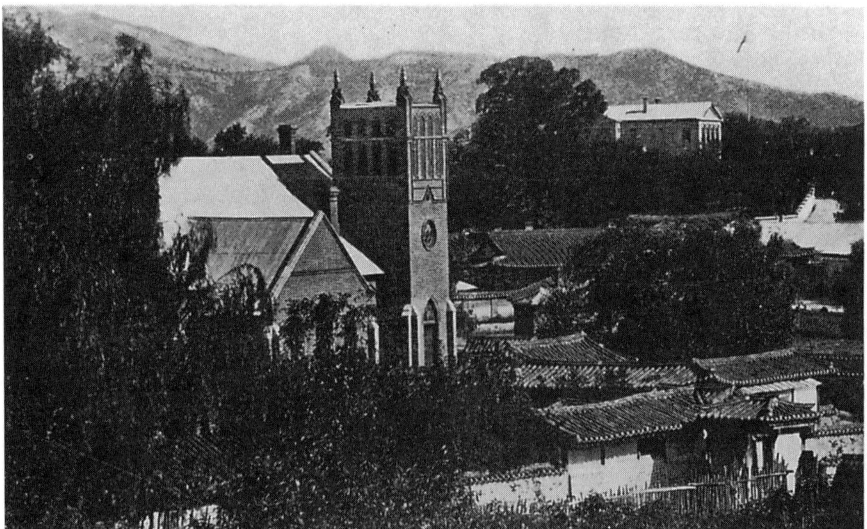

FROM HULBERT, "THE PASSING OF KOREA" (DOUBLEDAY, PAGE)

First Methodist Church, Seoul, and British Legation (background)

General Superintendent of the Korean Methodist Church, Dr. J. S. Ryang, delivered the opening address. Stressing the remarkable progress achieved during the half a century of Methodism in Korea he cited the following milestones:

> "It was the Methodist Mission which *established the first school for girls, the first and only college for women, the first women's hospital, the first school for* [the] *blind, the first kindergarten for children, ordained the first Korean pastors, and produced the first Korean woman M.D., the first trained nurse, the first trained kindergarten teacher, and the first Korean woman Ph.D.*"[1]

That anniversary year gave us all cause to realize anew that "*with God all things are possible*," and that His miracles continue even when the hour seems darkest. This truth I was to rediscover in an intensely personal way in the not so distant future.

---

[1] *Within the Gate*, Charles A. Sauer, Ed., Addresses delivered at the Semi-Centennial of the Methodist Church in Korea, Y.M.C.A. Press, Seoul, Korea, 1934.

CHAPTER 24

Family Crises

Chaisie, who had served as *amah* to both William and Joe, now confided to me that *wesa pooeen* (lady doctor, i.e. Marian) was often resting on the couch these days when I was away at the clinic.

"Yes, I know, Chaisie," I replied. "She is 'expecting.'"

Marian and I played the "name game" traditional to couples awaiting a new baby, although agreeing on a suitable name was not so easy. I suggested that if we had a girl, she should be called "Marian."

"No," came the reply, "I think I would like her to be called 'Phyllis,' after my dear college friend, Phyllis Crook."

After the customary battle of words, we laughingly settled for "Phyllis Marian." But the word battle was only half over.

This time Marian proposed "Sherwood" for a boy, and I suggested "Frank" after my uncle, the Methodist minister in Albany for whose sake my mother had returned early to America. He had always taken a deep interest in our family. So we settled for "Frank Sherwood."

Some time after that, while listening with my stethoscope over my wife's abdomen, Marian observed my puzzled look. She was quick to remark, "What's the matter?"

"I am hearing things," I replied. "I do believe I hear two distinct heartbeats, here and there." I pointed and handed her my stethoscope.

Marian listened intently and confirmed my findings. "Now I understand!" she exclaimed. "At times, I felt as though there were two football teams competing inside of me—one time the right side would win, and another time the left. Meanwhile, I've been feeling rather knocked out in the skirmish."

"It is no wonder you have not been your usual active self during this pregnancy. To think you are carrying twins!" This was indeed exciting news.

Although Marian had stood her other two pregnancies well, and had even continued her medical work until almost the last minute, this time she was finding it extra hard. There was increased pressure on her heart. It would act up at times and give us considerable alarm. I was not at all happy, given these developments, at the prospect of delivering my own babies, especially since no suitable nurse was presently available. I suggested, therefore, that we go to Seoul or Pyong Yang for the delivery. Marian felt the long trip would be too hard on her, and to this I was inclined to agree.

With difficulty, we did manage to secure a nurse, Mrs. Martin. However, she had been out of nursing for some time and I was not sure how she might handle an emergency should one develop. I knew I would have to focus my attention on Marian, and rely totally on the nurse to manage the twins after the delivery. I frankly told Marian of my concern.

Marian responded with a smile, "At Stetson Hospital you easily delivered triplets and even took time out for a coffee break in the process. You should have no difficulty at all this time, with one less to deliver."

I realized that I should not worry Marian with my apprehensions. I tried to give her a cheerful and encouraging smile, which I fear was rather superficial, for deep down I was quaking.

September in Korea is usually delightful. Since I felt that Marian needed a little change, we drove down to the Haiju harbor about five miles away to watch the colorful fishing boats come in with their catch. This proved interesting, but Marian did not enjoy the strong odor from the fish and seaweed drying on the seashore. She informed me that she also felt delivery might be imminent and so we hastened back.

Soon after our return home labor started. For awhile Marian watched our nurse begin the necessary preparations. When she felt all was going well, Marian turned the rest over to us and we were relieved, for we did not want her to have any last minute worries.

When Marian went into labor on that memorable day, September 12, 1934, all started off well. I checked on Marian's heart which had been giving me some concern. Her heart and the twins' hearts were reacting as well as could be expected, considering the strain and stress they were experiencing. The positions of the babies were also normal.

The delivery of the first twin went routinely, and as Marian had correctly predicted, this baby was a girl. I grew more relieved when she became a "cry baby," and I began to relax a bit, especially since Marian's heart seemed to be standing the strain well. It was a little wait before the second baby made an appearance, but this delay did not bother me, for I recalled the long wait between babies when I delivered the triplets in Philadelphia.

Then I suddenly sprang to attention, as I shouted the words, "Here it comes, nurse. Are you ready?"

She gave me a slow affirmative nod. The second baby was a boy. However, I heard no reassuring baby cry as he was delivered. Marian's condition was not good, so I turned the baby over to the nurse for his first spanking while I applied my stethoscope to Marian's chest. It was with difficulty that I could even hear her heart beat and her pulse had precariously weakened. I was becoming alarmed and was more than preoccupied, although I did manage to interject, "How is he?"

The nurse's cryptic reply was, "Not breathing."

"Call Dr. Kim at once!" I yelled.

Dr. Kim came in breathless. He had hurried up the hill to our brick house as soon as he had received the call. Immediately he sized up the situation and started to give artificial respiration. He continued for awhile, but finally announced sadly that our precious babe was dead. Dr. Kim then helped me with Marian, whose pulse, though still very weak, was beginning to respond to supporting treatment. It was some time before I dared tell her about Frank, as I well knew what a terrific blow it would be to her.

This loss made our daughter, Phyllis, doubly valued. Many babies would not take prizes in a beauty contest when first born, but Phyllis was to me beautiful from the first. Our sons were more than delighted to have a sister and, in their excitement, had little comprehension that they had lost a brother.

Our nurse had bathed and clothed Frank in the lovely hand embroidered dress which had been prepared for him to wear at his christening. Frank was certainly a perfect baby, and he seemed just innocently asleep, when he was shown to his heartbroken mother. Our Sanatorium carpenter built Frank's tiny coffin, which our hospital nurses beautifully lined with Korean raw silk cloth. After the casket was sealed, it was covered with white chrysanthemums which were just coming into bloom.

We had decided the appropriate burial place for Frank should be our family plot on the banks of the Han River near Seoul where my father and my little sister lay. So we telegraphed our dear friends, the Nobles, that I would be driving up to Seoul with Frank's body and would they kindly make the necessarv funeral arrangements. Of course, Marian was not physically able to travel yet, and that sad motor trip proved very hard for me.

The Nobles received me with understanding sympathy, for in their day they had been through a similar experience. We also discovered that our bereavement gave us a closer bond to our Korean friends, since there was hardly a Korean family that had not lost a child. Infant mortality was very high in Asia.

That night at the Nobles I had expected to have Frank's coffin with me, but they felt it should have a place of honor in their parlor. The small funeral service, to which our most intimate friends were invited, was held on September 20, 1934. Mr. Noble gave a most comforting message. I had wished Marian could have heard it.

The return journey was easier on me, for I was eagerly looking forward to getting better acquainted with our new daughter. When I reached home I imagined that she even greeted me with a welcoming smile, which our nurse was quick to inform me was due only to a gas pain. Later I had to admit that she probably had been right.

Marian had not felt strong enough to nurse Phyllis and we seemed unable to find a milk formula that suited her. Whatever we gave her resulted in severe colic. After feeding her, I used to pace up and down with her on my shoulder in a distant part of the house so that Marian would not be distressed by her pitiful cries. The poor baby finally would fall asleep from sheer exhaustion.

One time I overheated Phyllis' milk by mistake, as I thought, so I skimmed off the film that had formed on top. However, to my great and relieved surprise, there was no crying following this feeding but only a contented cooing. Unwittingly I had discovered what was causing her discomfort. Evidently that part of the casein I had skimmed off the milk was the cause of her problem. From then on we deliberately overheated the milk and removed the film that formed on top. Phyllis thrived on this new formula and became a happy baby. She was her fond daddy's pride and joy, as well as fun for the rest of the family, who all spoiled her terribly.

The Roman Catholic Sisters at the Convent did exquisite embroidery, so Marian had had a lovely, long, hand embroidered dress made especially for each of the twins for the occasion of their christening. Our good friend, Ethel Underwood, wrote us an unexpected and cordial invitation that whenever we wished to have

Phyllis christened, she would love to have us all as guests in her home. They asked us to select a date and give them a list of those we would like invited.

We gladly accepted and suggested that both the Reverend Horace Underwood and the Reverend W. Arthur Noble perform the ceremony. The affair was even lovelier than we had anticipated. Phyllis was already beginning to show the effects of her mother's careful training, for she did not cry when the water was placed on her head. Marian was showered with congratulations for having such a beautiful baby, although I felt I deserved a small share of the credit. Our visit was a happy one and did Marian a world of good. Once again she became her former cheerful self.

Japan marked the Twenty-fifth Anniversary of the Korea-Japan Annexation Treaty in the year 1935. One day the Governor informed me that an urgent request had been received from the Governor General of Chosen (Korea) for me to attend the special function that was to be held in the capital. I was to travel to Seoul where the Silver Jubilee Awards were to be given.

The Governor saw my bewilderment and hastened to inform me that I was to be the recipient of a Certificate of Merit for my pioneer contribution towards the conquest of TB in Korea. Two other Methodist missionaries were also to receive Certificates of Merit at the same time. The Reverend F. E. C. Williams, head of the Kongju

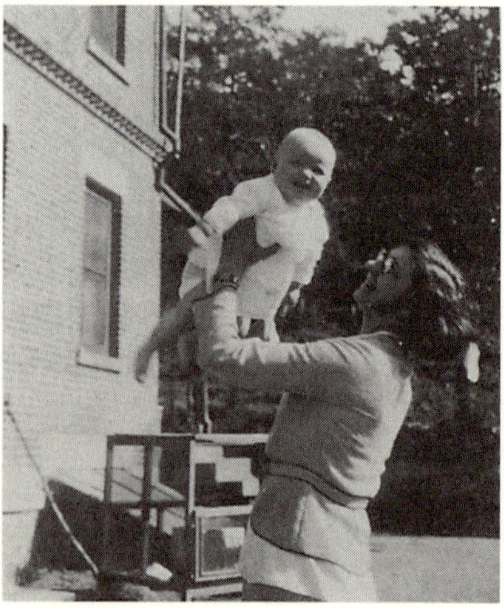

Marian and Phyllis

Agricultural Vocational School was to be honored for his rural educational work, and Dr. A. G. Anderson of Union Christian Hospital, Pyong Yang, for his eminent medical service. The latter served as one of the consulting physicians to our tuberculosis sanatorium.

The appropriate attire for this occasion was morning frock coat and striped trousers, the Governor advised. I hesitated, for I well knew that all who served so loyally in the TB cause were deserving of recognition. Noticing my hesitancy, the Governor smiled and said that this was not really an invitation but an order.

The function proved to be a grand affair indeed. The Japanese Government officially recognized our efforts, in the flowery language of the Orient. Many of the awards went to those who had shown marked bravery in the fighting in Manchukuo. In the citation given to me, it was noted that my fight had not been on the field of battle, but in waging war against TB. In addition to the award, a purse of 50 yen ($17.00) was donated to me for the furtherance of TB medical work.

This recognition from the government proved to be good for the cause. I found that I was being called upon frequently to address various gatherings, and was invariably introduced as "The Christmas Seal Doctor."

On one of our frequent trips to Seoul, the children were especially thrilled when we were invited to be guests of the Horace H. Underwoods. The special reason was that the Underwoods had recently acquired some purebred collies from America, and one of them had given birth to a litter of puppies. Our boys loved to roll on the Underwoods' luxurious green lawn while the puppies romped over them. The dogs would suck the children's ears which brought forth peals of laughter.

When Ethel saw how especially attached William was to the puppies, she kindly offered to give him one of them. William accepted with alacrity. We parents, knowing better the responsibility involved, were at first reluctant, but under his irresistible, "Please!" we finally gave in. We had been told that the puppy, whom William named "Mac," was too young yet to have his anti-rabies shots, but at this tender age, was not apt to get involved with other dogs.

One day in May, 1936, after our return to Haiju, Marian was teaching William his Calvert lessons on the upper verandah of our house. The Calvert School system was a well known boon to parents of children living abroad in areas where schooling was not available.

This home study program, conducted as a correspondence course from Baltimore, Maryland, enjoyed a justifiably fine reputation. Students tutored in it found they could make an easy transition to schools in the U.S.A.

Our two younger children wanted to play with Mac. Marian, not wishing to interrupt William's lesson, sent Joe and Phyllis to fetch the dog themselves. They both came back crying and saying that Mac had snapped at them.

Marian remarked, "Oh, that must be just puppy playfulness."

She sent William to bring Mac. He returned with the complaint that Mac had bitten him and had also bitten Chaisie when she tried to help. Marian felt that this was ridiculous and decided to go herself. (I was away at the Sanatorium clinic at the time.) Mac appeared very excitable and when Marian reached out to pick him up, he bit her forearm in two places.

She became alarmed and decided to put Mac outside in our large empty chickenwire pen in which we sometimes kept pheasants. When I returned from my work at the Sanatorium, I was told what had happened and immediately went out to take a look at Mac. He was excitedly running 'round and 'round in the pen, occasionally snapping at his tail. It was then I realized that there must be something radically wrong, and forbade anyone to touch Mac while he was in such an excited condition. However, I hoped that he would settle down, for I felt fairly sure no mad dog could have bitten him. However, on this assumption I was evidently sadly mistaken. William later reported that a stray dog had bitten Mac some weeks before, but had run off as soon as William yelled at him.

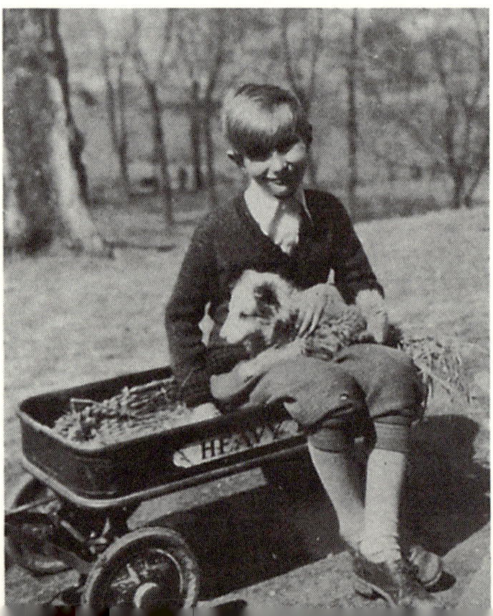

William and his collie, "Mac"

When Marian was holding her "Mothers' and Child's Welfare Clinic" the following day at the Middle House (where we had first lived), William rushed in, in great distress with Mac in his arms, crying, "Mac is trying to bite off his tail!"

Sure enough, Mac was bleeding freely. Marian, of course, ordered William to put the dog down immediately. She cleared the room at once of the children, but unfortunately, not before Mac had bitten one of them. Marian quickly wrapped Mac securely in her leather coat and took him back to his pen. She then treated the injury of the child who had been bitten. The family, however, insisted that they be given some of Mac's hair to burn on the wound according to an age-old custom of the Koreans.

Marian caught Mac again while the man servant, Kim Sa Bong, cut off some fur. The dog bit him before he managed to get the door to the pen closed.

Although Mac occasionally nibbled away at some food, he completely refused to touch water, evidently due to the painful spasm of his pharynx on swallowing, which resulted in a fear of drinking. Hence, our suspicions that he was suffering from hydrophobia now seemed substantiated. This gave me the emotional jitters when I realized how many people Mac may have infected with his deadly virus. If the special Pasteur inoculation treatment was not given in time, the most horrible and painful of deaths was the certain result of rabies.

I then announced that as soon as I could get the needed vaccine, all who had been bitten or even licked by Mac would have to be inoculated. To my horror, the Korean family whose child had been involved, gave me a flat, "No." They claimed they already had used the sure Korean remedy against mad dog bite. The hairs from the very dog which had done the biting had been burned over their child's wound.

Of course, I knew that this simple native remedy would not prevent the frightful death that awaited the victim of a rabid dog. This old-fashioned Korean treatment had some rationale, however, in that such cauterization might have prevented ordinary infection in the case of a non-rabid dog bite. It also had the advantage of searching out the vicious dog and securing its death. This was usually by stoning, which I had often seen in the streets when I was a boy. I realized in this instance, it did give me a good bargaining point.

"Very well then," I said, "they have carried out their method of treatment, and my wife has risked being bitten again in catching the dog to get its hair. Now it would only be fair to try our Western method of inoculations." They reluctantly conceded my point.

I telegraphed to the Government Public Health Department in Seoul for the special vaccine needed to inoculate the seven victims: the Korean child, Chaisie, Kim Sa Bong, Marian and William, all bitten; and Joe and Phyllis, possibly licked by the dog. We could not take chances with the latter two lest Mac's saliva may have entered any skin abrasion they might have had at the time.

What was my horror to receive the cryptic reply, "Out of stock." At once I cabled to Japan, only to receive the same response. By this time, I was frantic, as precious time was running out. I recalled the horrible pictures we had seen when we visited the Pasteur Institute in Paris. Only with the advent of the Pasteur treatment in 1885 had anyone been able to prevent such fearsome tragedies. Even then the inoculations had to be given within the month of the bite.

In the meantime, I had a few "Job's comforters" who tried to tell me that perhaps Mac was not mad after all, but just suffering from some canine nervous disorder. However, I brushed their well intentioned remarks aside, and took the precaution to allow Mac the freedom of his pen. I did not put him out of his misery, as my natural instincts otherwise would have dictated. Death took him in nine days, which was within the prescribed fourteen day limit for rabid dogs. Then I sent Mac's brain immediately for pathological examination to Dr. Douglas Avison, at Severance Union Medical College in Seoul. The report came back, "Positive for Negri bodies," (diagnostic of rabies). Now there was no doubt about it; my worst fears were confirmed.

By this time, although I had not been bitten, I felt as though I were going mad. Like a drowning man grasping for a straw, I sent a frantic cablegram to our pharmaceutical agent and good friend, Mr. Harvey Stokely, at Shanghai, China. I knew that he would try his best to locate and send the essential vaccine material from some laboratory in that vast land where there must be so much rabies. The need had now become more urgent and imperative than ever. I tried to conceal my anguish from my family, but I fear without much success.

After a few hours, which seemed almost like a lifetime to me, came the heavenly words by cable, "Available. Dispatching at once." My relief was short-lived, for it appeared that my troubles were far from over.

First, the material was in a very different form than the usual vaccine. The parcel that arrived at the Customs House contained specially treated spinal cords of rabbits, and the Customs Officer had never seen such before. He therefore questioned the customs declaration that had been given in Shanghai. I fervently assured him that the declaration was correct. I had to take precious time out to explain it in detail and convince him of how very urgently we needed it. My anxiety and sense of desperation must have finally registered with him, for after some delay, he reluctantly passed it. I could see that he was still baffled over why the spinal cords of rabbits could be used in the prevention of rabies, since it was not so listed in his book of words.

In those days the technique for the preparation of anti-rabietic vaccine was complicated and followed the meticulous scientific methods originally laid out by Louis Pasteur. The rabbits to be used were first infected with the virus of rabies by intracerebral inoculation. The resultant death of the rabbit after this infection with the virus occurred in 15 to 21 days. It was these spinal cords, and not their suspension material, that were then sent out to the doctors who needed them. The suspension to be injected into the patient had to be freshly prepared each day. This was done by macerating the rabbit cord by mortar and pestle, then by passing the suspension through a filter paper. (These days, all these complicated daily preparations are eliminated, for the vaccine is now supplied in 10 cc phenolized ampules.)

The first injection to be given the patient was from the suspension of the cord which had been dried for twelve days. This was the most attenuated, and so the weakest injection. Subsequently, daily fresh preparations from progressively more virulent nervous tissue were to be given in increasingly stronger injections, until a total of seventeen had been administered. This seemed like a month of Sundays to the poor patient, for each inoculation was more painful than the last, with increasingly greater reactions. Thus, if the injections had been given in time, and there had been no slip-up in the original preparation of the cord, nor the daily preparation and administration of the injections, immunity should have been achieved. However, there were still all these "ifs" all down the line. It was the "all or none law." Each step had to be perfect or all was spoiled.

I fear I had not given strict attention to all these details when I was a medical student, for at the time they seemed to hold merely academic interest. But now I suddenly came alive to their full significance and to the fact that this long chain was no stronger than its weakest link. Had not the medical books mentioned that besides the painful inoculation reactions, the injection sites would light up at precisely stated intervals? The sites, which were located on the back between the shoulder blades, did in fact light up and burn, itching unbearably. (Present day medical practice favors the abdomen as the area to receive the injections.)

Then later, when more and more injections had been given, all the sites joined in a grand tattoo chorus on the taut sensitive skin, causing such itching that scratching was uncontrollable. We had to keep the children's fingernails cut to prevent lacerations. In my nightmares, I would sometimes wake up with a start and feel sure I had heard my loved ones barking like dogs. I felt I was becoming a nervous wreck.

Grueling as this entire ordeal was proving to be, we found that one of the day's injections must have involved some impurities in the suspension material. There soon followed even more excruciating pain for my patients. The injection sites on Marian, William and Phyllis developed into abscesses which required opening surgically. The morphine and sleeping tablets did not put Marian under and Dr. H. C. Yi, our Sanatorium doctor, had to use a local anaesthetic. Marian still experienced much pain. Her suffering was compounded when she heard the cries of her children. Being helpless to alleviate their distress only added to her own. The infection left a large scar on each of its victims as evidence of the torture they had endured.

It seemed that neither science nor compassion were adequate to this situation, and I felt utterly powerless, knowing that the treatment must simply run its full course. I found myself turning to the Savior to ask for His healing for the stricken ones and His strength for me. The word "savior" comes from the Latin word, *salvare*, which means to save or to heal, and in those circumstances, calling upon the Great Healer took on new meaning for me. I experienced a feeling of assurance, and then, soon afterwards, I had cause to feel my prayers were answered.

After our ordeal had passed, one of the Haiju Elders shared with me what had been going on in the minds of the "City Fathers" when they learned of the incident. At first they had been inclined to be very critical and even resentful that three Koreans had been bitten by our *mitchin kae* (mad dog) even though these Koreans were poor and not *yangbans* (aristocracy). After all, they were still Koreans!

"This is what comes of allowing these unwelcome foreigners here and permitting them to try to convert us to their strange religion," he had said. "Who ever heard of putting under the skin some juice from the spinal cord of a rabbit, of all creatures? How ridiculous! Such gross ignorance and wild superstition should not for a moment be tolerated by us Koreans. They are just torturing our poor people needlessly by their cruel injections. We already have a perfect remedy that has stood unquestioned for centuries."

"But there is one thing that must be said in all fairness," another, who was more sympathetic, had interrupted. "They do give our Koreans the same care and consideration they give their own people, and in addition, they have shown respect for our remedy, at risk to themselves. They did catch their mad dog, cut its hair, and burned it on the wound of the Korean child."

"This act proved to be farsighted, Dr. Hall," the Elder said to me now in a congratulatory tone. "I believe it actually prevented a public disturbance."

With the series of inoculations finally at an end, I decided to take the family to the beach at Wonsan so that we could all unwind from the tensions of the preceding weeks. We stopped over in Seoul with our dear friends, Maud and Kris Jensen, who had recently returned from their furlough and had learned of our troubles. They proved to be a very special comfort to us.

Kris was always cheerful and a talk with him was far better than a tonic. Maud and Marian were kindred spirits, and our children enjoyed the two Jensen children, Clairlee and Philip. All in all, the effect of the Jensen family on us was like a breath of fresh air. They also spent their holidays at Wonsan Beach so that over the years we became very close. On this particular visit, we felt the restorative power of their love and understanding could only have been Heaven sent. From that point on, things began to get better.

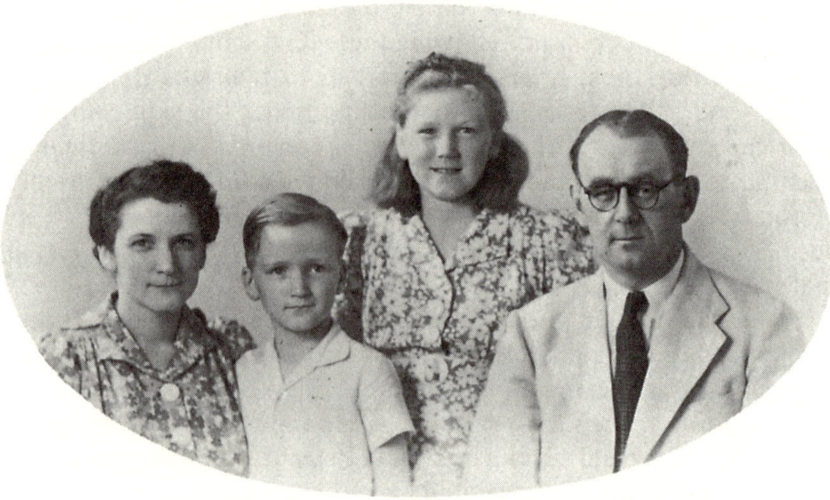

Maud, Philip, Clairlee and Kris Jensen

CHAPTER 25

The Visit

All through the ordeal of the anti-rabies inoculations, Marian had looked forward to a proposed visit by her sister, Emma Lineweaver, and Emma's son, John. John was eleven and although William was two years younger, it would mean that he would have a companion during the seven months that Marian's relatives hoped to stay in Korea on their round-the-world trip.

Emma's husband, the Reverend Norris A. Lineweaver, was at that time headquartered in Marion, Virginia and was serving as a chaplain in the Civilian Conservation Corps (C.C.C.). His service required considerable travel between camps. Their eldest son, Norris E. Lineweaver, then twenty, was attending Marion Junior College. It had seemed an ideal time for such a trip.

Emma and John sailed from Baltimore in late September, 1936 and, traveling by way of the Panama Canal, Los Angeles, and Yokohama, they arrived in Korea early in November. The Lineweaver visit was a morale booster for the Hall family.

Many years later, John shared with me the letters Emma had written home during that memorable year. Excerpts from Emma's correspondence, included here, offer a view of our life in Korea from another perspective.

November 15, 1936

"... Marian and William and Mrs. Barnhart met us in Seoul at the train and upstairs in the station were three more people, Mr. and Mrs. Henry Appenzeller (who start home on furlough in April) and Mr. Kris Jensen (who with his family have recently come back from furlough). The men folks attended to our baggage and we were whisked into a taxi and after a while made a turn into a street which Marian informed me was the only one of its kind in the world! Narrow and winding, full of Korean pedestrians and ox carts, with barely enough space for autos to pass, it wends its tortuous way out of the city and up a hill to the home of Dr. H. H. Underwood, president of Chosen Christian College. At this home, we were to be guests for a few days instead of going on immediately to Haiju. The Underwoods are members of the Underwood typewriter family, and have a very large well equipped modern home, steam heat, several bathrooms upstairs etc. John and I were ushered up to a lovely big room and a bath for our private use.

". . . We arrived just at the time of the monthly meeting of the Presbyterian missionaries in Seoul, and the meeting was being held in the Underwoods' home, in the library which is as large as many a Sunday School room. The Underwoods have five children: one son [Horace G.] in college in America, twin sons (James and John) in high school in Seoul, Dick, about John's age, and Grace, the baby and only girl (about 6 years old).

". . . We just had time to change our clothes and be ready for the afternoon meeting of the missionaries. After so many weeks on the boat without religious services, it was nice to be able to enjoy the brief devotional service preceding the business meeting. There was . . . discussion of . . . a recommendation that missionaries to Korea need now to study the Japanese language as well as the Korean. Officialdom in Korea is mostly Japanese, hence the wisdom of missionaries being able to speak their language.

"After the meeting, the Underwoods were hosts to the assembly for dinner. I was placed at a table with a group of especially jolly folks who called each other by their first names and from then on I have been 'Emma.' It was a pleasant experience to have for my first evening in Korea.

"The next morning was November 11 and the day we attended the meeting of the Korea Methodist missionaries . . . We had to slip away from this meeting early because of a luncheon invitation from a drug salesman, Mr. Harvey Stokely, . . . a friend of Marian and Sherwood. He entertained us at the Chosen Hotel . . . From there we went to the station to see if I could get to one of my trunks for my dinner gown, to wear at the dinner party being given by the

Underwoods in honor of Sherwood's birthday and our arrival. I was successful and able to find the box containing my velvet dress.

"I then went to get my hair curled in a Japanese Beauty Parlor. Neither Marian nor I could speak Japanese but we made motions and Marian left me there while she went again to the Chosen Hotel where the Methodist group were having a tea and reception. The Japanese operator brought me some magazines–printed in Japanese–to read while my hair was drying! Marian came to get me to take in some of the tea program (I was too late to take in the tea!) . . . . From there we went back to the Underwoods to get ready for the big dinner party.

"There were 24 guests including the British Consul and his wife and the American Consul. They were all interesting people. I was seated at the right of the host and Sherwood at the right of the hostess. At my left was Father Hunt of the English Church in Seoul. He was a most pleasant companion and his English accent was music in my ears. We played charades after dinner and other games and had a most happy evening.

"The next morning, November 12, we visited the Palace Gardens to see the chrysanthemum show. . . . There were of course a great many of the magnificent blooms that are native flowers of Japan. . . .

"We were entertained for lunch at the home of Dr. and Mrs. Avison of the Severance Union Hospital. The Avisons are Canadian Presbyterians, very pleasant people.

"In the afternoon the Underwoods took us to the Union Recreation Hall to bowl, and from there, I took them to a Japanese restaurant for eels and rice and sukiaki while Marian and Sherwood attended a meeting. When I say I took them, I mean I was hostess. Here I had my introduction to the Japanese custom of removing shoes. We stood before a little raised platform and discarded our street shoes for Japanese sandals. We were then shown to a little room with paper walls, at the door of which we left our sandals and went in our stocking feet. We sat on cushions on the floor before small tables that were about one foot in height.

"It was quite cold and the only heat was from a small brazier of charcoal. My feet nearly froze. I did *not* like the eels but managed to make a good meal from sukiaki . . .

"The next morning, November 13, Sherwood and the children went to Haiju but Marian and I stayed over a day so that Marian could finish her Christmas shopping.

"Since Mrs. Underwood lives so far out of the city, we two were invited to stay overnight with the Barnharts. Mr. Barnhart is a Y.M.C.A. secretary. It was while here that a Korean man came along selling the brass trimmed chests and I bought one for Norris. . . .

The next day, November 14, after spending the morning shopping, we had our lunch and packed up for home. Between us we had 9 good sized pieces of baggage! As you can imagine it was some job for two of us to handle. Koreans . . . simply run for the train as soon as the gates are opened, to get a seat in the train. We had a hard time finding a place to sit, but we finally did and got our suitcases and parcels stowed away. We knew we had to change once, so when a porter came through jabbering something in Korean and Marian said we had to change cars, I enthusiastically grabbed a couple of suitcases and got off the train. I was about to go after more packages when Marian called, 'Emma, where are you?' It seems that we were in a car that was going to be dropped, so all we had to do was walk back through the train —with nine pieces of baggage! And all this, fifteen minutes before we must change trains at Dojo! Well, we managed it somehow and arrived at long last at our final destination—Haiju. Sherwood was there to meet us with the Sanatorium car and in a few moments we were at Marian's home. Chaisie, the cook, had hot cocoa and sandwiches ready for us and a nice fire glowed in our bedroom stove.

"Our room faces north and west. Two large windows look out over the city and my first view was of course at night. The lighted city looked like an inverted sky full of stars. . . .

"From the east window, through the porch windows we get a glimpse of the W.F.M.S. house and the path leading to the Sanatorium. . . . To the right we see the driveway, down to the gate at the compound. . . . To the left we see the road which leads from town and winds around our compound up the hill back of our house and on to the Korean cemetery and the Sanatorium. About halfway up the hill another road branches off from this to the right and goes over the hill to a Korean village. It is over this hill that we see so much of the coming and going of Koreans . . .

"Beyond the lawn and the compound in front, is the Boys' School and the Hospital, and beyond them again, the city of Haiju. Still further beyond, rise the mountains which were the first thing I saw when I awoke the morning after my arrival. I do not even have to raise my head from the pillow to see the sun touch the tip of the highest peak early in the morning. The view of the mountains takes up half the window.

". . . The next event of interest . . . would be the Korean feast to which we were invited, to celebrate the birth of the first child of one of the Sanatorium doctors (Korean). The father entertained the whole staff of the Sanatorium and Sherwood and Marian and myself. The feast was held at a Korean restaurant—the home being too small. The host sat, legs akimbo, at the head of the table and Sherwood and Marian and I had the seats of honor next to him . . . For the first time I heard a prayer to God in another than my own language. It quite touched me . . . He was asking a blessing not only on the feast . . . but also upon the new-born child."

November 20, 1936

". . . I went with Sherwood to church on the first Sunday after our arrival . . . Sherwood took me by a short cut which led through an alley. Korean huts opened on the alley and the aspect on every side was one of poverty and filth. Garbage of every kind was simply thrown outside the doors.

"We went to the First Church . . . Everything was in Korean of course and I could not understand what was being said. There were many more women than men . . . In some respects the church building reminded me of our church at Damascus [Maryland] before it was done over.

"There are doors at either side and men enter on one side and women at the other . . . Sherwood pointed out to me the difference between women raised in the South and those raised in the North. The former were bareheaded while the latter had towels bound around their heads. Some few men wore American style business suits but most were in the costume of the country."

November 23, 1936

". . . On November 22, Mr. and Mrs. Sasaki entertained . . . Sherwood, . . . Marian, William, John and myself at their home for a Japanese feast. We went in a taxi and when we got there, we were admitted by their Japanese house boy to the hall which like all Oriental houses has two levels. . . . Sandals were provided for us to use. Mr. Sasaki's house is planned in both Japanese and Western style. We sat in chairs in the living room and visited with Mr. Sasaki, who had called at the house previously to meet us. Later, Mrs. Sasaki, a very charming Japanese lady, and their children (5 of them) came in to be introduced. Mrs. Sasaki does not speak English but Mr. Sasaki interprets for her.

"We went in to dinner through sliding paper paneled doors. For us they used a Western dining table and chairs. In front of each of us was placed a tray containing many small round covered bowls, and chopsticks, . . . but spoons were provided for the soup. . . . I always enjoy the rice, which is the bread and potatoes of the Oriental meal and which is here cooked so deliciously. There was fish, chicken soup and some very delicious bamboo shoot concoction which I liked very much. . . . The piece of devil fish I tried to eat . . . was horrid and I had a terrible time to get it swallowed. Some Westerners like this kind of fish. William does. To me it tasted like fishy rubber.

"Dessert consisted of fruit—apples and oranges; and candy; and bean paste cubes; and roasted chestnuts.

"As I said before, Mr. Sasaki is the Japanese vice-governor of this province (Yellow Sea Province). He and his family are very much devoted to our Hall family. Mr. Sasaki was the chief of police here before he was vice-governor."

November 28, 1936

"Father Carroll, an English Episcopal clergyman (high church) stationed at Pyong Yang, arrived on Wednesday evening to spend the holiday with us. He left last evening (Friday). Miss Barlow, also English, was a guest at dinner at noon on Thanksgiving Day.

"In the afternoon we played games and sang hymns. Miss Barlow brought an English Wesleyan Hymnal and I was carried back to the days of my girlhood when I sang the Thanksgiving hymns in the choir at Epworth at Harvest Festival. The weather was quite stormy—wind and rain. When we woke up on Friday morning it was snowing, much to John's and William's delight.

"We are all fearfully busy because of the Christmas Seal work which is still taking up much of our time. I must stop now for it is almost time for me to teach Spelling to John and William. Marian has them now for Arithmetic."

In addition to the educational benefits which the Lineweaver world travels were affording John, Emma was keeping up his formal schooling during the year by tutoring him with the aid of the Calvert School home study course. This was the same Calvert system that Marian had been using to teach William.

December 10, 1936

". . . More and more I am impressed with the loneliness of this station. Marian and Sherwood are the only married couple with children. The one other married couple are Salvation Army people . . . The only other white people are Father Beere, an Episcopal clergyman, . . . and Miss Barlow . . . I do not think the Board has any right to send, or allow to stay, only one family. There is work for several families and they should be here and paid decent salaries . . . This is the only Methodist station in Korea where there are not two or more families in residence . . ."

December 21, 1936

"I do not . . . think that I said much about the Christmas meeting at the Mothers' Club which I was invited to address on December 19. The meeting was held in First Church.

"When we arrived, the church was almost filled with mothers and children with a sprinkling of men and boys. Marian and I were escorted to seats of honor on the rostrum.

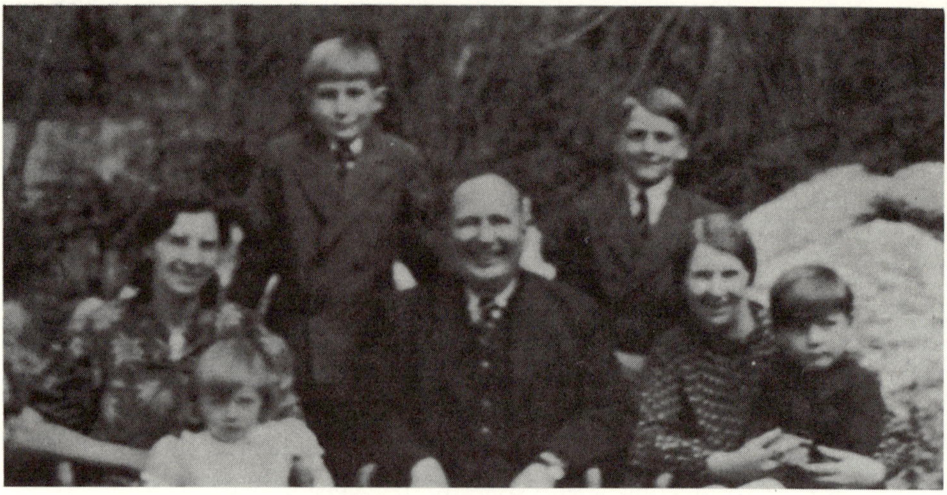

Emma Lineweaver and son John (2nd and 3rd from right) with Halls in Haiju, 1936

There was first a devotional service led by the woman doctor (Korean) at the hospital, all in Korean of course. Following the devotions there were a few numbers by children . . . After this part of the program, Marian, as founder of the Woman's Club, presented gifts to each mother whose child came up to a certain standard.

"It was here for the first time that I noticed the custom of Korean nursing mothers of having nothing to cover their breasts, but allowing them to dangle below the short jacket of the Korean woman's costume. Later I saw a woman on the street on a bitter cold day with breasts hanging down and almost wholly exposed to the freezing blast. Of course these people think no more of exposing their breasts or squatting by the roadside to perform the last act of digestion than we do at exposing our elbows. They think it is very shocking for adults to expose the arms and shoulders. Marian says that in summer the children run around the streets stark naked.

"Now to go on with the story of the Woman's Club. My speech came after the program. I had about ten minutes worth, but the translation (by Dr. Kim . . .) took about 20 minutes, so I decided if I was ever asked to speak again, I'd plan for three minutes.

"After me came a Korean minister with a speech . . . At the very end presents and candy were given to the children. . . .

"The thing that impressed me most was the difference between the mothers and children who had come under the influence of the missionary and those one sees on the street.

"Marian and Sherwood had a great disappointment yesterday. Their best donor to the work (who sends $500.00 . . . every Christmas) died suddenly. They have not only lost a helpful personal friend, who sent them checks for themselves occasionally, but the $500.00 for the work. Their basic pay is $1000.00 per year with $100 for each child, which is not adequate.

"I shall be thinking of you for Christmas . . . Marian and I are to sing a duet at the 'Sanatorium Christmas Eve' (tomorrow) and I must make a selection for us to practice as soon as I have finished this letter . . ."

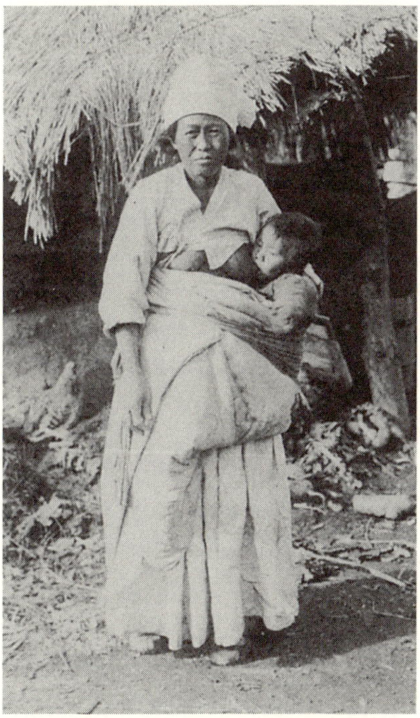

"Warm meals served at all hours"

January 2, 1937

". . . Shops here are filled with New Year gifts as those at home are at Christmas. Marian had the Sasakis here to Christmas dinner. They invited us for New Year Festivities but I was unable to go because of a bad cold . . ."

January 7, 1937

". . . Mr. Stokely, Parke-Davis drug salesman, arrived last night to stay all night and today. It seems that these American or English businessmen always stay at . . . missionary homes when travelling in territory where there are no hotels to accommodate them. Mr. Stokely is a very nice man, who operates out of the Parke-Davis headquarters in Shanghai. . . .

"Next month . . . the Korea Medical Association (of which Sherwood is president this year) has its annual meeting and I am urging Marian and Sherwood to go together for the two or three days it is in session and let me take care of the two younger children. Mrs. Underwood has invited William and John to stay with her Dick at that time and go to school with him."

January 14, 1937

". . . By the way it is best not to use War Department envelopes in sending mail to me. Sherwood says it is wiser for me not to mention your connection with the army even though you are a chaplain and in C.C.C. work. The government is very nervous, especially about Americans. Our every move is watched. When Marian and I went to Seoul after Christmas, the detective here wanted to know where we were going and when we got to Seoul station, another detective asked us where we were going to stay."

January 29, 1937

". . . Sherwood and Marian and I walked down to the vice-governor's office today to look at some samples of homespun cloth. We may buy some to make pants for William and John. It is very reasonable and a new project of the government to help encourage the sheep raising industry in Korea . . ."

February 11, 1937

". . . This is Korean New Year's Day and also a Japanese holiday. Korean children are passing up and down the road in their gayest dresses and Japanese flags are fluttering all over the town. It is very muddy underfoot or I would have walked with John down to the city to see the festivities. I haven't seen any kites flying yet.

". . . Sherwood was summoned to the Government Building to receive a gift of money from the Emperor to the Sanatorium. It will be presented by the Governor of this province. I will leave my letter open until he returns so that I may tell you how much the gift was . . .

"P.S. The gift was 300 yen (not quite $100)."

February 13, 1937

". . . I think I mentioned to you some time ago that the annual meeting of the Korea Medical Association is to be held in Seoul this coming week. Sherwood is president and Marian is to read a paper on 'Rabies.' Mrs. Underwood invited the boys to go and visit Dick. . . . Marian and Sherwood are to stay at the British Consulate.

"They leave tomorrow morning and return Friday or Saturday. I am so glad I can make it possible for Marian to go with Sherwood without the two younger children. The *amah* will stay in the house with us."

February 19, 1937

"Miss Barlow dropped in for a few minutes yesterday so I invited her . . . for tea this afternoon . . . We had a nice chat. The special winter Bible classes are now going on and Miss Barlow is very tired. She is getting up in years and the work begins to be wearing on her.

"She threw me into something of a quandary by telling me that both this part of Korea and Japan are fiercely hot in July. That is why the missionaries go up north for July and August. . . .

"Sherwood was talking to some missionaries in Seoul and they said that by all means John and I ought to be getting our passage booked as boats are crowded in the summer.

"I told him my thought of avoiding the hot months by leaving earlier than at first planned but I could see he did not like the idea very well. I think they are quite anxious for us to go with them to Wonsan Beach . . ."

February 23, 1937

"Not only have Marian and Sherwood had news of the death . . . of Mrs. Moore who built the Sanatorium chapel and who contributed $1000.00 per year towards the Sanatorium, but Mrs. Haskins (Emily's mother), who supports them on the field, died a few weeks later. Although the Board is now responsible for them, this loss will affect the possibility of their return to the work after furlough, for Sherwood does not think that Emily, although the only inheritor of her mother's wealth, will continue their support. The money did not come to them direct, but through the Board and they get only the same salary as other missionaries."

February 28, 1937

". . . Both from the north windows and the west of our room we can see the Korean world go by, up and down the road that goes by the missionary compound . . . Beyond the road to the left is the Korean cemetery which is always located on a hill. . . . A funeral just passed!

"A funeral procession here looks more like a parade. Several boys go ahead carrying gaily coloured banners (to scare the evil spirits away); then comes the box holding the tablets on which are recorded the doings of the deceased. This is carried by two men and looks like a palanquin but smaller. Then comes the body carried on a catafalque, supported on long poles on the shoulders of the bearers. The catafalque is gaily festooned with silk of many colours like a float, and over all floats a canopy. After this came the professional mourners with their weird wails, and then the family, dressed in white with high headdresses of white . . ."

March 18, 1937

"Here I am again at Seoul, and staying at the Jensens. Sherwood is at Sauers. . . . We came up . . . to meet Bishop

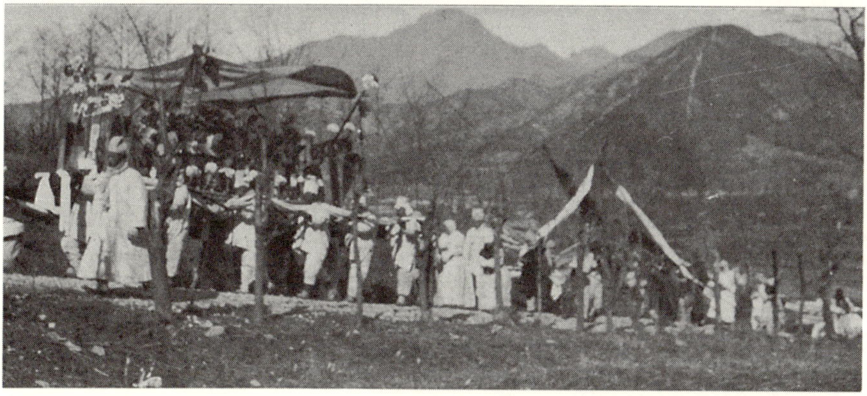

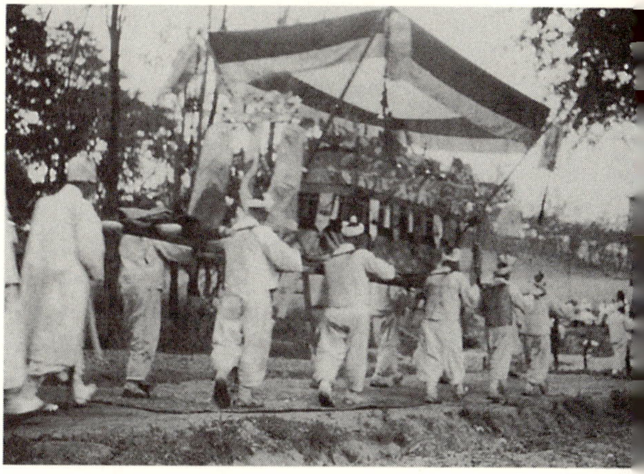

Korean funeral procession, Haiju, 1937

and Mrs. Baker on their arrival at the station. It was bitterly cold . . .

"The Bishop talked to us about the state of the church in America–quite encouraging . . . In the afternoon there was a reception at the Chosen Hotel for Bishop and Mrs. Baker with about 200 missionaries and Korean Christians in attendance. I chanced to be seated at the speakers table almost opposite the Bishop and near Miss Helen Kim, who is the president of Ewha College and one of the most outstanding Korean women. She made the speech of welcome to Bishop and Mrs. Baker and to my mind, made the real speech of the afternoon.

". . . I am . . . going ahead with my plans to go to China (Peiping) for 10 days . . . have found some people I can travel with. There remains only the purchase of the tickets, travelers checks and arranging to stay at the Methodist Compound in Peiping. It will take us two days and a night to get there. . . .

"Sherwood says that even if we should become millionaires within the next ten years, never again can we see Peking as well as now, for the old Peking of historic interest and beauty is fast falling into disrepair and ruin. . . . Everyone says I shall spend more than I intend to because beautiful things are so cheap in Peking, but I can't spend more than I have! John is real thrilled at the thought of going and I, too, of course. Imagine seeing the Great Wall!"

March 25, 1937

"The mail just came and there was a very nice letter from Mrs. W. C. Kerr for me saying she would be glad to have John and me join her on the trip to Peiping. She and her daughter and another young lady . . . will travel third class as far as Shanhaikwan. The return fare to this point and back is about $20.00 for John and me . . . From there we get a ticket (single) to Peiping since there is no reduction on round trip fare. . . . Third class fare from there on is about $2.00 . . . This is cheaper than I had anticipated and I am so happy to have the opportunity to travel with someone who knows the ropes and speaks both Japanese and Korean. The Kerrs are Presbyterian (North) and are doing missionary work with the Japanese.

"All I have to do now is to get a Japanese police permit to return to this country from China . . . I am not sure how long we shall stay there—perhaps ten days or two weeks. . . . John and I have been reading up . . . about China and especially about Peking, Marco Polo and Kublai Khan."

April 2, 1937

". . . John and I leave here on April 5 for Seoul. We are invited to visit the Phipps at the British Consulate for a few days and on April 8 at 3:35 P.M. we leave by train for Peiping, via Mukden. We shall get to Mukden early on the morning of the ninth and from there take another train (at 8:20 A.M.) to Shanhaikwan and Peiping, arriving at the latter city at 11:20 P.M. . . .

"We have all been writing letters like mad during the last three or four days because the government has increased the postage to foreign countries exactly twice."

"c/o Mrs. O. T. Krause
"Methodist Mission
"Peiping, China
"April 10, 1937

"Dear Sherwood and Marian,

"Here I am sitting at a desk in a comfortable bedroom at the above address. . . . We got in to Peiping last night at 12:20 P.M. Seoul time, 11:20 P.M. Peiping time. Mrs. Kerr's friends met us and we all came together (in rickshaws!) to this compound. Mrs. Krause had hot soup for us and then we tumbled into bed at once for we were practically exhausted. We came all the way third class and believe it or not the train from Mukden to Peiping was as clean if not cleaner than the one from Seoul to Mukden and far less crowded! The seats were padded with black oilcloth and were quite comfortable. No one pushed us about or crowded us. The meals were very good too. Our worst trouble was in getting seats at Seoul and the fact that our checked baggage has not yet arrived . . ."

April 15, 1937

"Dear Norris,

"Have just returned here weary from a day of sight-seeing and will start a letter to you . . . The pictures that are stamped on this paper were done at the stations in Manchukuo. The first one (of the Great Wall where it ends in the sea at Shanhaikwan) was done on the train soon after we left the latter city. The others John got off the train to get. A man would be on the platform with a table and stamp machine etc. all ready to do them. The Chinese collect them in albums made for the purpose. John was quite thrilled over it. Oriental people, especially Japanese and Chinese, are very fond of children, and everywhere John is treated with friendliness."

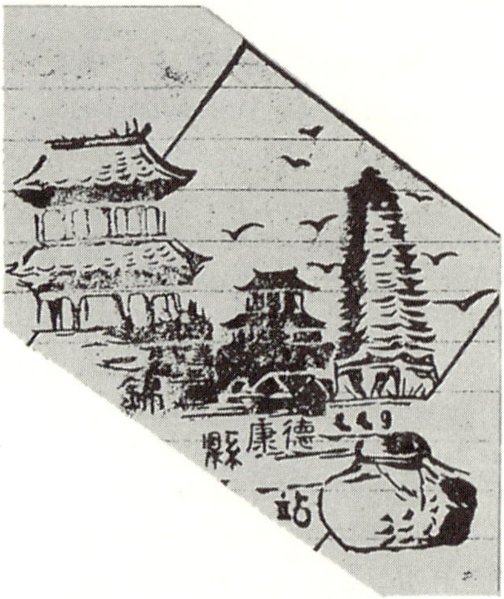

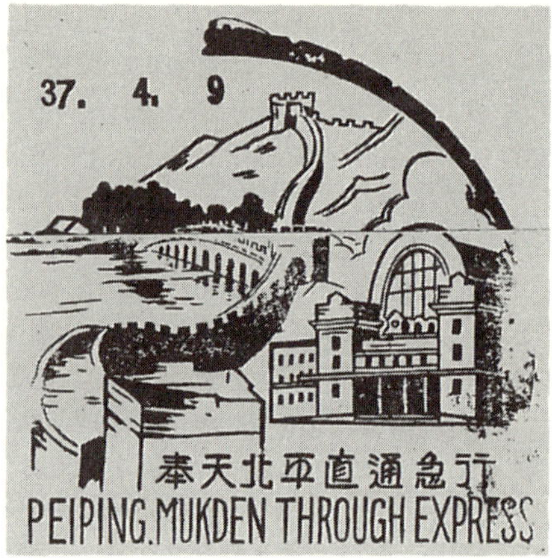

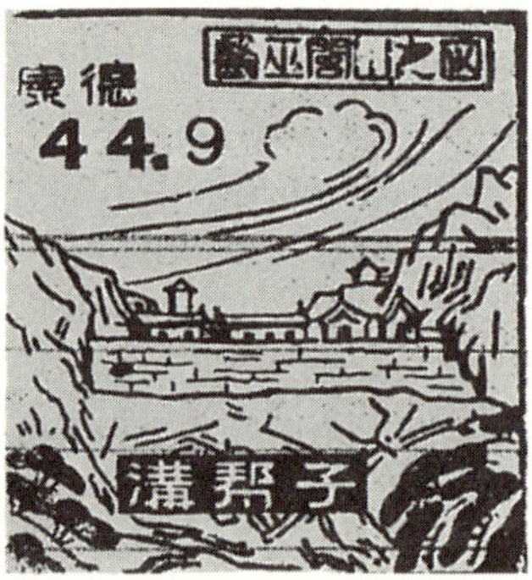

Pictures stamped on stationery during Lineweaver train trip from Mukden to Peiping, 1937

(Above–Great Wall ending in the sea at Shanhaikwan)

April 18, 1937

"... We leave on a train at 6 A.M. tomorrow ... Since we do not get our sleeper train until Mukden at about 12 P.M. and must be up for customs at Antung at 5 A.M., I expect we shall be very weary when we get to Seoul. We are to stay again at the British Consulate before going on to Haiju. We have been so weary and sleepy each evening after returning from our sight-seeing trips that writing has been almost impossible."

Years later, John recalled that memorable journey to Peking. He remembered that the train to Mukden was crowded with Japanese soldiers and that they seemed present in large numbers at every station along the way. Their uniforms, with ceremonial swords clattering at their sides, made quite an impression on John as a lad. As the train entered China proper, he recalled seeing Chinese soldiers from the train window. Dressed in white, quilted, pyjama-like uniforms, they were twirling machete-like knives over their heads and throwing them at targets. These military preparations struck John as being more primitive than some of the Japanese troop maneuvers he had observed in Haiju.

One day when taking a walk through the Korean cemetery on the hill behind our house, John had accidentally happened upon some Japanese soldiers. They were crawling among the grave mounds on their stomachs, with their rifles in hand. Undoubtedly the soldiers and John had both been equally startled. When John had returned to the house a little shaken, I told him that the missionary community had heard rumors that the Japanese military had plans for a wide-scale expansion of Japanese influence and control in Asia, and particularly in the northern portion of China.

We had certainly seen increased military activity in Haiju, such as the troop practice John had encountered, which suggested that the rumors bore some truth. We were also aware that our own whereabouts were always under careful scrutiny, and it was not unusual to be quizzed by detectives about one's travel plans.

Little did we then realize the extent to which these military ambitions would reach; or that in only a matter of months, a long war between Japan and China would be instigated at a site near the city John and Emma had so recently visited. At the Marco Polo Bridge at Lukouchiao just outside of Peking on July 7, 1937, Japanese troops on night maneuvers clashed with Chinese soldiers. This incident sparked the Sino-Japanese conflicts which continued through World War II. For technical reasons of international law, no formal declaration of war was made. We were to continue to feel the effects of these clashes. However, at the time of our relatives' visit to Peking, we all remained blissfully unaware of the state such political events had reached.

John's other vivid impression of that trip was that on their return through Manchukuo, he had seen the heads of bandits impaled on spikes along the railroad tracks. These were set out as ghoulish reminders to other bandits of the fate that awaited them if they were to attack the train. It apparently did not serve as a full determent, for the incidence of banditry on that line was extremely high.

Miss Barlow told us that she had heard reports that mines were being laid in the Mediterranean. Nevertheless, Emma decided that she and John would return to the United States by way of Ceylon, Aden, the Suez Canal and on to London, where they would transfer to the *Queen Mary* to sail to New York. Arrangements had to be made months ahead and by April they had been booked to sail on the *Terukuni Maru* of the N.Y.K. Line, the same Japanese line that had brought them from America.

Mr. Phipps of the British Consulate did not think they had anything to fear, for he noted many people had been traveling that way and the danger of a general conflict did not appear any more imminent than it had been the six months previous. They were scheduled to leave Seoul for Japan on May 25, 1937.

The visit all of a sudden seemed to be hastening too rapidly to an end. I had promised Emma that I would arrange for her and John to visit Pyong Yang before they left. Conveniently for our plans, Annual Conference was to meet at Pyong Yang in early May.

We journeyed to Pyong Yang by way of Chairyung, a flourishing Presbyterian mission where our friends, the Livesays and the Bairds were stationed. The Reverend William M. Baird, Jr. was the brother of my boyhood chum, John. His wife, Anna, was a nurse. The Reverend J. B. Livesay, whom we called "JL," was married to a Canadian, Muriel. Marian and Muriel, besides both hailing from Canada, shared many common interests. Since Chairyung was the nearest mission station to ours, we visited back and forth as the occasion permitted.

When the Chairyung missionaries learned of our plans to attend the Methodist Annual Conference in Pyong Yang, they extended us a warm invitation to stop en route. Emma's letter home described the trip:

May 6, 1937

"... We had a very pleasant visit with the folks in Chairyung. Marian and her three children and the *amah* and I went in the car. (Did I tell you that Sherwood has turned his car over to the Sanatorium, with the understanding that they have occasional use of it?) Sherwood and John went by train. We got there in time for tea with the Livesays. Sherwood and John arrived later and we all had dinner with Rev. and Mrs. W. M. Baird. Both the Livesays and the Bairds are Northern Presbyterians. Rev. Livesay comes from Waynesboro, Virginia.

"The Halls all stayed at the Livesays for the night and John and I slept at the Bairds. Mrs. Baird and I took quite a liking to each other . . .

"About noon next day, Sherwood and John and I said good-bye to the rest and the car took us to a station several miles distant to get the train for Pyong Yang. We arrived at our destination at about 3 P.M. Sherwood is staying with the Rev. and Mrs. W. E. Shaw (District Superintendent of our church) and John and I are staying with Dr. and Mrs. A. G. Anderson. Dr. Anderson has charge of the hospital built in memory of Sherwood's father. The Andersons lost a beautiful 22 year old daughter from spinal meningitis about two years ago—the first foreign person to die in the new isolation ward her father had built.

"There are two other children, a son and a daughter in America attending school. At home is Robert, age ten, and he and John have taken to each other right away."

May 7, 1937

"The Andersons are lovely hosts and we are having a most pleasant time. We attended the evening meeting of the conference on Wednesday. It was very inspiring to see that audience of over 500 Koreans. The girls of the high school were there in a body. Of course everything was in Korean and I could only catch the spirit of the service. It was thrilling to hear them sing, 'My Jesus I Love Thee.'

"The set-up was much like that of our conference at home—several small tables on the platform with potted plants and flowers around. I thought that a small table down in front was for the press, but I was told that it was for a member of the Government Intelligence Department. . . .

"On Thursday morning Mrs. Anderson took me with her to the shopping district where she had errands to do . . . In the afternoon we had a cup of tea at the W.F.M.S. House and in the evening I was invited to the Woman's Hospital to dinner. Other guests were Sherwood; Rev. Billings, president of our Theological Seminary in Seoul; and Rev. Norris, a teacher there; Dr. Block (a woman doctor); and Rev. Sauer of Seoul.

We had a lovely dinner with Miss Butts, Miss Payne and Miss Anderson (our host's sister) as hostesses.

"They live in one section of the hospital built by Sherwood and his mother. At 14 Sherwood was the foreman!

"Now it is Friday . . . and this evening Sherwood and John and I have dinner with Father Carroll (who was Marian's Thanksgiving guest). Tomorrow we go for a boat ride up the river (the whole conference) to have a picnic supper. On Sunday, of course, we shall go to church and some time on Monday go back to Haiju, finish packing up, and leave there on the fourteenth for Songdo, then Seoul and then on the twenty-fifth go to Japan."

May 10, 1937

"Between Pyong Yang and Haiju we passed through the famous apple country of Korea. It is the Shenandoah Valley of Korea! On every side we saw apple orchards. The blossoms were white, though, not pink like ours. I was told that apples from this region are sent all over the world, just as our Virginia ones are."

May 14, 1937

". . . We left Marian's home and Haiju less than an hour ago. Sherwood went to Seoul yesterday to meet . . . a donor who is making a world tour and . . . may return with him to visit the work, . . . so Marian and William saw us off. The whole family will come up to Seoul before we leave Korea on May 25.

"I was very touched to have two Japanese families come to the Haiju station to see us off. The wife and child of the doctor in charge of the children's department of the Japanese Government Hospital here, arrived first, and handed me a gift . . . Mrs. Iwafuchi apologized for her husband's absence because he had a very sick patient he could not leave. The vice-governor and his wife, Mr. and Mrs. Sasaki, also came . . .

"We are passing through a very different scene from that seen on our arrival. Then the harvest had been gathered and the land was bare and cold. Now the rice fields are alive with spring, and beast and man are trudging through the mud about the business of raising the staple food of this country. Here and there we see the tender green of the rice seedling beds. These are the sprouts which will later be transplanted. . . .

"Before long we shall be at Dojo where we change trains for Songdo (Kaijo) where we expect Miss Ellasue Wagner to meet us. We plan to stay there all night, and see the work in that station which is a stronghold of Southern Methodism. Then on the evening of tomorrow, we go on to Seoul when we shall be guests of the Underwoods until we leave for Japan."

May 27, 1937

"Marian and William came from Haiju last Thursday evening and Sherwood and the children on Saturday. . . .

"On Sunday we all went with the Underwoods and several other families to a mountain named Nam Han (Southern Fortress) for a picnic lunch. A Korean emperor once lived within this fortress and there is a wall all around it. It was a

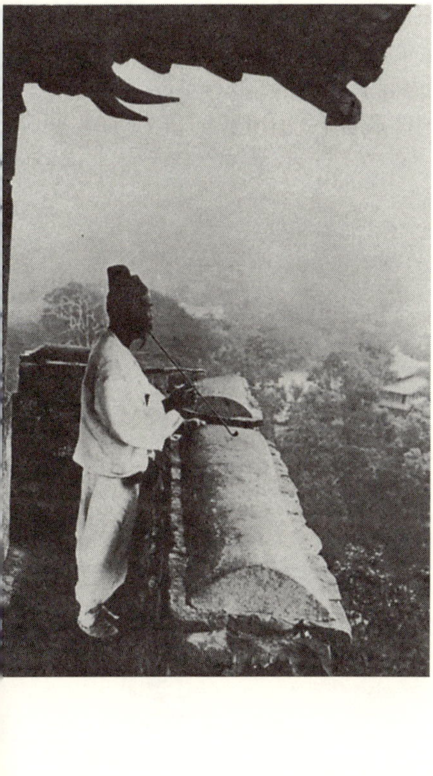

Pagoda and wall at Nam Han San (Southern Fortress Mountain)

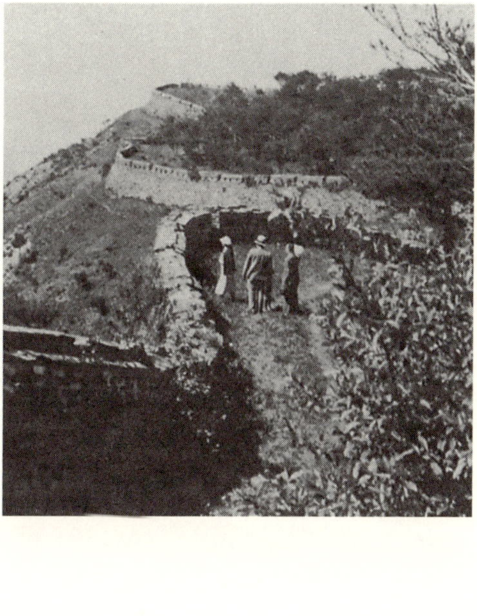

> most delightful experience to drive through the Korean countryside and then leave the cars and climb to the top of the mountain from which we got a magnificent view of the valley below. . . . This was one of the most memorable of our trips in Korea . . .
>
> "Monday, May 24, was Empire Day and we were invited to the British Consulate for the events and program, which included music and games for the children. There are quite a number of Britishers in Seoul and I felt quite at home . . . seeing the Union Jack and singing 'God Save the King'!"

Only a few more hours remained before the Lineweaver visit would be drawing to a close. Marian and I invited twenty guests to a farewell "*sukiaki* party" for Emma at a restaurant in Seoul. Emma was surprised and delighted to have this opportunity to say a personal farewell to these warm hearted people who had befriended her and John during their Korean sojourn.

From the restaurant we went to the Seoul Union Club House for ice cream, provided by Mrs. Underwood, and here the children joined us. Later that evening Emma and John bade us all *adieu* as their train pulled away from the Seoul station.

It had been a mutually enriching experience to have the Lineweavers with us for seven months. Filled with the memories of their visit, we turned back to Haiju and the reality of adjusting to their absence.

CHAPTER 26

The Castle at Wha Chin Po

As we resumed the happily interrupted normalcy of our lives, we were aware that the Japanese military had been taking a larger and larger role in the everyday life of Korea. Our preoccupation with our own personal crises and family events had tended to turn our attention away from what was happening in the rest of the world.

One day in the fall of 1937, word came over our radio that the summer resort at Wonsan Beach had been declared as being in the "Prohibited Zone"! All cottages there had to be dismantled or removed forthwith! Confirmation of this surprising news soon followed.

The Japanese military, although not noted for generosity, had given us an ideal campsite some 100 miles further down the coast, in lieu of the beach they were taking from us. It was located that much nearer to the famous Diamond Mountains, which could be seen looming up in the distance only a few hours trip away. The new beach had the rare combination of an ocean front, on the one hand, and a lake on the other, offering a choice to vacationers. At the southern extremity rose a hill, the western slope of which overlooked the lake. The eastern side dropped to the sea in a sheer cliff. The Japanese named this beach site "Kashinho," but the Koreans called it "Wha Chin Po" (Hwajinpo), which means literally, "Flower Lake Port." The lake was about three miles long and roughly in the shape of a cloverleaf and surrounded by mountains. It reminded many of us of Lake Lucerne in Switzerland.

Marian and I had been appointed to the Executive Committee of the Beach and were requested to proceed at once to the scene of the action. Marian had, in addition, been asked to serve as the official photographer of the new beach. She was to bring her movie camera with her.

The military offered to pay a fair compensation for each cottage at Wonsan Beach, or to pay for the cost of moving the house by boat and putting it up at the new beach. Most of us preferred the latter alternative, especially since many of the cottages were light wooden structures which could easily be taken apart and reassembled. First, we all gathered at Wonsan Beach where each family hastily packed their belongings at their respective cottage. Then we carefully numbered and labeled each section of our cottage, hoping that the parts would all fit back nicely when reassembled.

Because we had a time limit, it was necessary to call in local Koreans with no experience in carpentry to assist in the dismantling. Nothing was to be left standing. When the last house had been sent to the new location, either by rail or sea, the beach was dynamited so that not even a tree was left upright.

Although it was hard to bid good-by to our old beach, which had held many fond memories for us all, we became eager to explore the new campsite. As Marian and I were on the official committee, we were among the first to see it. This committee had the job of staking out and numbering the new plots. Marian busied herself taking pictures and movies of the beautiful campsites for those who could not be present. In due course, the lot numbers would be put in a hat and well shuffled and then the owners would draw for their lot.

The beach site proved to be even better than we had been led to believe. Fresh drinking water could be obtained simply by sinking a pipe several feet into the sand. When the ocean became too rough, there was always the alternative enjoyment of a sheltered lake just to the rear.

When we drew our plot number, it turned out to be on the lake front, so we arranged to have our wooden cottage assembled on it. Most of the cottage sections had arrived in correct number sequence, but the few that had somehow been mixed up had to be located. Eventually, like a jigsaw puzzle, the various sections were all neatly fitted together, and we had our cottage back, albeit on a new location.

If there had been no ocean front, we probably would have been content on the lake, but we had grown accustomed to the action of the roaring waves at Wonsan Beach and we began to miss them. So later, when we had an opportunity to acquire a site on the cliff, we jumped at the chance, for it seemed that most people did not want the climb. We were young and did not mind it, especially as I was able to put in a zigzag path with a fairly gentle slope through the pine trees leading to the site. This made ascent delightful, and one

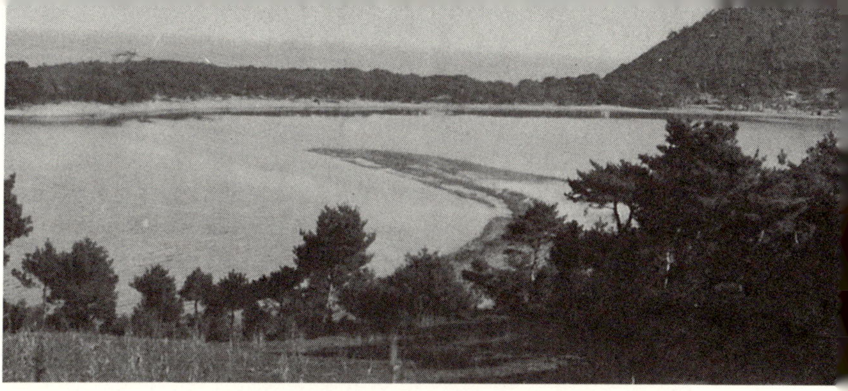

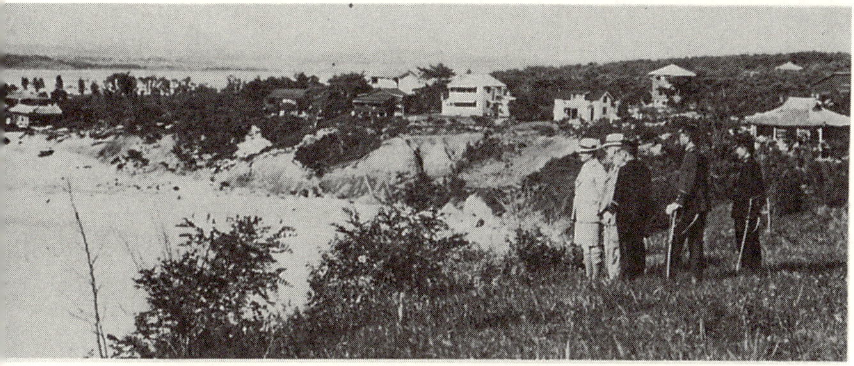

Wha Chin Po Beach (top) and vacation houses transplanted there from Wonsan Beach (bot.)

felt rewarded for the climb, for there was a superb view that could be obtained from there.

We began to build castles in the air and have a lot of fun making plans on paper for the cottage we would build on the new site. Such paper dreams cost us nothing.

During the Russian revolution of 1918-19, the missionaries in Korea had befriended some of the White Russian refugees who had had to flee from Russia for their lives. Similarly, when some of the Germans fled to Korea from the terror of Hitler, missionaries again found themselves befriending political refugees. Herr Weber was one of these. A young architect by training, he was eager to show his gratitude and his abilities. One evening in Haiju we happened to be toying out loud with some of our paper dreams and rough plans for a new cottage at Wha Chin Po. Herr Weber eagerly sprang to his feet and exclaimed that he would enjoy building it for us if we would only give him the chance.

This seemed like a good idea all around. I certainly had no notion of how I was ever going to get the time to supervise its construction, especially since we were then in the midst of a severe typhoid fever epidemic. These patients needed constant attention, for some had profuse hemorrhages.

The proposal by our German friend would give an outlet to his talents which he was anxious to use. Of course, the perennial problem was money for the undertaking, but Herr Weber told us not to worry on that score. He assured us that he would like to donate his services to us and even do much of the actual construction work himself. All he would expect would be money for materials and something toward his own living expenses. These latter, we realized, would not be much, for he lived very frugally.

I made a quick trip with Herr Weber to Wha Chin Po and showed him the actual site on the cliff overlooking the sea. I introduced him to a local Korean contractor there who had done a good and reasonably priced job of reassembling our wooden cottage. Because this was off season, the contractor promised to keep expenses down, which he assured me could easily be done for the stone could be procured right on the site. Furthermore, the farmers were not yet working their fields so they could be secured to help for a song. In fact, I did not even need to advance him a single yen until the cottage was completed and I was fully satisfied with his work.

In building at the Sanatorium, I had always been careful to take bids and draw up a written contract, legally attested. However, this seemed such a small affair, and the two men seemed so trustworthy, that I neglected to do for myself what I had always insisted must be done for others. From force of habit, I did have some misgivings at the time, but I was short of both time and money. I also knew the risk of paying in advance, so I had reluctantly agreed.

I had already talked over our plans with Herr Weber and left the rough sketch with him. He again assured me that I could safely entrust him with all the details, and that he and the contractor would keep costs down to a minimum. The latter two men appeared to get on well together, which augured well. They said that I need not return until the work was finished.

Although I had expected to come back and inspect the cottage while it was still in the process of being built, medical work detained me. When I did find time to break away to pay a visit to our "wee cottage," I was in for no small surprise. In fact, no word in the dictionary could adequately convey my astonishment. I was truly speechless! The contractor and Herr Weber, I could see, were both bursting with delighted pride over their creation, and it seemed almost cruel for me to even attempt to disillusion them.

There before my eyes, as incredible as anything out of Ripley's *Believe It or Not*, stood not a wee cottage, but a small castle! The grey stone walls contrasted with the green pine woods in the background. In fact, it looked just like one of those castles on the Rhine, parapet, tower and all, which Herr Weber had now faithfully repeated here in the "Land of the Morning Calm."

One could walk out on the flat roof of the castle and survey the grand scenery on all sides. In fact, the roof could readily lend itself to moonlight parties out-of-doors. The large round tower with its attractive window seats, seemed to be the special pride and joy of Herr Weber. He envisoned the lady of the castle pouring tea here and entertaining her friends. The tower had been built next to the cliff, looking out to sea, giving the illusion that one was on a ship actually on the ocean.

"On special occasions when your good *frau* wishes to throw larger parties, here is the spacious living room," announced Herr Weber as he led me into a room with bulging bay windows at one end, and at the other, a huge, dazzling fireplace built of rock crystals procured from a remote cave. "This will serve as the conversation piece," he declared with ill concealed pride. He lit a fire in the fireplace to show how nicely it drew. The crystals reflected the dancing flames and Herr Weber stood back to admire the sparkling beauty of his masterpiece.

While Herr Weber and the contractor were exhibiting the finer points of their workmanship to me with such pride and joy, my mind was racing at high speed. How on earth was I ever going to be able to pay the huge bill that shortly they would be presenting to me? This was most certainly a problem situation if ever there was one. I realized I had only myself to blame for not having insisted upon a formal written contract, and I tried to comfort myself that, at the time, it had hardly seemed necessary for such an insignificant little camp. But behold, here had developed the brainchild of Herr Weber's unfettered imagination which had completely outdistanced my wildest dreams. I had to admit that the two men had done an excellent job and that the general effect was striking. That, however, was poor comfort to me. I knew that Herr Weber had contributed largely of his own talents, tools and craftsmanship. Even so, I was sure that such a pretentious structure, this castle-on-the-Rhine that had somehow materialized at Wha Chin Po, would be no match for my poor slim pocketbook.

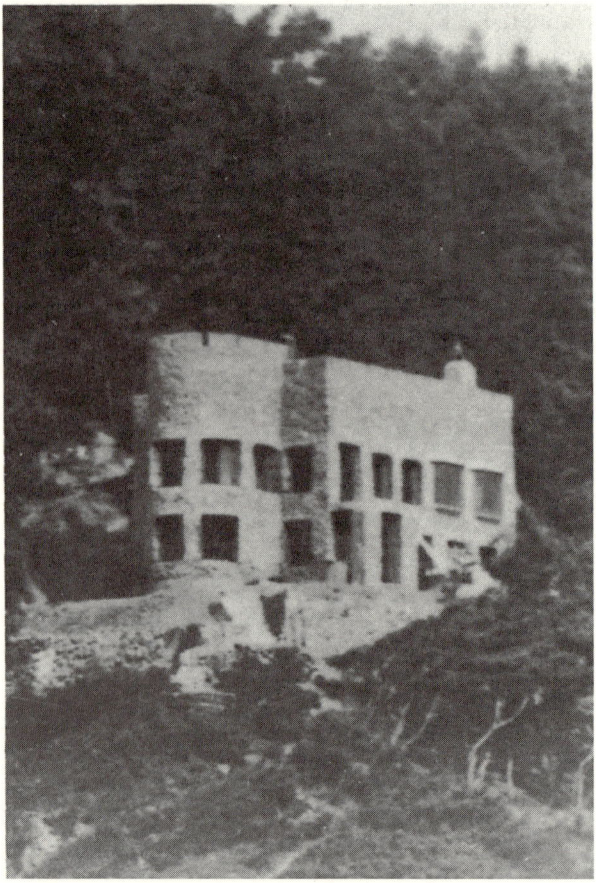

"The Castle" at Wha Chin Po

Although I was almost too stunned to speak, I finally screwed up courage to stammer out, "How much?"

The answer I heard was a surprise in the modesty of their demands, but still far more than I could afford, and to be candid, I simply did not have the cash for it. Since my predicament was really of my own making, I strongly felt that I could not let them down. I simply must somehow find a way out, although at the time I had not the faintest idea how. I asked them to please give me a chance to work out the financial arrangements, for this castle had taken me by surprise. Herr Weber hoped that it had been a happy one, but I was off before he could hear my reply.

It took me some time to recover from the shock, not that this was the first time I had been short of funds. I had become somewhat experienced at handling such situations. My formula, though not always easy, was simple. Where the matter was personal, I just tightened my belt until income caught up with outgo. Where the work was concerned, when emergencies arose, I would issue special appeals until enough funds came in to cover the emergency. But here was something entirely different.

On the one hand, no amount of belt tightening could help. On the other hand, I could hardly issue special appeals on a personal matter of this nature, even if my pride would let me, which of course it would not. It would be difficult to imagine that my friends and supporters would rush in to help me pay for a castle!

There appeared no way out of my self-inflicted dilemma. My mind remained a blank. Then there gradually drifted over my remorseful consciousness the familiar lines, "God works in mysterious ways His wonders to perform." Although it hardly seemed appropriate to bring God into the picture when the situation was so clearly my own fault, these lines continued to haunt me.

All of a sudden I found my thoughts turning back to my boyhood days at Pyong Yang and to my friend there, Susan Roe. She had been Nursing Superintendent at my mother's hospital but was now retired. Her sister, Lucy, had married a high official in the American gold mines (Oriental Consolidated Mining Company). The thoughts persisted until I had a strong compulsion to go right to Susan at Pyong Yang and talk over my problem with her. I recalled that she had always been good about money matters.

When I arrived in Pyong Yang, Susan greeted me warmly. She declared, "I am so glad you have come, for I was about to telegraph you. Now we can get the business all settled while you are here."

I gasped, "What business?"

"Why, that vacant plot of yours here in Pyong Yang which has lain dormant all these years," she replied with a smile, as she saw my astonishment. "Well, it has suddenly come to life," she continued, "for my sister, Lucy, tells me that the mining company officials claim that it is just the location and size they need for a distribution center. They are willing to pay spot cash for it, if your price is right."

I knew nothing of local real estate values but I knew what I needed to pay Herr Weber and the Korean contractor, so I blurted out that figure. Susan seemed to think that should satisfy them, and being an American firm, they were not likely to quibble over the price since the plot was just what they wanted. This proved to be the case. With a heartfelt prayer of gratitude to God, and hearty thanks to Susan and her sister Lucy, I was back with the needed funds in what seemed no time at all, and was able to pay in full for the construction of my castle.

To back track a little, my father had left me some life insurance money, you may remember, which as a boy I had invested in building a brick house. This house enabled our Mission to accommodate two missionary families, while the proceeds of this investment had helped me toward paying my college expenses. At the same time, I had put a small part of the investment into the purchase of a plot of land, which was then very cheap. This I had done with the idea that if and when I had children, it might help with their college expenses.

This latter part of the plan did not work out. Nevertheless, for a few happy seasons our family and friends did enjoy The Castle before it was summarily snatched from us, along with all its contents, by the cruel fate of war. All that remains to us of our castle is a photograph and an oil painting of it which Marian did. But the happy memories it gave to us can never be taken away, and each of our children was nonetheless, able to enjoy a college education without the benefit of its financial help.

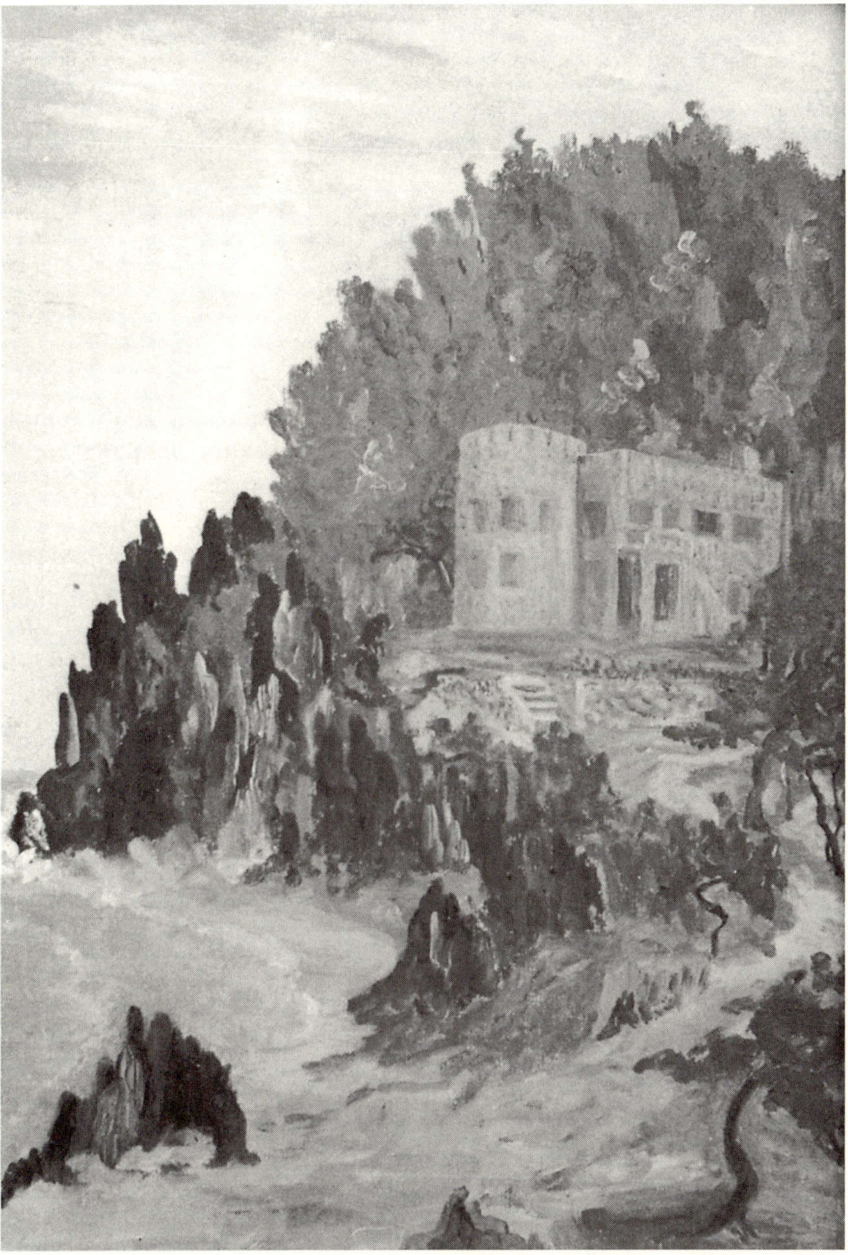

Marian's painting of "The Castle"

CHAPTER 27

Deputies

Our second furlough came due in the summer of 1938. We had booked passage on the *Empress of Japan*, a luxury liner that would take us to Vancouver, British Columbia, in Canada by way of Honolulu, Hawaii. We sailed from Japan on July 27, 1938.

Among the letters awaiting our arrival was a cordial invitation from our cousins, Louise and Arthur Symons, to journey a short distance south of the Canadian-U.S. border and visit them at their home on Hood Canal in the state of Washington. We accepted, and were soon enjoying the Symons' hospitality at their lovely ranch-style home on the scenic canal.

We discussed our plans for our furlough with the Symons one evening. We explained that in addition to some refresher courses, we would need to be doing deputation work among the various Methodist churches that might invite us to visit them. The Symons inquired as to why such activity was called "deputation work."

We had used the term so often that we had not really thought it might seem odd to someone unfamiliar with this missionary practice. Marian, with her characteristic taste for accuracy, asked to consult a dictionary. She reported her findings: A "deputy" was "a person empowered to act for another"; a "deputation" was "the act of appointing persons to represent others"; and to "depute" was "to appoint a substitute or agent and send with a special commission or authority to transact business in another's name."

Although we had not given it much thought before, we realized that in truth that was what we, as missionaries, were commissioned by the church to do—to act in its name as we went about the business of the church in another land. And in order to be "empowered," we needed the backing of those church members whom we represented, both in the spiritual sense of their prayers and interest to uphold us, and in the material sense of the funds that would make it possible for us to "transact the business" of our Christian mission. These were troubled times and the news of "*wars and rumours of wars*" that were reaching America from Europe and the Far East were not conducive to the task of fund raising which, as deputies, now lay before us.

The Symons suggested that before we begin our work, we should seize the opportunity of being this close to Alaska and take the scenic coastal trip there via the Inland Waterway. It did seem like a good idea, and Marian's Mount Union College Physical Education instructor, Jessie Glasse, now married to a minister, was living in Juneau. The Glasses had often asked us to come and see them. The Symons wished us a happy trip and we returned to Vancouver to catch the next sailing of the *Princess Louise* for Alaska.

The small coastal vessel seemed like a dwarf compared to the large trans-oceanic liner to which we had become accustomed. We found, however, that it was much cozier and we soon became well acquainted with nearly all the passengers. Frequent stops along the route afforded us plenty of opportunity to stretch our legs and visit interesting sights.

As we approached Juneau, we rushed to see the famous Mendenhall Glacier. It was said that a blast from the ship's horn would create sufficient vibration to cause a piece of the glacier to fracture and a huge chunk of ice would fall into the sea. Although we donned our raingear to protect us from the splash, the famed glacier failed to "perform."

Shortly thereafter, the *Princess Louise* docked at Juneau where we were met by the Glasses. Jessie and her husband, the Reverend John Glasse, drove us to the church parsonage where we were to stay for the two days the boat would be in port before continuing the trip up to the Lind Canal.

The Glasses were eager to show us the sights of Juneau and to drive to the Mendenhall Glacier for a first-hand look. Phyllis piped up that we had already seen it but that it did not break for us when the captain blew the whistle.

The Glasses laughed heartily. "Don't regret that, for we shall give you a little ice cutter and you can help break off enough ice from the glacier to make us some ice cream. We have an old-fashioned ice cream freezer and the boys can take turns cranking it by hand. We'll bring all the ingredients along with us."

This unique experience of glacier-made ice cream proved also to be delicious. We were beginning to wonder if the remainder of the trip could live up to this highlight. However, that evening Phyllis developed a soaring fever.

We were forced to cancel our plans for the northern part of the tour and stayed in Juneau until the ship stopped there on its return voyage. Fortunately by then Phyllis was well enough to travel. We took turns in the meantime seeing the sights around Juneau while either Marian or I stayed with Phyllis.

We particularly enjoyed our visit to an Alaskan gold mine and watched the molding of gold bricks. We were invited to dip our fingers very quickly in and out of this beautiful molten golden soup. We all declined, despite the assurances that we would not be burned.

Upon returning to Vancouver, we began our trans-Canada journey eastward. The trip through the Canadian Rockies proved enjoyable in more than one respect. We had a stopover at Banff and boarded a bus from the train station to the Banff Springs Hotel. Being a family of five, we could not all sit together, so William elected to find a seat beside a friendly looking lady. They were soon engaged in animated conversation.

Later we met his seat companion, Mrs. Herbert Greene (Beatrice), who was traveling with her husband's aunt, Mrs. Frederick McOwen (Louise). We shall always be grateful to Providence and William for thus beginning for us a warm friendship with Bee and Herbert Greene and with their Aunt Lou. Mrs. Greene had been charmed by William's conversation and later told us about it.

They had begun by finding out where each other lived. When William discovered that Mrs. Greene and Mrs. McOwen lived in Philadelphia, he grew very excited. He showed a considerable knowledge about their fair city and expressed a fervent wish to hear the Philadelphia Orchestra play. His new found friends promptly extended him an invitation to do just that should he ever find himself in Philadelphia.

As they conversed on other matters, William (then age eleven) apparently declared to his surprised and entranced audience, "I am a student of the classics, and I plan to improve on them."

Mrs. Greene and Mrs. McOwen asked William to introduce them to the rest of his family, and they cordially invited us to visit them if we should ever come to Philadelphia. It so happened that our immediate destination was Ventnor, New Jersey where we planned to stay in the cottages maintained by the Pennsylvania Medical Missionary Society as we had done on our previous furlough.

So it was that we stopped off in Philadelphia en route to Ventnor. There we met Herbert Greene, owner of a manufacturing and distributing company for rubber goods which were traded under the name of M. L. Snyder & Sons. We were most graciously entertained by this loving couple as we would be many times again through the years. William was taken to hear the Philadelphia Orchestra and amused the Greenes by expressing his shock that the harpist could receive such high pay for just sitting there and plunking a few strings from time to time. Mrs. McOwen took us all out to dinner at the exclusive Union League Club. She explained that the Union League was formed in 1863 to furnish money and men to uphold President Lincoln and the Union at the time of the Civil War. The entire visit was a memorable beginning to the year of study and deputation work that lay ahead of us.

Miss Josephine Zimmerman, who operated a school in Ventnor, remembered William from our last furlough when he attended her kindergarten. We enrolled both boys in her school and then looked for someone who could help to run the household and take care of the children while we were away at our deputation work and our post-graduate studies. Generous friends made it possible for us to hire Leona Porter and our children became very attached to her. She cared for them so lovingly and operated the household tasks so expertly that our children did not seem to mind our absences from home, even when it would sometimes be for several weeks. Leona was very interested in missions and we continued to correspond with her even after we returned to Korea.

Now that the Methodist Mission Board had embarked on its policy of assigning missionaries to specific churches, who contributed through the Board for their support, we looked forward to meeting our patrons in person. This system, known as the "Parish Abroad," had many advantages, not the least of which was that we came to know personally those whom we were representing on the mission field. Some of the churches had arranged with their key parishioners for us to stay a few days at each of their homes and this allowed us to get better acquainted.

In addition to the lasting friendships which developed and the great assistance to the mission work which resulted, we found that the churches involved remained interested in the mission work and in us even when the pastor was transferred. Since ministers are shifted from church to church rather frequently under the Methodist system, it was of great benefit to have this feeling of continuity remain because of these wider contacts among the congregation itself.

Of course this meant that our visits to the different churches were sometimes for a longer time than was the case with the usual single speaking engagement. These associations bore rich fruit in the years that followed. We were given the feeling that we were truly "empowered to act" in behalf of these supporters.

Two of the churches I had scheduled first on our itinerary were the Tabernacle Methodist Church in Binghamton, New York and the Methodist Church at Liberty. The former had established the Haskins Bible Class in memory of Mrs. Fred Haskins who, until her death, had contributed to our salary and to our work. This class was to later take up a share of our financial support and were always generous in their interest and concern for our work.

My mother had her office in Liberty for the small medical practice which she kept up after she retired from the mission field. I welcomed this early opportunity to visit her and to also thank those Liberty friends who had so generously supported both my mother's work and ours in Korea. During our furlough, my mother would come to Ventnor periodically and sometimes would help take care of the children for a few days when Marian and I had to be away.

After Marian had had a chance to take a graduate level refresher course in gynecology and obstetrics in New York City, I was able to take my turn. I enrolled in a course in advanced studies in tuberculosis offered by the Trudeau School of Tuberculosis. This was held from May 15 to June 10, 1939 at Saranac Lake in the Adirondack Mountains in New York State.

The Director of this school was none other than the brilliant son of Dr. Edward Livingstone Trudeau. The latter had founded the first sanatorium in the United States in 1885. It was at Saranac Lake that Dr. Edward Trudeau had conquered TB in himself and became the living demonstration to others of the importance of rest, good food, fresh air and graded exercises in combating this disease. The first cottage, afterwards known as "The Little Red," still stood as a reminder of its founder's valiant spirit.

The accepted treatment of Dr. Edward Trudeau's day had been to shut patients up in dark houses, protecting them from the air by tightly closing windows and doors. This airless, sunless treatment, which was designed to avoid aggravating the patient's coughing spells, actually served to hasten their demise. Dr. Trudeau had watched his brother die of TB and when he too contracted the disease, he resolved that if he was soon to leave this world, he would do so with God's pure air in his lungs and God's sunshine brightening his room.

Despite the dire predictions that he was inviting an early death by his life of hunting and fishing and ample exposure to the winter cold, the world now knows that he won his battle against TB. Later, the author, Robert Louis Stevenson, came to Saranac Lake to seek treatment for TB and he became a good friend of Dr. Edward Trudeau, although it was reported that Mr. Stevenson was not a very good patient. He disliked cold and preferred to shut himself in his cozy cottage with all the windows closed. But Dr. Trudeau insisted that he endure the cold and follow the regulations of the sanatorium.

Dr. Edward Trudeau died at the age of 67 in 1915 and the Adirondack Cottage Sanitarium he founded became known as the Trudeau Sanatorium after his death. Since then, other sanatoria were opened in this same vicinity, some small and humble and others luxurious. Some of these institutions stressed a medical treatment for TB and others specialized in a surgical approach to the disease.

The school directed by Dr. Trudeau's son, Francis B. Trudeau, M.D., took advantage of the nearness of these other institutions to expose its graduate students to the different methods of treatment then in vogue. These field trips were of particular interest to me for I could observe many varied approaches to conducting TB institutions.

One of the more lavish of the sanatoria we visited was that operated by the Theater Guild of America for actors and actresses who had been stricken with TB. It was apparent that no cost had been spared to provide everything possible for the comfort of each patient. Windows made of special glass to freely admit ultraviolet rays had been supplied and an ample nursing staff awaited the beck and call of the patients. A beautiful theater had also been provided for the enjoyment of those who were convalescing. Compared to the simpler institutions, one wondered if, after all, adequate provision had been made here for God's free pure air and natural sunshine.

Dr. Francis Trudeau led us in an intensive review of tuberculosis treatment and waxed eloquent when he described his father's great fight back to health and usefulness. We were also exposed to instruction from other authorities in the field, and I found that in addition to this formal aspect of the program, I gained much from conversing with my fellow students. There were about 100 students from all over the United States and Canada and different parts of the world, and we had much to learn from each other's experiences.

The Trudeau Sanatorium followed a fairly conservative approach to TB treatment, but their records of success seemed to justify this course. We did learn the newer techniques for staining the tubercle bacilli to better see them under microscopic examination. We also received some expert instruction in reading skiagrams (x-ray films and plates) to help us distinguish between TB foci and artifacts which closely resembled them but could lead to a false diagnosis if not recognized.

The most vigorous treatment debate of that day was on the use of pneumothorax treatment, which, when performed under careless or unsterile conditions, could render the cure worse than the disease. Cases of empyema (pus in the pleural cavity) would be the common result if the proper care were not taken. We had some heated discussions on this subject, I recall, but they tended to direct our attention to a more careful application of this method. We were fortunate in being able to see this technique performed especially skillfully by the doctors who used it at the Trudeau Sanatorium.

At the conclusion of this rich experience, I had a whirlwind trip out to Ohio and back to attend the twentieth anniversary of my graduating class at Mount Union College in Alliance and make some speeches to Ohio churches while there. I took this opportunity to visit another of our main support churches, The Church of the Saviour in Cleveland, which was our first "Parish Abroad" church and had been so generously supporting our work since April, 1931.

On June 14, 1939 my mother was to celebrate the fiftieth anniversary of her graduation from Women's Medical College. Marian and William and I joined her in Philadelphia to witness the ceremony. She was presented with a gold medal along with nine of her classmates of the Class of 1889, when the class had numbered 41 students, my mother being the youngest of them. My mother had brought with her a class picture and also photographs of all the professors who were there in 1889. One of those was Dr. W. W. Keen who had told an interesting story about my mother when she was a medical student:

> "A student who lives vividly in my recollection furnished me in May, 1887, a wholly unique surgical experience—unique, I fancy, even in the annals of Surgery. The student sought my advice for a number of tuberculosis glands in the neck. As they were on the point of becoming abscesses I advised their removal. To this she immediately consented, but added, 'Upon one condition.'
>
> "'And what is that?'

"'That I shall not take either ether or chloroform.'

"'But, my dear child,' I said, 'surely you do not understand. This operation will last probably an hour and a half. I must make an incision from your ear to the breast bone and then along the clavicle nearly to the shoulder, raise both flaps over a large area and dissect the glands most carefully from the jugular vein, carotid artery, probably the great sub-clavian vessels and certainly from all the numerous nerves in the neck. If you jump from sudden pain, I do not know where the point of my knife may go.'

"'Yes,' she replied, 'I quite understand. I will stand any amount of pain without budging, but I will not take either ether or chloroform.'

"'Why not?'

"'Because I have already had two operations for similar glands elsewhere, both done by Prof. Henry B. Sands of New York, one with ether and the other with chloroform, and I suffered so intensely from the after effects that I prefer to endure the pain of the operation. If I cannot have the glands removed without the anesthetic, I will not have the operation performed.'

"'Well,' said I, seeing her absolutely fixed determination, 'only within a few days I have seen an account of a new local anesthetic called cocaine, and if you are willing, I will try that, but I can't promise how much it will dull the pain.'

"'Anything except ether or chloroform,' was the quiet but decided answer.

"A few days later I operated. She never so much as winced. Now, however, comes the additional and unique surprise. I had made my incisions and had begun to dissect the flaps when she said to me, 'Would you mind if one of the residents (the operation was done in the Woman's Hospital and the residents, of course, were women) were to get me a hand glass and let me watch the operation?'

"For a moment I confess I was–if I may venture to use the word–'flabbergasted.' But I instantly made up my mind that anyone who could face fearlessly an hour and a half of pain without any anesthetic would be able to watch the operation without flinching. And so it proved. For over an

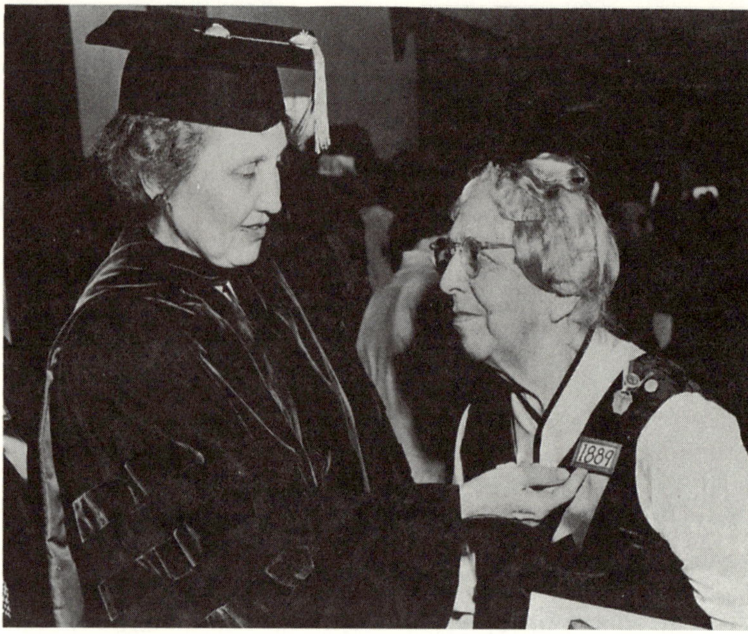

Dean Marion Fay of Women's Medical College of Pennsylvania greets alumna Dr. Rosetta Hall

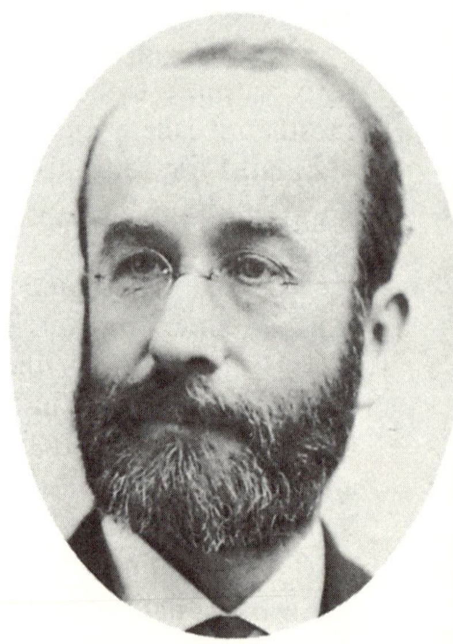

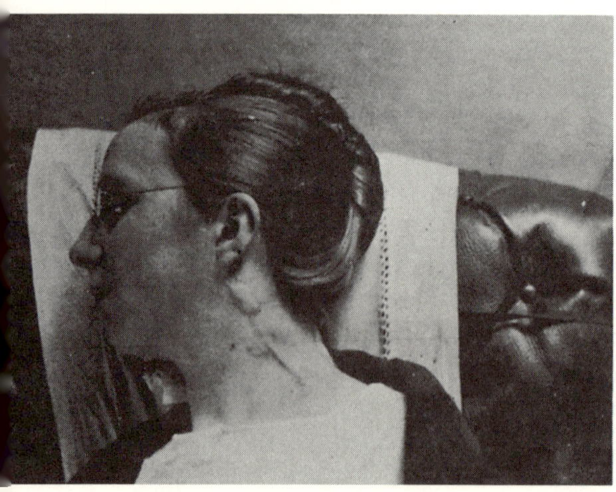

Rosetta Sherwood consults Dr. Keen about tubercular glands in her neck, 1887

hour she held the glass and watched every stroke of my knife even when shaving the great jugular and without a single movement of head, hand or foot."[1]

We were very proud of Mother and basked in the reflected glory of the honors and recognition she received that day. They were a great satisfaction to her. She was particularly happy that her husband's namesake, her grandson, was along for this occasion.

The New York World's Fair had opened on April 30, 1939. We took advantage of this unique opportunity to visit it and, along with many others, marveled at the improbable foretaste of the future which some of the exhibits projected. William and Marian had been so fascinated by watching television at the Fair, they were late to a gathering of the "Korea Klub" one evening where I was to meet them. The "Korea Klub" was a group of those who had lived in Korea at one time or another and this occasion was a reunion dinner in New York for some who were second and third generation "Korea-ites." My mother noted that she was the only first generation member there.

Our agenda all year had been crowded with reunions, courses, sightseeing, visits, and deputation work. Buoyed by our furlough experiences, we were eager to return to Korea. We knew, furthermore, that we had a real contribution to make, for word we received from Korea spelled out some of the crisis situations which were developing, in part, because of the Sino-Japanese conflict. Dr. Kim implored us to bring desperately needed supplies for both the hospital and the sanatorium, for during the past year they had been forced to "make-do" or do without what we had formerly considered essential materials.

A letter from Miss Lund also made us realize we should not delay in getting back. It seemed that the Japanese military was putting heavy pressure on the medical staffs of both institutions to leave and be rewarded with higher pay by working in military and government hospitals. Miss Lund seemed to feel that only my voice of protest would stem the pressure that was being placed on the staff and that the latter needed me to defend their right to remain.

---

[1] "Imperial Chalices From Korea Highlights Career of WMC's Oldest Alumna," *Germantown Courier*, Vol. 14 No. 27, June 15, 1950, Feature Page.

Miss Elizabeth Keith, the English artist, who had designed the Korean TB Christmas Seals for 1934-35 and 1936-37, wrote that she was planning to be in Korea on a visit. She offered to design a Christmas Seal for us for the 1940-41 campaign if I could arrange to meet her in Seoul by September.

With all these pressures to hasten our departure for Korea, we made reservations on the *SS President Pierce* to sail from San Francisco on August 11, 1939. My mother had agreed to come to "The Anchorage," the name of our Ventnor cottage, to help us with the last minute packing. We had arranged for our heavy trunks and the hospital supplies we were taking back to be sent on ahead to San Francisco. They were to be shipped by freighter from Philadelphia by way of the Panama Canal. We had been invited to visit Emily Haskins Luce and her minister husband, the Reverend Clayton Luce, who lived in the town of Street, Maryland.

From there we would stop to see Marian's sister, Emma Lineweaver, and family who were now serving at Ekhart Mines, Maryland, before we headed West. Our itinerary took us by way of Pittsburgh on July 16; Chicago, July 19; Ann Arbor, July 21; arriving in San Francisco in time for our August 11 sailing date. The *President Pierce* was due to arrive at Kobe, Japan on August 27.

We bade my mother good-by on July 8 and had just arrived at Cousin Emily's when we received a telegram from the Mission Board. It advised us to halt all preparations for leaving until we were able to raise our own travel expenses to Korea because the Board had found itself in financial difficulties and could not supply us our fare.

This put us in a quandary for we had already shipped the hospital supplies and our heavy trunks on to San Francisco. Marian and I prayed about our dilemma and felt that God would help us come to a decision.

We wondered if we should tell Cousin Emily about our problem, but decided against it, for her mother had always been so generous to us and our work down through the years, it didn't seem right for us to beg now. So we kept our concern to ourselves. While Cousin Emily was driving us to Eckhart Mines, little Phyllis, who was then four years old, began to sing enthusiastically a song she had learned in Sunday School, "The B-I-B-L-E." Cousin Emily seemed deeply touched by her singing.

As she dropped us off, Cousin Emily pressed a check into my hand. I was dumbfounded to see that she had given us $500.00. Whether or not it was Phyllis' singing that had prompted so generous an act in our moment of need, we did not know, but we gave her the credit for it, and certainly it was a vivid reminder to us of God's love. We took it to be an answer to our prayer, and that somehow, between Eckhart Mines and San Francisco, we would acquire the needed remaining amount to cover the cost of getting our family and the hospital supplies to Korea.

We wrote to friends and patrons in the cities and towns through which our transcontinental train would pass. We explained our situation to them frankly and told them that we were leaving according to schedule in the faith that by the time we reached San Francisco, we would be enabled to make the rest of the journey to Korea.

We were not disappointed. Friends met us at the station as our train passed through, or we would stop over for a brief visit. By the end of our "whistle stop" journey, we arrived in San Francisco with our passage money and enough over to pay the freight on the hospital supplies. In a very new and special way, we felt our responsibility to serve as deputies for those who expressed their faith in us by responding to this emergency.

After completing this chapter, I came across a volume of my mother's journals which had been mislaid. Most of the diary covered the period of my mother's first year in Korea and had been the source from which she wrote the long letter home, excerpts of which form Chapter Two of this book. However, I was particularly struck by the final entry, dated May 17, 1891. The subject seemed to afford a fitting conclusion to this present chapter, and I should like to share some of my mother's thoughts on the subject of "deputies" as she perceived the missionary's role back in 1891:

> "'*. . . And who knoweth whether thou art come to the kingdom for such a time as this?*' Esther IV:14
>
> "The above was the text of Rev. Bunker's sermon this morning. . . . The text and the sermon . . . remind me of a little study I have been making in John lately. In one of the

chapters in the book *Live Christ* that Dr. Hall gave me, it is suggested to look up the references in which Jesus uses the expression, '*My Father hath sent me*,' and I was surprised to find in the book of John alone, 30 verses expressing that idea.*

"*John: IV:34; V:24,30,37,38; VII:16,28,29,33; VIII:16,18,26,29,42; IX:4; XI:42; XII:44,45,49; XIII:20; XIV:24; XV:21; XVI:27,28; XVII:8,18,21, 23,25; XX:21.

"When I was a little girl I remember to have heard the conundrum, 'Why is a missionary like a penny?' As a rule I forget riddles and conundrums, but the answer to this always impressed me—'because he is *one sent*.'

"Jesus is our perfect example of a missionary. The consciousness that the Father sent Him was ever in His mind, and He wanted to tell everyone that He did not act for Himself but for Another . . . '*As my Father hath sent me, even so I send you*.'

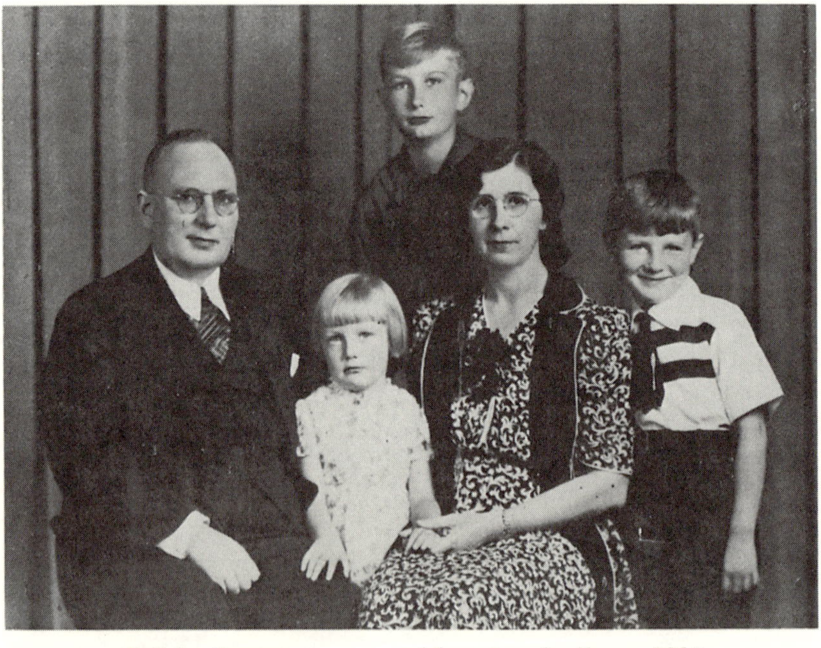

Hall family portrait on eve of departure for Korea, 1939

"Why did the Father send the Son? '*God so loved the world that He gave His only begotten son*'—it was to reveal the Father's love. '*As thou hast sent me into the world, even so have I sent them into the world,*'—our mission is like Christ's.

"It seems too high, too altogether great, but God does not ask anything He does not give the strength to perform; as Jesus said, '*I am not alone.*'—'*He that sent me is with me.*' So Jesus when He sent us, saying '*Go ye, therefore, and teach all nations . . . whatsoever I have commanded you,*' added the blessed surety, '*Lo, I am with you alway even unto the end of the world.*'

"There is one question that came to my mind in studying this that I think I never thought of before. Would Jesus have come if the Father had not *sent* Him? I have always thought of Him as a voluntary offering, and so in a sense he was, but was it the Father or the Son that first suggested saving us in this way? John 7:28 says, '*I am not come of myself.*' John 8:42 says, '*I proceeded forth and came from God; neither came I of myself, but He sent me.*' This makes me grasp John 17:21, 22, 23 as I never did before. '*Thou hast sent me, and* ***hast loved them, as thou hast loved me.***' I don't understand how or why the Father *could* love us so, but He must have done so or He never would have sent Jesus to suffer for us.

"The thought that God loves these Koreans as He loves His own Son stimulates me to want to tell everyone I meet of the 'Good news.'"

CHAPTER 28

Whispers of War through My Stethoscope

We sailed on schedule from the United States on August 11, 1939. Upon our arrival in Seoul, however, we found that the year 1939 had never come to Korea!

The Western calendar had been replaced by the Japanese calendar which reckoned time from the accession of the first Japanese Emperor, Meiji. On official documents, the year we knew as 1939 was the year 2599, the year of the reigning Emperor.

Koreans were being encouraged not only to adopt this Japanese system, but were considered unpatriotic if they did not do so. Although Westerners were still permitted to call the year 1939, the Koreans were being given the subtle message that to follow Western ways was equivalent to being disloyal to the Emperor. The Japanese military seemed to be intentionally trying to revive Korea's age-old historic suspicion of Western foreigners. We were soon to discover how this might begin to affect us in a more personal way.

In a letter to my mother dated September 12, 1939 just after our return to Korea, I wrote:

> "... We had a very hot trip from Kobe to Seoul and struck one of the worst hot spells in Seoul that we have ever experienced.
>
> "Joe had a heat stroke with high fever for three days which gave us some anxious moments. We all were prostrated with the heat. But on account of Joe's illness, we had to delay our coming to Haiju. Many failed to get the message and came down to the Haiju station for nothing, for which we were sorry.
>
> "Dr. Yi of the Sanatorium, and Dr. Kim of Norton Hospital, and the head teacher of the Boys School, all came up to

Seoul to greet us when we first arrived. A good turn-out of the Seoul foreigners were there too. Marian and the two smaller children were at Ruth's [Appenzeller] and William and I at Jensens when we were in Seoul. All were very good to us . . .

". . . There are practically no taxies for foreigners. The anti-foreign feeling in general, and the strong anti-British feeling in particular, had greatly subsided just before we came. Relations improved when Japan denounced Germany for her pact with the Reds. . . . Many of the missionaries still think it is not wise to go into the country, though we have met with no affront except the refusal of taxi service. Both Japanese and Koreans have been most friendly to us.

"It is the first time we have been faced with a shortage of food supplies. We have not been able to get butter and are so sorry we did not bring some from Miss Santee's in Kobe. Marian went to several stores and finally was able to get one pound of sugar. Flour is also hard to get and there are no rubber or leather goods or cotton goods available . . . Canned goods of all kinds are rapidly disappearing and prices are prohibitive. But rice and potatoes are plentiful and though we cannot get Klim [powdered milk], we can get milk from our Sanatorium farm which is proving a life saver. Also our missionary friends who laid in supplies in advance have offered to help us out, so there is no danger of starving. The fuel problem is perhaps our most acute problem but fortunately we have some coal left and we can still buy wood.

"Times and conditions have changed, but we believe with them there are still greater opportunities for service as the people are more eager than ever for the Gospel message, and our workers seem more cooperative. So we are glad we came back when we were needed most and could serve the best.

"The x-ray films we brought out for the Sanatorium proved a wonderful godsend as they had not been able to get any for a year; also the gauze and bandage material we brought out for the hospital, as they had been working with paper bandages which are far from satisfactory. We are unable to order x-ray films, gauze and bandages, Haliver-oil capsules and other medicines, as no money is allowed out of the country.

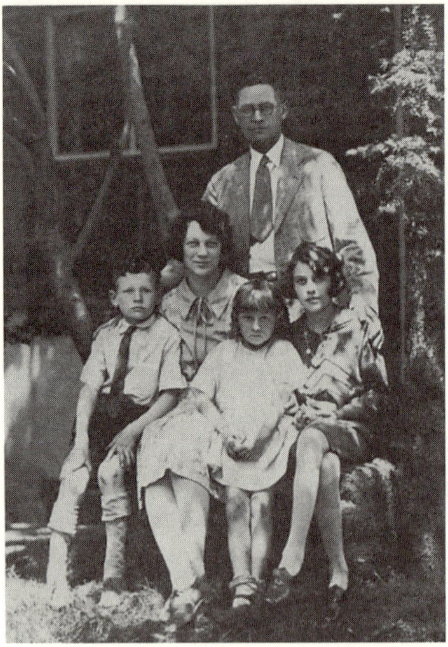

Henry and Ruth Appenzeller with children: Margaret (11), Richard (8), Carol (6)

"But of course we are allowed to receive gifts from our friends of all the above, as long as they do not come direct from the company, are wrapped with some old sheets or clothes and are distinctly marked—'Gifts for charity purposes for mission hospital—no commercial value.'

"On reaching Haiju, we were escorted to Miss Lund's and Miss Dalbey's, i.e. the W.F.M.S. home, and they kindly entertained us as paying guests until we could get settled to a certain extent in our house. This was a great help. Miss Dalbey is the new worker here who takes Miss Barlow's place. She seems quite nice . . . She is about as old as Miss Lund. They gave a birthday party for Phyllis which we all enjoyed . . .

"I was pleased to find the Boys' School, Hospital and Sanatorium all in excellent shape and better than when I left them, with increases in both students and patients as well as staff. So far they have all seemed glad for my return and resuming responsibility but are naturally disappointed that I did not bring any large gift for the work with me . . . I told them I still hoped to raise funds for the Boys' School chapel which is so greatly needed . . .

"The Sanatorium, hospital and school gave a very fine welcome party or feast for us shortly after our arrival. Miss Lund and Miss Dalbey were invited too. The School Board also gave a welcome party and there was a large evergreen welcome arch to greet us at the Sanatorium on our arrival . . .

"We found quite a lot of our stuff stolen, but I think your goods here escaped for the most part except some of the removable parts on your stoves . . . There are a lot of repairs and other things that need attention such as a leaky roof etc. and where all the money is coming from, I don't know. We bought a second-hand coal stove at San Francisco and found we could get one at Seoul for about the price it took to bring it out, as so many foreigners are leaving for one reason or another. . . ."

The whispers of war were slow to reach Haiju. The Japanese military had removed our shortwave wireless radio, which meant we were unable to pick up international news. Our longwave radio only blared forth propaganda: the great victories of Hitler in Europe, and Japan's glorious conquest of Manchuria and now, of China. U.S. and British loans to the Nationalist government in China had stirred up Japanese resentment and caused them to challenge foreign rights everywhere. Nothing must hinder the establishment of the "new order" in the Far East.

I knew that the victories for the Japanese that were touted by radio propagandists had been paid for at a heavy cost of lives. There was hardly a Japanese family in Haiju that had not lost a loved one, and many who had lost all their sons. The students of our Haiju Boys' School together with students from the other schools, and the prominent gentry, were asked to pay tribute to the warrior dead. As principal of our Haiju Boys' School, it was my painful duty to go with my students to the station when the trains came in bearing ashes of the war dead in urns contained in specially labeled little white boxes. These sad occasions were becoming more frequent, and each time the number of little white boxes increased.

The students were also summoned to the station from time to time to cheer the new Japanese recruits who were being sent to the front. I observed at this time that there were no Korean recruits. (At a later date, there were some Koreans whom the Japanese felt could be trusted who were pressed into army service.) As the war progressed, both the younger and older men were being drafted.

The Government Hospital was hastily building temporary extensions to receive wounded Japanese soldiers, and some of our staff doctors and nurses were being requisitioned to help out. Thus, our remaining staff had to do double duty. This kept us all on the jump, and my stethoscope was in greater demand than ever.

I was struck by the fact that all the glorious victories I heard about over the radio and in the newspapers seemed to be at variance with the increasing number of casualties who were arriving even in our small area. Our mail was being heavily censored, and whole pages were removed from the letters reaching us. It was very frustrating to be kept in the dark about events that might indeed affect our friends and us.

"Necessity," it is said, "is the mother of invention." I reasoned that if my stethoscope was able to pick up even faint sounds from the chest, not audible to the naked ear without this aid, why not try using my stethoscope on my longwave radio? I just might pick up something which was being broadcast from that independent American radio station in Shanghai which was reputed to broadcast accurate news, and not just propaganda.

So late one dark night, after I had carefully circled the outside of our home to make sure there were no intruders, I pulled down the black shades which were used in practice for possible bombing raids. Carefully locking all doors before turning off the lights, I tried my little experiment. At first, I seemed to get only local stations, which came through my stethoscope with greater clarity, even when dialed very low. Nothing, however seemed to come through from Shanghai.

I was almost going to give up, when suddenly, although as faint as a whisper, there came the voice of radio broadcaster Carrol Alcott out of Shanghai. The picture that emerged as I listened was quite a different one from that presented in the Japanese broadcasts. It was, nonetheless, black enough, especially as far as Hitler's war was concerned. Japan, however, was not as yet getting all her own way in China. It was still a boost to our morale to feel in touch with the truth of what was happening in the world outside.

Of course, except for Marian, I was careful to tell no one of this tapping of our radio for outside news. However, without consciously realizing it, perhaps I showed a more confident and assured attitude. The Japanese gendarmes would visit me from time to time to try to find out how much I knew about developments in China and Europe. I was careful not to divulge what I knew in any shape or form.

They often asked me silly questions, such as, whether I had heard that there had been an attempt on the Emperor's life. To this I would retort, why should they expect me to hear about any such conspiracy when they were so carefully censoring my letters? Anyway, this kind of news would hardly be conveyed to me, a foreigner in their midst.

Dr. Kim had once been called by the gendarmes to read one of my letters that I had sent to a friend, for the good doctor was more familiar with my rather illegible handwriting. Nothing incriminating was found in it. They also asked Dr. Kim and others whether I had at any time discussed the war situation with them or had made any inquiries about troop movements.

Dr. Kim replied, no, but that I had complained bitterly about not getting certain essential drugs for use on our own hospital patients. He was assured that the authorities would look into the matter.

Many ordinary items had also gone completely off the market. Even sugar was no longer available except at special stores in Seoul. Here one could get a maximum of one pound of sugar, only if one made a purchase of other commodities amounting to at least 100 yen ($20.00).

We had guests in to tea one afternoon and when they spied the sugar in a bowl on the table, their eyes almost popped. They each made a dive for it, and in less time than it takes to tell it, the sugar bowl had been completely emptied. After that experience, Marian prudently followed the example of the missionary ladies who only served pre-sugared tea, although she always felt apologetic about it.

The news that continued to come over our radio from Shanghai, amplified by my stethoscope, was far from reassuring. The theater of war in Europe was enlarging at an alarming pace. The commentator spoke of the terrible atrocities being committed by both sides in the Far East. Each side attempted to out-do the other in an ever rising crescendo of sadistic savagery. He narrated some of the incidents and ghastly details. Of course, I did not relay this part of the news to my family, but we could be thankful that the actual theater of war seemed to be receding from our location, and Korea, for the most part, still appeared to be the "Land of the Morning Calm."

Marian had thought it might be a good idea to try to bring some cheer to the wounded soldiers in the military hospital wing of the

Haiju Government Hospital. She set about to organize a work party among the more active of her "Mothers Club" members, and among the public spirited ladies of Haiju, both Korean and Japanese. All entered into the project with good will and enthusiasm. They rolled bandages and prepared sweets and other small gifts to distribute to the wounded. What was their consternation, therefore, when they were met at the military wards by the guard and turned back.

He told them, "Positively no admittance to civilians!" However, he did condescend to receive their token gifts for the wounded. He gave them not so much as a word of thanks. This impertinent rebuff was hard to understand at the time and was very disconcerting.

A few days later, while I was making my rounds at the Sanatorium, a Japanese military courier in a new uniform came to give me a message. The thought flashed through my mind that no doubt the chief medical officer had learned of Marian's good will mission and was sending an apology for the guard's rudeness.

I hastily tore open the official looking note, and to my surprise, read words to the effect that they had learned of my reputation as a chest specialist. They were baffled by a mysterious lung disease that was rapidly spreading among their wounded and the attendants. The disease was proving invariably fatal and they wished to consult with me on its cause. I was asked to keep this information in strictest confidence. The note ended with a request that I be so kind as to rush over to the military hospital at once as the matter was urgent.

It was hard for me to disrupt my ward rounds for my habit was to try to complete what I had begun. However, the S O S call seemed both urgent and mysterious. I excused myself to my staff and rushed off with the courier. All eyes were following me with more than a little curiosity.

It was fortunate that the courier accompanied me, for at the hospital entrance, I too was challenged by the guard and was told, "No civilians allowed." My guide was able to explain my presence and although the guard reluctantly waved me past him into the forbidden precinct, I could distinctly feel his animosity and suspicion.

I had long wanted to see this area. I had received no word from those of my staff who had volunteered for service here, and I was anxious to see how they were faring. When I spotted one of them near the entrance I greeted him.

He surprised me by saying in a low voice, "I am not allowed to talk, but please, please do get us out of here quickly. This place is worse than a jail. We are not even allowed to communicate with our relatives."

Before I could question him, the chief medical officer was coming forward to greet me, and my former staff member melted quietly into the background. The medical officer greeted me warmly, and I could not help but note the contrast between him and his guard at the entrance.

Within the medical fraternity the world over, there is a bond of friendship that knows no race nor national boundary. Besides, he was a naturally friendly type, so we were soon warming up to one another. I observed that he had a scar on his face, probably inflicted on the battlefield.

As we walked slowly down his ward, he said, "You will soon observe why civilians are strictly prohibited from entering here." He went on to say, "These are not just ordinary wounded soldiers, whom we should gladly have the public visit, but these wounded are different. They were received by our advance forces in the enemy prisoner of war camps near Mukden. All had been severely and most cruelly tortured and badly mutilated.

I was about to interrupt him and say, "Yes, I had heard of such atrocities over the radio news from Shanghai but never expected to see the results of them." Fortunately, I checked myself in time.

These actual cases had been ill treated even more brutally than I had imagined possible. I was shocked at what I saw. Some had had only their hands and ears cut off, but somehow, the human face seems hardly human without ears. Others were without a nose or feet. When a boy in Korea, I had seen women who had had their noses removed because of unfaithfulness, but this time was the first I had seen men in this condition. Perhaps what shocked me the most at the time was to see some with their eyes gouged out. It was all most pitiful to behold, and it did something to my emotions.

When I served at the emergency clinic in Philadelphia as an intern, I had given first aid to those who had been terribly mutilated by industrial accidents. However, in those cases, their condition was caused by a purely accidental circumstance. Here, I was stunned by the realization that these mutilations had been deliberately executed by fellow human beings—"Man's inhumanity to man."

For the most part, both parties to the conflict espoused the Buddhist doctrine of not willfully inflicting violence on any creature, let alone on humans. I could not help but reflect that the Christians had often been no better, especially at the time of the Inquisition. I also recalled having seen the "Iron Maiden of Nurenberg" whose spiked doors, I learned to my horror, were closed slowly on the poor victim who had been put inside this European instrument of torture.

The military ward was indeed a chamber of horrors and its memory haunted me for a long time. However, this was not what the medical officer had brought me in to see. At the end of this long ward there was a partition and a small temporary door over which should have read a caption, "Abandon hope all ye patients who enter here." Anyway, the fear expressed in the attendant's eyes seemed to indicate that he beheld such a caption, which was invisible to us, as he timidly swung open the door and then beat a hasty retreat.

All this aroused my curiosity and added to the air of mystery. I might have hesitated to enter the doorway myself had not the medical officer accompanied me. The door opened into a small dressing room, where we donned surgical outfits, masks, rubber gloves and all. I was asked to bring my stethoscope. Before passing through the next door, I was quickly briefed as to what this initiation-like procedure was all about.

It seemed that a few of these wounded and mutilated soldiers had also become desperately ill, with a mysterious malignant epidemic type of disease. After a very short while, their lungs became affected, soon after which, despite all that could be done, they departed this world to join their ancestors. Even a couple of the attendants had succumbed.

"This has made all the staff very apprehensive," sighed the chief medical officer, "and though they possess the qualities of discipline, courage, and honor, they have become so reluctant to attend the victims of this strange epidemic that I have had to call them here by lot. Of course I have thought of the possibility of bubonic plague, but there is no swelling nor tenderness of the lymphatic glands in the groin nor in the axilla, as certainly would be the case were it plague.

"The initial attack of this malady in our patients comes on suddenly, with severe headache, nausea and vomiting. The fever sometimes goes as high as 105 degrees Fahrenheit. These patients experience extreme prostration. But what I wish to especially point out to you, as a chest specialist, is that nearly all of them experience hurried breathing, cough and expectoration. However, their sputum is watery and frothy, and not viscid and rusty as one sees in pneumonia. They become almost black with cyanosis, and then it may be only a few hours before they expire.

"So you see, it is because of the special lung symptoms, we wish to consult you and obtain your expert opinion. We have taken every precaution to isolate the victims, but this malignant epidemic continues to spread at an alarming rate."

With this introduction, the army medical officer bowed me into the improvised isolation ward. Here I found the patients to be badly cyanosed and appearing desperately ill, almost moribund. The officer then requested me to please examine several of his patients. After a general physical examination, I particularly listened with my stethoscope over their blue, heaving and gurgling chests. Never before had I heard from a single chest such a variety of rales. They rasped on my sensitive ears, making me wince with a peculiar pain. These rales all pointed to a rare disease which I now was encountering for the first time.

While he was almost breathing down my neck, the officer expected me to come up with the immediate and correct diagnosis. I had to try to think rapidly. The suspense was getting worse by the minute. It was indeed a delicate situation, for I must not cause the medical officer to lose face, since then any opportunity I might have to show how this deadly epidemic could be controlled and checked would be lost.

He had made the matter all the more difficult for me by definitely ruling out plague. Now he was insisting on a quick answer, while I, on the other hand, needed time to gradually bring him around to my point of view, and so avoid direct confrontation.

Therefore, in order to cushion the blow, I told him frankly that this was the first time I had actually seen the disease. From all indications, nevertheless, it appeared to me that his patients were suffering from that rare illness caused by *Pasteurella pestis* about which I had studied while at the London School of Tropical Medicine. After I had given a little pause for this to sink in and he had had time to cogitate on its full implication, I could see he had never heard of *Pasteurella pestis*, which was all to the good. I commented that this, of course, was only my provisional diagnosis, but that I was confident that if a specimen of sputum from one of the victims was examined in his laboratory, the microscope would reveal typical gram negative bacilli, singly or in pairs, the stain appearing at the ends in a safety-pin pattern. (This was later confirmed.)

By this time, he had gathered his courage sufficiently to ask, "But what is the common name of the disease?"

At this point I had a strong urge to get out of this death ward "stat," as we say in medical parlance. I was convinced that the thin gauze mask over my mouth and nose was my chief protection against the microbe-laden droplets that filled the foul atmosphere of this death ward. I wondered how quickly the flimsy gauze would reach its saturation point.

Although I had been dealing with droplet infection in my TB work for the greater part of my medical career, and was a master in the fine art of breath-holding when an ignorant patient might cough in my face, this situation somehow seemed more subtle and menacing. Perhaps, for the first time, I understood the terror the attendants must have felt while caring for these adult "blue babies." One had to experience it to fully appreciate it.

Evidently the officer sensed the tone of urgency in my voice, although I had tried to appear cool, calm and collected. We quickly changed back into our clothes. Then I was shown into his large office, where, over handleless cups of clear green tea, I was able to discuss my diagnosis at some length, in a purer and more relaxed atmosphere.

I told the officer about a medical meeting I had recently attended in Seoul where the chief speaker was to be a physician from the Mukden Medical Mission Center. However, the speaker had not been able to attend due to the outbreak of a devastating epidemic that was raging in North Manchukuo (Manchuria). Later, unfortunately, the physician himself had become a casualty while attending the victims of this epidemic. Thus, I had been challenged by this tragic event to look up more details about the disease involved.

"Plague, as you know, is an ancient scourge," I reminded the medical officer, "for even in our own Scriptures there are several references to it. In the book of I Samuel, for example, there is a description of it following a war between Israel and the Philistines where thirty thousand bodies were left dead on the battlefield. In an attempt to be rid of the plague that ensued, the Philistines were advised by their priests to make golden images of the mice that were ravaging the land."

Up to this time the officer had listened very politely, but his patience, it seemed, was about exhausted. He blurted out almost rudely, "But, Doctor, I have already clearly told you that there has been no enlargement of the lymph glands, which always accompanies plague."

By now he was obviously very agitated and becoming almost bellicose. Then I sensed if ever a "*soft answer*" was needed to "*turn away wrath*," now was the time. So I said, "I agree with you most heartily, for my own findings confirmed that there were no enlarged glands. However, we must remember that there is not just one type of plague, but at least two. The more common bubonic plague occurs mostly in warmer climates. However, there is a much more dangerous type which occurs in colder climates. This variety is perhaps the most dangerous infection known to man, and has been vividly described by the ancients as 'the black death,' due to the accompanying cyanosis. This, undoubtedly, is the type of plague with which you are now confronted, since your patients have recently been in that northern, colder part of Manchukuo where this type of plague is endemic. Both types start with the diseased rodent.

"Usually the rat has fleas, which in turn become infected and may bite man, giving him plague. However, one reason why the pneumonic type is even more frightening, is that it often short-circuits the rat-flea route, and thus gives direct infection from man to man, like the cases you have here."

Meanwhile, I could see the officer's jaw gradually dropping, and the redness of his face slowly receding, to be replaced by marked blanching. He deeply sucked in his breath, saying only, "*Sodiska?*" (Is that so?) Then he requested, almost apologetically and humbly, "Please tell me what I should do."

When I saw that I had now won him over, I thought it was best not to belabor the matter more than necessary. So I simply replied, "The precautions you have already taken are all to the good, but for your own protection and that of your staff, you must at once increase the number of layers of gauze for your face to at least eight, and cover all by a deflection mask. Since the chance of infection through droplet nuclei is extremely high, it would be well to also use goggles."

It was now the officer's turn to try to conceal his fears by a pretended smile, but I could see he was petrified with fear. So I quickly switched my remarks to other matters, not quite so personal, relative to the patients and their protection. I suggested, further, that it would be well for the wounded soldiers not yet infected with the plague bacilli, to adopt a *neko* (Japanese word for cat) for their mascot, to serve as the guardian of their ward against rats.

The mascot idea highly amused the officer. I could see he was gradually relaxing and in a better humor, although still very attentive.

I went on to suggest, "On a broader scale, the Public Health Office of the city should be approached for a war on rats, and a bounty for rat tails could be offered. Also, it might be well if each section of the city adopted a *neko*."

The army medical officer seemed most grateful for my help with the diagnosis of his patients, and for my practical recommendations, particularly in regard to the increased protection for his medical staff. When I was on the point of leaving, he once again swore me to absolute secrecy, both about the fateful epidemic and the mutilated soldiers.

Since the incubation period for plague is about seven days, and I was not sure that the thin layer of gauze had adequately protected me, I had to act quickly. I decided it might be best for me to get away during this period, both for the protection of my family and all concerned. Therefore, I went to the Union Christian Hospital at Pyong Yang, on the pretext of going for a medical check-up. It was customary, in any event, for missionaries to submit an annual medical report to the Mission Board, so no suspicions were aroused by my sudden departure. This time for reasons of my own, I felt my examination should be done at Pyong Yang where, if I should come down with plague, I could have the benefit of their well equipped isolation ward without worrying or involving my family. However, as it turned out, all my precautions proved unnecessary.

Upon my return to Haiju, I had been half expecting to be met by the alley cats of the city, on the one hand, exultantly meowing that their mission had been accomplished. On the other hand, I could anticipate the attendant wrath of the rice merchants, over the fact that their old rice no longer smelled as if it had been inhabited by rats. It could therefore not fetch so high a price.

No such reception greeted me in reality. I was told later, confidentially, that since there had been no new cases of plague, the Chief

Medical Officer thought it best not to alarm the public. The war on rats, therefore, was never declared.

Haiju had been fast becoming an important port. Two branch railway lines now converged on this provincial capital although when we first came, there had not been even one. In the meantime, two other missions had decided to establish work in Haiju. Major G. S. Arndt and his wife were the representatives of the Salvation Army. The Church of England Mission had recently transferred Father E. I. Carroll from his former station in Pyong Yang to Haiju upon his return from furlough in England.

These were welcomed by all except the military, who were extremely suspicious of the newcomers. The military simply could not understand how England, engaged in a war for her survival, could allow a young man of military age and in good health to leave England. Further, the military titles and quasi-military uniforms of the Salvation Army always did annoy the Japanese High Command, although the civilians had become accustomed to it.

In due course, the Arndts were mysteriously transferred, though the reason was never disclosed. However, Father Carroll remained for a time, though he reported that strange characters, disguised as farmers, were pretending to work the fallow fields around his house. It was evident that the military were keeping their suspicious eye on him.

Some of the anti-foreign feeling and tightening of military controls made us feel that we were involved in a war of nerves if not of another variety. Some Occidentals felt they could take it no longer and so they left Korea. For this we could hardly blame them. Marian and I also talked over the matter, but we agreed that as long as we could be of service and not be too great an embarrassment to the Koreans, we should remain at our post. We also discussed it with our Korean friends. Without exception, they strongly urged us to stay. However, we suggested to them that they should visit us at our home as infrequently as possible, for we had heard that each visit was reported to the military and would be counted against them.

Since there were now too many peeping Toms around, I felt that it would be a wise precaution to forego listening with the aid of my stethoscope to the more authentic radio news from Shanghai. It was hard on us both not to know the true state of events in the world, but there seemed to be no other wise choice. Later, the Reverend

Arthur E. Chadwell, who was with the Church of England Mission in Pyong Yang, received a ten month prison sentence for listening to his shortwave radio.

We had also cautioned our friends in the homeland that it would be better for them not to refer to the war if they wanted their letters to reach us. As it was, many passages from their letters were being cut out by the censors, and we would play guessing games trying to imagine what may have been written. We had to learn the fine art of reading between the lines, which was not always easy. Later we found out to our amusement that we had made some rather ridiculous mistaken guesses. Likewise, others reading letters from us had sometimes missed the message we were trying to convey in a veiled form.

Nevertheless, on the whole, much of life and work went on as usual. We found the civilian Japanese to be friendly and very understanding. They went out of their way to show us various acts of kindness while on the other hand, the military were becoming more arrogant than ever. Had the city of Haiju been able to boast of the luxury of sidewalks, I feel sure we would have been rudely brushed off them as they passed.

One day we were saddened to learn of the death of the infant son of our friends, the Sasakis. When Mr. Sasaki called to give us the sad news, he did so with a smile. We were puzzled over this, but found out later that it was a Japanese custom to deliver such information with a smile so as not to inflict one's real sorrow on one's friends. Of course we were all sympathy. Marian went over at once to call on Mrs. Sasaki to offer her any help that might be needed.

Our other special Japanese friends were the Nagatas. Mr. Buitsu Nagata taught English in the Government High School and frequently came over to consult us. He discovered that we were also keen philatelists, so he braved the possible displeasure of the military to do stamps with us. In this pastime his family and ours spent many a pleasant evening together. (We continue to exchange stamps, by letter, to this day.)

Christmas was coming soon and we did not want bereavement nor war clouds to dim its joys, especially for the children. We made a special effort to make it a memorable one for our school, hospital, sanatorium and our own family. The children joined in the spirit of Christmas by helping Marian wrap packages for the patients.

We had decided to broaden our Haiju Christmas celebration by inviting our dear friends, JL and Muriel Livesay, to be with us. Their

Presbyterian mission station at Chairyung was only thirty miles north of Haiju and over the years we enjoyed many congenial visits with each other. Our youngsters eagerly looked forward to the prospect of JL's piggyback rides for he always found time to play with them.

We felt that it might also cheer the Sasakis if we invited them and their lively children to share our Christmas dinner. One of my former patients had presented us with a gift of pheasants so that everyone at our festive board was able to have a generous helping accompanied by cranberry sauce sent to us by friends in America.

Before we partook of the meal, I requested JL to give us a brief talk on the meaning of Christmas and what the coming of the Prince of Peace had meant to us all. Somehow, we had a strong intuition that this might be the last Christmas that we would be able to share together in Korea.

Both JL and the usually dignified Mr. Sasaki became boys again, and romped and played with the children to the delight of all. They seemed to enjoy the new toys fully as much as the children. A sweet smile lit up the delicate and beautiful features of Mrs. Sasaki as she

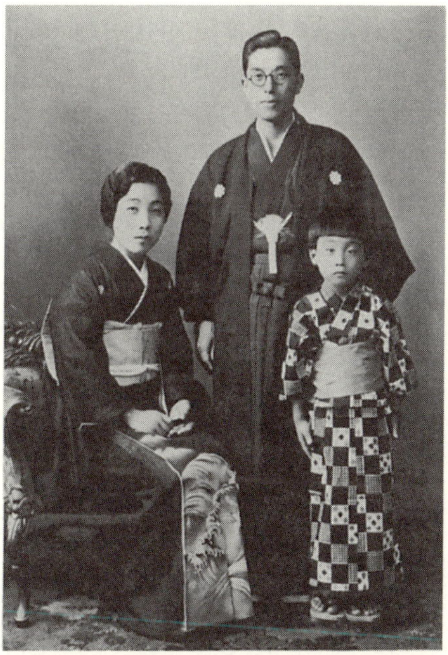

Mr. and Mrs. Buitsu Nagata and son

watched the fun and her previous sadness was for the moment forgotten. It was indeed a happy and memorable time for us all.

The subsequent experiences of our Christmas guests, however, were far from happy ones. This we learned many years later. After American forces occupied Korea at the conclusion of World War II, Mrs. Sasaki met an untimely death as a result of a grueling march which she and other prisoners of war were forced to take and which taxed her frailty beyond endurance. Mr. Sasaki, a man of peace, had joined the Red Cross service but he did not long survive his wife.

The Livesays subsequently were transferred to the Philippines only to find themselves again under Japanese military occupation. The Livesays escaped into the jungle, hidden by native Filipinos. Muriel was expecting a baby at the time. While visiting us at Charleston Lake in Canada years later and under more peaceful conditions, she described how she gave birth to her son in a cave during their flight. The newborn infant was taken by a Filipino woman who stained the baby's face with walnut juice so that he looked like a native baby. She cared for him while the Livesays resumed their escape from the pursuing Japanese forces. How they were eventually reunited with their son, Tomas, and their tales of many narrow escapes from their would-be captors was a story verging on the miraculous.

Our own experiences were also to have a happy ending, although that seemed doubtful at the time. Fear, like the sword of Damocles, for a long time was to hang over our heads.

CHAPTER 29

Gendarmes

In the summer of 1940 all sorts of wild rumors were afloat. One of these was that the Sanatorium was to be taken over by the military because of its commanding view of the harbor and the military activities there. Many of our staff members were reputed to be on the military's "wanted" list. It was feared that essential drugs would soon be impossible to procure.

What alarmed local residents most, however, was the persistent rumor that the self-exiled Koreans in Siberia were preparing to arm a Communist force to take over Haiju. The city had become a strategic port. It was said that since the Japanese military were now preoccupied with the war in China, their rear in Manchukuo and northern Korea had become exposed. So it was rumored that a "blitzkrieg-like" attack by the Korean Communists might give a crippling blow to the vulnerable Japanese rear positions.

There was just enough logic in the rumor to make it appear quite credible. It became more so when one of our doctors admitted to me that he had been approached by the projected Korean liberation front to help.

Excerpts from a letter I wrote to my mother on April 1, 1940 described the temper of the times:

> ". . . There has been quite a stir here over Hull's speech and it looks as though the Americans as well as the British are 'on the spot' now—misery loves company. There is a movement on foot now to take English out of the schools and to remove English from all signs, and those who have English Christian names have to change them.
>
> "Also, all Koreans are expected to change their Korean names and surnames into Japanese and already many of them have done so. The younger ones willingly but the older ones under protest, though they have not made it absolutely compulsory yet.

"We are certainly living in a changing world. Practically all the barbed wire had been removed from our two compounds and of course we can't replace it at any price. So we are fence-less and so that practically makes our gardens useless. There is also a great deal more stealing—they have removed all the electric wires from the middle house and just the other evening someone stole Joe's pet rabbit.

". . . We are to have our Sanatorium Board meeting on Saturday and so I am very busy in preparation for the same. It is so hard to get doctors or in fact anybody. So many have gone to Manchuria and China in anticipation of large incomes. The government pays them large salaries too and allows them to retire four times sooner than if they worked in Korea, on the grounds that their lives are in danger. But many are taking the risk and are hoping they may make their fortune and return alive.

"That accounts in part for the great increase of travel on the main line and another reason is that Korea was never so prosperous on the whole. Money is really cheap, there is so much of it. Land in Pyong Yang in some sections they say is selling at the rate of 170 yen a *pyung*.[1] How long this boom will keep up no one knows. It is hardest on the salaried men and the small merchant who can't get supplies to sell. They are hit hard; but the laborer, the farmer, the gold, coal and iron ore miners and the big merchants are making money in a big way now.

"William has been accepted by the Pyong Yang Foreign School for the high school course beginning this fall. Due to his excellent Calvert School record he will not be required to take the usual entrance examinations . . .

"Have just heard that the Bernheisels, who went to a church and spoke, were forcibly ejected from the church by the authorities as they had been told not to take part in the service and I believe not even attend as well. Mrs. Bernheisel was severely manhandled and one arm badly bruised . . . Hear that 6 of the leaders were arrested too . . .

---

[1] [One pyung is a little over four square yards.]

> ". . . I don't know the reason why the Canadian dollar is so good out here; but I understand that there has been no trouble with Canadian trade and they are anxious to get Canadian money here. I've heard that the Japanese who reside in Canada contributed generously to the Canadian War Fund so that evidently there is good spirit there. The British Ambassador in Tokyo made quite a conciliatory speech and there was quite a stir in the U.S. over it. Well I must not get on politics or I shall get in trouble . . ."

Unfortunately, we were not able to keep any written records of our experiences at the time. It was not safe to do so. As a matter of fact, it appeared that the only thing permissible to write about was the weather and some even felt that too might prove dangerous.

However, some months later, we were able to write in a fairly lengthy circular letter an account of our experiences to our friends and supporters in America. From this and what we have been able to recall from memory, I have tried to reconstruct the events of the summer and fall of 1940 as accurately as possible.

Father Carroll of the Church of England Mission at Haiju had been a rather frequent caller at our home. Our children loved him and he, in turn, was fond of them. He was spending all his spare time in language study and found that he grew very lonely for human companionship. It was then a rather natural thought for us to invite him to vacation with us at our castle at Wha Chin Po.

I was doubly glad when the summer of 1940 came and we could get away from all the vexing rumors at Haiju. The city was becoming a hot spot in more senses than one. However, it did not turn out that we could "pack all our troubles in our old kit bag" and be free from worries for long. Indeed, Father Carroll later laughingly remarked to us that our invitation to him that summer must have been, by far, the most costly and dangerous invitation we had ever issued. It was.

At the beach everything was quiet and peaceful. It was good to be out of the ear shot of the Haiju loudspeakers, which constantly blared forth news of real and imagined victories, of new restrictions in regard to rations, and the most recently concocted rumors calculated to keep the people on the alert. What few rumors came to the beach soon fell into proper perspective and were quickly forgotten.

Inspirational meetings with fine speakers were held at the beach to meet the general need for mental and spiritual refreshment of the local community. The normalcy and serenity of beach life made it almost hard to realize that a world war was being waged not too far from us. That this was only the calm before the storm was reflected in the letter Marian later wrote to our friends:

> "The first Sunday in August my husband, our guest, Father Carroll, and I were standing outside our cottage at Wha Chin Po Beach watching a gorgeous sunset reflected in lake and ocean. In the distance were the famous Diamond Mountains. From our vantage point halfway up the hill we could get one of the loveliest views in the world. Superficially all was peace and beauty but Father Carroll was telling us that Father Chadwell, the English church priest in Pyong Yang, was in jail. We'd read of Cox' suicide (?) in Japan and other arrests there. Father Chadwell's arrest was the beginning of the farcical spy round-up in Korea.
>
> "Next morning at 7 A.M. I heard someone prowling around our cottage and got up to investigate. It was two gendarmes in plain clothes and they had come to arrest our guest. They kept insisting to us that he was a good man, nevertheless they took him back to Haiju bag and baggage and put him into jail for four days, all at his own expense.
>
> "Our cottage being on a hill, is well above the 20 meter limit beyond which it is absolutely forbidden by military law to take pictures; yet before the gendarmes left they took Father Carroll up on the roof and tried to force him to take pictures. Just as they were getting ugly Sherwood stepped up and said he couldn't permit infraction of military regulations from his house, so they desisted but our guest was jittery from then on, and anxious to get down from the roof fearing he'd suffer the fate of Cox.
>
> "We were warned by the gendarmes to say nothing at all about our guest's leaving. I don't know how they expected us to explain his sudden disappearance but we didn't have to give information. In spite of their precautions they ran into the whole beach population for they left just as folks were gathering for the work of special meetings just beginning. Father Carroll passed friend after friend. The Seoul folks

> recognized the gendarme and knew what was up so that word of his arrest went to Bishop Cecil [Cooper] on the same train as he did."

The next day, I received what seemed to be a mysterious telegram saying I was needed urgently at Haiju on Sanatorium business. Some of our friends, fearing a ruse, urged me not to go. But I would never have forgiven myself if I had not gone, and then later found out I had really been needed. So I took the first train out, but not before we had figured out a code telegram for me to send back. If I found everything all right and could return right away, I would wire Marian, "Pets well."

I left with mixed feelings, but encountered no difficulty en route to Haiju. Everyone was surprised to see me back so soon, and wondered who could have sent the telegram summoning me, like the call of, "Wolf, wolf!" when there was no wolf. So I was able to send the telegram to Marian which we had previously arranged. When I was about to board the train back, two officers whom I recognized, stepped up and summarily announced, "Sorry to inform you that you are, as from now, under arrest! However, we shall not seize you here, where you are well known. We know you to be a gentleman of honor; just give yourself up at the Gendarmery in Seoul on your arrival."

I needed to play for time in which to inform my friends of my arrest. I mentioned in an offhand way that the hour would be late upon my arrival in Seoul, so would it be all right if I went to the Gendarmery (the term used for the military police station) in the morning?

They hesitated. Then one said, "Be sure to get there by 10:00 A.M."

The other added, "Have a good night's sleep. You will need it."

No one guarded me on my train journey and I was alone with my thoughts. I wondered how best to contact my friends. On reaching Seoul late that night, I went directly to the home of the Jensens. I found that they had already gone to the Beach, but fortunately for me, some of their friends had come in from the country to get supplies and were staying there for the night. I briefly explained my situation to them and asked them to contact Mr. Phipps, the British Consul General, and inform him of my problem. I felt that it would be better for me not to try to contact either him or Marian directly.

I asked that they send a note to Marian by someone going to the Beach, for I knew she would be worried when I failed to return.

The next morning I showed up at the Gendarmery right on time, taking nothing with me except a small inspirational book. I was ushered immediately into a small office. An officer there met me and said that even though the Haiju authorities had assured them that I would be certain to turn up, they hardly expected me to be on time. They had, therefore, taken the precaution to have me carefully watched. "But I see," he continued, "you are a man of your word, which is to your good."

With that hint of encouragement, I was motioned into a bare room, where there were two chairs placed opposite each other. I was asked to occupy one of them.

Presently, a rough looking, heavy set military officer came in and seated himself squarely in front of me. He apparently had a sheaf of questions to ask me. The first questions were general, such as date and place of birth and other routine questions easy to answer. He had been fairly civil, but when he got down to specifics, his manner abruptly changed.

He now assumed a threatening attitude and at times it seemed he might hit me. He shouted at me, "I know you to be a spy. If you will confess to it, there will be no need for further questioning, nor even torture, and all will be over in no time."

Then I replied, "Yes, I know it does not take long to shoot a self-confessed spy, but I emphatically deny that I am a spy, and you can never find evidence to prove your contention."

"This is a rude reply," he roared angrily, "and deserves a slap in the face." He feinted one. He waved his papers in front of me as he declared, "I have all the evidence right here, which proves you are a spy and it will be useless for you to deny it."

A sneer crossed his cruel face and with a note of triumph he continued, "You well know that a British spy, Father Carroll, was arrested the other day from your house. This proves that you consort with a spy, and by keeping company with a spy, it is clear you also must be a spy."

My reply was heated. "I strongly deny that Father Carroll is a spy, and I also earnestly deny that I consort with spies."

The officer lowered his voice and almost as if talking to himself, he said, "We shall have proof when we get Father Carroll's confession."

Then I knew he had been bluffing and I repeated, "I know full well that Father Carroll is no spy, and he will never confess to being one."

With an ugly look he responded, "You know we have ways of getting confessions out of people, and you will also be confessing soon. You had better do so now, as I told you, and save yourself a lot of suffering."

"Yes, I am only too well aware of your methods," I replied, "but remember this, a confession made under duress is no legal confession. Once and for all, I again strongly declare that I am not a spy."

He abruptly branched out on a new angle. "We have further evidence to prove you are a spy. Your wife has taken pictures of Kashinho Beach [Japanese rendering of "Wha Chin Po"] coast line, well above the prescribed 20 meter limit, as well as at Kaishu [Japanese for "Haiju"]."

"Yes, I agree in both instances that she did take the pictures you mentioned. But in the first instance, they were taken at the special request of the Beach authorities with military permission and a military officer present. This was on the occasion of the opening of the Beach, as also arranged by the military. These facts can easily be confirmed by your own files. In the second instance, the pictures were taken before Japan was at war and there are no recent structures shown in them. In peacetime, as you well know this limitation did not apply."

Evidently, I had taken the wind out of his sails, for at my refutation, he suddenly vanished in disgust. I was left alone with my inspirational book which, by this time, I sorely needed.

Another officer soon appeared and informed me that I was their paying guest.

"But neither a grateful nor a willing one," I responded.

He ignored my remark and told me I could write in an order which would be sent to a nearby restaurant. In this way I learned by chance that Bishop Cecil Cooper was also a prisoner. The messenger boy had somehow confused Bishop Cecil's order with mine and I received the dinner he had ordered. I knew then that I was in good company, albeit in separate cells. Later, I also learned that Mr. Phipps had sent me a good meal from his own table which I never did receive. No doubt it was enjoyed by my captors.

The second officer to interrogate me was quite different in his approach, and I could see was not at all happy in his role of inquisitor. At times he even seemed almost friendly and appeared to want to help me with the best way I should answer the questions he put to me. His questions centered largely around financial matters. For instance, he asked, "What foreign government is paying you?"

To this I simply replied, "No foreign government is paying me. I get my salary from the Methodist Mission Board, which our Mission treasurer, Mrs. Kris Jensen, here in Seoul can easily confirm."

What seemed to puzzle him most was why two physicians would work in Korea for such meagre pay, when they could command so much more in their own homeland and be near their relatives and friends. I saw that he had not the vaguest conception of religious motivation nor service, so it would be useless to try to get through to him on that angle. I attempted to do it in a way I hoped he might comprehend.

"You are a soldier. You serve your Emperor loyally, without consideration of pay, and would even be willing to give your life on the battlefield should the necessity arise."

He nodded agreement so I was encouraged to continue. "We also give our allegiance to our Lord and King, Jesus Christ, and try to serve Him loyally, without consideration of pay, and would also be willing to give our lives on the mission field should the necessity arise. Can you see the parallel?" I asked. "Do you expect us to be less loyal to our King, than you are to your Emperor?"

I could see that my illustration had registered. He ceased to press the matter further, but switched to a different subject.

"Do you know Dr. Douglas Avison?"

"Yes," I replied. "We both graduated in medicine from the University of Toronto, and we have always been good friends."

"So you must know why he made that trip to Peking?" he asked.

Then I saw that he was trying to trap me, so at once I replied, "I shall not involve my friends. If you have any questions to ask about him, then you must approach him directly."

He saw that I meant what I said and that he could not dissuade me. He did seem to be the more intelligent of my inquisitors and so I had hoped that I might be able to reason with him.

I was anxious to get word to Marian in regard to my safety, for I knew how worried she would be. Therefore, I was bold enough to ask this officer if he would be so kind as to send a telegram to my family, reassuring them of my safety. Surprisingly enough, he consented to do so, though I had no means then of knowing whether he would actually send it. Later, I found that he did, and that such a message had been delivered to Marian. Unfortunately it did not reassure her much for it was in Japanese and Marian knew that I would have wired in English.

The prospect of my getting out seemed to be far from bright. Indeed, from what I had heard of the way Father Chadwell had suffered, the chances of my being released looked very dim. When I was not being interrogated, there was a guard ever by my side. I could not even go to the toilet without him accompanying me there.

I was finally left alone in my cell where I had opportunity to read my inspirational book and to do some praying. I also brooded over how nice it would be to be back with my family. It grew too dark to read and I settled myself for an uncomfortable and anxious night.

It must have been afternoon when I heard heavy footsteps approaching, and the beat of my heart seemed to keep pace with them. Suddenly my cell door was flung open wide and a pompous looking officer appeared in the doorway with his aide and asked if I was Dr. Hall.

"Yes, I answer to that name," I replied.

"I have orders for your immediate release," he announced, "on the one condition that you tell no one of what transpired here."

"May I tell my wife?" I asked.

He hesitated for a moment, then replied, "I suppose so, but do not tell your children. Children have a hard time keeping secrets. If word comes to us that you have told anything, you will be brought right back here and will have real reason to be sorry for yourself. From now on you will be carefully shadowed."

Then he spoke to his aide, "Take this released prisoner to the railway station and see to it that he takes the night train to Kashinho Beach and that he speaks to no one.

He turned and left abruptly before I could express my gratitude for my release, even though I hardly felt any thanks was owed to him. I felt immensely relieved and thanked God. The aide told me to get moving although I hardly needed such admonition.

I asked my escort if I could collect my suitcase which I had left at a friend's home.

He looked surprised at my request. "You heard my instructions that I was not to allow you to contact anyone."

I reassured him that my friend's home would now be empty as they had gone to the Beach. He reluctantly conceded that in that event I could pick up my baggage.

What was my consternation, therefore, to find the house was not empty, for the shoppers, who, I thought, would surely have left by now, were still there. I quickly put my finger to my lips and pointed to the porch, as I noticed they were about to speak. I picked up my suitcase, and beat a hasty retreat.

My escort was simply furious. He commanded, "Drop that suitcase at once and come right back with me to jail. You have badly tricked me and you will sorely suffer for this."

Although my mouth had become dry, and I could hardly speak, I said, "Please let me explain. I honestly thought the house would be empty. These people are not the regular occupants, but evidently just their friends who had come up to Seoul to do some shopping. As I promised, I did not say a single word to them. Did you hear me say anything?"

He had to admit that he had not. By this time he had cooled down and evidently found my explanation satisfactory for we now headed in the direction of the train station. My heart resumed its normal pace and once again a sense of relief returned.

After purchasing my ticket, I boarded the train, clutching almost madly the suitcase which had nearly brought me to ruin. I bade my escort a glad farewell as he gave me a friendly smile. I concluded he was not such a bad fellow after all, even though he had given me quite a spell of momentary panic.

My trip back was without further incident and I landed happily in the bosom of my joyous family. Marian told me that special prayers had been offered in my behalf at the meetings and that the whole Beach community was deeply concerned and eagerly awaiting news of me.

When it was the traditional bathing time at the Beach, and nearly everyone was out for a dip or a swim, I felt it wiser not to join the others. We took our swim as a family separately. My worries seemed to wash off my brow with the waves, and I felt how wonderful it was to be with my family again. They never seemed more precious.

In the circular letter Marian wrote some months later she reported:

> "Sherwood returned to us Monday morning but he nearly didn't get back at all. It was only when he pointed out to the officials that they would cause much more comment by pre-

venting his return than by letting him come back, under promise not to talk, that they consented to his coming at all. . . .

"People understood why we couldn't talk and refrained from asking questions but he could talk freely to me. He looked haggard after the ordeal of two days and a night. The first day was devoted to trying to prove him a British spy. He was shouted at and called a liar numerous times, all of which seems to be part of the accepted procedure and you are not supposed to consider it unpleasant. . . .

"The second day's session was face-saving for the gendarmes. Someone told Sherwood that if the officials had realized all his U.S.A. connections they'd never have taken him but having started the machinery they couldn't stop it."

At the gendarmery I had been given a questionnaire form for Marian to fill out, which she sent in promptly. Since we heard nothing further, we thought that the affair had ended and that our worries were now happily over. We were just nicely beginning to relax when Marian received a telegram in Japanese from the gendarmery, calling her up to Seoul.

I had fervently hoped that Marian might be spared this ordeal but there was no alternative open to us. Carefully I went over with Marian all the facts I had given to the officers, to assure that our facts would agree. I fully realized that she would undoubtedly be able to clothe these bare facts better than I had done. Marian was always quick at repartee and they would have to be smart indeed to outwit her. At least, I found that I never could.

Marian's letter contained a description of her own experience at the gendarmery:

". . . I was met by an officer who courteously carried my small overnight bag and escorted me to a waiting taxi. (It is very difficult to get a taxi these days.) Two of our own missionaries were on the same train and naturally anxious about me for I was the first woman to be called up as far as we knew. One told me later they were watching me without seeming to and were relieved when they saw the gendarme carry my bag.

"I was taken direct to the gendarmery where I sat in a sort of reception room for 3 hours or more. We got in at 8 A.M. I was questioned until noon using a Japanese interpreter who spoke English quite well. I had to corroborate all Sherwood had told them and add some of my own and they wrote reams and reams about us in this day of paper shortage.

"Time out for lunch which I'd brought along with me as also I brought my Japanese language study books. We were taking the summer course at the beach and they were making me miss two expensive lessons so I used the interpreter to help me catch up.

"In the afternoon there were more questions but they never called me a liar and I never lost my temper which is what they try to make you do. Finally all the questions were asked and answered but they kept me just sitting waiting another hour before giving me my freedom. Then the gendarme who had questioned me called a taxi and, until it arrived, gave me some more instruction in writing Japanese characters—all very politely. When the car came at 6 P.M. he started to carry out my bag but some military officers came along and kidded him about it and he didn't have the courage and gallantry to go through with it so put it down for me to carry the rest of the way myself.

"I went to a friend's house for supper and as the gendarme had previously called another friend to get me reservations on the train back to the Beach, I was able to return to my anxious family by the night train.

"From then on detectives seemed to spring up like mushrooms anywhere and everywhere about the beach, especially as guests would be leaving a tea or chatting together before leaving. Their English is so meagre that I doubt if they ever learned anything but they were more than a nuisance. Our beach officers, Americans, were quizzed about all manner of things and the police went through the treasurer's books and kept him hours at a time for questioning.The whole atmosphere was tense and uncomfortable. Japanese friends who had earlier accepted invitations to various homes suddenly found excuses for not coming.

"Less than a week after my return another telegram came in Japanese. By this time a telegram in Japanese meant only bad news for us and we wondered what new trouble was ahead. This time it was the opposite. It was an invitation from the Governor of our province asking Dr. Sherwood to be a delegate to Japan on the occasion of the 2600th Anniversary celebration in Tokyo in November. What a relief! From their point of view this is a great honor.

"By the end of August we thought our personal troubles with the gendarmes were ended. I took William direct to Pyong Yang and settled him in the dormitory and high school there. Sherwood took the younger children home to Haiju. . . ."

Although Marian had encountered no problem on her trip, I soon found that our troubles were not over. The morning after our return home, Phyllis happened to be looking out of our front window. As she peered down the long approach road to our house, lined with poplar trees, her keen eyes spotted some bright glittering objects that shone in the early morning sunlight. These were slowly moving up our road. A more careful look revealed that the shiny objects were attached to five men.

Presently she yelled to me, "Look, Daddy, men with big knives [swords] are coming up our hill!"

I gave a hasty glance and sprang into immediate action. The first thing I had intended to do on our return was to burn the beautiful aerial photograph of Haiju and the harbor that included the sanatorium site which Mr. Sasaki had given to us some time back, but which now would be considered incriminating evidence. Fortunately, there was a good fire in the kitchen stove, and I was just able to get this photo map stuffed into it and consigned to the flames, when the officers landed on our front porch.

It was then that Phyllis called again, "Daddy, come quickly. The men with the big knives are wanting to come in. Shall I let them?"

"Yes," I shouted to her from the kitchen. "Be sure to greet them sweetly." I knew she would do that, but I was not so sure about myself.

The Chief Officer announced that they had been ordered to carefully search our house. "We have come to help you, so it is to your interest to cooperate fully with us."

"But, Officer," I protested, "we have already been fully cleared by the military in Seoul!"

"Yes," he replied, "but they have not yet searched your house. They are bound to do that."

Although I had not yet fully comprehended the significance of what he had said, I had no choice but to tell them to go ahead.

He added, "We are after three things in particular: any pictures or movies you may have taken over 20 meters, especially in the coastal area; any notebooks or letters that involve you with any government; and your bank books and any statements that show foreign payments to you."

This was indeed a tall order and was, I thought, bound to consume much searching and time. However, the way they handled it, the time element was relatively short.

Joe sensed that these men were not guests, but unwelcome intruders. He stoutly braced himself before the cabinets where his mother stored her movies and photographs in orderly fashion. Emphatically he announced, "You can't have these. Mother worked hard to take these pictures and won't even allow us children to touch them."

Although Joe's intentions were of the best, and this rough looking officer even smiled kindly at his protestations, they gently brushed him aside and bagged the whole lot.

As the officer did so, he said, "When the trouble has blown over, these will be returned to you."

They took longer about the other items on their agenda. The officer observed, "You don't seem to be as orderly as your wife. If you had everything filed, the way she has, we would all be through here more rapidly!"

"I agree," I responded with a smile, and added, "but it is lucky for you my wife did not see her precious pictures stuffed in your bag in such a disorderly way."

After this exchange, they settled down to serious business. Among the letters, they were extremely interested in one from the Korean Methodist Church in Honolulu which mentioned an enclosed contribution for the Sanatorium. The officer then asked me to show its entry in the bank statement, which I found for him.

He then said, "This could be very damaging to you, for you know Hawaii is a hot bed of the Korean Independence Movement. Any connection you may have with the Koreans there might be very unfavorable to you."

I protested, "This is just a church offering to our anti-TB work. There is nothing political about it. Your officials have made similar contributions."

He only smiled and pocketed what he considered to be incriminating evidence, assuring me that these would be returned in due course. He also took a letter I had received from our friend, Mr. H. V. Stokely, representative of Parke-Davis Company, stationed at their Shanghai office.

He then pounced on a notebook of Marian's, which he thought might be a code book and prove to be the most incriminating evidence of all. I was at pains to point out that these were just medical prescriptions, which my wife had jotted down while serving as an intern at Southside Hospital, Pittsburgh, and in no way could be interpreted as a code. Despite my explanation and assurances that any physician would confirm what I had said, they insisted on taking the book.

Finally, they departed. Although my study never did have the reputation of being in apple pie order, the officers certainly left it as though a cyclone had struck. The children assisted me in returning things to some semblance of neatness.

When Marian returned home, Joe and Phyllis rushed to greet her. Phyllis declared, "Mother, we're so glad you are back. Policemen were here and took away everything, but I hid my dolls."

Joe echoed, "And I hid my train and cars. After they went away, Daddy and we put everything back in shape-ship order."

Marian instinctively corrected, "You mean ship-shape order."

"No," Joe insisted. "Daddy says we got everything back, but the order may have been mixed up, so he called it shape-ship order! I tried to keep them from taking your nice movies, but they would not listen. You should have been here to stop them."

That afternoon Mr. Sasaki called, but he was not his usual self. He said how very sorry he was for all we had been through, but feared the worst was not over yet. He had good reason to believe that the military was planning to search our house.

Then I interrupted and announced that the police had already done so.

"Yes, I know," responded Mr. Sasaki. "They were really trying to protect you. I arranged for them to search your house before the military could do so, since we do not want them to find anything that might be used against you. Our police office is keeping everything in tight security until this trouble blows over."

Then it dawned on me just what the police officer meant when he had said, "We have come to help you!" although, of course, he could not have spelled it out to me at the time.

CHAPTER 30

Kangaroo Court

All letters to and from Korea were being heavily censored. We had once heard a story about an unacceptable Russian writer who had been sent to one of the notorious prison camps in Siberia. He had secretly promised to write to his family in green ink if his food and other items were scanty. When his family finally heard from him, they received an enthusiastic letter enumerating the abundant supplies procurable at the prison camp. At the close of his letter, however, there was a brief postscript to the effect that the only shortage he found was that of green ink.

I was reminded of this anecdote when I sat down to write a letter to my mother and wanted to relay to her some intimation of what we had experienced in recent weeks. I tried to allude to it in a similarly disguised manner as I wrote her on September 12, 1940:

> "You may remember a title of one of J. Fenimore Cooper's books which I enjoyed so much as a boy; but never dreamed it would come so close home to Marian and me. After a very severe storm here similar to the one we had at the Beach, the atmosphere is now clearing and I believe we can hope for clearer weather ahead. This evidently is the typhoon season here and one can never be sure how or when or in what form it will come.
>
> "Your card for the pastor arrived on Phyllis' birthday and we were glad to see by it that you were well. We had a simple party for Phyllis, but grateful we could have any at all—home and loved ones seem more precious than ever these days."

My mother had written a notation on the margin of this letter after she received it:

> "Sherwood took this way of telling his mother of their two sieges of being questioned as 'spies' but if I hadn't read a cable in a N.Y. paper, I'd not have guessed."

One area I did not feel concern about was the TB Christmas Seal campaigns. They were now better understood and seemed to be progressing well year after year. I was able to relax and had begun to delegate more of the details to the members of my enthusiastic committee. This had freed me to do more actual clinical work. However, my complacency proved short-lived.

Miss Elizabeth Keith, the famous English artist who had often painted the English royal family, had designed a most intriguing seal for our 1940-41 campaign. This depicted two adorable Korean children in colorful attire. In the background to lend contrast were the snow clad mountains. The scene was framed by a holly border with red berries which added a festive look. The design had been approved by the government and everyone seemed please with it. We had been given the green light to go ahead.

I said "everyone" had approved, but, as it turned out, there was one very unexpected and important exception. For there was now a power on the scene with which we had not reckoned—the Japanese military. Without warning, the gendarmes descended on our neatly piled parcels of seals, all ready for distribution, and confiscated the lot (though it seems, a few seals somehow escaped their eagle eyes).

This vandalism completely stunned me. When I had recovered sufficiently, I indignantly protested and demanded an explanation.

It seemed that the military considered the design in violation of a defense regulation. At first I could not imagine why the design could be considered threatening to military defense—just two innocent children. What harm could they possibly be to Japan's military might? Then the white mountains featured in the background of the design were savagely pointed out to me as the "villain" in the seal. Did I not know the military regulation that no height over the 20 meter limit could be shown? Surely I must realize that the mountains depicted must be higher than this limit.

If the seals had been sent out, they declared, it would have meant a court sentence for me. Thus they posed as my benefactors for having confiscated the seals before they had been distributed. Then, as if to add insult to injury, they informed me that the Christian date on the seals, 1940-1941, must be removed. They suggested the year

2600 be substituted for the Christian date. It had been that many years since the founding of the great Japanese Empire.

This last rejection I felt I could somehow handle, although I would not allow the year 2600 to be printed on our Korea seals. I was finally successful in getting around their objection by replacing the date with "Ninth Year" on the seal. It had been nine years since the first seals were issued.

A more difficult task now facing me was that of persuading a very sensitive artist like Miss Keith to change her design. It had already been accepted and was considered about perfect. Miss Keith had been a guest in our home once and had painted our cook's daughter while with us. The girl she painted was a lovely Korean bride, whose eyes had been pasted shut before the ceremony, as was the custom. I vividly recalled that on this occasion I had had quite a time procuring the background which Miss Keith considered would best set off her colorful bride. Eventually I hit on the idea of an antique Korean screen which fortunately met Miss Keith's criteria. So I knew from experience that it would be no easy matter to persuade Miss Keith to change the background of her seal design which she felt was so ideal.

As I had predicted, though I tried to use my most diplomatic approach, Miss Keith was simply furious. I experienced considerable difficulty in calming her. In fact, I was about to give up and secure another artist when she consented to change the background. She did so with the utmost reluctance and only for the sake of the cause. But she added emphatically, "I shall not allow my initials to appear on the revised seal design." To this I had to agree.

Actually, the new design was also very appealing. The gaily dressed girl and boy were depicted standing in front of an artistic, ancient Korean gateway. But to the discerning eye, distant mountains could be dimly seen through the gateway. This was Miss Keith's little joke, to which, fortunately, the military censor chose to turn a blind eye.

Now that I had appeased Miss Keith and satisfied the military censors, I was ready to tackle the printing press at the Y.M.C.A. at this eleventh hour and attempt to get the seals printed before the deadline. The "Y" responded valiantly and we were able to get the seals out in time for Christmas use. This printing proved to be the last seals of any kind to be issued in Korea for many years, for World War II was fast closing in on us. Had someone suggested that only a few missionaries would be left in Korea by Christmas, he would have been considered out of his mind.

Although Mr. Sasaki had forewarned us, I found myself startled when military gendarmes arrived on our doorstep. Again came the unceremonious announcement that they had come to search our house.

I assured them they would not find anything of interest, for the police had been there already and had found nothing rewarding. This news shook them like a thunderbolt. Their flushed cheeks appeared to reflect their mounting rage. Had the circumstances been different, I might almost have felt sorry for them. As it was, I could not help but rejoice privately at their discomfort, and above all, at their departure.

Soon afterward, Mr. Sasaki called on us again, but this time his face was beaming. He announced, "I have some bittersweet news for you. The military have finally dropped the spy charge against you and have turned over your case to the Kaishu (Haiju) Civil Courts. That is the sweet part, for it means that your lives are no longer in danger. However, the bitter part will be hard on your pocketbooks. Even before your court trial, the verdict has been determined. I believe you call this a 'Kangaroo Court.' Thus, no matter what, you two are to either have three months in jail or pay a fine of 5000 yen [$1000].

"Since the military have lost face pretty badly, for they now have no evidence to present, they have turned your case over to the Civil Court with reluctance. The judge fears that the military will call a retrial if the Civil Court should let you off too lightly; hence, the prison sentence or heavy fine."

This news was indeed startling to us. Grateful for our freedom, we were now confronted with the problem of how we were going to be able to raise such a huge sum. Most of the friends who might have helped us had been evacuated from Korea. We were not free to choose that option, for our case was still pending, and according to Japanese law, we were guilty until proved innocent. In fact, we had been serving under a modified form of arrest and had not been allowed to leave the District of Haiju.

Twice we were called to the Prosecutor's office. The military had turned their files over to him and we had to go over many papers to verify their accuracy. Then a week later we received a call to appear at the courtroom. After waiting there awhile, the Judge, the Prosecu-

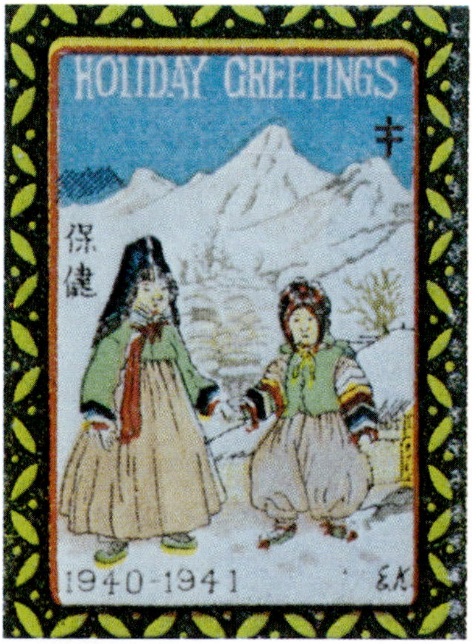

Original design by Elizabeth Keith–distribution prohibited by Japanese government

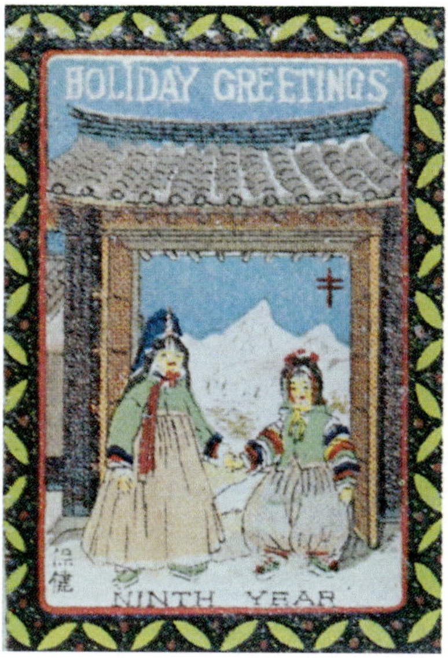

Revised design by Elizabeth Keith

Christmas Tuberculosis Seals of Korea, 1940-1941

Photographs courtesy of Smithsonian Institution

Magnification 2X.

tor and the Clerk formally filed in and took seats above us in chairs upholstered in blue velvet.

At first, we were seated. Marian had crossed her legs and before she knew it, an orderly seemed to appear from nowhere and roughly slapped her knee down. After that, Marian took the hint. We were then told to stand before the august group with our heads bowed. This irked Marian no end, especially since we had done no wrong.

Now the clerk briefly read out the salient points, as reviewed by the military, and the Prosecutor solemnly announced that our case was to be tried October 25, 1940. The Judge then declared that we could defend ourselves verbally, in writing, or hire a lawyer to defend us.

We decided to take no chances and hired a lawyer, a Mr. Pak. He was tall, slim, and in his late forties and had a fine reputation for winning difficult cases. He agreed to accept our case.

We expected Mr. Pak would want to thoroughly quiz us to ascertain all the facts, but we were rather disappointed and somewhat apprehensive because he did not do so. He evidently had his own means of ferreting out the material.

When we approached Mr. Pak and volunteered our help and suggestions, he simply said, "You need have no worry about the outcome. Just leave it all to me, and I shall successfully see you through the trial. Be at peace and enjoy good sleep."

October 25, the day of our trial, finally came. It was true, we might just as well have had a good night's sleep, for worry would not have changed the predetermined events of that day. Mr. Pak put up a wonderful defense for us. We heard an eloquent plea in our behalf and wondered how Mr. Pak had learned so many facts without consulting us, and that he was able to marshall them so forcefully.

Among the arguments Mr. Pak presented was the fact that my father had given his life on the battlefield of Pyong Yang while treating Japanese soldiers. So was it reasonable to suspect his son of now being a spy against other Japanese soldiers? His son, Dr. Sherwood Hall, possessed as much filial loyalty as a Korean, for he was born in Korea, so he would never betray a cause espoused by his father.

Mr. Pak had then referred to my mother as beloved by both Japanese and Koreans, who called her the "Mother of Pyong Yang." She had been a founder of hospitals, a school for the blind and deaf, as well as the founder of Korea's first medical school for training women doctors in modern medicine. Could the son of such a mother betray his mother's deep love for Oriental people? Never in a thousand years!

As a climax, Mr. Pak spoke beautifully of Dr. Marian Hall. At the risk of her own life and that of her unborn babe, she had taken a very hazardous night call in the cold of winter, which most men doctors would have refused. By her skill as a surgeon, on that occasion she had saved the life of a poor young man in a remote country village. She had also been called up to Seoul by Dr. Mary Stewart to help operate on a female patient of the ancient Royal Korean household. Never in ten thousand years would such sacrificial deeds be forgotten.

Mr. Pak concluded his eloquent defense by asking the military a rather embarrassing question. "How does it happen that Dr. Sherwood Hall has been singled out by the Governor of this great Province of Whanghai to represent us at the 2600th Anniversary of the founding of the Empire of Japan? And on this glorious occasion, we are given to understand, the Emperor wished to honor my client for his great achievements in the field of tuberculosis control. This dread disease, thanks to my client, is no longer the 'great white plague' in this land. In fact, before my client's efforts, this fatal disease was fast becoming the 'great yellow plague' and would have been a menace to each of you in this courtroom."

Our lawyer then countered point by point what he considered the flimsy accusations that had been put forth, which in view of his clients' background, were absolutely without foundation. It was felt that Mr. Pak's spirited performance had, at least, prevented the danger of a retrial by the military, and had thus spared us that ordeal.

In offering his rebuttal to the military accusations, Mr. Pak remarked, "I understand that the United States of America claims that anyone born there is a citizen of their country, no matter what the nationality of his parents. By the same token, I claim my client is citizen of 'Tai Han' (Korea). The military have classified my client as British spy and enemy alien. I strongly refute this, and I have clearly shown that he is neither enemy nor alien. My client has often said that as he listens with his stethoscope to our people's hearts, that he finds our heartbeats are one with his. He feels and holds a common bond of love and affection, uniting him with us. Our clients have been told to appear here in this courtroom with bowed heads. Instead, those who have so unjustly accused them, should now appear with bowed heads of shame!"

The military observers in the courtroom stared out of the window, pretending they had not heard.

Mr. Pak's defense had served us well. Had it not been for the insistence of the military, we were later told, the judge would have excused the case. As it turned out, just as Mr. Sasaki had previously informed us, we were given a judgement of three months in jail, or paying a fine of 5000 yen ($1000).

Not a word of the trial appeared in the local papers, which seemed to want to play it down, but some time afterwards it was written up in the Western press as a "Kangaroo trial." Indeed it was! The whole affair was a farce. This was especially demonstrated when the Emperor of Japan gave gifts to Korea on the occasion of the 2600th Anniversary; and, coincidentally, the largest single gift of 5000 yen, the same amount as our fine, was given to our Haiju Sanatorium. I had not been able to attend the formal ceremonies because our court case was not over, and I was not allowed to leave the Haiju District even for an event of this import.

Although the Emperor's gift did not help us personally, it did greatly benefit our beloved Sanatorium. It showed how very unpopular and distasteful to the civil authorities the whole affair had been.

CHAPTER 31

Exodus

A message from the State Department of the United States was received by radio on October 9, 1940 and was confirmed by Mr. O. Gaylord Marsh, U.S. Consul-General. It urged the evacuation of all Americans, especially women and children and announced that two passenger ships would be sent to Chemulpo on November 16, 1940 to provide passage back to America. The *SS Mariposa* and the *SS Monterey* were to be diverted from their Honolulu–San Francisco route for this purpose. By the end of the month the British Consul-General, Mr. Gerald Phipps, was advising British nationals to evacuate and return to their homeland.

Having been accused of being British spies and then handed the sentence of the Court, we felt that we should at once consult Mr. Phipps in Seoul. I could not leave Haiju without a permit and someone to meet me at the other end. However, I was able to see Mr. Phipps and asked him if he felt it advisable for us to pay the fine. Sometimes the paying of a fine is considered an admission of guilt, so it might be better to be jailed than to get into that trap.

Mr. Phipps left us in no doubt, however, as to which course of action to take. He had already consulted Mr. Oda of the Foreign Affairs Department along with our Methodist Mission representative, Mr. Charles A. Sauer. Mr. Oda was a Christian and a Methodist and had always been very helpful to me in our Christmas Seal matters. Mr. Oda had confirmed that only undue pressure from the military could have accounted for the judge laying down such an obviously unjust sentence. Any further appeals would only run into the same pressure and likely make matters worse. Mr. Phipps told us that we had been shown the handwriting on the wall. Even though there was nothing legal about our trial, he strongly advised us to pay the fine and leave the country as soon as possible.

By mid-November the *SS Mariposa* had left with 219 American citizens aboard, 74 of them Methodists and 24 W.F.M.S. missionaries.

We were not free to leave, for we had yet to raise the required sum of money to purchase our freedom. Acting promptly on Mr. Phipps' good advice, we busied ourselves at once to try to sell off personal effects, household goods, coal *et cetera*. These all brought a fairly good price, for due to the war there was a great scarcity of consumer goods.

A few of the more wealthy Christians, like Mr. Chuni Chell, offered to sell some of their rice fields to help us out, but fortunately, with what we had sold and could borrow, we did not need to call upon their aid. However, towards the end, the military did try to make it difficult by threatening anyone who purchased from "enemy aliens," as they continued to call us. Despite this handicap, we succeeded in raising the entire amount within the prescribed time limit. In order to do so, however, we had to sell most of our warm clothing and blankets, which later we were to need.

When I showed up at the Prosecutor's office with the whole of our "ransom money," I announced that I had come to buy back our freedom. I cheerfully deposited the entire amount before the Prosecutor's astonished eyes.

"I never thought you could make it!" he exclaimed. Only this morning I had ordered disinfectant from the hospital to clean up your two cells, for you know they have an unbearable stench and are infested with vermin. I had also ordered traps for the rats which often run over the sleeping prisoners and bite them. It is difficult to get a good night's rest in these circumstances.

"As a special consideration, I had ordered a couple of our office chairs to be delivered to your cells. I know that you Westerners are not accustomed to sitting on the floor, especially a cold damp one, for a long time. However, there was not room to put in any cots, so you would have had to sleep on the floor. Now, what a pity, after all my careful preparations, I find such will not be necessary."

I told the Prosecutor that I was impressed by all his thoughtfulness, but was now more than glad we would not need to avail ourselves of his hospitality.

He did concede in parting, "After all, I am really happy you won't have to be our 'special guests.'"

Later we heard stories of Americans, like Dr. E. W. Koons, who had chosen not to be evacuated, and who were cruelly tortured by the Japanese. Dr. Koons had received the special "water cure" which was effected by forcing water into the stomach so that it was stretched almost beyond the point of human endurance. This left no evidence or mark of torture as would the torture of removing fingernails by the roots. Fortunately, most Americans got out of Korea before this kind of severe treatment had been meted out to them.

When I reached home I gave a shout of joy, as I hugged Marian and the children and told them we were free at last.

Marian then asked, "May I begin packing now?"

I nodded a vigorous yes and started towards my study with the intent of sitting right down to write a letter to our good friend, Mr. H. W. Davidson, a businessman in Seoul, who could arrange for our passage to America. But before my letter could be written, a telegram arrived.

For a moment, I hardly dared to open it. The children, however, were clamoring, "Read it, read it, read it!" My first glance revealed that it was not written in Japanese but was a cablegram from our Mission Board in New York. It read as follows:

"Would you consider immediate transfer to tuberculosis work at Ajmer, India? Cable reply."

Much relieved, we went into a family huddle. Originally, India would probably have been our last choice. However, we had both dedicated ourselves to a lifetime of service on the mission field. Since the door in Korea was definitely closing, and the door to India was opening, we took it to mean God's choice for us. Our cabled reply to the Mission Board was in the affirmative.

Some time afterward, we learned that the Mission Board had been extremely pleased with our decision to go directly to India. An article later appeared in the magazine, *World Outlook*, entitled "Tuberculosis Control in Two Lands." It featured our transfer and was illustrated with pictures of our work in both countries.

Having made this decision, I went to my office to pen a different letter to Mr. Davidson from the one I had originally intended. I requested him to secure for us the first possible booking on a ship to India.

He wrote right back that passenger service was very difficult to obtain these war days, but that the *SS President Jackson* was on her maiden voyage around the world and was due to dock at Kobe, Japan the first week in December. He would try to get us reservations on it to Bombay. Things were apparently working out well.

Our children were all excited about going to the land of elephants and camels, but they were not so sure about the cobras. In the meantime, we received notice that due to the war situation, the Pyong Yang Foreign School would have to close. Marian had been planning to go to Pyong Yang to bring William home anyway, but this advanced that time considerably.

Meanwhile, I wanted to make the appropriate arrangements to put our Sanatorium on a sound financial basis and to give it permanence and lasting tenure. Therefore, I had been trying to form a holding body called a *Zaidan Hojin* which, I believe, is a system unique to Korea. Upon the formation of an administrative body of trustees, the *Zaidan Hojin*, the government agreed to take the responsibility of assuring that the Sanatorium land, buildings and properties would continue to be used as a tuberculosis institution. As previously, the day-to-day affairs of the Sanatorium would continue to be administered by a Board of Governors.

This procedure turned out to be a difficult and complicated business. Fortunately I had the strong backing of the Governor and some concerned high officials in Seoul. With their help, it was accomplished in record time. Of course, the *Zaidan Hojin* was entirely dependent upon the stability of the government and whether or not it remained in power. In time of war one could only assure the probability, and not certainty, of the government's ability to guarantee the continuance of the Sanatorium. The Norton Memorial Hospital, being an older institution and well established, was felt to have more secure prospects for its future and was, therefore, not in need of these special legal arrangements.

We had received a proposal from a flourishing Southern Methodist school at Songdo, about fifty miles distant, to join forces with our Haiju Boys' School. The missionary formerly in charge had been evacuated and undesirable elements wanted to take control of it. Since I was now free to travel outside of the District of Haiju, I was asked to go and appraise the situation. This I did and was able to bring back a favorable report. Our Haiju Boys' School Board decided to assume responsibility for the school which would keep it in Christian hands and also enhance the prestige of the Boys' School at Haiju.

Fortunately, Marian was able to find a good Korean woman doctor to take over her medical work and the Child Welfare Clinic. So the stage was now all set to begin packing in earnest. It was made relatively simpler for Marian in view of the fact that so many of our things had been sold. There were still items to be sorted out, nonetheless. We were unable to take with us mother-of-pearl inlaid chests and other priceless heirlooms left to me by my parents which were precious to me for their sentimental value. We never saw these again.

We were in a quandary as to just what should be taken. Some of those en route to Japan had been stripped of everything, while others seemed to get through unscathed. If we took what might be considered too much in this time of scarcity, it might be just the excuse needed to confiscate everything. We concluded, therefore, that we would only pack what might be viewed as essential. In a sense, we now shared the sad lot of refugees the world over, and it increased our appreciation of the ordeals they had to endure.

The days were more crowded than ever. In addition to keeping up with the regular work, I had to try to find suitable Board members for our three institutions and replace staff members who had been commandeered by the military. Good workers were difficult to find, while opportunists and some very shady characters seemed to abound. I was concerned that the latter not slip in and spoil the work we had been able to build. With much searching and prayer we were eventually able to locate staff and Board members who impressed us as being well qualified and dedicated. We could now leave with the comforting assurance that God would continue to work things out for the best.

As is the custom in the Orient, it is proper before leaving to call on various officials and important people. These numerous farewells were often taxing both physically and emotionally. One day when I was on such a round of calls, a rumor reached Marian while she was in the midst of packing, that someone had seen me go into the Prosecutor's office. Since no one had seen me come out, it must be assumed that I had been arrested.

"Oh, not again!" Marian exclaimed.

By this time her nerves were so on edge that she broke down and wept. I returned soon after and was most disturbed to see her distress. I reassured her that all was well; that I had just paid a farewell call on the Prosecutor and had had a long talk with him.

In the course of our conversation, the Prosecutor had revealed to me that among the sins the military had listed against us was that we were friends of the Saitos. Viscount Saito had served as Governor-General of Korea from 1919 to 1927. When serving as Prime Minister of Japan and afterwards, he had been strongly anti-military.

Viscount Saito had resigned as Premier on July 3, 1934 because one of his cabinet ministers had been arrested in connection with a financial scandal. However, a cabinet of loyal Saito followers was formed. The Viscount was assassinated on February 26, 1936 as part of a number of assassinations carried out against prominent statesmen by two regiments of the Tokyo military garrison. These had mutinied under the leadership of some junior officers. While the rebellion against the Saito adherents was obscure as to origin, it was a time when the military began to dominate Japanese political life.

The Prosecutor reported that among the items searched at our house, a personal letter from Viscountess Haru Saito had especially interested the military investigators. It was a reply to our letter of sympathy on the death of her husband. (She had been wounded in her vain attempt to shield her husband from the assassin.) It was dated May 15, 1936, written on black-bordered stationery from her residence at Nakacho, Yotsuya, Tokyo, and signed in her own hand. The Prosecutor showed me the part of her letter which had been viewed as incriminating:

> ". . . I appreciate what you have to say about my late husband and of the memory in which he is held. . . . I shall always remember with happiness your kindness to my late husband during his days here on earth. With kindest regards,
>
> "Sincerely yours,
> "Haru Saito"

The Prosecutor said that the military had taken the last paragraph, especially, to confirm that I, too, must be strongly anti-military. He reported that they were not at all happy therefore that the Haiju Civil Court had only made us pay a fine and had seen fit to free us. He concluded by saying that he was very glad that I was leaving soon before more trouble might arise.

Prominent people of Haiju had arranged a farewell party for us, but had proceeded to make the arrangements in secrecy because of the military presence. However, the supposedly well kept secret somehow got out, and two uninvited military guests showed up at the party. Fortunately, they had not arrived before the flag of old Korea had been formally presented to us, and I had had time to carefully tuck it away inside my coat pocket. The representatives lost no time in finding out and jotting down the names of all those present, which was rather disconcerting to say the least. This also had the effect of putting a damper on the speeches, which were shortened considerably from their prepared length. In the midst of all this, an express telegram was delivered to me from Mr. Davidson.

It contained distressing news. "Sorry—no vacancies available on *SS President Jackson*."

This was indeed a bad blow to our plans and we went immediately into another family huddle. We then announced to the gathering that we would leave Korea anyway, as per schedule, for we felt that we would have a better chance of getting the first available ship out of Kobe, Japan, than we would by waiting an indefinite period of time in Haiju. So we told them that we would proceed on faith, for we were confident God would find a way. (This proved to be the case, for after many uncertain days in Kobe, we ended up sailing on the *SS President Jackson* after all.)

When the party finally broke up, we warmly thanked our friends and told them we were saying our "good-bys" now for we did not want anyone to be embarrassed at the station. We earnestly requested that no one come to see us off.

Then I turned to the uninvited guests, saying, "You see that this party is no conspiracy against the might of the military, so please do not send in the names of those present. Simply tell the authorities about the telegram and our determination to leave for India as planned. They can be assured there will be no incidents resulting from this party." Perhaps this request would not be heeded, but I felt it needed to be made anyway and would be a comfort to our friends.

It was decided to have the official farewell function for us at the Sanatorium chapel with all three of our Christian institutions participating. This memorable affair went off quietly, as far as we could see, with no uninvited guests present. At the close, the Reverend Y. S. Kim, our Sanatorium Chaplain, made a very eloquent plea for our return as soon as conditions would allow. At the end he broke down crying. Many were weeping quietly and I, too, was close to tears as I gave our response. I had a strong feeling that we could never return to dear Haiju, and it was hard to say such a final farewell.

I was relieved when several patients came up to me right afterwards with the concrete request that I go over their chests with my stethoscope, to which they attributed magical healing power. They did not consider it just a diagnostic tool as I had always stoutly maintained. I knew that these particular patients had all improved so I could at least give them this comfort and encouragement.

The departure from the Haiju station was without incident, although tears flowed freely from Phyllis and her beloved *amah*, Chaisie. Mr. Buitsu Nagata, teacher at the Government High School, and his family came to see us off and we were touched by this act of friendship at such a time.

When we arrived in Seoul, it seemed wiser to divide forces, for I knew we were being carefully watched by the plain clothes detectives. Marian and the children had accepted a gracious invitation to stay at the Phipps, while I went to stay with our good friend Charlie Sauer. He had remained behind to wind up the Mission's business in Seoul, while the J. Z. Moores were holding the Mission fort, so to speak, in Pyong Yang. Eventually all of them had to leave.[1]

Overnight, it seemed, Seoul had joined the wartime capitals of the world. The streets were comparatively empty. Instead of the many white clad pedestrians, there were a few drab grey ones, for this was the prescribed color these war days. They mingled with the dull khaki of the uniformed soldiers, while women and children could hardly be seen anywhere at all.

Many of the Korean shops were boarded up for the long night of war. As I passed the forlorn empty houses of our friends, I was startled anew by the realization that these friends had already left. I recalled them to mind and the delightful times we had spent in their homes. I felt saddened by the realization that such occasions were not likely to come again. All this put me in a pensive mood, but the worst was yet to come.

Passing through the formerly gay and busy Chinatown section of the city, I was stunned to see it had become so desolate. In the good old days, Chinatown, in the heart of Seoul, was particularly gay. During the traditional New Year festival, it would be lit with picturesque Chinese lanterns. The noise of firecrackers would tickle the ears of the

---

[1] Less than ten percent of the Protestant missionaries remained in Korea by Christmas, 1940. Those who elected to stay were placed under custody on December 8, 1941, following Japan's attack on Pearl Harbor the day before. Some were placed under house detention, while others, like Dr. Koons, were jailed and tortured. In June, 1942, all British and American missionaries and businessmen were released, and expelled from the country.

children, and deafen the ears of the adults. Gaily dressed "sing-song girls" would make a Western country fair seem drab by comparison.

Now there were no signs of life in this section of the city, with the exception of the scampering, brazen rats that no longer had to fear being turned into soup. When I thought of the fate of the former happy inhabitants of this area, I shuddered involuntarily.

I did not care to linger, and from this depressing scene, I wandered into the Japanese sector of the city. Here there was certainly much life and activity, but none of the customary smiling, happy faces. What immediately struck the ear was the "clack-it-clack" on the hard pavement of the *geta* (wooden shoes) that nearly everyone was now wearing. This was to save precious leather for shoes for their soldiers.

While I was taking in the changed scene, I was startled by the sudden appearance, seemingly out of nowhere, of a plain clothes detective. As he approached me, I wondered, "What have I done now?" For an instant it flashed over my apprehensive consciousness that perhaps I had unwittingly entered a prohibited zone. However, to my immense relief, he greeted me quite courteously.

With a smile he said, "We have been watching you carefully from a distance. We note that you have not tried to make any improper contacts so we think now it might be safe to turn back to you some 16 m.m. movie film which someone has brought to our Police Office. If you will come right over with me now, we shall be glad to return it to you.

Could this be bait for some sort of trap, I wondered? Was this a devious way of taking me into custody? I fear I was no longer the trusting soul I had once been, but despite my suspicions, I had no choice but to follow my captor or benefactor, whichever the case might be.

As I entered the Police Office, I could feel at once that the atmosphere was friendly. I was greeted by smiles, and began to regret my previous unjust suspicions.

The officer in charge announced, "Here is some home movie film we should like you to identify." He motioned me to a chair and said, "Please examine them at your leisure. We don't want to hurry you."

I lost no time, nonetheless, in picking out various scenes from the film that was undoubtedly ours. The officer peered over my shoulder. He was genuinely interested in the scenes and said that he was sure that my wife would be glad to get back these films of our children.

"It is good to know that you love children as we Japanese do," he commented. "At heart we are really one."

"For your own protection we have destroyed some of the scenery footage taken from high places. Those scenes can be taken again after the war."

He seemed in a conversational mood, although I was eager to be off. He talked at length about the military and suggested that although the military appeared to be on the way up, they did not yet feel firm in the saddle. (Later, they would not care about world opinion, but apparently at this time they still felt the need to be careful.)

"The military officials were furious when you were freed by the Civil Court," the police officer volunteered. "But, here is the important point. When they learned that you were not returning to your homeland, but were going to India, they felt they had saved face. They boast, as you know, that under the plan for establishing the Greater East Asia Co-Prosperity Sphere, they will eventually emancipate even India. Evidently they think that you will be in the reception committee to receive them there."

He concluded by giving me the good news that he did not think that they would now cause us any more trouble. "That is why we think it is now safe to return your films to you."

He then called an orderly and told him to carry the heavy package of films for me. I offered the Chief Police Officer more than the usual perfunctory *aregoto* (thanks), for my gratitude was heartfelt.

I believed now that it was more important than ever for me to make the routine official farewell calls as I had done in Haiju. At first, I had not intended to call on the Chief of the Gendarmery, for I had built up considerable resentment against him during our recent difficulties, which almost verged on hatred I am sorry to say.

However, in my calmer moments I realized that not all Japanese civilians were "good guys" nor all military personnel "bad guys." As a Christian, I further realized, I must "hate the sin and love the sinner," for Jesus, even while suffering in his death agony on the cross, had made that sublime appeal of the ages, "*Father, forgive them; for they know not what they do*." Thus, on sober second thought, I could not do otherwise than to call on the Chief.

It felt wonderful to be able to walk right into the Gendarmery as a free man and not as a prisoner. The Chief of the Gendarmery greeted me pleasantly. I told him that I had come to say farewell and to tell him that I held no hard feelings against him. (I omitted mentioning what a struggle it had been for me to reach this point.) I also assured him that I had not come to ask any favors, nor did I expect any.

He apparently chose to ignore my mention of "hard feelings," and simply replied that both Mr. Oda and Mr. Sasaki had spoken highly of my work for TB sufferers in Korea, and he also wanted to personally thank me for the service I had rendered this cause. (His remark confirmed what I had felt all along, that we must have had "friends in court!")

He then asked the date and time of our departure from Seoul, telling his secretary to make note of it. This, I thought at the time, was just a routine check. Then I took my leave, feeling at least I had done my Christian duty, albeit perhaps not as cheerfully as I should have.

At last the stage was set for our departure: our official calls had been made, our account in the bank closed, the proper visas entered on our passports, our train, ferry and hotel reservations made. As in Haiju, we had requested our Korean friends in Seoul not to see us off at the station. This was for their own protection. However, some did not heed our advice and came anyway.

There were very few Occidentals left in Seoul, but these few had turned out in force. A number of our Japanese friends also were awaiting our arrival on the station platform, among them the Odas and the Sasakis. Mr. Sasaki had very recently taken a position with the Red Cross in Seoul. Each person there, in their own way, had helped our work and us personally during our time in Korea.

What astonished us most, however, was to see none other than the Chief Officer of the Gendarmery and his aide at the station platform. It would, indeed, be a rare occurrence for such a high ranking military officer to want to thus honor a former prisoner. Both our friends and we were beginning to wonder, "What next?"

However, our fears were soon allayed when they greeted us cordially. The Chief Officer announced that they had come to wish us a safe and pleasant journey to India. More significant than his just giving us this friendly send-off, were his words of assurance that he had issued firm orders that both we and our baggage would be well protected, and there would be no further molestation by the military on our trip to Kobe and while in Japan. His word proved good, and we remembered with regret the many precious things we had left behind.

Amid the farewells, I found myself cornered by the Chief Officer's aide in an embarrassing situation. His question revealed that he was still smarting over a sense of rivalry and loss of face. He wanted to know which had accorded us better treatment, the police or the military. I tried to fend off a direct answer by simply saying that we were grateful to both for having freed us. He was not satisfied with my response and was still trying to pin me down when his superior officer called him off, fortunately, to allow us to speak to a number of friends before the train left.

We had just time to board. The train slowly pulled away from the station as we waved good-by. Our friends and the city of my birth soon faded into the distance, but not from our memory or affection.

CHAPTER 32

Mansei

When we reached the port of Fusan, we were happy to learn that there would be considerable time before the departure of the ferry to Japan. We decided to set off on a sentimental journey.

Our children had often heard us refer to the cherry tree garden by the sea where their mother and I had been given such a warm and colorful welcome when we first arrived in Korea in April, 1926. There the children would be free to run and have a chance to work off some of the energy which the confinement of the train ride had pent up.

When we reached the garden that bleak November day, it had none of the warmth and color of the beautiful, charming spot we had remembered. Instead, the garden had a forlorn, drab appearance. Of course there were no blossoms, and at this time of the year, the trees were even bare of leaves.

Marian and I sat down on one of the garden benches, where William soon joined us, while Joe and Phyllis raced happily over the garden paths. Those of us on the bench were in a rather pensive mood, for we were recalling all that had happened to us in recent weeks. It was really the first opportunity we had had to gather up our thoughts.

William, being thirteen years old and realizing what might have been our fate, had suffered a greater traumatic experience than our two younger children, although all of us had been affected. For awhile he did not seem to want us out of his sight. He finally did decide to join his brother and sister playing tag, tempted by the fact that his long legs could easily overtake and outdistance them.

Marian, I imagined, was silently going over meaningful memories, some happy and others not so happy. I was quietly reliving in my mind's eye the sixteen wonderful growing-up years of my boyhood in Korea, and then my return to the land of my birth with my doctor wife. The past fourteen and a half years that had marked our life together on the mission field had been full and rich, for all the crises we had weathered. I felt a special bond to this country, where so much of my family history was enacted, and in whose service two generations of physician partners had given and received so much love.

With deep emotion I recalled the "Quadruple Anniversary" celebration of May 7, 1938 in Haiju. It was a day that stood out, especially for me. At that time, we commemorated 35 years of service of the Haiju Boys' School, founded by the Reverend Carl Critchit. We had also honored the Norton Memorial Hospital built 30 years previously by Dr. A. H. Norton whose vision and work were responsible for erecting that building. It had replaced a small and inadequate dispensary that had served the community for many years.

The Mothers' and Children's Welfare Club had been founded by Marian in 1928. That eventful anniversary day, it had more than 60 mothers enrolled who were learning better ways of caring for their over 100 children. At the May 7 ceremony each mother was given a gift of infant's clothing and I could see the radiance of their faces before me now. The fourth "anniversary" to be celebrated that day was that of the founding of the Haiju School for the Tuberculous ten years before.

I looked fondly at Marian as I called to mind the words she had written of that occasion in an article for the *Korea Mission Field*:

> "Eleven years ago my husband and I went for a walk over the hills between our residence and the sea. We stopped here and there to admire the view. I saw only rice fields and sea and the beauty of the pine clad hills. My husband saw the same, but saw it all as the setting for the fulfillment of a boyhood dream. For him the hills were dotted with cottages housing men and women whose future was menaced by the disease, tuberculosis. He saw these sufferers coming in ill and with fear in their hearts. He saw them going out well and with a new hope in life.
>
> "No fairy godmother appeared with magic wand to change the scene which he saw, but a year later we celebrated the opening of the first wing of what is now the central building around which cluster an ever increasing number of cottages. As I attended the tenth anniversary of that occasion and looked back in memory over the few years intervening, it

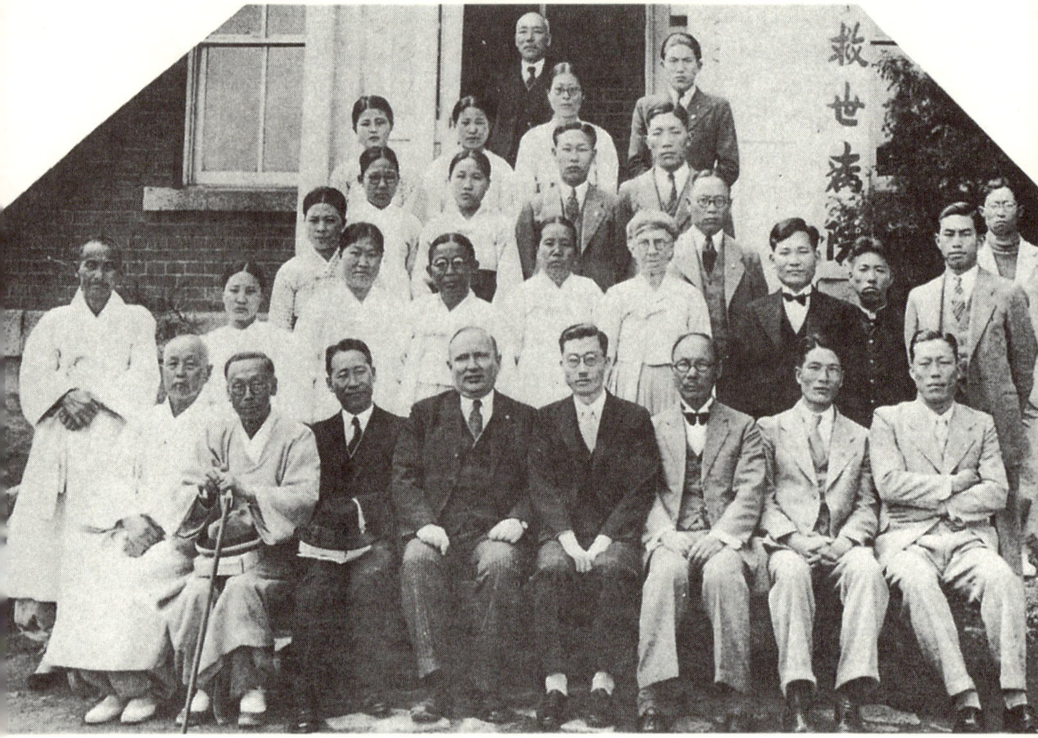

Norton Memorial Hospital Staff

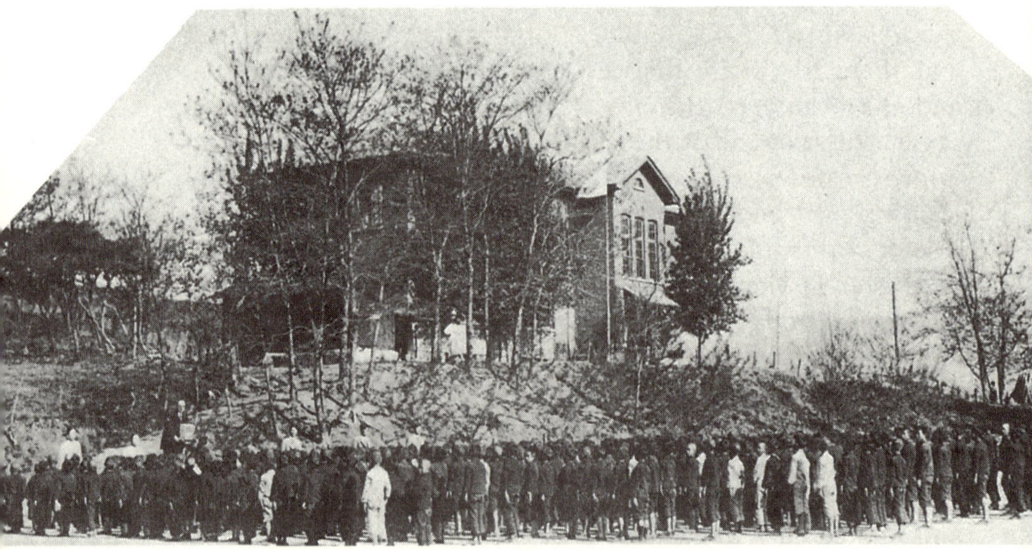

Haiju Christian Boys' School 35th Anniversary, 1938

seemed that magic had been at work. I knew it to be the magic of a deep rooted faith that the dream was God given and that He would find the way to its realization, if the dreamer had the faith and perseverance to keep on dreaming. Friends have been given in unexpected places, difficulties of all kinds have been met and overcome until the institution which began in a small way ten years ago is now filling a considerable place in the lives of many for whom there was otherwise little hope.

"The services were held outdoors under an awning erected in the yard of the Sanatorium Chapel. Following congratulatory speeches by Governor Kang and Vice Governor Sasaki of our province, Dr. H. H. Underwood of the Chosen Chirstian College made the address of the day. While those who had spoken before him wished for the sanatorium long years of increasing service, Dr. Underwood expressed quite an opposite sentiment by hoping that the institution would soon find itself unnecessary because tuberculosis, due to the efforts of this institution and others, would be wiped from the land.

"Amongst the congratulatory letters and telegrams received and read was one which particularly touched our hearts because it expressed so well the aims of the institution and appreciated so sympathetically the difficulties which have had to be overcome. It ran as follows:

> "'Dear Friend,
>
> "'Congratulations! Although we cannot be there, we rejoice with you over the fact that Haiju Sanatorium has given ten years of Christian ministry to the healing of the bodies and souls of men in the same manner, we believe, as Christ would have done it had He been walking the earth with men during these years of toil.
>
> "'First, you had to drive out fears and superstitions and instill in their stead a faith in your power to heal that would last through years of slow recovery. Next, it was imperative that you gather together for your staff of doctors and nurses, men and women of just the highest type of Christian character lest by

some act or word the patient's hope be discouraged. The financial difficulties, as we well know, have not been the least of your burdens. In remaining faithful to your task you yourselves, have become almost segregated from the helpful association of fellow missionaries. Surely there has been no more acceptable ministry in Chosen than yours!

"'It is a way we have on the mission field of being completely occupied with our own sphere of work so that we do not often encourage each other with helpful suggestions and praise. We want you to know at this time, we both have the highest regard for you and do not cease to pray for the success of your undertakings.

"'Yours in a common cause, . . .'

"The following letter was sent to Dr. Hall from the patients along with a handsome gift of silverware:

"'Dear Dr. Sherwood Hall,

"'What a holy and great enterprise you have begun! Who does not praise brilliant and great merit? Today is the glorious tenth anniversary of our Haiju Sanatorium. Its wonderful development we owe to you. It is the crystal of your blood and sweat.

"'It is evident today that tuberculosis is the enemy of mankind, and it ruins all countries and all nations. But ten years ago in Korea, we Korean people could not understand the above facts. You have established our Sanatorium; nevertheless, the lack of knowledge about tuberculosis has hindered the people in fighting many difficulties. You have cured many people who had wept in deep despair because of tuberculosis.

"'Not only cured, but you have raised the first banner of prevention against tuberculosis in Korea and have done your best as the leader of our Korean anti-tuberculosis society. You have given the best years of your life and many people can sing and enjoy their happiness and bliss because of you. Your love is

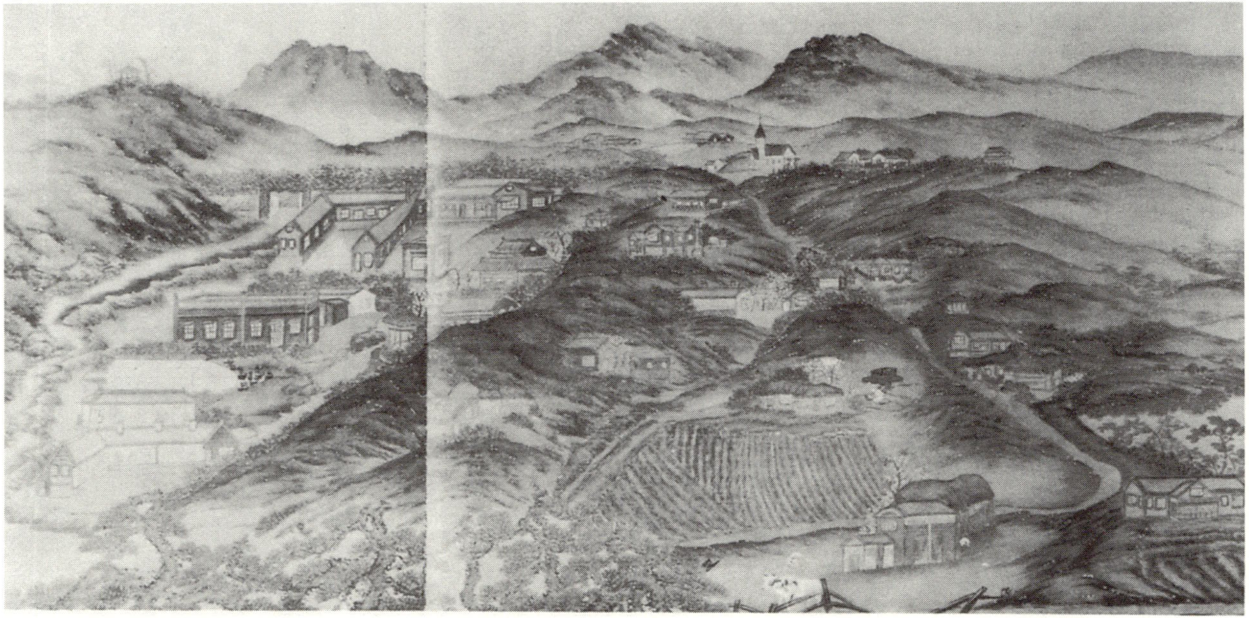

Korean artist's sketch of Sanatorium, chapel, farm, and rehabilitation center

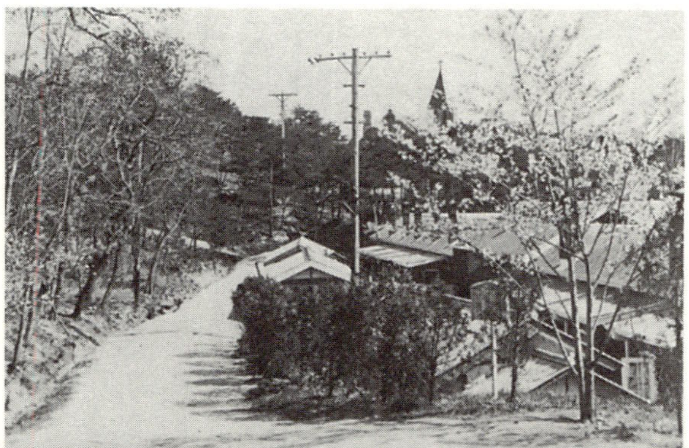

Sanatorium with chapel in background

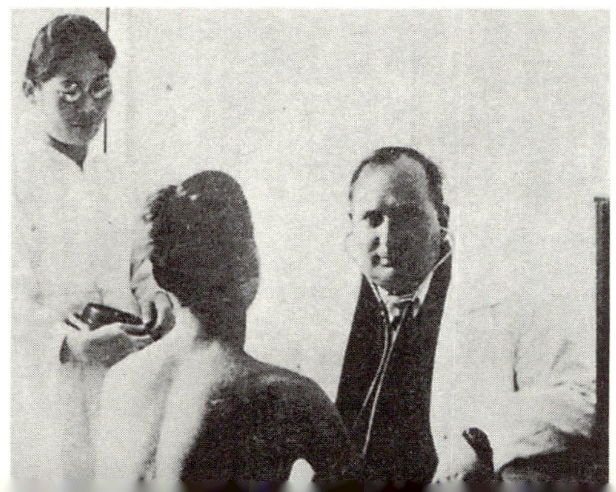

Dr. Hall, patient, and nurse

higher than the Taishan [the highest mountain in North China] and deeper than the Yellow Sea.

"'On the glorious tenth anniversary of our Sanatorium, we who have been embraced in your meritorious love and passionate kindness, cannot refrain from thanking you in every way. We present only a little gift as a symbol of our gratitude. If you receive our present in memory of our thanks, it is the highest honour for all of us patients.

"'Yours faithfully,'

"(Signed by all patients)"

These had indeed been some twenty-four eventful and exciting years for me, in total, in the "Land of the Morning Calm," which at that moment could hardly claim for itself such a title. Yes, it was hard to leave Korea, with all its meaningful associations for us, but I was realist enough to know that it would have been harder for us, and for the Koreans we loved, for us to have stayed.

I emerged from my reverie and called to the children. From my inside coat pocket I took out the beautifully hand embroidered Korean flag, so recently given to us as a loving remembrance at that touching party of farewell in Haiju. I unfurled the flag and hung it, for the time being, on a branch of a nearby tree as our family gathered around it.

A traditional Korean toast or cheer is "*Mansei!*" which in literal translation means, "May it live 10,000 years!" Now I suggested that we all give a fond salute to our Korean flag, the ancient flag of the land where four of us present had been born, and where Marian had given in loving dedication some of the best years of her life. In unison we shouted, "*Mansei!*" and we saluted the real flag of Korea.

Then I took out of my other pocket a scrap of paper on which I had copied some lines from Minnie L. Haskins' lovely poem, "Gate of the Year." As we clasped hands, I asked my family to repeat the lines after me as I read:

"I said to the man, who stood at the gate of the year,

"'Give me a light, that I may tread safely into the unknown.'

"And he replied,

"'Go into the darkness, and put your hand into the hand of God.

"'That shall be better to you than light, and safer than a known way.'"

In this fashion did we leave our "garden of memories" and Korea.

Epilogue

While another volume is needed to cover the remaining years of our Christian medical work in India, certain events which followed our departure from Korea on December 9, 1940, pertain especially to this volume.

My mother, Dr. Rosetta Sherwood Hall, continued to remain active in medical practice until she moved to the Bancroft-Taylor Rest Home in Ocean Grove, New Jersey in 1943. This was a home for deaconesses and missionaries of the Methodist Woman's Division of Christian Service.

Always an ardent advocate of peace, my mother lived to see Korea involved in four wars during the course of her lifetime. Her deep love for the Korean and Japanese people made it extremely difficult for her to comprehend the missionary exodus from Korea in the early 1940's, and the role assumed by the Japanese militarists, even where her own son was involved.

While at Ocean Grove, she participated actively in the many medical societies and church connected groups to which she belonged, and wrote articles on the Far East. When a flu epidemic created excessive demands on the infirmary of the Rest Home, she gave her assistance. She apparently became vulnerable herself to the virus, and passed away in her sleep to her heavenly home on April 5, 1951 at 9:20 P.M. She was 85.

Her grandson, William James Hall, came from Canada to attend the funeral service conducted by my brother-in-law, the Reverend Norris A. Lineweaver and her pastor at the St. Paul's Church in Ocean Grove, the Reverend B. Harrison Decker. My mother's ashes were buried beside my father, sister and son, on the banks of the Han River in Seoul.

Marian and I were still serving on the mission field in India at the time of my mother's death. Later, when we were privileged to revisit Korea in 1960, we toured the Seoul Women's Medical College which

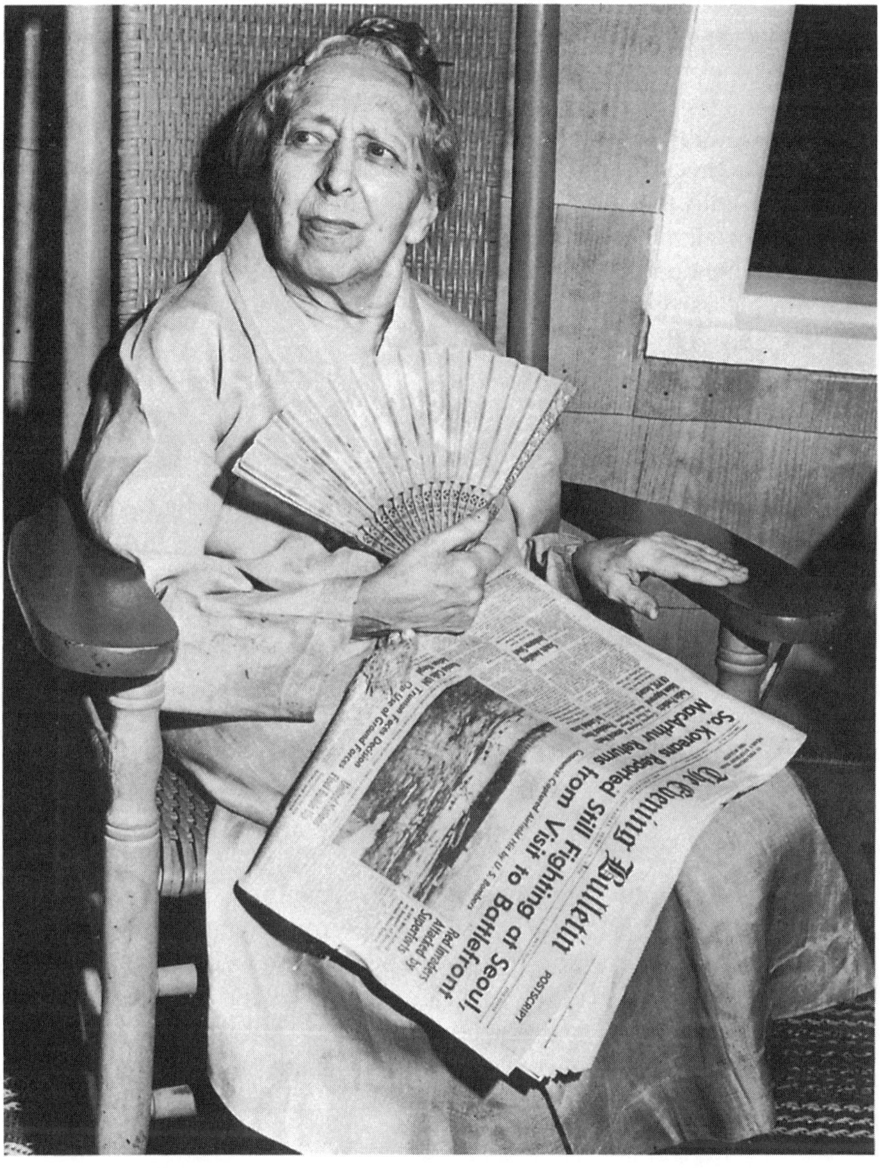

Dr. Rosetta Hall in retirement reads of the fourth war involving Korea in her lifetime, Sept. 19, 1865–April 5, 1951

had been founded by my mother as the Woman's Medical Institute in 1928. It had been endowed in 1938 by Mr. Kim, Chong-Ik of Soon Choon (Sunchon), South Chulla Province (Chollanamdo), and that same year had received full government recognition. The college was now housed in a fine new building.

On the occasion of this memorable return visit, we were invited to the Headquarters of the Korean National TB Association in Seoul. Here, at a special ceremony, Marian and I were each honored with a beautiful gold insignia on which was engraved the "Yang" (the symbolic male element, indicative of the source of life) and the "Yin" (the complementary female element). Superimposed on these was the double-barred Cross of Lorraine, the international symbol of the fight against TB.

The Association President, Dr. K. C. Chung, presented me with a "Certificate of Merit." It was inscribed in Korean (*hangul*) characters, and roughly translated read:

> "In recognition of your selfless and distinguished contribution rendered to tuberculosis control in Korea, this is to honor you.
>
> "Especially commendable are your pioneer achievements, not only in founding Korea's first TB sanatorium in 1928, but in issuing Korea's first TB Christmas Seals, 1932-1941.
>
> "With grateful acknowledgement of what you have done for Korea, we are very proud to present this Certificate of Merit, as a token of our appreciation to you."
>
> (Stamped with their official seal.)

I was very moved by this gracious recognition. After expressing my appreciation, I congratulated them for founding the Korean National TB Association on November 6, 1953. I also mentioned how glad I was that the TB seal campaign had been resumed in 1949 and that it continued to be successful.

During our visit we were told that the Haiju Sanatorium had continued to function despite two wars. When the institution was built so close to the 38th Parallel, we little dreamed that a geographer's imaginary line would one day come to hold either political or personal significance. Yet this 38th degree of north latitude in Korea had already played an important though little known role in history and in politics.

While attending the University of Toronto (Ontario College of Education) in 1950, my son, William, had met Nicholas Ignatiev (then warden of the Graduate School social center, Hart House). Mr. Ignatiev learned that William had grown up in Korea and that he had just returned from a "Summer Internship" experience at the United Nations. Here he had observed the sessions at which the U.N. decided to send forces to support South Korea in response to the invasion by North Korea across the 38th Parallel. In the course of their conversation, Mr. Ignatiev pointed out that the division of Korea along the 38th Parallel after World War II had had historical precedent. In 1896, Russia and Japan had divided Korea into spheres of influence. This agreement, first proposed by his father, Count Nicholas Pavlovich Ignatiev, gave Russia influence north of the 38th Parallel and the Japanese influence to the South.

Russia was enjoying special favor with the Korean King in 1896 and had obtained timber and logging concessions in the North along the Tumen and Yalu Rivers. The Russian Maritime Province, which shared a common boundary with Korea along the Tumen River, was another of Count Ignatiev's diplomatic triumphs. While an envoy at Peking, he had concluded a successful treaty with China in 1860, in which this territory was ceded to Russia and made possible the construction of a seaport for eastern Russia, Vladivostok. Later, it was served by the Trans-Siberian Railway line which the Chinese had permitted Russia to extend across northern Manchuria.

Less than a decade after the tacit agreement to divide Korea into spheres of influence, Japan observed with alarm that the Russian "sphere" seemed to be expanding rapidly beyond Korea into southern Manchuria. The Russians had obtained a 25-year lease from China to build a naval base at Port Arthur and to construct a South Manchurian Railway line from the Russian-built Chinese Eastern Railway at Harbin. This was to run down the Liaotung Peninsula to convey supplies to the ice-free ports on the southern tip, Dalny (Dairen) and Port Arthur. Directly across the Korea Bay at the mouth of the Yalu the Russians were adding to their naval strength by settling the port of Yogampo, despite Korean objections, on the pretext of needing a log-shipping point. Vigorous Japanese opposition had stymied an earlier attempt by Russia to secure a naval base at Masanpo, across the Korea Strait from Japan.

This attempted expansion south of the 38th Parallel into the Japanese sphere of influence was contrary to both public and private agreements between Russia and Japan. The accumulating evidence that Russia's further encroachments along the northern Korean frontier had in mind permanent occupation aroused the military might of Nippon. In 1904, in action similar to that taken at Pearl Harbor years later, Japan launched a surprise attack on Port Arthur and the Russo-Japanese war was begun. Japan emerged as victor, the first Oriental nation of modern times to conquer a Western power, and Asia presented a new look.

It was at the close of World War II, in 1945, that the fateful 38th Parallel again gained prominence. This time it was Japan who was defeated. Again the Parallel became the dividing line for spheres of influence, although now it was between Russia and the U.S.A. The choice of the 38th Parallel was made as a practical means for dividing the location of Russian and U.S. responsibility in accepting the surrender of Japanese troops. Perhaps unaware of the historical precedent set by Russian Count Nicholas Ignatiev, U.S. Rear Admiral Matthias Gardner is credited with suggesting the 38th Parallel as the demarcation line.[1] The U.S., in using this device, viewed it merely as a convenience. It had no way of foreseeing that the Russians would begin at once to seal off the border along the 38th Parallel, effectively creating two distinct zones.[2]

What had seemed innocuous enough at the time, lead to disastrous results both to Korea and the rest of the world. It had the effect of dividing Korea, and shattering that nation's ideal of a united country. The North aligned with Communism and became the Democratic People's Republic of Korea (North Korea). The South was oriented to democracy and the political ideals of the United States and became the Republic of Korea (South Korea). Furthermore, the natural economy of Korea was now disrupted, for the North had most of the mining and industry, while the South was largely agricultural.

The 38th Parallel again appeared in the international limelight with the advent of the Korean War on June 25, 1950. The probing attacks, by North Korean troops who crossed the line, blossomed into a full-scale war with United Nations forces coming to the aid of the South Koreans. The Armistice, concluded at Panmunjon on June 8, 1953, fixed a Military Demarcation Line across Korea, running

---

[1] Robert Leckie, *Conflict, the History of the Korean War, 1950-53,* pp. 31-32.
[2] *Conflict,* pp. 32-33.

below the 38th Parallel in the West, and above it in the East, with a buffer zone of two kilometers on either side of the line known as the Demilitarized Zone (DMZ).

One former member of our Haiju Sanatorium staff, Dr. M.K. Moon, was captured by the Communists during the Korean War (as was our good friend, Kris Jensen). Dr. Moon's experiences were related to us when we were in Seoul in 1960.

Dr. Moon had served as a lecturer during our Christmas Seal Campaigns, so we were particularly interested in his story. The Communists had forced him to work for them at Wonsan Harbor (not far from where the U.S. Naval vessel, the *USS Pueblo*, was seized in 1968). Dr. Moon was ordered to build a model sanatorium near Wonsan.

He told his captors, "If you will allow me to return to the Haiju Sanatorium, I can copy there those plans and bring them back here, for that is just the kind of facility you need in this place."

Reluctant to let him go at first, they finally agreed. He worked hard copying the layout of the Haiju Sanatorium for he was being carefully guarded. The gradual relaxation of the guard's vigil was directly proportional to the increase of the magnetic attraction which the 38th Parallel had for Dr. Moon. So on one dark night, while at the lower part of the Sanatorium grounds, he slipped away and through the lines to the South.

Following the end of World War II we were offered the opportunity to return to the mission field in Korea. The work of the Methodists in Korea had been primarily in the North, and there existed much confusion in the post-war establishment of Methodist Mission work. Because of this confusion in the Mission program in Korea, and the fact that we were needed for the work in India, we elected to stay in the latter country.

My mother was puzzled by our decision not to return to Korea. A letter I wrote to her after the Communist attack on Songdo (Kaesong) on June 25, 1950 revealed how fortunate we were in having made the decision that we did.

> "The mother of Mrs. Jensen wrote us a very thrilling account of the escape of the Korea missionaries as well as a very sad and touching account of the capture of Mr. Jensen and the other missionaries in Songdo, including that of the doctor and his wife in charge of the Mission hospital there. . . . You remember they wanted us to go to this very hospital.

"We have been always grateful to Bishop Ryang for giving us timely warning and strongly advising and urging us *not* to come back to Korea; because they loved us and did not want the fate to befall us that he predicted would befall the Songdo missionaries. How right his predictions were. I don't suppose there is any possibility of them ever getting out alive and they were probably killed on the spot. I see the Communists are now threatening to exterminate *all* the Korean Christians both Catholic and Protestant."

Ironically, Kris Jensen had been as opposed to the opening of the Songdo mission as had Bishop Ryang. Although Kris was not killed, as I had feared, he was interned by the Communists along with the five missionaries of that station whom he had gone to visit. Kris was released three years later via Siberia and Russia and arrived in New York along with four of the surviving missionaries on May 13, 1953. He returned to South Korea in September, 1953, slightly over three months after his release. He died in Korea in November, 1956, a well known Christian and greatly beloved by people of all ranks.

In the August, 1973 issue of *Decision* magazine, Sherwood E. Wirt described Korea as "a new superpower of the spiritual world" in his article entitled, "Korea: God's loving cup." He went on to say:

". . . Korea, a nation beleagured for centuries by mighty powers . . . has become a powerhouse of God. A land of missionaries has become a land of mission. A persecuted remnant has become a pacesetting church."

The truth of this had been foreseen by the missionaries who were forced to leave Korea in the late fall of 1940. It seems a fitting conclusion to this volume to quote from a memorandum addressed to the Foreign Department of the Woman's Foreign Missionary Society of the Methodist Church. It was written aboard the *SS Mariposa* en route from Kobe to San Francisco on November 22, 1940 and was signed by Marion L. Conrow, Secretary of the Executive Committee, Korea Mission Council.

"In spite of the apparent yielding of organized Methodism to overwhelming forces, our last conversations with individual

Christians showed us again how unconquerable is their faith, how patient and forgiving their love, and how great their courage as they add our burdens to their own. They know that we are not abandoning them, but that we will continue to work for them all our days, and hope to see them again some time. We leave Korea in the full confidence that the Christian Church there cannot be overcome by principalities and powers, and that nothing can separate them from the love of Christ.

"Since leaving Korea, the following hymn has come from the heart of one of our number. Tune: "Vesper" Methodist Hymnal No. 593.

"1. Bless all sick and suffering
In this troubled time;
In the darkest prison
Shed Thy light divine.

"2. May thy tortured children
Be supremely blest,
Knowing Thou art watching
Every cruel test.

"3. When, all trials over,
They at last are free,
May they tell the story,
Magnifying Thee."

References

Andrews, Roy Chapman. *Ends of the Earth*. New York: G. P. Putnam's Sons, 1929.

------"Exploring the Unknown Corners of the 'Hermit Kingdom.'" *National Geographic Magazine*, v. 36, July 1919: 25-48.

Baker, Frances J. *A Woman Doctor in the Land of Morning Calm; A Sketch of Dr. Rosetta Sherwood Hall*. Boston: Woman's Foreign Missionary Society [Methodist Episcopal Church, n.d.] 8 p. pamphlet.

Bratton, Fred G. *Friends Unique; Two Personality Sketches*. [n.p.: n.d.] 27 p.
Privately printed booklet.

Bishop, Isabella L., and Osbert John Radcliffe Howarth. "Korea." In *Encyclopaedia Britannica*. 11th ed. v. 15. Cambridge: Cambridge University Press, 1911. p. 908-913.

Caldwell, John C. and Elsie F. Caldwell. *Our Neighbors in Korea*. New York: John Day, 1961.

Centre for East Asian Cultural Studies, comp. *A Short History of Korea*. Tokyo: 1963.
"Distributed outside Japan by East West Center Press, Honolulu."

Chetelat, Enzo de. "Roaming Korea South of the Iron Curtain." *National Geographic Magazine*, v. 97, June 1950: 777-808.

Choi, Woonsang. *The Fall of the Hermit Kingdom*. Dobbs Ferry: Oceana, 1967.

Chung, Kyung Cho. *Korea Tomorrow, Land of the Morning Calm*. New York: MacMillan, 1956.

Clare, Kenneth G., and others. *Area Handbook for the Republic of Korea*, by Kenneth G. Clare, Gerald J. Foster, Robert C. Hannus, William Hrabko, Carolyn Knapp, Kyung Lee, Robert T. Mott, and Yung Park; prepared for American University by Westwood Research, Incorporated. Washington: U.S. Govt. Print. Off., August 1969.
"DA Pam 55-041."

Clark, Allen D. *History of the Korean Church*. Seoul: Christian Literature Society of Korea, 1961.

Clyde, Paul H. *The Far East; A History of the Impact of the West on Eastern Asia*. New York: Prentice-Hall, 1948.

Conrow, Marion L. *To the Foreign Department of the Woman's Foreign Missionary Society of the Methodist Church*, by Marion L. Conrow, Secretary of the Executive Committee, Korea Mission Council. Memorandum written aboard *SS Mariposa* en route from Kobe to San Francisco: November 22, 1940. 6 p. mimeographed.

"Corea and the Gospel." *Christian Herald*, v. 17, August 8, 1894: 497-499.

Crane, Paul S. *Korean Patterns.* Seoul: Hollym, 1967.
Opposite title page: "Royal Asiatic Society, Korea Branch, Handbook Series Number 1."

Curzon, George Nathaniel Curzon, 1st Marquis. "In the Diamond Mountains: Adventures Among the Buddhist Monasteries of Eastern Korea," by the Marquess Curzon of Kedleston. *National Geographic Magazine,* v. 46, Oct. 1924: 353-374.

Deering, Mabel Craft. "Chosen–Land of Morning Calm." *National Geographic Magazine*, v. 64, Oct. 1933: 421-448.

Dewey, Thomas E. *Journey to the Far Pacific.* New York: Doubleday, 1952.

Donohugh, Thomas S., ed. *Methodist Overseas Missions Gazatteer and Statistics.* New York: Board of Missions and Church Extension of the Methodist Church, 1948.

"Dr. Rosetta S. Hall To Mark 50 Years of Medical Practice." *Liberty Register* (New York), March 9, 1939. reprint.

Durant, Will. *Our Oriental Heritage.* New York: Simon and Schuster, 1954. (Durant, Will and Ariel Durant. *The Story of Civilization*, Part 1).

Evans, M. Filmer. *The Land and People of Korea.* London: Adam & Charles Black; New York: MacMillan, 1962.

Ewing, Ethel E. *Far Eastern Society, Our Widening World.* Chicago: Rand McNally, 1963.

Fairbank, John K., Edwin O. Reischauer and Albert M. Craig. *East Asia: The Modern Transformation.* Boston: Houghton Mifflin, 1965. (Their *A History of East Asian Civilization*, v. 2).

—————— *East Asia: Tradition and Transformation.* Boston: Houghton Mifflin, 1973.

Federal Council of Korea, and the Interchurch World Movement of North America. *Korea Hand Book of Missions, 1920.* [n.p.] 1920.
"Printed by The Fukuin Printing Co., Ltd., Yokohoma, Japan."
Foreword signed by "M. L. Swinehart, Kwangju, Korea."

Federal Council of Missions in Korea. *The Korea Missions Year Book*, ed. by F. E. C. Williams and Gerald Bonwick; statistician, M. L. Swinehart. Seoul: Christian Literature Society of Korea, 1928.

Gale, James S. *A History of the Korean People.* Seoul: Christian Literature Society of Korea, [n.d.]

"Published Serially in 'The Korea Mission Field,' July 1924 to Sept. 1927."

End paper inscription in Sherwood Hall's copy: "Dr. Rosetta Sherwood Hall's copy, 1928 the year she opened the Women's Medical Institute which had Dr. Gale's approval."

------ *Korea in Transition*. Nashville: Publishing House of the Methodist Episcopal Church, South, 1909.

------ *Korean Sketches*. New York: Young People's Missionary Movement of the United States and Canada, [and Fleming H. Revell] 1898.

Gosfield, Frank, and Bernhardt J. Hurwood. *Korea: Land of the 38th Parallel*. New York: Parents' Magazine Press, 1969.

Includes earliest known European description of Korea by a Dutch sailor shipwrecked on the Korean coast and a captive for thirteen years. (Published in 1653 by Hendrick Hamel.)

Greene, Fred. *The Far East*. New York: Rinehart, 1957.

Gurney, Gene, and Clare Gurney. *North and South Korea*. New York: Franklin Watts, 1973.

Hakwon-sa, Ltd. *Korea: Its Land, People, and Culture of All Ages*. Seoul: 1960.

Hall, Marian (Bottomley). "Quadruple Anniversaries." *Korea Mission Field*, [n.d.]

Believed to be 1938; cited from a reprint.

Hall, Rosetta (Sherwood). "The Deaf and Blind in Korea." *The Christian Herald*, May 10, 1911: 474.

------ "Early Medical Work for Women in Korea." *Woman's Missionary Friend*, v. 68, Feb. 1935: 51-53.

------ "The Edith Margaret Memorial." *Children's Missionary Friend*, v. 13, Dec. 1902: 140.

------ "Foreign Medical Women in Korea." *Journal of the American Medical Women's Association*, v. 5, Oct. 1950: 404-405.

------ "Glimpses of Women's Medical Work in Korea." *Woman's Work in the Far East*, Dec. 1913.

Cited from a reprint.

------, ed. *The Life of Rev. William James Hall, M.D., Medical Missionary to the Slums of New York; Pioneer Missionary to Pyong Yang, Korea*. New York: Press of Eaton & Mains, [1897]

------ "The Use of White Clothes, the Year Round." *Korea Mission Field*, v. 32, Dec. 1936: 263-264.

------ "Woman's Medical Institute." *Korea Mission Field*, v. 30, Jan. 1934: 15-16.

------ "The Woman's Medical Training Institute, Ella Anthony Lewis Memorial, Seoul." *Korea Mission Field*, v. 24, Sept. 1928.

Hall, Sherwood. "Application of Sanatorium Methods to Korean Patients." *China Medical Journal*, v. 44, July 1930: 662-778.

------ *Mother and Her Work*. Alliance: Burton's Print Shop, 1916. 15 p. pamphlet.

Privately printed by Sherwood Hall when a student at Mount Union College, Alliance, Ohio. Includes reprint: "A Korean Instance; An American Woman's Work for the Blind and Deaf," *American Review of Reviews*, Dec. 1914: 717-718; and reprint: Hall, Rosetta S., "Annual Report of Hospital of Extended Grace to Women and Children," Pyongyang, Mar. 1, 1916.

------ "The Story of Korea's First Christmas Seals." *Korea Mission Field*, v. 29, May 1933.

Cited from a reprint: 4 p.

Hapdong News Agency. *Korea Annual, 1971*. 8th ed. Seoul: 1971.

Han, Woo-Keun. *The History of Korea*, translated by Lee Kyung-shik and edited by Grafton K. Mintz. Honolulu: East-West Center Press, 1971.

Hatada, Takashi. *A History of Korea*, translated and edited by Warren W. Smith, Jr. and Benjamin H. Hazard. Santa Barbara: American Bibliographical Center, Clio Press, 1969.

Henthorn, William E. *A History of Korea*. New York: Free Press, 1971.

Hinton, Harold C. *The Far East and Southwest Pacific*. Washington: Stryker-Post, 1974.

"Annually revised."

Hodous, Lewis, "Confucianism." In *Encyclopaedia Britannica*. v. 6. Chicago: Encyclopaedia Britannica, 1953. p. 236.

Hulbert, Homer B., and others. "Korea." In *Encyclopaedia Britannica*. v. 13. Chicago: Encyclopaedia Britannica, 1953. p. 485-491.

------ *The Passing of Korea*. New York: Doubleday, Page, 1906.

Hyun, Judy. *The Korean Cookbook*. Chicago: Follett, 1970.

"With an introduction by Nika Standen Hazelton."

Initial chapter, "A Welcome to 'The Land of Morning Calm,'" p. 7-40, offers brief description of Korea and its food customs.

"Imperial Chalices from Korea Highlights Career of WMC's Oldest Alumna." *Germantown Courier*, v. 14, June 15, 1950: Feature Page.

International Publicity League of Korea. *Pictorial Korea*. Seoul: 1953-54.

Annual pictorial review.

Japanese Chamber of Commerce of New York. *The Sino-Japanese Crisis, 1937*. New York: 1937. 62 p. booklet.

Jensen, A. Kristian. *Internment, North Korea*. [New Cumberland, Pa.: The Author, 1953] 18 p. pamphlet.

Johnston, Richard J. *Getting to Know the Two Koreas*. New York: Coward McCann, 1965.

Keister, Gertrude (Oren). "The Miraculous Escape of 900 Korea Missionaries (including their families) from the Communists." *Indian Witness* (Lucknow), v. 80, Sept. 14, 1950: (1) 365.

Kim, H. Edward. "Rare Look at North Korea." *National Geographic Magazine*, v. 146, Aug. 1974: 252-277.

Kim, Hyontay. *Folklore and Customs of Korea*. Seoul: Korea Information Service, 1957.

King, Phyllis (Hall). "'Christmas Seal Doctor's' Collection Donated to Smithsonian." In *Korea Illustrated* (Washington), v. 1, No. 4, Spring 1973: 4-7, 12-14.

"Korea." In *Encyclopedia of World Travel*, ed. by Nelson Doubleday and C. Earl Cooley. Garden City: Doubleday, 1961. 268-272. (Their *Europe, Africa, The Middle East, Asia, The Pacific*, v. 2).

"Korea." In Gt. Brit. Foreign Office. *British and Foreign State Papers*. v. 74; 1882-83. London: William Redgway, 1890.

"Korea." In Gt. Brit. Foreign Office. *British and Foreign State Papers*. v. 84; 1891-92. London: William Redgway, 1898.

"Korea." In Gt. Brit. Foreign Office. *British and Foreign State Papers*. v. 85; 1892-93. London: William Redgway, 1899.

"Korea." In Gt. Brit. Foreign Office. *British and Foreign State Papers*. v. 86; 1893-94. London: William Redgway, 1899.

"Korea." In U.S. Dept. of State. *Foreign Relations of the United States*. 1883. Washington: Govt. Print. Off., 1884.

"Korea." and "Appendix I." In U.S. Dept. of State. *Foreign Relations of the United States*. 1894. Washington: Govt. Print. Off., 1895.

Korea Week. v. 1+ No. 1+ April 17, 1968+ Washington: Po Sung Philip Kim (797 National Press Bldg., 14th & F Sts., N.W.) semimonthly.

"The Land of the Morning Calm." In *Lands and Peoples, the World in Color*. v. 4. New York: Grolier Society, 1951. p. 373-384.

Langer, William L., comp. and ed. *An Encyclopedia of World History*. rev. ed. Boston: Houghton Mifflin, 1948.

Lattimore, Owen and Eleanor Lattimore. *China: A Short History*. rev. ed. New York: W. W. Norton, 1947.

New and rev. ed. of former title, *The Making of Modern China*, 1944.

Latourette, Kenneth S. *A Short History of the Far East*. 3d ed. New York: MacMillan, 1959.

Lee, Jai Hyon. *Korean Lore*. Seoul: Office of Public Information, Republic of Korea, 1954.

Leckie, Robert. *Conflict, the History of the Korean War, 1950-53*. New York: G. P. Putnam's Sons, 1962.

Legge, James, and others. "Confucius." In *Encyclopaedia Britannica.* v. 6. Chicago: Encyclopaedia Britannica, 1953. p. 236-239.

Lowell, A. Lawrence. *Biography of Percival Lowell.* New York: MacMillan, 1935.

Lum, Peter. *Six Centuries in East Asia, China, Japan and Korea from the 14th Century to 1912.* New York: S. G. Phillips, 1973.

MacNair, Harley F., and Donald F. Lach. *Modern Far Eastern International Relations.* 2d ed. New York: D. Van Nostrand, 1955.

Mathews, William H. *Korea in Pictures.* New York: Sterling, 1968.

McCune, George M., and Arthur L. Grey, Jr. *Korea Today.* Cambridge, Mass.: Harvard University Press, 1950.

Moffett, Samuel Hugh. *The Christians of Korea.* New York: Friendship, 1962.

Moore, Arthur J., Bp. *Christ After Chaos, the Post-War Policy of the Methodist Church in Foreign Lands.* New York: Board of Missions and Church Extension, The Methodist Church, 1944.

Moore, Ivan, ed. *Japan 1931-1945, Militarism, Facism, Japanism?, Problems in Asian Civilization.* Boston: D. C. Heath, 1963.

Mosier, Robert H. "The GI and the Kids of Korea." *National Geographic Magazine*, v. 103, May 1953: 635-644.

National Federation of Business and Professional Women's Clubs. "A Century of Medical Education for Women." *Independent Woman*, April 1950.

New York. Methodist Episcopal Church. Board of Foreign Missions. Korea Quarter-Centennial Movement. *Sir Launfal of Korea, Nathan Lounsbury Rockwell.* New York: [1909?].
"Reprinted from 'The Christian Advocate.'"

New York. Methodist Episcopal Church. Board of Foreign Missions. *World Outlook.* Korea Number; July 1916: 32 p.

Noble, Mattie W. *Victorious Lives of Early Christians.* Seoul: Christian Literature Society of Korea, 1927.

Osgood, Cornelius. *The Koreans and Their Culture.* New York: Ronald Press, 1951.

Paik, Lak-Geoon George. *The History of Protestant Missions in Korea, 1832-1910.* [2d ed.] Seoul: Yonsei University Press, 1971. (No. 6 of a series of reprints of Western books on Korea.)
"First edition, 1927, by Union Christian College Press, P'yongyang, Korea."

Pak, Rhoda Kim. "Medical Women in Korea." *Journal of the American Medical Women's Association*, v. 5, Mar. 1950: 116-117.

Palmer, Spencer J. *Korea and Christianity.* Seoul: Hollym, 1967.

Park, Chung Hee. *To Build a Nation.* Washington: Acropolis, 1971.

Phil, Marshall R., ed. *Listening to Korea*. Washington: Praeger, 1973.

"A Pioneer Missionary Called Home." *Christian Herald*, v. 39, no. 46, November 15, 1916: 1,247.

Price, Willard. "Jap Rule in the Hermit Nation." *National Geographic Magazine*, v. 88, Oct. 1945: 429-451.

Reischauer, Edwin O. *Japan, Past and Present*. 3d ed., rev. New York: Alfred A. Knopf, 1967.

Rhodes, Harry A., ed. *History of the Korea Mission Presbyterian Church U.S.A., 1884-1934*. Seoul: Chosen Mission Presbyterian Church U.S.A., 1934.

Rosinger, Lawrence K., and others. *The State of Asia, A Contemporary Survey*. New York: Alfred A. Knopf, 1953.

Republic of Korea. Korean Overseas Information Service. *History, Korea Background Series*. Seoul: 1972.

Republic of Korea. Ministry of Culture and Information. *Facts About Korea*. Seoul: June 1971.

Republic of Korea. Ministry of Transportation. *Welcome to Korea*. Seoul: 1958.

Roy, Andrew T. *On Asia's Rim*. New York: Friendship, 1962.

Sauer, Charles A. *Methodists in Korea, 1930-1960*. Seoul: Christian Literature Society, 1973.

------, ed. *Within the Gate*. Seoul: Korea Methodist News Service, 1934.
"Comprising the addresses delivered at the Fiftieth Anniversary of Korean Methodism, First Church, Seoul, Korea, June 19th-20th, 1934."
"And an historical play, 'At the Hermit's Gate, A Presentation of Some Events of 1883-1884,' by Ellasue Wagner."

Seoul. Methodist Episcopal Church. Woman's Foreign Missionary Society. *Fifty Years of Light*, prepared by their missionaries in commemoration of the completion of fifty years of work in Korea. Seoul: [printed by Y.M.C.A. Press] May 1938.

------ *First Annual Meeting of the Woman's Conference of the Methodist Episcopal Church in Korea*. Seoul: May 13-19, 1899.

Seoul. Methodist Episcopal Church. Korea Mission. *Korea Methodist*. v. 1, no. 10; Aug. 10, 1905: 129-144.

------ *The Korean Work of the Woman's Foreign Missionary Society of the Methodist Episcopal Church, 1897-1898*, reports presented to 14th annual meeting of Korea Mission. Seoul: Aug. 25–Sept. 1, 1898.

Simpich, Frederick. "Manchuria, Promised Land of Asia." *National Geographic Magazine*, v. 56, Oct. 1929: 379-428.

[Snyder, Helen Young] *The Mother of Pyong Yang*, by Mary Wilton [pseud.] [n.p.: n.d.] 12 p. pamphlet.

Sochurek, Howard. "South Korea, Success Story in Asia." *National Geographic Magazine*, v. 135, Mar. 1969: 301-344.

Solberg, S. E. *The Land and People of Korea*. Philadelphia: Lippincott, 1966.

Thomas, Edward J. "Buddha and Buddhism." In *Encyclopaedia Britannica*. v. 4. Chicago: Encyclopaedia Britannica, 1953. p. 325-327.

Time Inc. *The World's Great Religions*, [by the editors of "Life"] New York: 1957.

Appeared in "Life" in six parts during 1955: Feb. 7, Mar. 7, Apr. 4, May 9, June 13, Dec. 26.

Trudeau, Edward L. *An Autobiography*. New York: National TB Association and Doubleday, 1951.

Underwood, Horace H. *Modern Education in Korea*. New York: International Press, 1926.

Unger, Frederick W., and Charles Morris. *Russia and Japan and a Complete History of the War in the Far East*. [n.p.: W. E. Scull, 1905]

U.S. Dept. of Defense. Office of Information for the Armed Forces. *A Pocket Guide to Korea*. Washington: U.S. Govt. Print. Off., 1962.

"DoD PG–8A; DA Pam 360-414; NAVPERS 92960A; AFP 216-24; NAVMC 2579."

U.S. Dept. of the Army. *Communist North Korea, a Bibliographic Survey*. Washington: U.S. Govt. Print. Off., Feb. 1971.

"DA Pam 550-11."

U.S. Dept. of State. Bureau of Public Affairs. Historical Office. *A Historical Summary of United States–Korean Relations, with a Chronology of Important Developments 1834-1962*. Dept. of State Publication 7446. Washington: U.S. Govt. Print. Off., Nov. 1962.

Van Dusen, Henry P. *Methodism's World Mission, the Report of a Non-Methodist*. New York: Board of Missions and Church Extension, The Methodist Church, 1940.

Vinacke, Harold M. *A History of the Far East in Modern Times*. 5th ed. New York: Appleton-Century-Crofts, 1950.

Vreeland, Nena and others. *Area Handbook for North Korea*, by Nena Vreeland, Rinn-Sup Shinn, Peter Just, and Philip W. Moeller. 2d. ed. Washington: U.S. Govt. Print. Off., May 1976.

"DA pam 550-81."

"One of a series of handbooks prepared by Foreign Area Studies of the American University."

Weems, Clarence Norwood, ed. *Hulbert's History of Korea*. New ed. New York: Hillary House, 1962. 2 v.

Homer B. Hulbert's *The History of Korea*, 2 v., was first published in 1905 by The Methodist Publishing House, Seoul. Clarence Weems' new ed. adds Introduction, Notes and Bibliography.

White, Peter T. "South Korea: What Next?" *National Geographic Magazine*, v. 148, Sept. 1975: 394-427.

Welch, Herbert. *As I Recall My Past Century*. New York: Abingdon, 1962.

White, John A. *The Diplomacy of the Russo-Japanese War*. Princeton: Princeton University Press, 1964.

Wilbur, Donald N., ed. *The Nations of Asia*. New York: Hart, 1966.

Wirt, Sherwood E. "Korea: God's Loving Cup." *Decision*, v. 14, Aug. 1973: 6-9.

Zirkle, Helen K. *The Christmas-Tuberculosis Seals of Korea*. Miami, Fla.: David G. Phillips (P.O. Box 37842, Buena Vista Station) for the Korea Stamp Society, 1966, 28 p.

Index

Sino-Japanese war (1894-1895), 146-154, 309

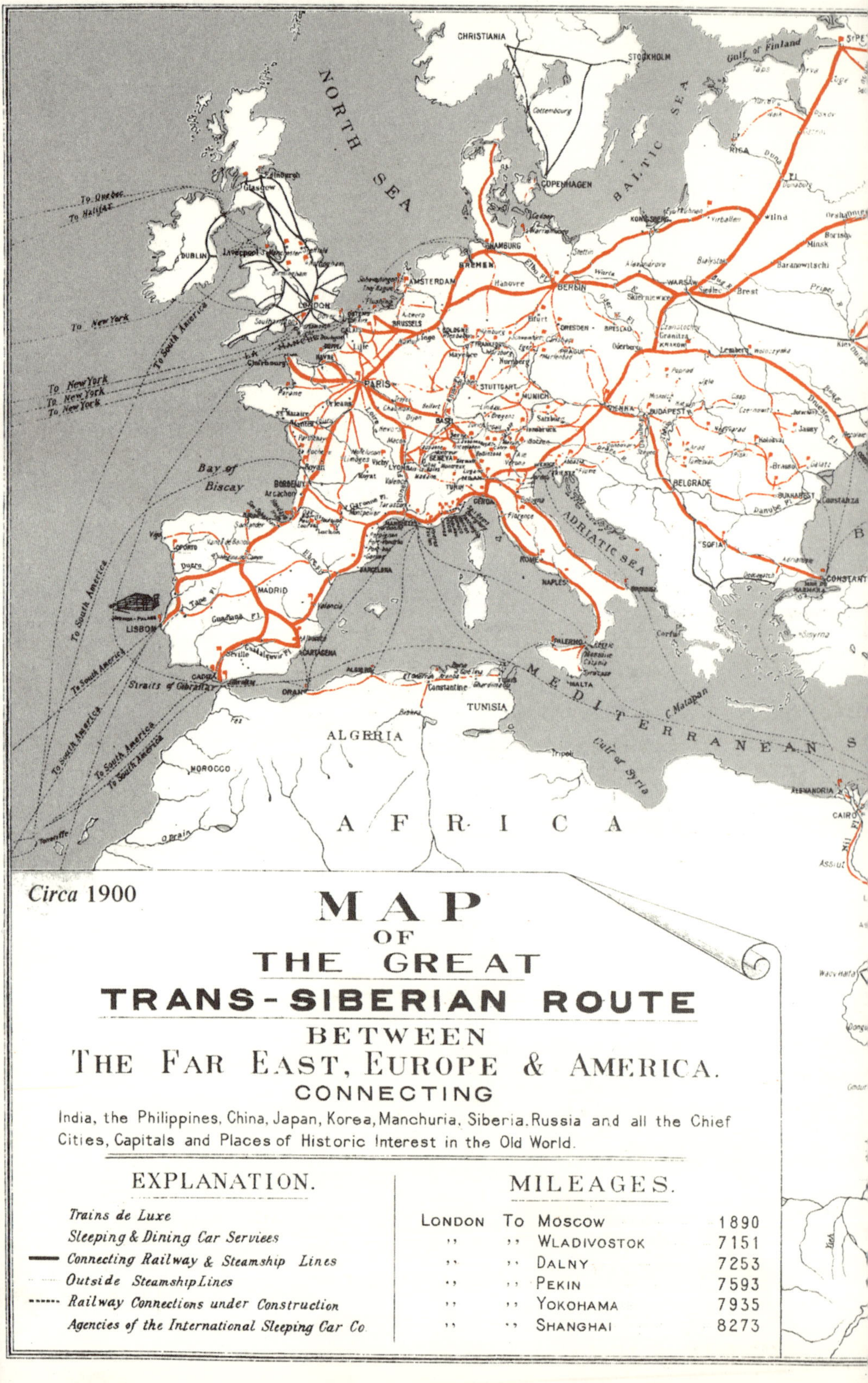
Circa 1900
MAP
OF
THE GREAT
TRANS-SIBERIAN ROUTE
BETWEEN
THE FAR EAST, EUROPE & AMERICA.
CONNECTING
India, the Philippines, China, Japan, Korea, Manchuria, Siberia, Russia and all the Chief Cities, Capitals and Places of Historic Interest in the Old World.
EXPLANATION.
Trains de Luxe
Sleeping & Dining Car Services
Connecting Railway & Steamship Lines
Outside Steamship Lines
Railway Connections under Construction
Agencies of the International Sleeping Car Co.
MILEAGES.
LONDON To MOSCOW 1890
" " WLADIVOSTOK 7151
" " DALNY 7253
" " PEKIN 7593
" " YOKOHAMA 7935
" " SHANGHAI 8273
NORTH SEA
BALTIC SEA
Gulf of Finland
ADRIATIC SEA
MEDITERRANEAN S
Bay of Biscay
Straits of Gibraltar
AFRICA
ALGERIA
MOROCCO
TUNISIA
CHRISTIANIA
STOCKHOLM
COPENHAGEN
RIGA
HAMBURG
BREMEN
BERLIN
WARSAW
AMSTERDAM
BRUSSELS
LONDON
DUBLIN
PARIS
DRESDEN
STUTTGART
MUNICH
VIENNA
BUDAPEST
BELGRADE
SOFIA
GENEVA
TURIN
GENOA
ROME
NAPLES
PALERMO
MALTA
MADRID
BARCELONA
CARTAGENA
LISBON
CADIZ
ALEXANDRIA
CAIRO
Constantine
To Quebec
To Halifax
To New York
To New York
To New York
To New York
To South America